Bates'

NURSING GUIDE
to PHYSICAL
EXAMINATION
and HISTORY
TAKING SECOND EDITION

Beth Hogan-Quigley, MSN, RN, CRNP

Family and Community Health Department
University of Pennsylvania School of Nursing
Philadelphia, Pennsylvania

Mary Louise Palm, MS, RN

Associate Clinical Professor Emerita
University of Rhode Island College of Nursing
Kingston, Rhode Island

Lynn S. Bickley, MD, FACP

Clinical Professor of Internal Medicine
University of New Mexico School of Medicine
Albuquerque, New Mexico

Wolters Kluwer

Philadelphia · Baltimore · New York · London
Buenos Aires · Hong Kong · Sydney · Tokyo

Acquisitions Editor: Kelley Squazzo
Product Development Editor: Annette Ferran
Director of Product Development: Jennifer Forestieri
Editorial Assistant: Dan Reilly
Production Project Manager: Cynthia Rudy
Design Coordinator: Stephen Druding
Illustration Coordinator: Jennifer Clements
Manufacturing Coordinator: Karin Duffield
Prepress Vendor: Aptara, Inc.

2nd edition

9 8 7 6 5 4 3

Printed in China

Library of Congress Cataloging-in-Publication Data

Names: Hogan-Quigley, Beth, author. | Palm, Mary Louise, author. | Bickley, Lynn S., author.
Title: Bates' nursing guide to physical examination and history taking / Beth Hogan-Quigley, Mary Louise Palm, Lynn S. Bickley.
Other titles: Nursing guide to physical examination and history taking
Description: 2nd edtion. | Philadelphia : Wolters Kluwer, [2017] | Includes bibliographical references and index.
Identifiers: LCCN 2016035739 | ISBN 9781496305565 (hardback)
Subjects: | MESH: Nursing Assessment | Physical Examination | Medical History Taking
Classification: LCC RC76 | NLM WY 100.4 | DDC 616.07/54–dc23
LC record available at https://lccn.loc.gov/2016035739

CCS0518

*Heartfelt appreciation to my family, friends, colleagues, and students
who inspire me to continue to grow and reach new horizons.
Special recognition to:
My husband, Peter, and daughters, Colleen and Megan, for their love and
support.
My parents, Jim and Betty, for their dedication and unconditional love.*

BETH HOGAN-QUIGLEY

*With much appreciation and thanks to my family:
My husband, William J. Palm, for his support and love during this project.
My children, Aileene, Bill, and Andy, with love.
Special thanks to my colleagues and students, who encouraged and
supported me throughout my teaching career.*

MARY LOUISE PALM

Carrie Bailey, PhD
Assistant Clinical Professor
The University of Tennessee Knoxville
Knoxville, Tennessee

Emily Barnes, DNP, FNP-C
Clinical Associate Professor
West Virginia University
Morgantown, West Virginia

Monte Beane, MSN, RN
Nursing Professor
Keiser University
Jacksonville, Florida

Patricia Birchfield, APRN, PhD
Professor Emeritus
Eastern Kentucky University
Richmond, Kentucky

Cheryl Blanche, DNP, APRN, FNP-BC
Adjunct Assistant Professor
Eleanor Wade Custer School of Nursing
Shenandoah University
Winchester, Virginia

Alice Blazeck, DNSC, RN
Assistant Professor
University of Pittsburgh
Pittsburgh, Pennsylvania

James Bockeloh, DNP, RN, FNP-BC
Clinical Assistant Professor
University of Wisconsin—Milwaukee
   College of Nursing
Milwaukee, Wisconsin

Rebecca Bodan
California State University, Fullerton
Fullerton, California

Joan Boyd, MS, RN
Professor of Nursing
Florida State College at Jacksonville
Jacksonville, Florida

Judi Brittingham, MSN, FNP-C, CNE, BSN
Assistant Professor of Nursing
Baptist College of Health Sciences
Memphis, Tennessee

Jill Buterbaugh, MSN, CRNP, FNP-BC
Assistant Professor of Nursing
Frostburg State University
Frostburg, Maryland

Tina Campbell, MSN, RN
Adjunct Faculty
Central Texas College
Killeen, Texas

Lindsey Carlson, MSN, FNP-BC
Assistant Professor of Nursing
William Jewell College
Liberty, Missouri

Pamella I. Chavis, RN, BSN, MSN, EdD
Clinical Associate Professor
North Carolina Agricultural Technical
   State University
Greensboro, North Carolina

Darlene Clark, MS, RN
Senior Lecturer in Nursing
The Pennsylvania State University
University Park, Pennsylvania

Susan Clark
Tennessee Technological University
Cookeville, Tennessee

Sophia Clarke, MSN
Adjunct Lecturer
Adelphi University
Garden City, New York

Terri Clifton
Assistant Clinical Professor
Auburn Montgomery
Montgomery, Alabama

Lola Coke, PhD, ACNS-BC, RN-BC, FAHA, FPCNA
Associate Professor
Rush University College of Nursing
Chicago, Illinois

De Anna Cox, FNP
Clinical Associate Professor
Nursing
University of South Carolina
Columbia, South Carolina

Sandra Croasdell, PMC, APRN, FNP-BC, CEN
Division Chair
Bay College
Escanaba, Michigan

Kathy E. Davis, PhD, MSN
Associate Professor
Gordon State College
Barnesville, Georgia

Maria De Los Santos, DNP, ARNP, MPH
Clinical Assistant Professor
Florida International University
Miami, Florida

David J. Derrico, RN, MSN
Clinical Assistant Professor
University of Florida
Gainesville, Florida

Lucie Dlugasch, PhD, MSN, ARNP-BC
Clinical Assistant Professor
Florida International University
Miami, Florida

Stacy Drake, PhD, MPH, RN
Department Systems
The University of Texas Health Science Center at
  Houston
Houston, Texas

Hobie Etta Feagai, EdD, MSN, BSN, FNP-BC, APRN-Rx
Professor of Nursing
Undergraduate and Graduate Nursing
College of Nursing and Health Sciences
Kaneohe, Hawaii

Shiela Ford, MSN-Ed, RNC
Department Chair of Nursing
San Jacinto College South Campus
Houston, Texas

Jami Fulwider, RN, MSN
Instructor
University of Nebraska Medical Center—
  Lincoln Division
Lincoln, Nebraska

Tracy George, DNP, APRN-BC, CNE
Assistant Professor
Francis Marion University
Florence, South Carolina

Rhonda Goodman, PhD, ARNP, FNP-BC, NCSN, AHN-BC
Assistant Professor
Christine E. Lynn College of Nursing
Florida Atlantic University
Boca Raton, Florida

Carmeka Greene, RN, MS, BSN, BA
Georgia Baptist College of Nursing
  of Mercer University
Atlanta, Georgia

Lisa Gurley, MSN, RN, CNE
Assistant Professor
Samford University
Birmingham, Alabama

Regina Hanchak, RN, MS
Adjunct
Erie Community College
Buffalo, New York

Kelli Hand, DNP, MBA, RN
Assistant Professor
University of Tennessee at Chattanooga
Chattanooga, Tennessee

Tammy Harris, MSN, RN
Clinical Instructor of Nursing
Stephen F. Austin State University
Nacogdoches, Texas

Kathy Haugh, PhD, RN, CNE
Associate Professor
Acting Director, Mary Morton Parsons Clinical
 Simulation Learning Center
Coordinator, RN to BSN Program
University of Virginia
Charlottesville, Virginia

Janice Hausauer, MS, FNP, APRN-BC
Assistant Clinical Professor
Montana State University
Bozeman, Montana

Lori Hendrickx, RN, EdD, CCRN, CNL
Professor
South Dakota State University
Brookings, South Dakota

Barbara A. Hoglund, EdD, FNP-C, CNE
Professor of Nursing
Bethel University
St. Paul, Minnesota

Stephanie Huff
Southern Union State Community College
Opelika, Alabama

Mark Jaffe, DPM, MHSA
Associate Professor
Halmos College of Natural Sciences and
 Oceanography
Nova Southeastern University
Davie, Florida

Carrie Johnson, DNP, RN
Professor
University of Mary Hardin Baylor
Belton, Texas

Pamela Johnson, DNP, RN
Assistant Professor Adult Health Nursing
University of South Alabama
Mobile, Alabama

Laly Joseph, DVM, DNP, RN,C, MSN, ARNP, ANP, B.C.
Assistant Professor of Clinical
University of Miami, School of Nursing
 & Health Studies
Coral Gables, Florida

Jeannette Kates, PhD, MSN, GNP-BC, CRNP
School of Nursing and Allied Health Professions
Holy Family University
Philadelphia, Pennsylvania

Donna Keeler, MSN, RN, CPAN
Instructor of Nursing
Moravian College
Bethlehem, Pennsylvania

Andrea Knesek, DNP, RN-BC
Professor, Nursing
Macomb Community College
Clinton Township, Michigan

Christine Krause, MSN, CPNP
Associate Director
Aria School of Nursing
Bensalem, Pennsylvania

Bonnie Laurent, MSN, RN, CPNP
Assistant Professor and Laboratory Manager
Massachusetts College of Pharmacy and Health
 Sciences University
Worcester, Massachusetts

Ramona B. Lazenby, EdD, RN, FNP-BC, CNE
Professor and Associate Dean of Nursing
Auburn University Montgomery
Montgomery, Alabama

Jane Leach, PhD, RNC-CNE
Midwestern State University
Wichita Falls, Texas

Jamie Lee, MSN, RN, CNL
Assistant Professor
Undergraduate Testing Coordinator
James Madison University
Harrisonburg, Virginia

Susan Lindner, RNC-OB, MSN
Clinical Assistant Professor
Family and Community Health Nursing
Virginia Commonwealth University,
 School of Nursing
Richmond, Virginia

Jeanne Linhart, RN-C, FNP-BC
Professor
Nursing
Rockland Community College
Suffern, New York

Shirley MacNeill, MSN, RN, CNE
Upward Mobility LVN to ADN Nursing
    Program Coordinator
Lamar State College—Port Arthur
Port Arthur, Texas

Phyllis Magaletto, RN, MS, BC
Department Nursing
Cochran School of Nursing
Yonkers, New York

Jane F. Marek, DNP, MSN, RN
Assistant Professor Case Western Reserve University
Frances Payne Bolton School of Nursing
Cleveland, Ohio

Tammie McCoy, RN, PhD
Professor and Chair
Mississippi University for Women
Columbus, Mississippi

Barbara McGraw, MSN, RN, CNE
Nursing Faculty
Central Community College
Grand Island, Nebraska

Carolyn Meehan, RN, PhD
Assistant Professor of Nursing
West Chester University
West Chester, Pennsylvania

Carrie D. Michalski, JD, RNC, MSN
Associate Professor
Department of Nursing
Southern Connecticut State University and
    Quinnipiac University
New Haven, Connecticut

Anne Bradley Mitchell, PhD, ANP-BC
Assistant Professor of Nursing
West Chester University
West Chester, Pennsylvania

Heather Mitchell, PhD, RN
Assistant Professor
University of Louisville
Louisville, Kentucky

Lynn Mohr, PhD, APN, PCNS-BC, CPN
Assistant Professor
Director Pediatric & Neonatal CNS Programs
Department of Women, Children, & Family Nursing
Rush University
Chicago, Illinois

Tamra Mohs, DNP, ARNP, FNP
Assistant Professor
St. Ambrose University
Davenport, Iowa

Loretta Moreno, RN, MSN
LVN Program Director
Schreiner University
Kerrville, Texas

Evelyn Parrish, PhD, APRN-BC
Professor
Eastern Kentucky University
Richmond, Kentucky

Jessica Parrott, DNP, RN, CPNP-PC, CNE
Department Chair/Associate Professor
Department of Nursing and Allied Health
Norfolk State University
Norfolk, Virginia

Karla Parsons, DNP, RN, FNP-BC
Assistant Professor, School of Nursing
California State University, Fullerton
Fullerton, California

Cynthia Ploutz, MS, RN, FNP
Hartwick College
Oneonta, New York

Robin J. Poedel, PhD, RN, FNP-BC
Clinical Assistant Professor
The University of Arizona
Tucson, Arizona

Colleen Quinn, EdD, MSN, RN
Professor of Nursing
Pembroke Pines, Florida

Susan M. Randol, MSN, RN, CNE
Semester Coordinator and Master Instructor
University of Louisiana at Lafayette
Lafayette, Louisiana

Jacquelyn Reid, MSN, EdD, CNM, APRN
Professor Emeritus
Louisville, Kentucky

Joli B. Reising
Firelands Regional Medical Center
    School of Nursing
Sandusky, Ohio

Shirley Retzlaff, MSN
Assistant Professor
Nursing
Bryan College of Health Sciences
Lincoln, Nebraska

Kerry Risco, PhD, CRNP, NP-C, WCC
Slippery Rock University
Slippery Rock, Pennsylvania

Lisa Roberts, DrPH, MSN, RN, FNP-BC, CHES
Associate Professor—PhD Program
Loma Linda University
Loma Linda, California

Teresa Roberts, PhD, RN, ANP-BC
University of Massachusetts
Boston, Massachusetts

Toni Roberts, DNP(c), RN, CHSE
Lecturer, Whitson-Hester School of Nursing
Tennessee Tech University
Cookeville, Tennessee

Shona Rue, MSN, CPNP, CNE
Lecturer/Clinical Instructor
University of Nevada Las Vegas
Las Vegas, Nevada

Whitney Shanley, MSN, BSN, RN, FNP-C
Nursing Instructor
George Washington University
Ashburn, Virginia

Joyce Shanty, PhD, RN
Nursing and Allied Health Professions
Indiana University of Pennsylvania
Indiana, Pennsylvania

Debra Shelton
Associate Professor
Northwestern State University
Shreveport, Louisiana

Mary Shortreed, DNP, RN, CNE
Assistant Professor
Youngstown State University
Youngstown, Ohio

Jeanann Sousou, DNP, RN, CNM-FA, CNE
School of Nursing
Rutgers, the State University of New Jersey
Camden, New Jersey

Ann St. Germain, MSN, ANP, WHNP
Associate Clinical Professor
Texas Woman's University
Houston, Texas

Ruth Swart, EdD, MHS, BN, RN, BSc
Senior Instructor, Faculty of Nursing
University of Calgary
Calgary, Alberta

Cheryl Swayne
Associate Professor
Advanced Nursing Studies
Northern Kentucky University
Highland Heights, Kentucky

Susan Terwilliger, EdD, MS, RN, PPCNP-BC
Clinical Associate Faculty
Binghamton University
Binghamton, New York

Ayasha Thomason, MNSc, APRN, WHNP-BC
Clinical Assistant Professor
University of Arkansas for Medical Sciences
Little Rock, Arkansas

Christina Tomkins, MSN, RN, CRNP, PHRN
Assistant Professor
Misericordia University
Dallas, Pennsylvania

Bates' Nursing Guide to Physical Assessment and History Taking is designed for undergraduate nursing students. In this ever-changing and diverse health care arena, nurses are at the forefront in coordinating and providing holistic care for the patient in many venues. Assessment is a key nursing function that ensures the patient receives optimal care. The text provides assessment tools to assist the student to obtain a thorough history and perform a comprehensive physical examination of each patient. The student will learn how to ask pertinent questions and recognize verbal and nonverbal cues while eliciting information related to patient complaints in each body system. The student will then use these history findings and critical thinking skills to prioritize and guide the physical examination. The subjective and objective findings obtained during the assessment will provide the basis for the nursing diagnoses and patient plan of care. Health promotion and disease prevention are highlighted for nurses to incorporate when educating patients, families, and communities.

Bates' Nursing Guide helps students build on their knowledge of human anatomy and physiology, as the lifelong and timeless skills of patient assessment are acquired. Throughout the book, the focus and emphasis is the "healthy" patient with common findings or diseases rather than the rare or obscure disorder. Occasionally, physical signs of rare disorders are included if they hold a solid niche in classic physical assessment or represent a disorder that is critical to the life of the patient. Each chapter explicitly reflects a strong evidence-based perspective, listing key citations that closely align content with new evidence from the health care literature. Color helps readers find chapter sections and tables more easily and highlights insets of key material and special tips for challenging aspects of examination such as examining the eye or assessing the jugular venous pressure.

BATES' NURSING GUIDE: HIGHLIGHTS

The book is divided into three units: *Foundations, Body Systems,* and *Special Lifespan Considerations.*

- *Unit 1, Foundations. Chapter 1, Introduction to Health Assessment,* presents the concept of health and what defines a "healthy" individual. The indicators and purpose of Healthy People 2020 are identified, as are the components of a health assessment and the role of the nurse in assessment. *Chapter 2, Critical Thinking in Health Assessment,* focuses on how to think "like a nurse," utilizing a case study approach to implement the nursing process. *Chapter 3, Interviewing and Communication,* leads the nursing student through therapeutic communication techniques, shares mnemonics for assessment questions, and identifies strategies for handling difficult patients. *Chapter 4, The Health History,* describes the different types of health histories, the purpose for each, and the components of a comprehensive health history. *Chapter 5, Cultural and Spiritual Assessment,* explains why culture and spirituality are important in the health assessment and case studies demonstrate cultural humility. *Chapter 6, Physical Examination: Getting Started,* introduces a logical sequence of the physical examination with an explanation of the techniques and visualization of the equipment. *Chapter 7, Beginning the Physical Examination: General Survey, Vital Signs, and Pain,* and *Chapter 8, Nutrition and Hydration,* continue the process of data collection and expand the process of clinical reasoning for nurses.

- *Unit 2, Body Systems.* This unit encompasses Chapters 9 through 21, which are devoted to the techniques of the regional examination of each of the body systems. These chapters are arranged in a "head-to-toe" sequence, just as the patient examination should flow. Each of the chapters contains:

  - A review of relevant anatomy and physiology

  - Key questions for a relevant nursing health history

  - Updated information for health promotion and counseling

  - Well-described and well-illustrated techniques of examination

  - Samples of documentation in DocuCare for each system

  - Extensive citations from the clinical literature

  - Tables to assist nursing students recognize and compare normal and abnormal findings

  The unit concludes with *Chapter 22, Putting It All Together,* which assists the student nurse to perform a "head to toe" examination following a sequence in which systems are integrated. Students frequently need this step-by-step guidance as they learn new skills and process how the objective data is collected in a systematic manner.

- *Unit 3, Special Lifespan Considerations.* In this unit, *Chapter 23, Assessing Children: Infancy Through Adolescence,* and *Chapter 24, Assessing Older Adults,* relate to special ages in the life cycle and how the assessment techniques and physical examination findings may differ.

This textbook has been written for the undergraduate nursing student. The initial project ensued as faculty and students requested a textbook that was geared to generalist nurses. The focus of the book continues to be **nursing** physical examination and history taking. The health history and the physical examination are both essential for patient assessment and care. Updates include the addition of the electronic health record (EHR), DocuCare.

Students are advised to return to chapters, especially in the *Foundations* unit, as they gain additional experience with patients. Each patient brings a unique background and set of abilities, ideas, issues, coping mechanisms, and family and community dynamics to the health care setting. These attributes mixed with a disease process can be confounding to even the seasoned nurse.

Students may study or review the Anatomy and Physiology sections according to their individual needs. They can study the Physical Examination sections to learn how to perform the relevant examination, practice it under faculty guidance, and review the section again afterward to consolidate their learning. Students and faculty will benefit from identifying common abnormal findings, which appear in two places. The right-hand column of the Physical Examination sections presents possible abnormal findings. These are highlighted in red and placed directly adjacent to the relevant text. Distinguishing these findings from the normal improves learners' observations and clinical acumen. Students will learn how to clearly recognize "normal" when assessing a patient and will recognize abnormal findings. Student nurses will learn to perform inspection, palpation, percussion, and auscultation as well as to utilize the findings in the nursing plan of care.

As students progress through each body system, they should study the documentation for the sample patient, Mrs. N, found in Chapter 2, *Critical Thinking in Health Assessment*. Students should make frequent references to the sections in each of the body systems chapters titled "Recording Your Findings" that display samples of the patient record. This cross-checking will help students learn how to describe and organize information from the interview and physical examination into an understandable documentation format. Furthermore, studying Chapter 22, *Putting It All Together,* will help students integrate the body systems examinations into a coordinated head-to-toe physical examination.

Close scrutiny of the Tables of Abnormalities will deepen students' understanding of important clinical conditions, what they should be looking for, and why they are asking certain questions. However, they should not try to memorize all the detail that is presented. As students work to master the skills of assessment, they should return to the related signs and remember the "normal." Students should use this book to analyze the concern or finding and make use of other clinical texts or journals to pursue the patient's problems in as much depth as necessary.

STUDENT AND INSTRUCTOR RESOURCES

Student Resources

Student resources to accompany this text are available online at thePoint.

Resources include journal articles, NCLEX-style review questions, a Spanish–English audio glossary, Watch and Learn video clips, and Concepts in Action animations.

Instructor Resources

The instructor resources are available on thePoint and include the following:

- Test Generator containing over 400 multiple-choice questions

- PowerPoint presentations

- Image Bank featuring all of the figures from each chapter

- Guided Lecture Notes for presenting key information to your students

- Assignments and Quizzes for gauging student understanding

- Discussion Topics to encourage critical thinking

- Case Studies providing real life application of concepts

A FULLY INTEGRATED COURSE EXPERIENCE

We offer an expanded suite of digital solutions to support instructors and students using *Bates' Nursing Guide to Physical Examination and History Taking*, 2nd edition, that elevate the learning experience. To learn more about any of these solutions, please contact your local Wolters Kluwer representative.

Lippincott CoursePoint and CoursePoint+: An Adaptive Learning Experience

Lippincott
CoursePoint

Lippincott CoursePoint is a fully adaptive and integrated digital course solution for nursing education. CoursePoint synthesizes adaptive learning tools and content with an electronic version of the text and a wide array of integrated learning aids—all in one convenient location.

At the heart of CoursePoint is our adaptive learning system, powered by prepU. In numerous studies, prepU has demonstrated improved student performance in both nursing courses and on the NCLEX. CoursePoint extends prepU's adaptive tools by connecting students to the resources that will help them understand the correct answers, with quiz results linked to relevant sections of the Nursing Health Assessment integrated eBook as well as videos, animations, interactive tutorials, audio tutorials, and interactive case studies via SmartSense links.

As the instructor, you have everything you need to develop your course, with easily accessible resources, organized by type or chapter, including the following:

- A thoroughly revised Test Generator, containing more than 400 NCLEX-style questions

- Strategies for Effective Teaching

- PowerPoint presentations, Guided Lecture Notes, and Prelecture Quizzes

- Image Bank

- Discussion Topics and Assignments

- Case Studies

CoursePoint's instructor reporting tools enable you to monitor individual student and class progress and strengths and weaknesses.

Lippincott
CoursePoint+

Lippincott CoursePoint+ takes learning one step further by integrating additional skills and simulation tools within the CoursePoint platform. Specifically, CoursePoint+ integrates vSim for Nursing: Assessment to provide students with a complete skills experience.

Simulation and EHR Resources

vSim *for Nursing*

- vSim for Nursing: Assessment is Lippincott's new computer simulation platform (available in Lippincott CoursePoint+ or via the Point). Co-developed by Laerdal Medical and Wolters Kluwer, vSim for Nursing: Assessment helps students develop clinical competence and decision-making skills as they interact with virtual patients in a safe, realistic environment. vSim for Nursing records and assesses student decisions throughout the simulation, then provides a personalized feedback log highlighting areas needing improvement.

Lippincott
DocuCare

- Lippincott DocuCare (available via the Point). Lippincott DocuCare combines web-based electronic health record simulation software with clinical case scenarios that link directly to much of the material presented in *Bates' Nursing Guide to Physical Examination and History Taking*. Lippincott DocuCare's nonlinear solution works well in the classroom, simulation lab, and clinical practice.

Additional Media

prepU

- prepU for *Bates' Nursing Guide to Physical Examination and History Taking*, 2nd edition, includes personalized, adaptive quizzes linked to the textbook content that foster formative assessment for students and instructors.

- Lippincott PassPoint for the NCLEX, powered by prepU, is an online, adaptive learning NCLEX preparation resource that allows students to take practice quizzes and comprehensive NCLEX-style examinations.

We appreciate the many professionals at Wolters Kluwer who provided guidance throughout the writing of the second edition of *Bates' Nursing Guide to Physical Examination and History Taking*. To Kelley Squazzo, who coordinated a seamless team, including Cassie Berube, Jennifer Forestieri, Cynthia Rudy, and Dan Reilly.

Special thanks to Annette Ferran for taking the lead on the team and for her attention and involvement. Her dedication in providing timely guidance and insight throughout the project is very much appreciated.

We would also like to thank the team at Aptara, with a special thank you to Karan Rana, project manager, who orchestrated the page proofs.

To all our colleagues, who provided expertise and support for our endeavor and helped make this text a reality.

To Connie Scanga, PhD, who provided additional clarification on various aspects of Anatomy and Physiology.

To Megan Quigley, who provided assistance with photography and computer graphics, at a moment's notice.

To our "models" who eagerly volunteered to be photographed.

To our students, past and present, who are the reason we teach and who inspire us to create and use better teaching tools.

UNIT 2
Body Systems   171

CHAPTER 9
The Integumentary System   173

CHAPTER 10
The Head and Neck   211

CHAPTER 11
The Eyes   236

UNIT

3

Special Lifespan   807

CHAPTER 24
Assessing Older Adults   925

UNIT 1

Foundations

Introduction to Health Assessment

The student will:

1. Define health and health assessment.
2. Explain the components of the health assessment.
3. Identify the health indicators and purpose of Healthy People 2020.
4. Define the nurse's role in assessment.

Health assessment is an integral part of nursing practice. Regardless of which career path in nursing you follow, assessment techniques are essential. Astute attention to details, use of appropriate questions, and a keen awareness of what a person says and does shape the plan of care to optimize each individual's health status throughout the lifespan.

HEALTH

Health is a relative state in which a person is able to live to his or her potential and includes the "7 Facets": physical health, emotional health, social well-being, cultural influences, spiritual influences, environmental influences, and developmental level. Health is the sum of these facets and is not solely defined as the absence of disease or eating right, but rather by the contributions of all dimensions.

- Physical health: how the body works and adapts

- Emotional health: positive outlook and emotions channeled in a healthy manner

- Social well-being: supportive relationships with family and friends

- Cultural influences: favorable connections to promote health

- Spiritual influences: living peacefully, morally, and ethically

- Environmental influences: favorable conditions to promote health

- Developmental level: how one thinks, solves problems, and makes decisions

Health is influenced by all these dimensions. A person's ability to adapt while not compromising the facets is important for health maintenance. Health is not a constant and cannot be taken for granted. The ability to juggle and align the facets in a harmonious network leads to a healthy state for an individual.

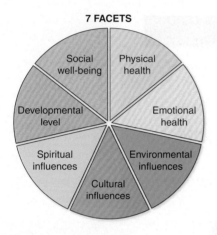

7 FACETS

HEALTH ASSESSMENT

The nursing health assessment entails both a comprehensive health history and a complete physical examination, which are used to evaluate the health status of a person. The ability to solicit information, understand the findings, and apply knowledge can initially be daunting to the new nurse. The nursing health assessment involves a systematic data collection that provides information to facilitate a plan to deliver the best care for the patient.

The first part of the health assessment is the health history, which also incorporates the "7 Facets". The nurse asks pertinent questions to gather data from the patient and/or family. Past medical records may also be used to collect additional information. Learning about the patient's physical and psychological issues, social and cultural associations, environment, developmental level, and spiritual beliefs contributes to the history.

The second component of the health assessment is the physical examination. The nurse uses a structured head-to-toe examination to identify changes in the patient's body systems. An unusual or abnormal finding may support the history data or trigger additional questions.

The purpose of the nursing health assessment is to determine a patient's health status, risk factors, and need for education as a basis for developing a nursing plan of care. The ability of the nurse to extrapolate the findings, prioritize them, and finally formulate and implement the plan of care is the overall goal. This is called "the Nursing Process." The information obtained

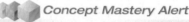 *Concept Mastery Alert*

When determining the type of health assessment to complete, the nurse needs to consider the patient's current situation and condition. A focused assessment is completed on a patient who has already had a comprehensive examination and is being seen for a follow-up visit. A patient who presents with a new problem of a serious or critical nature would require an emergency assessment to determine the patient's current status. However, if this patient is now stable and the acute condition has subsided, the nurse needs to complete a comprehensive health assessment to evaluate all body systems to better decide which system is contributing to the patient's current problem.

throughout the health assessment should be documented in a clear, concise manner. This information is collated in the patient's medical records.

The health assessment is similar to a puzzle. When the nurse meets a patient, it is like opening the puzzle box and dumping out the pieces. Each piece of the history and examination data represents a different aspect of the patient's life, which form a picture of who the patient is. The review of systems in the health history is like the corner and edge pieces of a puzzle that form the frame, in this case the basis for the assessment and how to proceed with the physical examination. Once the frame is in place it is easier to complete the puzzle. Listening and understanding a patient is key to having the pieces fit. The health assessment assists the nurse discover a patient's needs. As a rapport with the patient develops, more details are acquired. As the information is collated, actual health risks emerge, and eventually those last hard-to-fit puzzle pieces are found, which represent the potential health risks. This intricate puzzle is a person's life, and the pieces need to fit correctly for the person to maintain health and quality of life. As the puzzle takes shape, a picture is formed. Likewise, the nurse is able to see the patient as an individual more clearly and is able to create a specific nursing plan of care.

The assessment is typically performed on the patient's arrival to a health care facility. The extent of the health assessment is determined by the acuity of the patient's condition and the site of the care. For example:

- The patient in critical condition brought into a busy emergency department would be asked basic questions revolving around the event that precipitated the admission and whether the patient is on medications, has any allergies, or has any adverse reactions. The thorough health history would be completed when the patient was stable and able to answer questions.

- The patient who has a professional relationship with the nurse and had a thorough health assessment at the initial meeting does not need to have a health history repeated on each visit. Updates based on new events would be added as necessary.

- The nursing home admission of a patient with dementia may require the health assessment information to be supplemented with information from the family, past health care providers, and/or medical records, based on the ability of the patient to remember information.

Each person needs a complete health assessment. Ideally this is done on admission, but extenuating circumstances may prohibit its completion in detail at this time. The sooner the health assessment is completed fully, the better the nurse knows the patient, and more holistic care can be provided to ensure health promotion and quality of life.

Nursing and medical professionals both perform health assessments, and although the assessment techniques may be similar, the use is different. The medical focus is on diagnoses and treatment of the disease, whereas the nursing focus is on diagnoses and treatment of the actual or potential human responses to disease or life events (e.g., the birth of a child). The nursing assessment identifies many contributing factors to the individual's health and wellness, including all "7 Facets". The health assessment allows data to be collected that is specific to the patient. As the nurse spends time with the patient, he or she can identify concerns or changes. Any deviation is noted, as are the coping mechanisms and resources the patient has available. This information is used to determine health problems or other potential problems the patient has. Development of the nursing care plan and working with the individual patient are paramount in health promotion.

Once the plan is in place, evaluation continually occurs and reconfiguring the plan may be necessary. The health care team meets to collaborate on patients and decide the best overall care. This occurs throughout the lifespan, from the inception of life until death. The health care team is a partnership and includes the nurse, physician, nutritionist, social worker, physical therapist, occupational therapist, speech therapist, and/or dentist. They all work together on the same team for the benefit of the patient.

Through the health assessment, nurses detect areas of concern, *requiring immediate attention,* as well as health maintenance or improvement needs. Nurses have taken the lead in health promotion and disease prevention and are to assist patients to change behaviors and lifestyles to obtain optimal health. Such changes enable individuals to increase control of and improve their overall health. Selecting the level of care and teaching is governed by the nurse as care is rendered. During the overall assessment of the patient, the nurse uses the findings to decide the areas that take precedence.

Health promotion and disease prevention are essential areas of patient education. Maintaining health is a balancing act influenced by behaviors and choices. Health education is a vital component of nursing practice. The nurse assists people in making connections between a healthy lifestyle and disease prevention. Additional components that contribute to health include the individual's personality and attitude, resilience, family dynamics, access to health care and resources, nutrition, exercise, culture, and beliefs.

Healthy People 2020 is a framework that identifies risk factors, health issues, and diseases of concern in the United States. The goals and objectives serve to improve the health of individuals and communities, targeting 10-year increments. The overall goal is to increase quality of life by creating guidelines for a healthy lifestyle as well as educating people and cultivating an awareness that will assist in the elimination of health disparities. Healthy People 2020 promotes health and disease prevention as it improves the quality and length of a person's life.

The national health objectives determined by Healthy People 2020 are broad and take into consideration the results of the Healthy People 2010 outcomes. These are based on current data, new developments, and challenges that are prevalent or emerging in the United States. The U.S. Department of Health and Human Services provided the data online and invited health care leaders and the community to voice their opinions regarding the focus for the next decade.

The Healthy People 2020 indicators pertinent to each individual will be determined as the nurse completes the health assessment on each patient. Using the website (http://www.healthypeople.gov), the nurse can identify health indicators, appropriate interventions, and resources.

Role of the Nurse in Assessment

Nurses deliver care across the lifespan, in a variety of practice arenas. A small sample of the groups served are pediatrics, geriatrics, medical, surgical, mental health, maternity, and community health. Nurses assess patient needs, develop interventions, and educate and counsel individuals, families, groups, and communities toward higher levels of health and wellness. Nurses view health as the focus, with the patient, the environment, and the nurse all influencing the health status of the patient. It is crucial to use all "7 Facets" that affect the patient's health, as this guides the nursing plan of care. Also important is the patient's view and definition of health. One person may view health as being free of disease. Another may indicate health as good control of diabetes and blood glucose. One person has a chronic disease and the other does not, but they both see themselves as healthy. When meeting with the patient, ask what his or her goals and views are:

"What would you like to accomplish during this visit?"
"Tell me how you see yourself in regards to health."
"Tell me why you are here today."

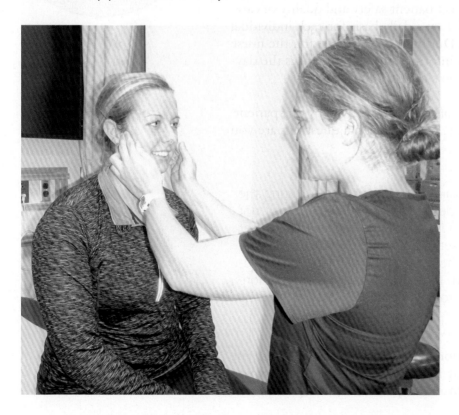

Focusing on the answers (verbal) and the actions (nonverbal) of the patient, the nurse is constantly assessing and formulating a plan of care so that the patient can achieve the best possible health.

Health goes beyond the individual patient. It also encompasses the community. Nurses are involved in the shaping of public policy and in social, economic, and workplace decisions. In order for the nurse to assist a patient with health, a healthy environment must also be nurtured. The community and the environment need to be defined and realistic goals set for possible change (e.g., nurses may promote healthy diets in school cafeterias). This marks the path for prevention of illness and maintenance of health and wellness. Nurses may assess the individual, family, or community; however, the focus of this text will be the assessment of the individual.

Nurses are instrumental in the care of patients. They oversee the holistic care of each patient. The nurse's initial role in health assessment is to collect data. Constant observation and attention to details and nuances are critical. Each person comes with a vast array of information and is influenced by his or her surroundings, including the physical, emotional, cultural, and spiritual environment. This extensive body of knowledge and the responsibility that each patient encounter requires can seem overwhelming to the new nurse. As the nurse becomes more proficient and comfortable in his or her role, the knowledge base and expertise increase and foster confidence.

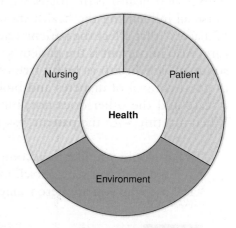

As a nurse, it is vital to sift through all the patient information and make decisions on what information will impact patient safety and quality of care. The ability to identify what is important on a daily basis for each individual patient is paramount for nursing care. During the health history, the nurse asks questions to determine the health information that influences the day-to-day care and how it affects the person's quality of life.

This brief encounter depicts the wealth of information given by one patient. During this short interaction with Mr. P, what additional questions are you forming related to his health needs?

Mr. P arrives at the clinic with complaints of blurred vision. During the health history, the patient also confides to the nurse that he has not been able to make it to the bathroom in time and has been incontinent frequently. He verbalizes that he is upset that he is unable to see well and that has slowed down his mobility. The decrease in mobility and incontinence have limited his social life with friends and he is becoming more irritable and feeling lonely. He admits to feeling like he wants to sleep all the time.

The nurse is already formulating additional questions to correlate with the standard health history based on what the patient has disclosed. As you read through this book, you will learn more questions to ask, those that are system specific as well as those regarding overlapping systems. How you interpret this nurse–patient interaction will be much different after you learn how to do a health assessment.

As a student nurse, you might take the encounter at face value and attribute Mr. P's downward spiral to his initial blurred vision. However, after a thorough assessment, you may uncover additional issues and determine that his vision problem is not the root of his irritability and fatigue.

There is too little information available in the scenario to judge what is going on with this patient. It is important to allot a sufficient amount of time to do a detailed health assessment. Once more details are uncovered, more possibilities arise. Mr. P could potentially have multiple issues, such as diabetes, a brain tumor, depression, blurred vision, or benign prostatic hypertrophy. However, this discovery will not be unearthed without more information.

Accurate health history taking and physical assessment are the foundation of nursing practice. Nurses rely heavily on these skills in all aspects of nursing. The puzzle will be pieced together during the nursing history and assessment. For example, the patient recovering from an illness or surgery needs to be carefully assessed each shift, with changes noted that may indicate potentially dire consequences.

Assessing the patient by using the "7 Facets" is at the forefront of the nurse's responsibilities. Physically, the nurse may discover a change in vital signs, nausea, difficulty swallowing, or incontinence. Mentally, the patient may be experiencing changes in the level of consciousness and not know where he or she is or even who he or she is. Emotionally, is the patient more subdued, angry, or crying after a particular family member visits? The nurse will pursue the reason behind this change in the patient. Could there be abuse, money concerns, or a fear of abandonment? The nurse has developed a rapport with the patient and is now able to delve into territory that may have been off limits previously. Once these issues are acknowledged, the patient can develop a healthier life with appropriate interventions and options. Developmentally, a patient may need guidance in areas such as problem solving or moral understanding. Socially, the patient may be isolated from his or her support system in the hospital and need additional outlets. Providing information about self-help groups or health resources can provide additional avenues for people socially. Spiritually, it is best to let the patient take the lead on how he or she wants to handle spiritual care, as this dimension is very personal. If the patient wishes, connecting him or her with clergy of the same denomination while in the hospital may be welcomed, or assisting with transportation to worship services when at home may be reasonable. In all aspects it is best to work with the patient to enable partnering in choices. This allows the patient to make decisions regarding health care. The more a patient participates in these decisions, the better the outcomes are in the long term toward a healthier lifestyle.

Teaching opportunities for the patient and family present themselves during health assessments. The nurse uses information detected in the assessment to work with the patient to enhance quality of life. For example, the person who is overweight and has an increased body mass index (BMI) might need assistance with setting up a plan to lose weight. A plan that includes the family may be the best solution for one individual, but another may do better with an outside support group. A mutually agreed upon plan will assist the patient in maintaining autonomy and the highest level of wellness.

The nurse's ability to detect a change in a patient's physical, mental, emotional, developmental, social, or spiritual self, whether slight or significant, is instrumental in providing the best care. Just as a detective asks questions, the nurse finds clues and follows up on information in order to solve patient problems. Knowing how to facilitate the nursing health assessment by asking appropriate questions to obtain more information helps solve the mystery and create a nursing care plan. The care plan is evaluated periodically and changes made to update the plan. The nurse, like a detective, is always reassessing the patient or case for changes in order to achieve the best results. Each relies on both the science and art of their respective profession.

The nursing process will be explained in detail in Chapter 2, Critical Thinking in Health Assessment.

REFERENCES

American Association of Colleges of Nursing. *The Essentials of Baccalaureate Education for Professional Nursing Practice.* Washington, DC: American Association of Colleges of Nursing; 2008. Available at: http://www.aacn.nche.edu/education-resources/BaccEssentials08.pdf. Accessed November 14, 2015.

American Nurses Association. *Nursing: Scope and Standards of Practice.* 2nd ed. Washington, DC: American Nurses Association; 2010.

Babb M. Clinical risk assessment: identifying patients at high risk for heart failure. *Assoc Periop Reg Nurse J.* 2009;89(2): 273–274, 277–288.

Dawood M, Gallini A. Using discovery interviews to understand the patient experience. *J Nurs Manage.* 2010;17(1): 26–31.

Healthy People 2020. Available at: http://www.healthypeople. gov. Accessed November 14, 2015.

Hoffman K, Aitken L, Duffield C. A comparison of novice and expert nurses' cue collection during clinical decision making: verbal protocol analysis. *Int J Nurs Stud.* 2009;46(10): 1335–1344.

Mosby's Medical Dictionary. 9th ed. Philadelphia, PA: Elsevier; 2013.

Critical Thinking in Health Assessment

The student will:

1. Define subjective and objective data.

2. Identify appropriate subjective questions for the health history.

3. Explain the Nursing Process.

4. Explain the clinical reasoning process and its relationship to the Nursing Process.

5. Identify a patient's problems prioritized by severity.

6. Create a nursing care plan for a patient.

7. Analyze a written patient history and physical examination findings to identify patient problems and develop a nursing care plan.

8. Evaluate and revise a care plan based on a simulation of a patient.

The goal of health assessment by the nurse is the development of an individualized plan of care for each patient. The nurse uses the Nursing Process (*a problem solving process*) to identify patient problems; set a goal and develop an action plan; implement the plan; and evaluate the outcome (i.e., did the interventions resolve or improve the patient's problem? or does the plan need to be revised?).

The Nursing Process steps are Assessment, Diagnosis, Planning, Implementation, and Evaluation. During the assessment phase, the nurse gathers patient data via the health history and examination of the patient. A *clinical reasoning* process is then used to analyze the patient data and develop hypotheses as to the patient's problem or problems. Once the problems are defined, the nurse develops the plan of care and implements and evaluates it. During the process, the nurse records the patient assessment findings and the plan of care in the patient record to communicate the patient's story and the nurse's clinical reasoning and plan to the other health care team members. This chapter will discuss types of patient data, the clinical reasoning process, and the Nursing Process.

Critical thinking is ongoing, as is assessment of the patient. The two are intricately intertwined; neither exists in isolation. The health assessment is the discovery and collation of facts from both the health history and physical examination. The comprehensive health history and physical assessment build the foundation of the clinical assessment.

TYPES OF PATIENT DATA

Through skilled interviewing, the nurse will gather the history from the patient or the family; this is the **subjective data**, which is also known as *symptoms*. After the interview and collection of subjective data, the nurse will perform either a head-to-toe physical examination or a systems-specific examination based on the patient's information. The **objective data** is the information gathered from the physical examination and the laboratory tests. This is primarily factual and descriptive and is also known as *signs*.

As you learn the techniques of history taking and physical examination, remember the important differences between *subjective information* and *objective information*. These distinctions are equally important for organizing written and oral presentations about patients into a logical and understandable format.

Differences Between Subjective and Objective Data	
Subjective Data: Symptoms	**Objective Data: Signs**
What the patient tells you	What you detect during the examination
The history, from Chief Complaint through Review of Systems	All physical examination findings
Example: Mrs. G is a 54-year-old hairdresser who reports pressure over her left chest "like an elephant sitting there," which radiates to her left neck and arm.	*Example:* Mrs. G is an older, overweight white female, who is pleasant and co-operative. Height 5'4", weight 150 lb, BMI 26, BP 160/80 right arm, sitting, HR 96 and regular, respiratory rate 24 and regular, temperature 97.5°F oral

Obtaining Subjective Data

During the history, a rapport develops between the nurse and the patient and a mutual trust begins. As the fact-finding mission of the health history proceeds and data are collected, the nurse is putting pieces of the patient's puzzle together. By asking questions, the nurse clarifies the patient's problems and teaching needs. Each time the patient has a positive response to a question, the topic should be addressed further. As a new nurse, the questions you need to ask may seem endless, and the use of the mnemonic "OLD CART" is instrumental in assisting you to formulate the questions. Remember to ask one question at a time to insure a thorough understanding on both the patient's and the nurse's parts. The patient needs to understand the specific question and not hear a rapid fire list, and the health care provider needs to be able to illicit which answer pertains to the specific question.

Remember to open the chief complaint (CC) interview with a broad, open-ended question; for example, "Tell me about your headache from when it began to now." Then use OLD CART to identify missing data.

Mr. C. is a 57-year-old male who presents to the clinic with complaints of a headache. During questioning you refer to "OLD CART":

OLD CART
Onset
Location
Duration
Characteristic symptoms
Associated manifestations
Relieving factors
Treatment

Onset: when the sign or symptom began.
When did the headache begin?
Location: where the sign or symptom is located.
Where exactly is the headache? Can you point to it?
Does it radiate?
Duration: how long the sign or symptom has been going on.
Does the headache come and go? Is it continuous? What time of day is it most severe?
Characteristic symptoms: what the symptom feels like, how it is described, and the severity.
How does the headache feel? Is it throbbing? Sharp? Stabbing? Describe it. Rate it on a scale of 1 to 10, with 10 being the worst pain you have felt in your life.
Associated manifestations: what else is going on when the patient experiences the sign(s) or symptom(s).
Does anything else happen when you get the headaches? Blurred vision? Nausea? Vomiting? Seizures?

Relieving factors: anything the patient has tried to relieve the headache.
What have you tried to make your headache subside? Cool compresses? Rest in a dark room? Did it work?

Treatments: any interventions the patient has previously tried.
Has the patient seen a health care provider? Tried any remedies: medications (prescription, over the counter, or herbal), acupuncture to make the headache go away? Does it work?

NURSING PROCESS

The nurse collects patient information and synthesizes it (assessment), decides what is most important (nursing diagnosis), develops a plan (goals/plan), implements the plan (interventions), and determines whether it is working for the patient (evaluation). This occurs in a multitude of sites and settings with all types of people. For example:

At the community clinic, while assessing height and weight, you note that a 2-month-old has gained 7 lb in the past month.
At the senior center, you note that the blood pressure reading of one of the members is 192/104, R arm, sitting.
Postoperatively you assess your patient and find him crying uncontrollably.

These scenarios can have different outcomes based on how the nurse and patient handle the situation. As a student nurse, you may find yourself in a quandary, uncertain of how to handle a situation or what to tackle first. Developing your knowledge base and diagnostic reasoning skills will assist the problem solving process. The nursing process assists you to logically and efficiently structure the patient's care.

The nursing process is the broad systematic framework that provides a methodical base for the practice of nursing. This problem solving approach addresses the human responses and needs of each patient, family, and community. The nursing process is also the scaffold that the American Nurses Association uses to develop the Standards of Nursing Practice.

The patient is the focus in the nursing process, with the nurse assisting the patient to achieve optimal health using individualized interventions. This is a mutually agreed upon plan of care which contributes to the patient's involvement and increased success.

Assessment, Diagnosis, Planning, Implementation, Evaluation: ADPIE

The five steps of the nursing process are all incorporated into the patient's plan of care and revised as the patient's health status changes.
The first step is assessment. **Assessment** is the subjective and objective data gathered during the initial health history and physical examination and collected on each patient encounter. This data is instrumental

in devising a plan of care for the patient. Therapeutic communication is essential to elicit pertinent information about the patient, the family, and the community in order to provide the best care for the patient. As you document your findings, cluster key points and relevant pieces of information together. This will help you formulate the preliminary problem list. The assessment phase continues throughout the entire patient encounter, which provides the potential for updates in the plan of care based on new assessments and data.

The second element is the diagnosis. **Diagnosis** has a nursing focus and is based on real or potential health problems or human responses to health problems. The nurse uses clinical reasoning to formulate diagnoses based on the assessment data and the patient's problem list. The diagnosis sets the stage for the remainder of the care plan.

The third element is planning. **Planning** is devising the best course of action to address the patient's diagnoses. During planning, the nurse and patient select goals for each diagnosis in order to alleviate, decrease, or prevent the problems addressed in the nursing diagnosis. There should be a short-term goal (STG) and a long-term goal (LTG) with realistic timeframes incorporated. Developing a successful plan requires good interpersonal skills and sensitivity to the patient's goals, economic means, competing responsibilities, and family structure and dynamics. Interventions are then developed for each goal.

The fourth element is the implementation of interventions. **Implementation** of the interventions can be completed by the patient, the family, or members of the health care team. The interventions should clearly relate to the nursing diagnosis and the planned goals. The interventions are individualized for each patient and will be modified as the patient's status or environment changes to support positive outcomes.

The fifth and final element is evaluation. **Evaluation** is a continuing process to determine if the goals have been attained. The nursing care plan is revised based on the patient's condition and whether the goals are realistic or appropriate for the patient. The intervention and evaluation process is ongoing and confirms that the nursing care is relevant.

"A nursing diagnosis is a clinical judgment concerning a human response to health conditions/life processes, or a vulnerability for that response, by an individual, family, group, or community. A nursing diagnosis provides the basis for selection of nursing interventions to achieve outcomes for which the nurse has accountability." (Approved at the ninth NANDA Conference; amended in 2009 and 2013.)[1]

ASSESSMENT AND DIAGNOSIS: THE PROCESS OF CLINICAL REASONING

The process of clinical reasoning may seem mysterious to beginning students. Assessment appears to take place in the experienced nurse's mind. These expert nurses often think quickly, with little overt or conscious effort. They differ widely in personal style, communication skills, clinical training, experience, and interests. Some nurses find it difficult to explain the logic behind their clinical thinking. As an active learner, it is expected that you will ask teachers and clinicians to elaborate on the fine points of their clinical reasoning and decision making.[2-4] Using the nursing process and care planning as a student is instrumental in learning to think like a nurse. This framework is concrete and organized. Using the step by step approach, facilitates the learning process.

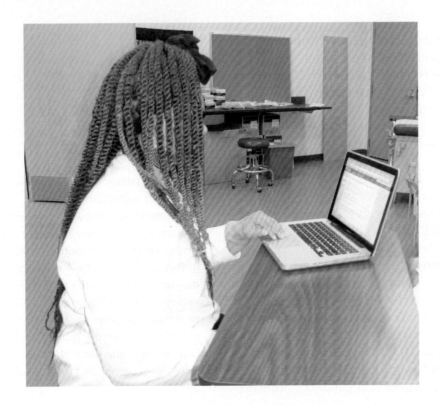

Cognitive psychologists have shown that clinicians use three types of reasoning for clinical problem solving: pattern recognition, development of schemas, and application of relevant basic and clinical science.[5-8] As you gain experience, your clinical reasoning will begin at the outset of the patient encounter, not at the end. The novice nurse needs to see all the pieces and the plan of care in a systematic fashion where they are able to evaluate the situation, whereas, the experienced nurse seems to figure out the plan from the onset. Ultimately, as students gain experience over the first few years in practice, this acumen will be acquired, too.[9,10]

Identifying Problems and Making Nursing Diagnoses: Steps in Clinical Reasoning

- Identify abnormal or positive findings.
- Cluster the findings.
- Interpret the findings.
- Make hypotheses about the nature of the patient's problem.
- Test the hypotheses and establish a working nursing diagnosis.
- Develop a plan agreeable to the patient.

- **Identify abnormal or positive findings.** Make a list of the patient's *symptoms*, the *signs* you observed during the physical examination, and any laboratory reports available to you. Also, identify the positive responses during the health history. For example, the patients living in a community with a high crime level is important when organizing the issue/problem list and in development of the plan.

- **Cluster the findings.** This step may be easy. The symptom of a scratchy throat and the sign of an erythematous inflamed pharynx, for example, clearly localize the problem to the pharynx. A complaint of headache leads you quickly to the structures of the skull and brain. However, do not forget to include information on the patient's stress level due to being laid off work and lack of income. Other symptoms may present greater difficulty. Chest pain, for example, can originate in the coronary arteries, the stomach and esophagus, or the muscles and bones of the chest. If the pain is exertional and relieved by rest, either the heart or the musculoskeletal components of the chest wall may be involved. If the patient notes pain only when carrying groceries with the left arm, the musculoskeletal system becomes the likely culprit.

  When localizing findings, be as specific as your data allows, but bear in mind that you may have to settle for a body region, such as the chest, or a body system, such as the musculoskeletal system. On the other hand, you may be able to define the exact structure involved, such as the left pectoral muscle. Some symptoms and signs cannot be localized, such as fatigue or fever, but are useful in the next set of steps. In addition, obtaining more information regarding psychosocial issues may add more depth when trying to pinpoint the "real" problem.

- **Interpret findings in terms of probable process.** Patient problems stem from different causes, including changes: disease processes, relationships, nutritional, immunologic, infectious, congenital, traumatic, toxic, economic, or cultural causes, and many other possibilities exist. Analyze the data to evaluate the patient's health status. It is important to differentiate a problem that should be treated by a nurse versus one that should be referred to another health discipline.

- **Make hypotheses about the nature of the patient's problem.** Draw on all the knowledge and experience you can muster, and it is here that reading is most useful for learning about patterns of abnormalities, diseases, and issues that help cluster your patient's findings. You may need to gather more data to rule in or out your hypotheses.

  By consulting the clinical literature, you embark on the lifelong goal of **evidence-based decision making**.[11,12]

Until you gain broader knowledge and experience, you may not be able to develop highly specific hypotheses, but proceed as far as you can with the data and knowledge you have. The following steps should help:

- Nursing diagnoses are based primarily on changes in a person's life, altered processes, and specific causes. You will frequently see patients whose complaints do not fall neatly into these categories. Some symptoms defy

 Concept Mastery Alert

Diagnostic reasoning involves a step-by-step process. In the first step, the nurse gathers data to identify what is and is not normal for the patient. In the second step, the nurse uses this information to look for cues that suggest or indicate whether or not the findings from the first step are related, thus clustering the data. From there, the nurse analyzes the data and applies knowledge and experience to make hypotheses about the patient's problem.

analysis and are medically unexplained. You may never be able to move beyond simple descriptive categories such as "fatigue" or "anorexia." Other problems relate to stressful events in the patient's life. Events such as losing a job or loved one may increase the risk for subsequent illness. Identifying these events and helping the patient develop coping strategies are as important as managing a headache or a duodenal ulcer.

- Another increasingly prominent category on problem lists is *Health Maintenance*. Routinely listing Health Maintenance helps track several important health concerns more effectively: immunizations, screening measures (e.g., mammograms, prostate examinations), instructions regarding nutrition and skin or testicular self-examinations, recommendations about exercise or use of seat belts, and responses to important life events.

- **Develop a plan agreeable to the patient.** Develop and record a *Plan* for each patient problem. Your *Plan* flows logically from the problems or diagnoses you have identified. Specify which steps are needed next. These steps range from monitoring daily weights, to consultation, to timing of dressings or IVs, to arranging a family meeting. You will find that you will follow many of the same nursing diagnoses over time; however, the *Plan* is often more fluid, encompassing changes and modifications that emerge from each patient encounter. The *Plan* should reference the diagnosis, therapy, and patient education for each individual. The nursing diagnosis may be the same; however, the remainder of the care plan is much different.

- Before finalizing your *Plan*, it is important to share your assessment and clinical thinking with the patient and seek out his or her opinions, concerns, and willingness to proceed with the interventions. Remember that patients may need to hear the same information multiple times and ways before they comprehend it. The patient should always be an active participant in the plan of care.

Clinical Reasoning: Developing Hypotheses About Patient Problems

The Nursing Process

1. Assessment

   Select the most specific and critical findings to support your problem list. At the community clinic while assessing length and weight on infants, you note that a 2-month-old has gained 7 lb in the past month. The mother reports that the child does not sleep through the night and the family of seven is living in a hotel room. The baby's crying is waking everyone up, so she has started feeding him more so that he will hopefully sleep when he is full. On further questioning, you find out that the 2-month-old baby is eating rice cereal six to seven times a day. This information is critical in building a thorough assessment.

2. Diagnosis

Use your inferences as multiple options for this child and family. The top nursing diagnosis would be:

Ineffective infant feeding patterns related to excess food intake

or

Overweight

Other choices on the list but not the best or top priority include:

Deficient Knowledge

Risk for deficient fluid volume

Disturbance in sleep pattern: Risk for sleep deprivation

Risk for constipation

3. Planning/Outcomes

Develop goals for the nursing diagnosis that are realistic and timely.

Nursing Diagnosis: Ineffective infant feeding patterns related to excess food intake.

The goals for this child might be:

STG: The infant will receive adequate nutrition for growth appropriate to age within 1 day.

LTG: The infant will maintain current weight over the next month.

4. Implementation/interventions:

The nursing interventions should help to achieve the goals stated.

a. Record daily weights and weekly length in a journal.

b. Educate the family regarding the importance of formula/breast milk only at this age for development and nutrition. Feeding the baby cereal at this age is not recommended as the baby's digestive tract is not ready to digest the cereal. The baby will get all the nutrients necessary for growth and development from formula/breast milk.

c. Assist the family to find alternative ways to calm the baby rather than using food. An example might be to take a walk outside as this will relax the baby and maintain quiet in the room. Another solution is to go into the bathroom and run the shower as the water may be calming to the child and separate him from the siblings so they are able to sleep, and it will limit distractions to both groups.

d. Record the sleep/wake cycle and include when and what the baby is eating. Once this is recorded, develop a schedule that will support healthy patterns for the family.

5. Evaluation

The child and family should continue to be monitored to determine if adjustments or additional teaching is necessary. Assess the child's length and weight every week and ask the family if they are obtaining more sleep.

See section on Evaluating Clinical Findings, p. 33.

RECORDING YOUR FINDINGS: THE CASE OF MRS. N

Now turn to the case of Mrs. N and scrutinize the history, physical examination, assessment, and plan.

The Case of Mrs. N

1/12/16 11:00 AM

Mrs. N is a pleasant, 54-year-old widowed saleswoman residing in Amarillo, Texas.

Referral. None.

Source and Reliability. Self seems reliable.

Chief Complaint: "My head hurts."

Present Illness: Mrs. N reports over the past 3 months, increasing problems with frontal headaches. These are usually bifrontal, throbbing, and mild to moderately severe. She has missed work on several occasions because of associated nausea and vomiting. Headaches average once a week, related to stress, and last 4 to 6 hours. Relieved by sleep and putting a damp towel on forehead. Little relief from aspirin. No associated visual changes, motor-sensory deficits, or paresthesias.

"Sick headaches" with nausea and vomiting began at age 15, recurred through her mid-20s, decreased to one every 2 or 3 months and almost disappeared.

Patient reports increased pressure at work from a new and demanding boss and worried about daughter (see *Personal and Social History*). Thinks headaches similar to headaches had in the past. Wants to be sure because mother died of a stroke. Concerned they interfere with work, make her irritable with family. Eats three meals a day, drinks three cups of coffee per day; cola at night.

Medications. Aspirin, 1 to 2 tablets every 4 to 6 hours as needed. "Water pill" in the past for ankle swelling, none recently.

Allergies. Ampicillin causes rash.

Tobacco. About 1 pack of cigarettes per day since age 18 (36 pack-years).

Alcohol/drugs. Wine rarely. No illicit drugs.

Past History

Childhood Illnesses. Measles, chickenpox. No scarlet fever or rheumatic fever.

Adult Illnesses. **Medical:** Pyelonephritis, 2006, with fever and right flank pain; treated with ampicillin; developed generalized rash with itching several days later. Reports kidney x-rays normal; no recurrence of infection. **Surgical:** Tonsillectomy, age 6; appendectomy, age 13. Sutures for laceration, 2009, after stepping on glass. **Ob/Gyn:** G3 P3–0–0–3, normal vaginal deliveries.

Menarche age 12. Last menses 6 months ago. Little interest in sex, not sexually active. No concerns about HIV infection. *Psychiatric:* None.

Health Maintenance. **Immunizations:** Oral polio vaccine, year uncertain; Tdap, 2009; flu vaccine, 2015, no reaction. **Screening tests:** Last Pap smear, 2012, normal. No mammograms to date.

Gravida (G) is the number of times the patient has been pregnant including current pregnancy.

Para (P) is broken down into:
T: term births
P: preterm births
A: abortions
L: living children
or TPAL

Family History

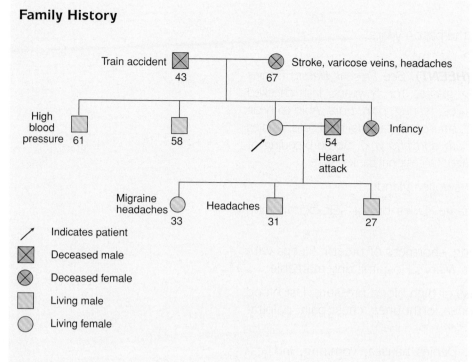

The *Family History* can be recorded as a diagram or a narrative. The diagram is more helpful than the narrative for tracing genetic disorders. The negatives from the family history should follow either format.

/   Indicates patient

⊠   Deceased male

⊗   Deceased female

▨   Living male

◯   Living female

OR

Father died at age 43 in train accident. Mother died at age 67 from stroke; had varicose veins, headaches.

Brother, 61, hypertension; brother, 58, mild arthritis; sister, died in infancy of unknown cause.

Husband died, 54 of heart attack.

Daughter, 33, with migraine headaches; son, 31, headaches; son, 27, well.

Denies family history of diabetes, tuberculosis, heart or kidney disease, cancer, anemia, epilepsy, or mental illness.

Personal and Social History. Born and raised in Lake City, finished high school, married at age 19. Worked as sales clerk for 2 years, moved with husband to Amarillo, had 3 children. Returned to work 15 years ago because of financial pressures. Children all married. Four years ago Mr. N died suddenly of a heart attack, leaving little savings. Mrs. N has moved to a small apartment near daughter, Dorothy. Dorothy's husband, Arthur, has an alcohol problem. Mrs. N's apartment is a haven for Dorothy and her 2 children, Kevin, 6 years, and Linda, 3 years. Mrs. N feels responsible for helping them; feels tense and nervous but denies depression. She has friends but rarely discusses family problems: "I'd rather keep them to myself. I don't like gossip." No church or other organizational support. She is typically up at 7:00 AM, works 9:00 to 5:30, eats dinner alone.

Exercise and Diet. Gets little exercise. Diet high in carbohydrates.

Safety Measures. Seat belt regularly. Sunblock SPF 15. Medications in unlocked medicine cabinet. Cleaning solutions in unlocked cabinet below sink. Shotgun and box of shells in unlocked closet.

Review of Systems

General. Has *gained* about 10 lb in the past 4 years.

Skin. Denies rashes or other changes.

Head, Eyes, Ears, Nose, Throat (HEENT). See *Present Illness.* Denies history of head injury. *Eyes:* Reading glasses for 5 years, last checked 1 year ago. Denies diplopia, blurring, halos, tearing, pain. *Ears:* Able to hear. Denies tinnitus, vertigo, infections. *Nose, sinuses:* Occasional mild cold. Denies hay fever, sinus trouble. *Throat (or mouth and pharynx):* Some bleeding of gums recently. Last dental visit 2 years ago. Occasional canker sore.

Neck. Denies lumps, goiter, pain. No swollen glands.

Breasts. Denies lumps, pain, discharge. Does breast self-examination sporadically.

Respiratory. Denies cough, wheezing, shortness of breath. Sleeps with one pillow. Last chest x-ray, 1994, St. Mary's Hospital; unremarkable.

Cardiovascular. Denies heart disease or high blood pressure; last blood pressure taken in 2010. Denies dyspnea, orthopnea, chest pain, palpitations, electrocardiogram (ECG).

Gastrointestinal. Appetite "good"; Denies nausea, vomiting, indigestion. Bowel movement about once daily, hard stools when tense; denies diarrhea, bleeding, pain, jaundice, gallbladder, or liver problems.

Urinary. Denies frequency, dysuria, hematuria, or recent flank pain; nocturia × 1, large volume. Occasionally loses some urine when coughs hard.

Genital. Denies vaginal, or pelvic infections or dyspareunia. Last Pap smear 2012, negative results.

Peripheral Vascular. Varicose veins appeared in both legs during first pregnancy. For 10 years, has had swollen ankles after prolonged standing; wears light elastic pantyhose; tried "water pill" 5 months ago, but didn't help; denies history of phlebitis or leg pain.

Musculoskeletal. Mild, aching, low back pain, often after a long day of work; no radiation down the legs; back exercises in past, none currently. No other joint pain.

Psychiatric. Denies history of depression or treatment for psychiatric disorders. See also *Present Illness* and *Personal and Social History.*

Neurologic. Denies fainting, seizures, motor or sensory loss. Memory intact.

Hematologic. Except for bleeding gums, denies easy bleeding, anemia.

Endocrine. Denies thyroid trouble, temperature intolerance, symptoms or history of diabetes. Minimal sweating.

Physical Examination

Mrs. N is a short, overweight, middle-aged woman. Animated and responds quickly to questions. Somewhat tense, with moist, cold hands. Hair fixed neatly, clothes immaculate, color is tan, and lies supine without discomfort.

Vital Signs. Ht (without shoes) 157 cm (5′2″). Wt (dressed) 65 kg (143 lb). Body mass index (BMI) 26. Blood pressure (BP) 164/98 right arm, supine; 160/96 left arm, supine. Heart rate (HR) 88 and regular. Respiratory rate (RR) 18. Temperature (oral) 98.6°F.

Skin. Cool, moist, tan. Scattered cherry angiomas over upper trunk. Nails without clubbing, cyanosis.

Head, Eyes, Ears, Nose, Throat (HEENT). *Head:* Hair coarse, full, brown. Scalp without lesions, normocephalic/atraumatic. *Eyes:* Distant Vision 20/30 in each eye. Visual fields full by confrontation. Conjunctiva pink; sclera white. PERRLA. EOMs intact. Disc margins sharp, without hemorrhages, exudates. No arteriolar narrowing. *Ears:* Soft, light brown cerumen partially obscures right TM; left canal clear, TM with cone of light. Acuity hears whispered voice at 1 foot BL. Weber midline. 2AC > BC. *Nose:* Mucosa pink, septum midline. No sinus tenderness or polyps. *Mouth:* Oral mucosa pink. Several interdental papillae red, slightly swollen. Dentition intact. Tongue midline, with 3 × 4-mm shallow white ulcer on red base on undersurface near tip; tender but not indurated. Tonsils absent. Pharynx without exudates.

Neck. Neck supple. Trachea midline. Thyroid isthmus barely palpable, lobes not felt.

Lymph Nodes. Small (<1 cm), soft, nontender, and mobile tonsillar and posterior cervical nodes bilaterally. No axillary or epitrochlear nodes. Several 0.5-cm inguinal nodes bilaterally, soft, equal nontender, mobile.

Thorax and Lungs. Thorax symmetric with equal excursion. Lungs resonant. Breath sounds vesicular with no added sounds. Diaphragm descends 4 cm bilaterally.

Cardiovascular (CV). JVP 1 cm above the sternal angle, at 30 degrees. Carotid upstrokes brisk, without bruits. Apical impulse discrete and tapping, barely palpable in the 5th left interspace, 8 cm lateral to the midsternal line. S_1, S_2; no S_3 or S_4. A II/VI medium-pitched midsystolic murmur at the 2nd right interspace; does not radiate to neck. No diastolic murmurs.

Breasts. Pendulous, left slightly larger than right. No dimpling, retractions, rashes, masses; nipples without discharge.

Abdomen. Protuberant. Well-healed 5 cm × 0.25 cm scar, right lower quadrant. Bowel sounds active. No tenderness or masses. Liver span 7 cm in right midclavicular line; edge smooth, palpable 1 cm below RCM. Spleen and kidneys not felt. No CVAT.

Genitalia. External genitalia without lesions. Internal examination deferred. Vaginal mucosa pink.

Rectal. Stool brown, negative for occult blood.

Extremities. Warm without edema. BL calves supple, nontender.

Peripheral Vascular. Trace edema at both ankles. Moderate varicosities of saphenous veins, both in lower extremities. No stasis pigmentation or ulcers.

PERRLA
Pupils
Equal
Round
React to
Light
Accommodate

EOM
Extra
Ocular
Movements

TM
Tympanic
Membrane

JVP
Jugular
Venous
Pressure

RCM
Right
Costal
Margin

CVAT
Costo
Vertebral
Angle
Tenderness

BL
Bi**L**ateral

	Radial	Femoral	Popliteal	Dorsalis Pedis	Posterior Tibial
RT	2+	2+	2+	2+	2+
LT	2+	2+	2+	Absent	2+

FROM
Full
Range
Of
Motion

See Muscle Strength Grading, p. 576

Musculoskeletal. No joint deformities. FROM in hands, wrists, elbows, shoulders, spine, hips, knees, ankles.

Neurologic. *Mental Status:* Tense but alert and cooperative. Thought coherent. AA&O × 4. *Cranial Nerves:* II to XII intact. **Motor:** Equal intact muscle bulk and tone. Strength 5/5 throughout. **Cerebellar:** RAMs, point-to-point movements intact. Gait stable, fluid. *Sensory:* Pinprick, light touch, position sense, vibration, and stereognosis intact. Romberg negative. *Reflexes:*

AA&O × 4
Awake
Alert
Oriented (person, place, time, situation)

RAM
Rapid
Alternating
Movements

	Biceps	Triceps	Brachioradialis	Patellar	Achilles	Plantar
RT	2+	2+	2+	2+	1+	↓
LT	2+	2+	2+	2+	1+	↓

Recording reflexes uses a grading system. 2+/4 = normal. See p. 704 for grading system.

Laboratory Data

None currently. See Plans.

Generating the Problem List

Now that you have completed your assessment and written record, you will find it helpful to generate a *Problem List* that summarizes the patient's problems. *List the most active and serious problems first, and record their date of onset.* Some nurses make separate lists for active or inactive problems; others make one list in order of priority. On follow-up visits the *Problem List* helps you remember to check the status of problems the patient may not mention. The *Problem List* also allows other members of the health care team to review the patient's health status at a glance.

A sample *Problem List* for Mrs. N is provided. You may wish to give each problem a number and use the number when referring to specific problems in subsequent notes.

Problem List: The Case of Mrs. N From Assessment Date		
Date Entered	**Problem No.**	**Problem**
1/12/16	1	Headaches
	2	Elevated blood pressure
	3	Overweight
	4	Family stress
	5	Tobacco use since age 18

6	Low back pain
7	Health maintenance
8	Occasional incontinence
9	History of right pyelonephritis 2001
10	Varicose veins
11	Allergy to ampicillin

The list illustrated here includes problems that need attention now, such as Mrs. N's headaches, as well as problems that need future observation and attention, such as her blood pressure. Listing the allergy to ampicillin warns you not to distribute medications in the penicillin family. Some symptoms such as canker sores and hard stools do not appear on this list because they are minor concerns and do not require attention during this visit. Problem lists with too many relatively insignificant items diminish in value. If these symptoms increase in importance, they can always be added at a later visit.

The Challenges of Clinical Data

As you can see from the case of Mrs. N, organizing the patient's clinical data poses several challenges. The beginning student must decide whether to cluster the patient's symptoms and signs into one problem or into several problems. The amount of data may appear unmanageable. The quality of the data may be prone to error. Guidelines to help you address these challenges are provided in the following paragraphs.

- **Clustering data into single versus multiple problems.** One of the greatest difficulties facing students is how to cluster clinical data. Do selected data fit into one problem or several problems? The patient's *age* may help—young people are more likely to have a single disease, whereas older people tend to have multiple diseases. The *timing* of symptoms is often useful. For example, an episode of pharyngitis 6 weeks ago is probably unrelated to fever, chills, pleuritic chest pain, and cough that prompt a visit today. To use timing effectively, you need to know the natural history of various diseases and conditions. A yellow penile discharge followed 3 weeks later by a painless penile ulcer suggests two problems: gonorrhea and primary syphilis. In contrast, a penile ulcer followed in 6 weeks by a maculopapular skin rash and generalized lymphadenopathy suggests two stages of the same problem: primary and secondary syphilis.

- Involvement of *different body systems* may help to cluster the clinical data. If symptoms and signs occur in a single system, one disease may explain them. Problems in different, apparently unrelated systems often require more than one explanation. Again, knowledge of disease patterns is necessary. You might decide, for example, to group a patient's high blood glucose and blurred vision together and place them in the Head, Eyes, Ears, Nose, and Throat system, and label the constellation "hyperglycemia." You would develop another explanation for the patient's mild fever, left lower quadrant tenderness, and diarrhea.

- Some diseases involve more than one body system. As you gain knowledge and experience, you will become increasingly adept at recognizing *multisystem conditions* and building plausible explanations that link together their seemingly unrelated manifestations. To explain cough, hemoptysis, and weight loss in a 60-year-old plumber who has smoked cigarettes for 40 years, you probably even now would rank lung cancer high in the problem list. You might support your list with your observation of the patient's cyanotic fingernails. With experience and continued reading, you will recognize that his other symptoms and signs can be linked to the same diagnosis. Dysphagia would reflect extension of the cancer to the esophagus, pupillary asymmetry would suggest pressure on the cervical sympathetic chain, and jaundice could result from metastases to the liver.

- **Sifting through an extensive array of data.** It is common to confront a relatively long list of symptoms and signs and an equally long list of potential explanations. One approach is to *tease out separate clusters of observations and analyze one cluster at a time*, as just described. You can also *ask a series of key questions* that may steer your thinking in one direction and allow you to temporarily ignore the others. For example, you may ask what produces and relieves the patient's chest pain. If the answer is exercise and rest, you can focus on the cardiovascular and musculoskeletal systems and set the gastrointestinal system aside. If the pain is substernal and burning and occurs only after meals, you can logically focus on the gastrointestinal tract. A series of discriminating questions helps you form a decision tree or algorithm that is helpful in collecting and analyzing clinical data and reaching logical conclusions and explanations[13-15].

- **Assessing the quality of the data.** Almost all clinical information is subject to error. Patients forget to mention symptoms, confuse the events of their illness, avoid recounting embarrassing facts, and often slant their stories to what they think the nurse wants to hear. Nurses may misinterpret patient statements, overlook information, fail to ask "the one key question," jump prematurely to conclusions and diagnoses, or forget an important part of the examination, such as the funduscopic examination in a woman with a headache. You can avoid some of these errors by acquiring the habits of skilled nurses, summarized below.

Tips for Ensuring the Quality of Patient Data

- Ask open-ended questions and listen carefully and patiently to the patient's story.
- When a patient answers "yes" to a question, continue further using "OLD CART" for additional details.

- Craft a thorough and systematic sequence to history taking and physical examination.
- Keep an open mind toward both the patient and the data.
- Always include "the worst-case scenario" in your list of possible explanations of the patient's problem, and make sure it can be safely eliminated.
- Analyze any mistakes in data collection or interpretation.
- Confer with colleagues and review the pertinent literature to clarify uncertainties.
- Apply principles of data analysis to patient information and testing.

Compose the record as soon after seeing the patient as possible, before your findings fade from memory. Record key points from each segment of the health history during the interview, leaving spaces for filling in details later. A sample progress note based on this patient's case is presented below.

Sample Progress Note

A month later, Mrs. N returns for a follow-up visit. The format of the office progress note is quite variable, but it should meet the same standards as the initial assessment. The note should be clear, sufficiently detailed, and easy to follow. It should reflect your clinical reasoning and delineate your assessment and plan. Be sure to learn the documentation standards for billing in your institution, because this can affect the detail and type of information needed in your progress notes.

The note below follows the SOAP format: Subjective, Objective, Assessment, and Plan. You will see many other styles, some focused on the "patient-centered" record. The terms for SOAP are often not listed, but implied. Frequently nurses record the history and physical examination, then document the plan with the listing of each problem and its assessment.

The Case of Mrs. N–Progress Note

2/12/16

Mrs. N returned to the clinic for follow-up of her migraine headaches. She stated that she has fewer headaches since avoiding caffeinated beverages. She is now drinking decaffeinated coffee and has stopped drinking colas. She has joined a support group and started exercising to reduce stress. She is still having one to two headaches a month with some nausea, but they are less severe and generally relieved with nonsteroidal anti-inflammatory drugs (NSAIDs). She denies any fever, stiff neck, associated visual changes, motor-sensory deficits, or paresthesias.

She has been checking her blood pressure at home. It is running about 150/90. She is walking 30 minutes three times a week in her neighborhood and has reduced her total daily calorie intake. She has been unable to stop smoking. She has been doing the Kegel exercises but still has some leakage with coughing or laughing.

Medications: Motrin 400 mg up to three times daily as needed for headache

Allergies: Ampicillin causes rash

Tobacco: 1 pack per day since age 18

Physical Examination: Pleasant, overweight, middle-aged woman, who is animated and somewhat tense. Ht 157 cm (5′2″). Wt 63 kg (140 lbs). BMI 26. BP 150/90. HR 86 and regular. RR 16. Afebrile.

Skin: No suspicious nevi. **HEENT:** Normocephalic, atraumatic. Pharynx without exudates. **Neck:** Supple, without thyromegaly. **Lymph nodes:** No lymphadenopathy. **Lungs:** Resonant and clear. **CV:** JVP 6 cm above the right atrium; carotid upstrokes brisk, no bruits. S_1, S_2. No murmurs. No S_3, S_4. **Abdomen:** Active bowel sounds. Soft, nontender, no hepatosplenomegaly. **Extremities:** Without edema.

Labs: Basic metabolic panel and urinalysis from 1/25/16 unremarkable. Pap smear normal.

Impression and Plan

1. Migraine headaches—now down to one to two per month due to reductions in caffeinated beverages and stress. Headaches are responding to NSAIDs.
   a. Affirm need to stop smoking and to continue exercise program
   b. Affirm patient's participation in support group to reduce stress
2. Elevated blood pressure—BP remains elevated at 150/90.
   a. Educate on newly prescribed diuretic
   b. Patient to take blood pressure three times a week and bring recordings to next office visit
   c. Affirm need to exercise, lose weight, and stop smoking
3. Cystocele with occasional stress incontinence—stress incontinence improved with Kegel exercises but still with some urine leakage. Urinalysis from last visit—no infection.
   a. Educate on newly prescribed vaginal estrogen cream
   b. Patient to continue Kegel exercises
4. Overweight—has lost ~3 lbs.
   a. Patient to continue exercise
   b. Review diet history; affirm weight reduction.
5. Family stress—patient handling this better. See Plans above.
6. Occasional low back pain—no complaints today.
7. Tobacco use—see Plans above.
8. Health maintenance—Pap smear sent last visit. Mammogram scheduled. Colonoscopy recommended.

The box below details the nursing process in the case of Mrs. N. Included are the problem list, which has been developed from the assessment; the nursing diagnoses, formulated from the problem list; the plan, including the STG and the LTG; the interventions/implementation; and the evaluation. Each of the nursing care plans would be individualized and updated for the specific patient.

The Case of Mrs. N–Nursing Process

1. Headaches

Assessment: A 54-year-old woman with a history of migraine headaches since childhood, with a throbbing vascular pattern and frequent nausea and vomiting. Headaches are associated with stress and relieved by sleep and cold compresses. There is no papilledema, and there are no motor or sensory deficits on the neurologic examination. The differential diagnosis includes tension headache, also associated with stress, but there is no relief with massage, and the pain is more throbbing than aching. There is no fever, stiff neck, or focal findings to suggest meningitis, and the lifelong recurrent pattern makes subarachnoid hemorrhage unlikely (usually described as "the worst headache of my life").

Nursing Diagnosis: Acute pain related to pain/headaches.

Plan:
STG: The patient will have decreased severity and frequency of headaches within 1 week as evidenced by journal/ phone app entries.
LTG: The patient will have acceptable relief options as evidenced by her return to activities of daily living and work within 2 weeks.

Interventions:
- Log headaches—onset, location, duration, characteristic symptoms, associated manifestations, relieving factors, and treatment.
- Discuss biofeedback and stress management.
- Advise patient to avoid caffeine, including coffee, colas, and other carbonated beverages.
- Start NSAIDs for headache, as needed and prescribed by nurse practitioner or physician.
- Follow-up appointment in 2 weeks and call physician/nurse practitioner sooner if signs/symptoms increase.

Evaluation*: Ideally, the patient will no longer have headaches; however, if they do persist, then the plan and goals need to be revised and/ or the interventions adjusted.

*Evaluations will be completed for each nursing diagnosis based on the individual patient and will be updated accordingly.

2. Elevated blood pressure

Assessment: Systolic hypertension with wide cuff is present. May be related to obesity, and/or to anxiety from the initial visit or white coat hypertension. No evidence of end-organ damage to retina or heart.

Nursing Diagnosis: Deficient knowledge related to the relationship between increased blood pressure and increased weight and/or stress.

Plan:

STG: The patient will verbalize understanding within 5 days of importance of decreasing blood pressure and how to begin the process of diet changes, exercise, and stress reduction to assist in lowering blood pressure.

LTG: The patient will have decreased blood pressure to below 140/90 within 1 month.

Interventions:

* Discuss standards for assessing blood pressure.
* Recheck blood pressure in 2 weeks, using wide cuff.
* Check basic metabolic panel; review urinalysis.
* Introduce weight reduction, exercise, and stress reduction techniques.
* Reduce salt intake.

3. Overweight

Assessment: Patient 5′2″, weighs 143 lbs. BMI is ~26.

Nursing Diagnosis: Ineffective health maintenance related to increased food consumption in response to stressors and insufficient energy expenditure for intake.

Plan:

STG: The patient will verbalize commitment to a weight loss program within 2 days.

LTG: The patient will decrease weight by 5 lbs within 1 month (143 to 138 lbs).

Interventions:

* Explore diet history; ask patient to keep food intake diary or use app for tracking food intake.
* Explore motivation to lose weight; set target for weight loss by next visit.
* Schedule visit with dietitian.
* Discuss exercise program, specifically, walking 30 minutes 5 to 6 days a week.

4. Family stress

Assessment: Son-in-law with alcohol problem; daughter and grandchildren seeking refuge in patient's apartment, leading to tension in these relationships. Patient also has financial constraints. Stress currently situational. No current evidence of major depression.

Nursing Diagnosis: Caregiver role strain related to daughter/grandchildren situation.

Plan:
STG: Mrs. N will verbalize a plan to decrease strain within 5 days.
LTG: Mrs. N will partake in the plan and have decreased signs/symptoms of stress within 1 month.

Interventions:
* Explore patient's views on strategies to cope with stress.
* Explore sources of support, including Al-Anon for daughter and financial counseling for patient.
* Continue to monitor for depression.

5. Tobacco use

Assessment: 1 pack per day for 36 years.

Nursing Diagnosis: Ineffective health maintenance related to insufficient knowledge of effects of tobacco use and resources available to quit.

Plan:
STG: The patient will verbalize plan to quit within 2 days.
LTG: The patient will decrease or quit smoking within 1 month.

Interventions:
* Educate patient on short- and long-term effects of smoking on self and grandchildren.
* Identify benefits of quitting smoking (e.g., money savings, health).
* Devise strategies to decrease/eliminate smoking.
* Offer referral to tobacco cessation program.

6. Occasional musculoskeletal low back pain

Assessment: Usually with prolonged standing. No history of trauma or motor vehicle accident. Pain does not radiate; no tenderness or motor-sensory deficits on examination.

Nursing Diagnosis: Impaired comfort related to back pain.

Plan:
STG: The patient will demonstrate abdominal exercises that will strengthen back within 4 days.
LTG: Patient will rate back pain as 1 to 2 on pain scale within 1 month of using interventions.

Interventions:
* Rate pain on scale of 1 to 10.
* Use heating pad to decrease pain.
* Review benefits of weight loss and exercises to strengthen low back muscles.
* Continue daily exercises to strengthen abdominal muscles.
* Refer to exercise therapist for evaluation and additional exercises as needed.

7. Health maintenance

Assessment: Last Pap smear 2012; has never had a mammogram.

Nursing Diagnosis:

Ineffective health maintenance related to insufficient knowledge of screening and prevention.

Plan:
STG: The patient will verbalize importance of health and prevention within 1 day.
LTG: The patient will have scheduled/completed all preventative screenings within 1 month.

Interventions:
- Teach Mrs. N breast self-examination if she would like to learn.
- Schedule mammogram.
- Send Pap smear today.
- Provide three stool guaiac cards; discuss screening colonoscopy at next visit.
- Update immunizations.
- Suggest dental care for mild gingivitis.
- Gun lock and store shells in a separate area.
- Advise patient to move medications and caustic cleaning agents to locked cabinet, if possible, above shoulder height.

8. Occasional stress incontinence

Assessment: Incontinence reported with coughing, suggesting alteration in bladder neck anatomy. No dysuria, fever, flank pain. Not taking any contributing medications. Usually involves small amounts of urine, no dribbling, doubt urge or overflow incontinence. Patient is perimenopausal.

Nursing Diagnosis: Stress incontinence related to loss of muscle tone.

Plan:
STG: Mrs. N will verbalize understanding of stress incontinence and exercises within 2 days.
LTG: Mrs. N will report decreased or elimination of stress incontinence within 2 months.

Interventions:
- Explain cause of stress incontinence.
- Review urinalysis.
- Teach Kegel exercises.

The remaining problems on the list do not need a care plan; they are provided as points to be aware of, such as the allergy to ampicillin, or to observe and incorporate into the patient's plan of care if they come into the forefront as more of an issue.

9. History of right pyelonephritis, 2006

10. Varicose veins, lower extremities

No complaints currently.

11. Ampicillin allergy

Developed rash but no other allergic reaction.

EVALUATING CLINICAL FINDINGS

Symptoms, physical findings, tests, and x-rays should help reduce uncertainty about whether a patient does or does not have a given condition. Clinical data, including laboratory work, however, are inherently imperfect. Learn to apply the principles of *reliability, validity, sensitivity,* and *specificity* to your clinical findings.

Principles of Test Selection and Use

Reliability

Indicates how well repeated measurements of the same relatively stable phenomenon will give the same result, also known as *precision*. Reliability may be measured for one observer or for more than one observer.

Example: If on several occasions one nurse consistently percusses the same span of a patient's liver dullness, *intraobserver reliability* is good. If, on the other hand, several observers find quite different spans of liver dullness on the same patient, *interobserver reliability* is poor.

Validity

Indicates how closely a given observation agrees with "the true state of affairs," or the best possible measure of reality.

Example: Noninvasive blood pressure measurements by sphygmomanometers are less valid than intra-arterial pressure tracings.

Sensitivity

Identifies the proportion of people who test positive in a group of people known to have the disease or condition, or the proportion of people who are *true positives* compared with the total number of people who actually have the disease. When the observation or test is negative in people with the disease, the result is termed *false negative. Good observations or tests have a sensitivity of more than 90% and help rule out disease because there are few false negatives. Such observations or tests are especially useful for screening.*

Example: The sensitivity of the Homan sign in the diagnosis of deep venous thrombosis (DVT) of the calf is 50%. In other words, compared with a group of patients with deep vein thrombosis confirmed by phlebogram, a much better test, only 50% will have a positive Homan sign, so this sign, if absent, is not helpful because 50% of patients may have a DVT.

To help remember this, experts state "when the **Se**nsitivity of a symptom or sign is high, a **N**egative response rules **out** the target disorder, and the acronym for this property is "*SnNout.*"[16]

Specificity

Identifies the proportion of people who test negative in a group of people known to be *without* a given disease or condition, or the proportion of people who are *true negatives* compared with the total number of people without the disease. When the observation or test is positive in people without the disease, the result is termed *false positive*. Good observations or tests have a specificity of more than 90% and help "rule in" disease because the test is rarely positive when disease is absent, and there are few false positives.

Example: The specificity of serum amylase in patients with possible acute pancreatitis is 70%. In other words, of 100 patients without pancreatitis, 70% will have a normal serum amylase; in 30%, the serum amylase will be falsely elevated.

Likewise, when the **Sp**ecificity is high, a **P**ositive test result rules *in* the target disorder. The acronym is "***SpPin***."[16]

LIFELONG LEARNING: INTEGRATING CLINICAL REASONING, ASSESSMENT, AND ANALYSIS OF CLINICAL EVIDENCE

Nurses make use of many assessment tools. These tools are used in areas of prevention such as falls, malnutrition, and skin breakdown. Screening tests for alcohol dependence (CAGE) or developmental delay (Denver II) are examples of additional tools. The concepts of sensitivity and specificity help in both the collection and the analysis of data. They even underlie some of the basic strategies of interviewing. Questions with high sensitivity, if answered in the affirmative, may be particularly useful for screening and for gathering evidence to support a hypothesis. For example, "Are you confined to bed?" is a highly sensitive question for detecting risk of skin breakdown. For patients who are immobile, there would be few false-negative responses. Thus, it is a good first screening question. However, because there are indicators other than activity and mobility that determine skin breakdown, it is not highly specific. Decreased sensory perception, friction, malnutrition, and increased moisture each is a reasonably sensitive attribute of skin breakdown and would add importantly to the growing evidence.

Data also come from the physical assessment and examination of the skin. Combining data from the history and physical examination allows screening of patients at risk for skin breakdown.

Skilled nurses use this kind of logic to generate tentative nursing diagnoses as soon as the patient describes the *Chief Complaint*, then build evidence for one or more of these diagnoses and discard others as they continue with the history and examination. The nurse searches explicitly for other possible manifestations of skin breakdown such as history of cerebrovascular accident or diminished lower extremity pulses of atherosclerotic peripheral vascular disease. By generating diagnoses early and testing them sequentially, experienced nurses improve their efficiency and enhance the relevance and value of the data they collect. Once the diagnoses have been identified the nurse develops appropriate nursing care plans.

This sequence of collecting data and testing hypotheses is diagrammed below.

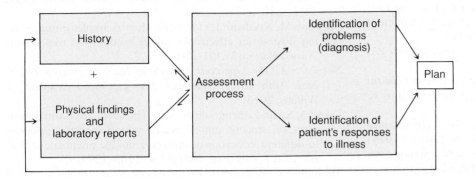

After the plan has been implemented, the process recycles. The nurse gathers more data, assesses the patient's progress, modifies the problem list if indicated, and adjusts the plan accordingly. As you gain experience, the interplay of assessment, data collection, and knowledge from the clinical literature will become increasingly familiar. You will come to value the challenges and rewards of clinical reasoning and assessment that make patient care so meaningful.

BIBLIOGRAPHY

CITATIONS

1. Herdman TH, Kamitsuru S, eds. *NANDA nursing diagnosis: definitions and classifications 2015–2017*. Oxford: Wiley Blackwell; 2015.
2. Benner P, Tanner C, Chesla C. *Expertise in Nursing Practice: Caring, Clinical Judgment, and Ethics.* 2nd ed. New York, NY: Springer; 2009.
3. Lyneham J, Parkinson C, Denholm C. Expert nursing practice: a mathematical explanation of Benner's 5th stage of practice development. *J Adv Nurs.* 2009;65(11):2477–2484.
4. Peterson MC, Holbrook JH, Von Hales DE, et al. Contributions of the history, physical examination, and laboratory investigation in making medical diagnoses. *West J Med.* 1992;156(2):163–165.
5. Bowen J. Educational strategies to promote clinical diagnostic reasoning. *New Engl J Med.* 2006;355(21):2217–2225.
6. Bowen J. Educational strategies to promote clinical diagnostic reasoning. *New Engl J Med.* 2006;355(21):2217–2225.
7. Coderre S, Mandin H, Harasym P, et al. Diagnostic reasoning strategies and diagnostic success. *Med Educ.* 2003;37(8):695–703.
8. Norman G. Research in clinical reasoning: past history and current trends. *Med Educ.* 2005;39(4):418–427.
9. Benner P. *From Novice to Exoert: Excellence and Power in Clinical Nursing Practice, Commerative edition.* New Jersey: Prentice Hall; 2000.
10. Abdoli S, Safavu S. Nursing students' immediate response to distressed clients based on Orlando's theory. *Iran J Nurs Midwifery Res.* 2010;15(4):178–184.
11. Schneiderman H. *Bedside Diagnosis. An Annotated Bibliography of Literature on Physical Examination and Interviewing.* 3rd ed. Philadelphia, PA: American College of Physicians; 1997.
12. McGee S. *Evidence Based Physical Diagnosis.* 3rd ed. Philadelphia, PA: Saunders; 2012.
13. Polit D, Tatano Beck C. *Nursing Research: Generating and Assessing Evidence for Nursing Practice.* 8th ed. Philadelphia, PA: Lippincott Williams & Wilkins; 2008.
14. LoBiondo-Wood G, Haber J. *Nursing Research: Methods and Critical Appraisal for Evidence-Based Practice.* 8th ed. St. Louis, Missouri: Elsevier; 2014.
15. Guyatt G. *Users' Guide to the Medical Literature: A Manual for Evidence-Based Clinical Practice.* New York, NY: McGraw-Hill Medical; 2008.
16. Sackett D. A primer on the precision and accuracy of the clinical examination. *JAMA.* 1992;267(19):2638–2644.

ADDITIONAL REFERENCES

Alfaro-LeFevre R. *Critical Thinking, Clinical Reasoning and Clinical Judgment.* 5th ed. St. Louis, MO: Saunders; 2013.

Bartlett R, Bland A, Rossen E, et al. Evaluation of the outcome-present state test model as a way to teach clinical reasoning. *J Nurs Educ.* 2008;47(8):337–344.

Carnevali D. *Diagnostic Reasoning in Nursing.* Philadelphia, PA: J. B. Lippincott Co.; 2007.

Carpenito-Moyet LJ. *Nursing Diagnosis: Application to Clinical Practice.* 14th ed. Philadelphia, PA: Lippincott Williams & Wilkins; 2012.

Cherry B, Jacob SR. *Contemporary Nursing: Issues, Trends, and Management.* 6th ed. St. Louis, MO: Mosby–Elsevier; 2014.

Cholowski K, Chan L. Diagnostic reasoning among second-year nursing students. *J Adv Nurs.* 2006;17(10):1171–1181.

Fletcher RH, Fletcher SW. *Clinical Epidemiology: The Essentials.* 5th ed. Philadelphia, PA: Lippincott Williams & Wilkins; 2014.

Innui TS. Establishing the doctor–patient relationship: science, art, or competence? *Schweiz Med Wochenschr.* 1198;128:225.

Laditka JN, Laditka SB, Mastanduno MP. Hospital utilization for ambulatory care sensitive conditions: health outcome disparities associated with race and ethnicity. *Soc Sci Med.* 2003;57(8):1429–1441.

Lee TT. Nursing diagnoses: factors affecting their use in charting standardized care plans. *J Clin Nurs.* 2005; 14(5):640–647.

MüStaub M, Needham I, Odenbreit M, et al. Implementing nursing diagnostics effectively: cluster randomized trial. *J Adv Nurs.* 2008;63(3):291–301.

Nettina SM. *The Lippincott Manual of Nursing Practice Handbook.* 10th ed. Philadelphia, PA: Lippincott Williams & Wilkins, 2013.

Palese A, Saiani L, Brugnolli A, et al. The impact of tutorial strategies on student nurses' accuracy in diagnostic reasoning in different educational settings: a double pragmatic trial in Italy. *Int J Nurs Stud.* 2008;45(9):1285–1298.

Thompson C, Bucknall T, Estabrookes CA, et al. Nurses' critical event risk assessments: a judgement analysis. *J Clin Nurs.* 2009;4:601–612.

Westfall U, Tanner T, Putzier D, et al. Activating clinical inferences: a component of diagnostic reasoning in nursing. *Res Nurs Health.* 2009;9(4):269–277.

Interviewing and Communication

The student will:

1. Use therapeutic communication techniques during the patient interview.
2. Describe the phases of the nurse–patient interview.
3. Identify environmental elements that support successful interviewing.
4. Begin the interview with broad open-ended questions then move to focused questions to clarify topics.
5. Demonstrate increased comfort when interviewing patients on sensitive subjects.
6. Discuss strategies for handling difficult patients.

The health history interview is a conversation with a purpose. As you learn to elicit the patient's history, you will draw on many interpersonal skills that you use every day, but with important differences. Unlike social conversation, in which you can freely express your own needs and interests, the primary goal of the nurse–patient interview is to improve the well-being of the patient. At its most basic level, the purpose of conversation with a patient is threefold: to establish a trusting and supportive relationship, to gather information, and to offer information.

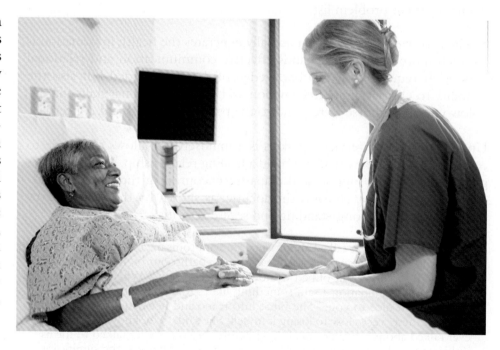

Relating effectively with patients is among the most valued skills of nursing care. Using techniques that promote trust and convey respect allows the patient's story to unfold in its most full and detailed form. Establishing a supportive interaction helps the patient feel more at ease when sharing information and becomes the foundation for therapeutic nurse–patient relationships.[1] Illness can make patients feel scared and isolated. A strong nurse–patient relationship can reduce feelings of isolation and fear.

This chapter introduces the essentials of interviewing. It emphasizes interviewing techniques, but covers fundamental communication skills that will be continually used in conversations with patients. The chapter covers the phases of interviewing, important therapeutic communication techniques, and strategies for interviewing special patients.

The process of interviewing patients requires sensitivity to the patient's feelings and behavioral cues and is much more than just asking a series of questions. This process differs from the *format* of the health history as presented in Chapter 4, The Health History. Both are necessary to care for patients but serve different purposes.

- The *health history format* is a structured framework for organizing patient information in *written, electronic, or verbal form* to communicate effectively with other health care providers. The patient's information is concisely organized into categories of present, past, and family health. The format identifies the specific information that must be obtained from the patient. As noted in Chapter 2, Critical Thinking in Health Assessment, the health history provides data for the nurse to generate an initial patient problem list.

- The *interviewing process* that actually generates the health information is much more fluid and demands effective communication and relational skills. It requires not only knowledge of the data needed but also the ability to elicit accurate information and the interpersonal skills that allow you as the nurse to respond to the patient's feelings and concerns.

Underlying these interviewing skills is a mindset that allows the nurse to collaborate with the patient and build a healing relationship. If the patient's greatest need is for support and empathy, encouraging the patient to discuss the *experience of illness* is therapeutic, as shown by the words below from a patient with long-standing and severe arthritis:

> The patient had never talked about what the symptoms meant to her. She had never said: "This means that I can't go to the bathroom by myself, put my clothes on, even get out of bed without calling for help." When we finished the physical examination I said something like: "Rheumatoid arthritis really has not been nice to you." She burst into tears, and her daughter did also, and I sat there, very close to losing it myself. She said: "You know, no one has ever talked about it as a personal thing before. No one's ever talked to me as if this were a thing that mattered, a personal event." That was the significant moment in the encounter. I didn't really have much else to offer. ... But something really meaningful had happened between us, something that she valued and would carry away with her.[2]

PHASES OF INTERVIEWING

Phases of the Interview

1. Pre-interview: set the stage for a smooth interview
   • Self-reflection
   • Review patient record
   • Set interview goals
   • Review own clinical behavior and appearance
2. Introduction: put the patient at ease and establish trust
   • Greet the patient and establish rapport
   • Establish the agenda for the interview
3. Working: obtain patient information
   • Invite the patient's story
   • Identify and respond to emotional cues
   • Expand and clarify the patient's story
   • Generate and test diagnostic hypotheses
   • Negotiate a plan, including further evaluation, treatment, education and self-management support and prevention
4. Termination:
   • Summarize important points
   • Discuss plan of care

Phase 1: Pre-Interview

Interviewing patients requires planning. There are several preliminary steps that are crucial to success: taking time for self-reflection, reviewing the patient record, setting goals for the interview, reviewing your behavior and appearance, adjusting the environment, and being ready to take brief notes.

Take Time for Self-Reflection

As nurses, we encounter a wide variety of patients, each one unique. Establishing relationships with people from a broad spectrum of ages, social classes, races, ethnicities, and states of *health or illness* is an opportunity and privilege. Being consistently respectful and open to individual differences is one of the nurse's challenges. Because we bring our own values, assumptions, and biases to every encounter, we must look inward to clarify how our own expectations and reactions may affect what we hear and how we behave. *Self-reflection is a continual part of professional development in clinical work. It brings a deepening personal awareness to our work with patients, which is one of the most rewarding aspects of patient care.*[3]

Review the Medical and Nursing Records

Before seeing the patient, review the medical and nursing records. This information helps identify areas to explore with the patient. Review identifying data such as age, gender, address, and health insurance, and peruse the problem list, the medication list, and details such as the documentation of allergies. The chart often provides valuable information about past diagnoses and treatments, but do not let previous documentation bias your problem solving or prevent you from developing new approaches or ideas. Remember that information in the record comes from different observers and that standardized forms reflect different institutional norms. Details and nuances of patient information can be lost in electronic charting programs with drop-down menus. Data may be incomplete or even disagree with what you learn from the patient—understanding such discrepancies may prove helpful to the patient's care.

Set Goals for the Interview

Before talking with the patient, clarify the goals for the interview. Goals range from following up on health care issues, identifying new problems, and completing forms for health care institutions to obtaining a basis for developing a plan of care. *A nurse must balance these provider-centered goals with patient-centered goals.* There can be discrepancies between the needs of the nurse, the needs of the institution, and needs of the patient and family. If you take a few minutes to think through the goals ahead of time, the interview will be smoother.

Review Clinical Behavior and Appearance

Just as the nurse carefully observes the patient throughout the interview, the patient will be watching the nurse. Consciously or not, the nurse sends messages through both words and behavior. Posture, gestures, eye contact, and tone of voice all convey the extent of interest, attention, acceptance, and understanding. The skilled interviewer appears calm and unhurried, even if time is limited. Reactions that indicate disapproval, embarrassment, impatience, or boredom block communication, as do behaviors that condescend, stereotype, criticize, or belittle the patient or family. Professionalism requires the nurse maintain equanimity.

Personal appearance also affects the clinical relationship. Patients find cleanliness, neatness, conservative dress, and a name tag reassuring. Remember to keep *the patient's perspective* in mind in order to build the patient's trust.

Adjust the Environment

Make the interview setting as private and comfortable as possible. A proper environment improves communication, though a hospitalized patient may need to be interviewed in a two-bed room or an emergency department. If there are privacy curtains, ask permission to pull them shut. Suggest moving to an empty room instead of talking in a waiting area. Adjust the room temperature for the patient's comfort when needed, for example, an elderly patient may appreciate a warmer room. *As the nurse, it is part of your job to make adjustments to the location and seating that make the patient and you more comfortable.* These efforts are always worth the time.

Take Notes

No one can remember all the details of a comprehensive history. Write down short phrases, specific dates, or words, but do not let note taking or written or electronic forms distract you from the patient. Maintain eye contact and note when the patient points to a body part, when describing a symptom. Whenever the patient is talking about sensitive or disturbing material, put down your pen or move away from the keyboard and focus solely on the patient. Most patients are accustomed to note taking, but for those who find it uncomfortable, explore their concerns and explain your need to make an accurate record. When using an electronic health record, review the patient's record before entering the room; elicit the patient's story while directly facing the patient, maintaining eye contact, and observing all nonverbal behavior; and address the viewing screen only after the establishment of the relationship and with the patient included in the process.[4–6]

The interview moves through the introduction, working, and termination phases. *Throughout this sequence, the nurse must be attuned to the patient's feelings, help the patient express them, respond to their content, and validate their significance.*

As a beginning student, concentrate primarily on gathering the patient's story and creating a shared understanding of the problem. As you become a practicing nurse, reaching agreement on a plan for further evaluation and treatment becomes more important. Whether the interview is comprehensive or focused, you should move through this sequence with close attention to the patient's feelings and affect, always working on strengthening the relationship.

 Concept Mastery Alert

To facilitate any patient interview and promote optimal communication, it is important that the nurse ensures that the environment for conducting the interview is comfortable and private. This may require interviewing the patient in an empty room, such as a conference room or exam room. This is done even before the nurse meets with the patient in phase 2.

Phase 2: Introduction

Greet the Patient and Establish Rapport

The initial moments of an encounter with the patient lay the foundation for an ongoing relationship. How you greet the patient and other visitors in the room, provide for the patient's comfort, and arrange the physical setting all shape the patient's first impressions.

As you begin, *greet the patient* by name and introduce yourself, giving your own name. If possible and culturally appropriate, shake hands with the patient. If this is the first contact, explain your role, including your status as a student and how you will be involved in the patient's care.

Using a formal title to address the patient—Mr. O'Neil or Ms. Washington, for example—is always best.[7] Except with children or adolescents, avoid first names unless you have specific permission from the patient or family. Addressing an unfamiliar adult as "granny" or "dear" can depersonalize and demean. If you are unsure how to pronounce the patient's name, do not be afraid to ask. You can say: "I am afraid of mispronouncing your name. Could you say it for me?" Then repeat it to make sure that you heard it correctly.

When visitors are in the room, be sure to acknowledge and greet each one in turn, inquiring about each person's name and relationship to the patient. Whenever visitors are present, *you are obligated to maintain the patient's confidentiality.* Let the patient decide if visitors or family members should remain in the room, before conducting the interview. For example, "I am comfortable with having your sister stay for the interview, Mrs. Jones, but I want to make sure that this is also what you want" or "Would you prefer if I spoke to you alone or with your sister present?"

Consider the best way to *arrange the room* and distance from the patient. Remember that cultural background and individual taste influence preferences about interpersonal space. Choose a distance that facilitates conversation and allows good eye contact, probably within a few feet of the patient, close enough to be intimate but not intrusive. Pull up a chair and, if possible, sit at eye level with the patient. Move any physical barriers, such as desks or bedside tables, out of the way. Avoid arrangements that convey disrespect or inequality of power, such as interviewing a patient on a bedpan. Such arrangements are unacceptable. Lighting also makes a difference. Sitting between a patient and a bright light or window may make the patient squint uncomfortably to see you.

Provide the patient with undivided attention. Spend enough time on small talk to put the patient at ease, and avoid looking down to take notes, read the chart, or scan a computer screen. In a first meeting, demonstrate interest in the patient as a person.[8]

Establish the Agenda

Once rapport has been established, the nurse is ready to pursue the patient's reason for seeking health care. This reason is traditionally designated the *chief complaint,* but when there are three or four reasons for the visit, the phrase *presenting problems* may be preferable. Begin with **open-ended questions** that allow full freedom of response: "What concerns bring you here today?" or "How can I help you?" Helpful open-ended questions include "Are there specific concerns that prompted you to schedule this appointment?" and "What made you decide to come in to see us today?" Note that these questions encourage the patient to express any possible concerns and do not restrict the patient to a problem per se. Sometimes patients do not give a specific problem; they ask for "just a check-up." An important fact to remember is that the first problem the patient brings up is not necessarily the most important one. In fact, when the chief reason for coming is psychosocial, it is usually *not* the first reason the patient mentions. The order in which problems are related is not connected to their clinical importance.

Identifying all the concerns at the beginning of the interview allows the patient and the nurse to negotiate which concerns are most pressing for the visit, and which can be postponed to a follow-up appointment. Questions such as "Is there anything else?" or "Have we got everything?" help elicit the patient's complete list of reasons for coming to the health care facility. The nurse may also have concerns such as blood pressure management or diabetic diet maintenance. Identifying the full agenda or even the "real reason" for the visit at the outset makes use of the time available more meaningful, facilitates time management, and reduces the short shrift given to late-emerging concerns, although negotiating the agenda at the outset still does not always avert the "hand on the doorknob syndrome"[9]—when the patient mentions a new problem as he or she is leaving.

Phase 3: Working Phase

Invite the Patient's Story

Once the agenda has been decided, invite the patient's story by asking about the patient's foremost concern, saying, "Tell me more about ..." Encourage the patient to tell his or her story in his or her own words.[10] Avoid biasing the patient's story. That is, *do not add new information* and *do not interrupt.* Instead, use active listening skills, such as leaning forward as you listen and using continuers such as nodding your head and offering phrases like "uh huh," "go on," or "I see." *Follow the patient's lead.* Asking specific questions prematurely or suggesting solutions before the patient's story is complete risks losing the very information being sought. Once interrupted, patients rarely return to telling their stories. After the patient completes the initial description of each problem, use *focused questions to explore the patient's story in more depth.* For example, *"How would you describe the pain?" "What happened next?" "Did you notice this occurs at a certain time?"* Using guided questioning allows the nurse to obtain a complete picture of the patient's concern.

See p. 50 for discussions of *continuers.*

See p. 49 for discussions of *guided questioning.*

Identify and Respond to the Patient's Emotional Cues

Emotional distress is frequently associated with illness.[9,11] Patients may withhold their true concerns in up to 75% of acute care visits[12] but offer various clues to their concerns that may be direct or indirect, verbal or non-verbal, and expressed as ideas or emotions.[13] Acknowledging and responding to these clues help build rapport, expand the nurse's understanding of the illness, and improve patient satisfaction.

If the patient has not mentioned his or her perspective on illness during the open-ended portion of the interview, explore this perspective prior to the directive. Probe the personal context of the illness by asking, "How has this affected you?" "What do you make of this?" or "How did you feel about that?" or stating, "Many people would be frustrated by something like this." In addition, explore the patient's ideas about the effect of the illness on his or her life.[10] See the box below for a taxonomy of the clues about the patient's perspective on illness.

Clues to the Patient's Perspective on Illness[14]

- Direct statement(s) by the patient of explanations, emotions, expectations, and effects of the illness
- Expression of feelings about the illness
- Attempts to explain or understand symptoms
- Speech clues (e.g., repetition, prolonged reflective pauses)
- Sharing a personal story
- Behavior clues indicative of unidentified concerns, dissatisfaction, or unmet needs such as reluctance to accept recommendations, seeking a second opinion, or early return appointment

---

Respond immediately when you hear an emotional cue. Appropriate response techniques include reflection, synonyms, and feedback indicating support and partnership. A mnemonic for responding to emotional cues is *NURS:* *N*aming—"That sounds like a scary experience"; *U*nderstanding or legitimization—"It's understandable that you feel that way"; and *ReS*pecting—"You've done better than most people would with this."

N—Naming
U—Understanding
ReS—Respecting

Expand and Clarify the Patient's Story

After eliciting the patient's story as fully as possible in a nondirective manner and exploring the patient's lived experience of the illness, guide the patient to elaborating on the areas of the health history that seem most significant. Clarify the attributes of each symptom, including context, associations, and chronology. For pain and many other symptoms, understanding these essential characteristics, summarized below as the seven key attributes of a symptom, is critical.

To pursue the seven attributes, two mnemonics may help:

- **OLD CART,** or **O**nset, **L**ocation, **D**uration, **C**haracteristic Symptoms, **A**ssociated Manifestations, **R**elieving/Exacerbating Factors, and **T**reatment, or

- **OPQRST,** or **O**nset, **P**alliating/**P**rovoking Factors, **Q**uality, **R**adiation, **S**ite, and **T**iming

The Seven Attributes of a Symptom

1. **O**nset. When did (does) it start? Setting in which it occurs, including environmental factors, personal activities, emotional reactions, or other circumstances that may have contributed to the illness.
2. **L**ocation. Where is it? Does it radiate?
3. **D**uration. How long does it last?
4. **C**haracteristic Symptoms. What is it like? How severe is it? (For a subjective symptom like pain, ask the patient to rate it on a scale of 1 to 10.)
5. **A**ssociated Manifestations. Have you noticed anything else that accompanies it?
6. **R**elieving/Exacerbating Factors. Is there anything that makes it better or worse?
7. **T**reatment. What have you done to treat this? Was it effective?

See p. 13 (Chapter 2, Critical Thinking in Health Assessment) for more symptom attribute questions using OLD CART.

Whenever possible, *use the patient's words,* making sure you clarify their meaning. Do not use medical jargon, because it confuses and frustrates patients. Be aware of how quickly jargon like "take a history" and "work you up" can creep into discussions. Choose instead plain English words such as "I'd like to learn more about your illness" or "Doing these examinations can help us understand what's causing your illness."

It is important to establish *the sequence and timing* of each patient symptom, if you are to arrive at accurate assessments. Encourage a chronologic account by stating, "Please describe the *symptom* from when it began to now" or "Please start at the beginning, or the last time you felt well, and go step by step" or asking such questions as "What then?" or "What happened next?" To fill in specific details, guide the patient's story by employing different types of questions and the techniques of skilled interviewing. Use focused questions to elicit information that the patient has not already offered. *In general, an interview moves back and forth from open-ended questions to increasingly focused questions and then on to another open-ended question, returning the lead in the interview to the patient.*

See the Techniques of Skilled Interviewing and discussion of focused questions, pp. 48–54.

Generating and Testing Diagnostic Hypotheses

The skills of diagnostic reasoning are developed over time with practice. As the history is gathered, one develops and tests hypotheses about the patient problem or problems. Identifying the attributes and details of the patient's symptoms is fundamental to recognizing patterns of problems and generating nursing diagnoses.

Some students visualize the process of evoking a full description of the symptom as "the cone":

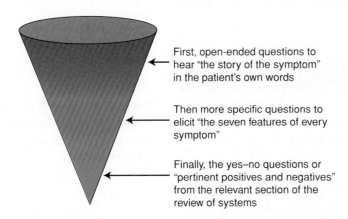

First, open-ended questions to hear "the story of the symptom" in the patient's own words

Then more specific questions to elicit "the seven features of every symptom"

Finally, the yes–no questions or "pertinent positives and negatives" from the relevant section of the review of systems

For example, in a patient with a cough, these questions would come from the Respiratory section of the Review of Systems, Chapter 4, The Health History, p. 77.

Each symptom has its own "cone," which is documented in the History of Present Illness section of the written record.

Appropriate questions about symptoms are also suggested in each of the chapters on the regional physical examinations. This is one way to build evidence for and against various diagnostic possibilities. The challenge is not letting this kind of inquiry dominate the interview and displace learning about the patient's perspective, conveying concern for the patient's well-being, and building the relationship.

See also Chapter 2, Critical Thinking in Health Assessment, pp. 11–36.

Create a Shared Understanding of the Problem

The literature makes it clear that delivering effective health care requires exploring the deeper meanings patients attach to their symptoms. Although the "seven attributes of a symptom" add important details to the patient's history, the **disease/illness distinction model** helps to understand the full impact on the patient.[12] This model acknowledges the very different yet complementary perspectives of the nurse and the patient. *Disease* is the explanation that the *nurse* uses to account for the symptoms. It is the way that the nurse organizes what is learned from the patient that leads to a nursing diagnosis. *Illness* can be defined as how the *patient* experiences the disease, including its effects on relationships, function, and sense of well-being. Many factors may shape this experience, including prior personal or family health, the effect of symptoms on everyday life, individual outlook and style of coping, and expectations about medical and nursing care. The melding of these perspectives forms the basis for identifying nursing diagnoses and creating a plan of care. *The interview needs to incorporate both these views.*

Even a chief complaint as straightforward as sore throat can illustrate these divergent views. The patient may be most concerned about pain and difficulty swallowing, missing time from work, or a cousin who was hospitalized with tonsillitis. The nurse, however, may focus on specific points in the history that differentiate streptococcal pharyngitis from other causes, or on a questionable history an allergy to penicillin. To understand the patient's expectations, the nurse needs to go beyond just the attributes of a symptom. Learning about the patient's perception of illness means asking patient-centered questions in the four domains listed below. This information is crucial to patient satisfaction, effective health care, and patient follow-through.[10]

A mnemonic for the patient's perspective on the illness is *FIFE—Feelings, Ideas, effect on Function, and Expectations.*

Explore the Patient's Perspective

- The patient's **F**eelings, including fears or concerns, about the problem
- The patient's **I**deas about the nature and the cause of the problem
- The effect of the problem on the patient's life and **F**unction
- The patient's **E**xpectations of the disease, of the clinician, or of health care, often based on prior personal or family experiences

To uncover the patient's feelings, the nurse might ask,

> "What concerns you most about the pain?"
> "How has this been for you?"

To explore the patient's thoughts about the cause of the problem, the nurse could say,

> "Why do you think you have this stomachache?"

Because self-treatment suggests the patient's thinking, you may ask,

> "What have you tried?"

A patient may worry that the pain is a symptom of serious disease and want reassurance. Alternatively, the patient may be less concerned about the cause of the pain and just want relief.

To determine the effect of the illness on the patient's lifestyle and function, particularly for patients with chronic illness, ask,

> "What can't you do now that you could do before?"
> "How has your backache (shortness of breath, etc.) affected your ability to work? Your life at home? Your social activities? Your role as a parent? Your function in intimate relationships? The way you feel about yourself as a person?"

You need to find out what the patient expects from you, the nurse, or from health care in general ... "I am glad that the pain is almost gone. How specifically can I help you now?" Even if the stomach pain is almost gone, the patient may need a work excuse to take to an employer.

Negotiate a Plan

Learning about the effects of the illness gives the nurse and the patient the opportunity to create a complete and congruent picture of the problem. This multifaceted picture then forms the basis for planning further evaluation (e.g., physical examination, laboratory tests, consultations) and negotiating a nursing care plan. It also plays an important role in building rapport with your patient.

See also Chapter 2, Develop a plan agreeable to the patient, p. 18.

Phase 4: Termination

Summarize Important Points and Discuss Plan

Let the patient know that the end of the interview is approaching to allow time for the patient to ask any final questions. Make sure the patient understands the mutual plans you have developed. For example, before gathering your papers or standing to leave the room, you can say, "We need to stop now. Do you have any questions about what we've covered?" As you close, summarizing the patient's problems and reviewing the plan of care and follow-up are helpful. "So, you will take the medicine as we discussed, check your blood glucose daily, and make a follow-up appointment for 4 weeks. Do you have any questions about this?" Address any related concerns or questions that the patient raises.

The patient should have a chance to ask any final questions; however, the last few minutes are not the time to bring up new topics. If that happens and the concern is not life-threatening nor requires immediate attention, assure the patient of your interest and make plans to address the problem at a future time.

THERAPEUTIC COMMUNICATION TECHNIQUES

This section describes the skills that form the basic tools of interviewing. The nurse employs these interviewing skills to achieve the tasks described in the Phases of Interviewing (see pp. 39–48) more effectively. Practice improves interviewing skills. Being observed and recorded during an interview allows for feedback from an experienced interviewer.

The Techniques of Skilled Interviewing

- Active listening
- Guided questioning
- Nonverbal communication
- Empathic responses
- Validation
- Reassurance
- Summarizing
- Transitions
- Empowering the patient

Active Listening

Underlying all the techniques is the habit of *active listening*. Active listening is the process of paying close attention to what the patient is communicating, being aware of the patient's emotional state, and using verbal and nonverbal skills to encourage the speaker to continue and expand.[15] This takes practice. It is easy to drift into thinking about the next question or the nursing diagnoses.

Guided Questioning: Options to Expand and Clarify the Patient's Story

There are several ways you can ask for more information from the patient without interfering with the flow of the patient's story. The goal is to facilitate the patient's fullest communication. Learning the following techniques encourages patient disclosures while minimizing the risk for distorting the patient's ideas or missing significant details. This is how one avoids asking a series of specific questions, which takes more time and makes the patient feel more passive.

- Moving from open-ended to focused questions
- Using questioning that elicits a graded response
- Asking a series of questions, one at a time
- Offering multiple choices for answers
- Clarifying what the patient means
- Encouraging with continuers
- Using reflection

Moving From Open-Ended to Focused Questions

Your questioning should proceed from general to specific. Think once again about the "cone," open at the top then tapering to a focal point. Start with the most general questions like "How can I help?" to still open but focused ones like "Tell me more about your experience with the medication." Then pose closed questions like "Did the new medicine cause any problems?" Begin with a truly open-ended question that does not inadvertently include an answer. A possible sequence might be

"Tell me about your chest pain." (Pause)
"What else?" (Pause)
"Where did you feel it?" (Pause) "Show me."
"Anywhere else?" (Pause) "Did it travel anywhere?" (Pause) "To which arm?"

Avoid *leading questions* that include the answer in the question or suggest a desired response: "Has your pain been improving?" or "You don't have any blood in your stools, do you?" If you ask, "Is your pain like a pressure?"

and the patient answers yes, your words may turn into the patient's words. Use the more neutral "Please describe your pain." Also avoid asking the patient *why* something was not done.

Questioning That Elicits a Graded Response

Ask questions that require a *graded response* rather than a single answer. "How many steps can you climb before you get short of breath?" is better than "Do you get short of breath climbing stairs?"

Asking a Series of Questions, One at a Time

Be sure to *ask one question at a time.* "Any tuberculosis, pleurisy, asthma, bronchitis, pneumonia?" may lead to a negative answer out of sheer confusion. Try "Have you had any of the following problems?" Be sure to pause and establish eye contact as you list each problem.

Offering Multiple Choices for Answers

Sometimes patients seem quite unable to describe their symptoms without help. To minimize bias, *offer multiple-choice answers:* "Which of the following words best describes your pain: aching, sharp, pressing, burning, shooting, or something else?" Almost any specific question can provide at least two possible answers. "Do you bring up any phlegm with your cough, or is it dry?"

Clarifying What the Patient Means

At times, patients use words that are ambiguous or have unclear associations. To understand their meaning, *request clarification,* as in "Tell me exactly what you meant by 'the flu'" or "You said you were behaving just like your mother. What did you mean?"

Encouraging With Continuers

Without specifying content, you can use posture, gestures, or words to encourage the patient to say more. Pausing with a nod of the head or remaining silent, yet attentive and relaxed, is a *cue for the patient to continue.* Leaning forward, making eye contact, and using phrases like "Mm-hmm," "Go on," or "I'm listening" all maintain the flow of the patient's story.

Reflection

A simple repetition of the patient's last words, reflecting or echoing back the patient's words, encourages the patient to express both factual details and feelings, as in the following example:

> Patient: "The pain got worse and began to spread." (Pause)
> Response: "Spread?" (Pause)

Patient: "Yes, it went to my shoulder and down my left arm to the fingers. It was so bad that I thought I was going to die." (Pause)

Response: "Going to die?"

Patient: "Yes, it was just like the pain my father had when he had his heart attack, and I was afraid the same thing was happening to me."

This reflective technique has helped to reveal not only the location and severity of the pain but also its meaning to the patient. It did not bias the story or interrupt the patient's train of thought.

Nonverbal Communication

Communication that does not involve speech occurs continuously and provides important clues to feelings and emotions. Becoming sensitive to nonverbal messages allows the nurse to both "read the patient" more effectively and send messages. Pay close attention to eye contact, facial expression, posture, head position and movement such as shaking or nodding, interpersonal distance, and placement of the arms or legs—crossed, neutral, or open. Be aware that some nonverbal language is universal and some is culturally bound.

Matching your position to the patient's position can signify increased rapport, just as mirroring your position can signify the patient's increasing sense of connectedness. One can also mirror the patient's *paralanguage,* or qualities of speech, such as pacing, tone, and volume, to increase rapport. Moving closer or physical contact like placing your hand on the patient's arm can convey empathy or help the patient gain control of difficult feelings. Sensitivity to the patient's culture must guide the use of nonverbal communication.

Empathic Responses

Conveying empathy greatly strengthens patient rapport. As patients talk they may express—with or without words—feelings they may or may not have consciously acknowledged. *To provide empathy, first identify the patient's feelings.* At first, this may seem unfamiliar or uncomfortable. When you sense important but unexpressed feelings from the patient's face, voice, words, or behavior, inquire about them rather than assuming that you know how the patient feels. You may simply ask, "How did you feel about that?" Patients may hold back their feelings, unsure of how they will be received. Unless you let patients know that you are interested in feelings as well as facts, you may miss important insights.

Once you have identified the feelings, respond with understanding and acceptance. Responses may be as simple as "I understand," "That sounds upsetting," or "You seem sad." Empathy may also be nonverbal—for example, offering a tissue to a crying patient or gently placing your hand on the patient's arm. For a response to be empathic, it must reflect a precise understanding of what the patient is feeling. If your response acknowledges how upset a patient must have been at the death of a parent when in fact the death relieved the patient of a long-standing financial and emotional burden, you have misunderstood the situation. Instead of making assumptions, you can ask directly about the patient's emotional response. "I am sorry about the death of your father. What has that been like for you?"

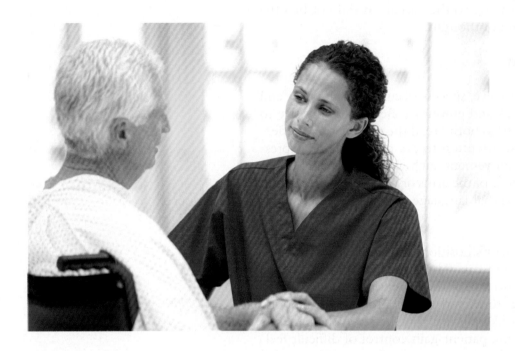

Validation

Another important way to make a patient feel affirmed is to validate or acknowledge the legitimacy of the emotional experience. A patient who has been in a car accident but has no physical injury may still be experiencing significant distress. Stating something like, "Being in that accident must have been very scary. Car accidents are always unsettling because they remind us of our vulnerability and mortality. That could explain why you still feel upset," reassures the patient. It helps the patient feel that such emotions are legitimate and understandable.

Reassurance

When you are talking with patients who are anxious or upset, it is tempting to try to reassure them. Saying, "Don't worry. Everything is going to be all right" may reassure the patient about the wrong thing and provide false reassurance. Moreover, premature reassurance may block further disclosures, especially if the patient feels that the nurse is uncomfortable with the anxiety or has not appreciated the extent of the patient's distress.

The first step to effective reassurance is simply identifying and acknowledging the patient's feelings. This promotes a feeling of connection. The actual reassurance comes much later after the interview, the physical examination, and perhaps some diagnostic studies have been completed. At that point, you can interpret for the patient what you think is happening and deal openly with expressed concerns. True reassurance comes from conveying information in a competent manner, making the patient feel confident that problems have been fully understood and will be addressed.

Summarizing

Giving a capsule summary of the patient's story during the course of the interview serves several different functions. It communicates to the patient that you have been listening carefully. It identifies what you know and what you do not know. "Now, let me make sure that I have the full story. You said you've had a cough for 3 days, that it's especially bad at night, and that you have started to bring up yellow phlegm. You have not had a fever or felt short of breath, but you do feel congested, with difficulty breathing through your nose." Following with an attentive pause or asking, "Is there anything else?" lets the patient add other information and correct any misunderstanding.

Summarizing can be used at different points in the interview to structure the visit, especially at times of transition (see below). This technique also allows you to organize your clinical reasoning and to convey it to the patient, making the relationship more collaborative. *It is also a useful technique for learners when they draw a blank on what to ask the patient next.*

Transitions

Patients have many reasons to feel vulnerable during a health care visit. To put them more at ease, tell them when you are changing directions during the interview. Just as clear signs along the highway give a sense of confidence, this "sign-posting" gives patients a greater sense of control. As you move from one part of the history to the next and on to the physical examination, orient the patient with brief transitional phrases like "Now I'd like to ask some questions about your past health." Make clear what the patient should expect or do next. "Before we move on to reviewing all your medications, was there anything else about past health problems?" "Now I would like to examine you. I will step out for a few minutes. Please undress and put on this gown." Specifying that the gown should close in the back protects the patient's modesty and can make examiners more comfortable.

Empowering the Patient

Patients have many reasons to feel vulnerable. They may be in pain or worried about a symptom. They may be unfamiliar or overwhelmed with accessing the health care system. Differences of gender, ethnicity, race, or class may also contribute to power differentials. However, ultimately, patients are responsible for their own care.[16] Patients who are self-confident and understand the recommendations are most likely to adopt offered advice, make lifestyle changes, or take medications as prescribed.

Listed next are principles that help you share power with your patients. Although many of them have been discussed in other sections of this chapter, the need to reinforce patients' primary responsibility for their health is so fundamental that it is worth summarizing them here.

Empowering the Patient: Principles of Sharing Power

- Evoke the patient's perspective.
- Convey interest in the person, not just the problem.
- Follow the patient's leads.
- Elicit and validate emotional content.
- Share information with the patient, especially at transition points during the visit.
- Make your clinical reasoning transparent to the patient.
- Reveal the limits of your knowledge.

ADAPTING THE INTERVIEW FOR SPECIAL PATIENTS

Some patients are challenging to interview due to their behavior or a disability. Your proficiency handling these situations will develop throughout your career. *Always remember the importance of listening to the patient and clarifying the patient's concerns.*

The Silent Patient

Novice interviewers are often uncomfortable with periods of silence and feel obligated to keep the conversation going. Silence has many meanings and many purposes. Patients frequently fall silent for short periods to collect thoughts, remember details, or decide whether you can be trusted with certain information. The period of silence usually feels much longer to the nurse than it does to the patient. The nurse should appear attentive and give brief encouragement to continue when appropriate. During periods of silence, watch the patient closely for nonverbal cues, such as difficulty controlling emotions.

Silence may be part of the patient's culture or be the patient's response to how you are asking questions. Are you asking too many short-answer questions in rapid succession? Have you offended the patient in any way by signs of disapproval or criticism? Have you failed to recognize an overwhelming symptom such as pain, nausea, or dyspnea? If so, you may need to ask the patient directly, "You seem very quiet. Have I done something to upset you?"

Patients with depression or dementia may lose their usual spontaneity of expression, give short answers to questions, and then fall silent. If you have already tried guiding them through recent events or a typical day, try shifting your inquiry to the symptoms of depression or begin an exploratory mental status examination.

See Chapter 19, Mental Status, pp. 650–663.

The Confusing Patient

Some patients present a confusing array of *multiple symptoms*. They seem to have every symptom that you ask about. With these patients, focus on the meaning or function of the symptom, emphasizing the patient's perspective (see p. 47), and guide the interview into a psychosocial assessment. There is little profit to exploring each symptom in detail. Although the patient may have several illnesses, a psychological disorder may be present.

At other times, you may feel baffled, frustrated, and confused because you cannot make sense out of the patient's story. The history is vague and difficult to understand, ideas are poorly connected, and language is hard to follow. Even though you word your questions carefully, you cannot seem to get clear answers. The patient's manner of relating to you may also seem peculiar, distant, aloof, or inappropriate. Symptoms may be described in bizarre terms: "My fingernails feel too heavy" or "My stomach knots up like a snake." Perhaps there is a mental status change like psychosis or delirium, a mental illness such as schizophrenia, or a neurologic disorder. Consider delirium in acutely ill or intoxicated patients and dementia in the elderly. Such patients give histories that are inconsistent and cannot provide a clear chronology about what has happened. Some may even make up information to fill in the gaps in their memories.

See Table 24-1, Delirium and Dementia, p. 975.

When you suspect a psychiatric or neurologic disorder, do not spend too much time gathering a detailed history. Shift to the mental status examination, focusing on level of consciousness, orientation, memory, and capacity to understand. You can work in the initial questions smoothly by asking, "When was your last appointment at the clinic? Let's see … that was about how long ago?" "Your address now is … ? … and your phone number?" You can check these responses against the chart or seek permission to speak with family members or friends and then obtain their perspectives.

See Chapter 19, Mental Status, The Mental Status Examination, pp. 650–663.

The Patient With Altered Capacity

Some patients cannot provide their own histories because of delirium from illness, dementia, or other health or mental health conditions. Others are unable to relate certain parts of the history, such as events related to a febrile illness or a seizure. Under these circumstances, you need to determine whether the patient has "*decision-making capacity*," or the ability to understand information related to health, to make health choices based on reason and a consistent set of values, and to declare preferences about treatments. The term *capacity* is preferable to the term "*competence*," which is a legal term. You do not need to consult a colleague in psychiatry to assess capacity unless mental illness impairs decision making. For many patients with psychiatric conditions or even cognitive impairments, their ability to make decisions remains intact.

For patients with capacity, obtain their consent before talking about their health with others. Even if patients communicate only with facial expressions or gestures, you must maintain confidentiality and elicit their input. Assure patients that any shared history will be kept confidential, and clarify what you can discuss with others. Your knowledge about the patient can be quite comprehensive, yet others may offer surprising and important information. A spouse, for example, may report significant family strains, depressive symptoms, or drinking habits that the patient has denied. Consider dividing the interview into two segments—one with the patient and the other with both the patient and a second informant. Each interview has its own value. Information from other sources often gives you helpful ideas for planning the patient's care, but remains confidential. Also learn the tenets of the *Health Insurance Portability and Accountability Act (HIPAA)* passed by Congress in 1996, which sets strict standards for disclosure for both institutions and providers when sharing patient information.[17]

For patients with impaired capacity, you will often need to find a *surrogate informant or decision maker* to assist with the history. Check whether the patient has a *durable power of attorney for health care* or a *health care proxy*. If not, in many cases, a spouse or family member who can represent the patient's wishes can fill this role.

Apply the basic principles of interviewing to your conversations with patients' relatives or friends. Find a private place to talk. Introduce yourself, state your purpose, inquire how they are feeling under the circumstances, and recognize and acknowledge their concerns. As you listen to their versions of the history, assess the quality of their relationship with the patient because it may color their credibility. Establish how they know the patient. For example, when a child is brought in for health care, a grandparent who provides daily day care, while parents work, may have the most inclusive knowledge of the child's course of illness. Always seek the best-informed source. Occasionally, a relative or friend insists on being with the patient during your evaluation. Try to find out why, and assess the patient's wishes.

The Talkative Patient

The garrulous, rambling patient may be difficult to interview, especially when faced with limited time and the need to "get the whole story." Several techniques are helpful. Give the patient free rein for the first 5 or 10 minutes, listening closely to the conversation. Perhaps the patient simply needs a good listener and is expressing pent-up concerns, or the patient's style is to tell stories. In some cultures, social conversation of various lengths before "getting down to business" is considered polite. Does the patient seem obsessively detailed? Is the patient unduly anxious or apprehensive? Is there flight of ideas or a disorganized thought process that suggests a thought disorder?

Focus on what seems most important to the patient. Show your interest by asking questions in those areas. Interrupt only if necessary, but be courteous. Learn how to set limits when needed. Remember that part of your task is structuring the interview to gain important information about the patient's health. A brief summary may help you change the subject yet validate any concerns. "Let me make sure that I understand. You have described many concerns. In particular, I heard about two different kinds of pain, one on your left side that goes into your groin and is fairly new, and one in your upper abdomen after you eat that you have had for months. Let's focus just on the side pain first. Can you tell me what it feels like?"

See Summarizing, p. 53.

Finally, do not show your impatience. If time runs out, explain the need for a second meeting. Setting a time limit for the next appointment may be helpful. "I know we have much more to talk about. We will continue after lunch. We will have a full hour then."

The Crying Patient

Crying signals strong emotions, ranging from sadness to anger or frustration. If the patient is on the verge of tears, pausing, gentle probing, or responding with empathy gives the patient permission to cry. Usually crying is therapeutic, as is your quiet acceptance of the patient's distress or pain. Offer a tissue and wait for the patient to recover. Make a supportive remark like "I am glad you were able to express your feelings." Most patients will soon compose themselves and resume their story. Aside from an acute grief or loss, it is unusual for crying to escalate and become uncontrollable.

Crying makes many people uncomfortable. If this is true for you, you need to learn how to accept displays of emotion so that as a nurse you can support patients at these moving and significant times.

The Angry or Disruptive Patient

Many patients have reasons to be angry: they are ill, they have suffered a loss, they lack their accustomed control over their own lives, and they feel powerless in the health care system.[18] They may direct this anger toward the nurse. It is possible that this hostility is justified ... were you late for your appointment, inconsiderate, insensitive, or angry yourself? If so, acknowledge the fact and try to make amends. More often, however, patients displace their anger onto the nurse as a reflection of their frustration or pain.

Accept angry feelings from patients. Allow them to express such emotions without getting angry in return. Avoid joining such patients in their hostility toward another provider or the agency, even when privately you may feel sympathetic. You can validate their feelings without agreeing with their reasons. "I understand that you felt very frustrated by the long wait and answering the same questions over and over. Our complex health care system can seem very unsupportive when you are not feeling well." After the patient has calmed down, help find steps that will avert such situations in the future. Rational solutions to emotional problems are not always possible, however, and people need time to express and work through their angry feelings.

Some angry patients become overtly disruptive. Few people can disturb the clinic, nursing unit, or emergency department more quickly than patients who are angry, belligerent, or out of control. Before approaching such patients, alert the security staff—as a nurse, maintaining a safe environment is one of your responsibilities. Stay calm, appear accepting, and avoid being confrontational in return. Keep your posture relaxed and nonthreatening and your hands loosely open. At first, do not try to make disruptive patients lower their voices or stop if they are haranguing you or the staff. Listen carefully. Try to understand what they are saying. Once you have established rapport, gently suggest moving to a different location that is more private and will cause less disruption.

The Dying Patient

Nurses care for dying patients of all ages in many settings, including hospitals, nursing homes, hospices, and the patient's home. Interviewing and caring for the dying patient can be challenging for all nurses and must be addressed, especially with the student or new nurse. Many students avoid talking about death because of their own discomfort or anxiety. It is important to work through your feelings. Courses, books, and discussion groups on the care of the dying patient help novices understand their feelings as well as the needs of the patient. Basic communication concepts related to the dying patient and appropriate for beginning students are presented below to begin learning.

Dying patients rarely want to talk about their illnesses at every encounter, nor do they wish to confide in everyone they meet. Give them opportunities to talk, and listen, but if they choose to stay at a social level, respect their preference. Remember that illness—even a terminal one—is only a part of the total person. A smile, a touch, an inquiry about a family member, a comment on the day's events, or even some gentle humor affirms and sustains the unique individual you are caring for. Communicating effectively means getting to know the whole patient; that is part of the helping process. Frequent symptom assessment is also important to ensure the appropriate comfort measures are carried out in a timely fashion.

Kübler-Ross described five stages in a person's response to loss or the anticipatory grief of impending death: denial and isolation, anger, bargaining, depression or sadness, and acceptance.[19] Later researchers discovered that these stages may occur sequentially or overlap in any order or combination. At each stage, follow the same approach. Be sensitive to the patient's feelings about dying; watch for cues that the patient is open to talking about them. Make openings for the patient to ask questions: "I wonder if you have any concerns about your illness? your treatment? and what it will be like when you go home?" Explore these concerns and provide the information the patient requests. Setting up a meeting with the physician, therapist, and other team members will help everyone understand the patient's issues and develop a cohesive plan of care. Avoid false reassurance. Accepting the patient's feelings, answering questions truthfully, and being present during difficult times will reassure the patient.

Understanding the patient's wishes about treatment at the end of life is an important nursing responsibility. Failing to establish communication about end-of-life decisions is viewed as a flaw in nursing care. Patients at admission to the hospital or other health agencies are usually asked whether they have *Advance Directives* or *A Durable Power of Attorney for Health Care*. Review the patient's medical record to see if this information has been collected. If there is no record of the patient's wishes, the condition of the patient often determines what needs to be discussed. For patients who are acutely ill and in the hospital, discussions about what the patient wants to have done in the event of a cardiac or respiratory arrest should be initiated with the patient and/or family. Often this is led by the attending physician, but the nurse may need to begin the process with the health team as well as helping the patient or family understand what each option means.

Asking about *Advance Directives, A Durable Power of Attorney for Health care,* or *Do Not Resuscitate (DNR) status* is difficult when you have no previous relationship with the patient or lack knowledge of the patient's values and life experience. Ask about the patient's perception of resuscitation, because the media give many patients an unrealistic view of its effectiveness. "What do you know about cardiopulmonary resuscitation (CPR)?" Work with the physician to educate the patient and family about the likely success of CPR and its side effects (e.g., fractured ribs). Assure the patient that relieving pain and taking care of other spiritual and physical needs will be a priority.

An **Advance Directive** is a document by which a person makes provision for health care decisions in the event that, in the future, he/she becomes unable to make those decisions. These may include the use of cardiopulmonary resuscitation (CPR), artificial feeding and/or hydration, and antibiotics.

A **Durable power of attorney for health care** is a legal document that designates an agent or proxy to make health care decisions, if the patient is no longer able to make them.

Hospice offers palliative care at the end of life. Hospice nurses help the patient and family make end-of-life decisions, complete tasks, and provide pain relief and nursing care. Patients with a terminal disease who only have months to live may benefit from the continuity of care that hospice services provide. Many patients and families are unaware of these services. Investigate hospice services in your area so you can explain how hospice can help your patient.

The Interview Across a Language Barrier

More than 46 million people in the United States do not speak English as their primary language, and the command of English for approximately 21 million is less than fluent.[20] Such people are less likely to have regular primary or preventive care and more likely to report problems with care or even experience medical errors. Learning to work with qualified interpreters is not only cost-effective but also important for optimal care.[21-24]

If your patient speaks a different language, make every effort to find an interpreter. A few broken words and gestures are no substitutes for the full story. The ideal interpreter is a neutral person who is familiar with both languages and cultures. Recruiting family members or friends to serve as interpreters can be hazardous—confidentiality and cultural norms may be violated, meanings may be distorted, and transmitted information may be incomplete. Untrained interpreters may try to speed up the interview by telescoping lengthy replies into a few words, losing much of what may be significant detail.

As you begin working with the interpreter, establish rapport and review what information would be most useful. Explain that you need the interpreter to translate everything, not to condense or summarize. *Make your questions clear, short, and simple.* You can also help the interpreter by outlining your goals for each segment of the history. After going over your plans, arrange the room so that you have easy eye contact and nonverbal communication with the patient. Then speak directly to the patient ... "How long have you been sick?" rather than "How long has the patient been sick?" Having the interpreter close by the patient, or even behind you, keeps you from moving your head back and forth as though you were watching a tennis match.

When available, bilingual written questionnaires are invaluable, especially for the review of systems. First, however, be sure that patients can read in their language; otherwise, ask for help from the interpreter. In some clinical settings, there are speakerphone translators; use them if there are no better options.

Guidelines for Working With an Interpreter: *Interpret Tool*[23]

I **Introductions:** Make sure to introduce all the individuals in the room. During introductions, include information as to the roles individuals will play.

N **Note Goals:** Note the goals of the interview: What is the diagnosis? What will the treatment entail? Will there be any follow-up?

T **Transparency:** Let the patient know that everything said will be interpreted throughout the session.

E **Ethics:** Use qualified interpreters (not family members or children) when conducting an interview. Qualified interpreters allow the patient to maintain autonomy and make informed decisions about his or her care.

R **Respect Beliefs:** Limited English Proficient (LEP) patients may have cultural beliefs that need to be taken into account as well. The interpreter may be able to serve as a cultural broker and help explain any cultural beliefs that may exist.

P **Patient Focus:** The patient should remain the focus of the encounter. Providers should interact with the patient and not the interpreter. Make sure to ask and address any questions the patient may have prior to ending the encounter. If you don't have trained interpreters on staff, the patient may not be able to call in with questions.

R **Retain Control:** It is important as the provider that you remain in control of the interaction and not allow the patient or interpreter to take over the conversation.

E **Explain:** Use simple language and short sentences when working with an interpreter. This will ensure that comparable words can be found in the second language and that all the information can be conveyed clearly.

T **Thanks:** Thank the interpreter and the patient for their time. On the chart for next time, note that the patient needs an interpreter and who served as an interpreter this time.

Source: USDHHS: Office of Minority Health. Communication Tools: Available at: https://www. thinkculturalhealth.hhs.gov/Content/communication_tools.asp. Accessed August 4, 2015.

The Patient With Low Literacy

Before giving written instructions, assess the patient's ability to read. Literacy levels are highly variable, and marginal reading skills are more prevalent than commonly believed. Explore the many reasons people do not read: language barriers, learning disorders, poor vision, or lack of education. Some patients feel uncomfortable about disclosing their reading deficits. Asking about educational level may be helpful, but practical approaches are more fruitful. Ask, "How comfortable are you with filling out medical forms?" or ask the patient to read whatever instructions you have written. (This will also address any difficulty with handwriting.) Another rapid screen is to hand the patient a written text upside down—most patients who read will turn the page around immediately. Lack of reading skill may explain why the patient has not taken medications as prescribed or adhered to recommended treatments. Respond sensitively, and do not confuse the degree of literacy with level of intelligence.[25]

The Patient With Impaired Hearing

Communicating with a person who is deaf can present many of the same challenges as communicating with patients who speak a different language. Even people with partial hearing may define themselves as deaf, a distinct cultural group. Find out the patient's preferred method of communicating. Patients may use American Sign Language, a unique language with its own syntax, various other combinations of signs, and speech. Thus, communication is often truly cross-cultural.

Ask when the hearing loss occurred relative to the patient's development of speech and what schools the patient attended. These questions help determine whether the patient identifies with the deaf culture or the hearing culture. If the patient prefers sign language, find an interpreter and use the principles identified earlier. Written questionnaires are also useful. Time-consuming handwritten questions and answers may be the only solution, although literacy skills may also be an issue.

Hearing deficits vary. If the patient has a hearing aid, make sure the patient is using it and it is working. For patients with unilateral hearing loss, sit on the hearing side. A person who is *hard of hearing* may not be aware of the problem, a situation you will have to tactfully address. Eliminate background noise such as television or hallway conversation. For patients who have partial hearing or can read lips, face them directly, in good light. Patients should wear their glasses to better see visual cues that help them understand you.

Begin by getting your patient's attention. Speak at a normal volume and rate. Use facial expressions and gestures. Avoid letting your voice trail off at the ends of sentences, covering your mouth or looking down at papers while speaking. Even the best lip readers comprehend only a percentage of what is said, so having patients repeat information back is important. At the end of the interview, write out instructions for them to take home.

The Patient With Impaired Vision

When meeting a patient who is blind or has low vision, shake hands to establish contact and explain who you are and why you are there. If the room is unfamiliar, orient the patient to the surroundings and report if anyone else is present. If you leave the room and return, announce yourself again. If the patient has a guide dog, ask permission before petting or greeting the animal. Direct questions and comments to the patient and not to a third party. Walk over to the side of the bed or chair and continue conversation with the patient, staying in one place while obtaining the patient history. It may be helpful to adjust the light. Encourage visually impaired patients to wear glasses whenever possible. Use more verbal explanations because postures and gestures are unseen. Read aloud what you write or enter in the medical record. Ask the patient what format is best for handouts or take home materials (recorded, large print [18-point type], via e-mail, etc.). Say "goodbye" before leaving the room so the patient is not left talking to himself or herself.

The Patient With Cognitive Disabilities

Patients with moderate cognitive disability can usually give adequate histories. If you suspect a disability, however, pay special attention to the patient's school record and ability to function independently. How far have such patients gone in school? If they did not finish, why? What kinds of courses have they taken? How did they do? Has any testing been done? Are they living alone? Do they need assistance with activities such as transportation or shopping? The sexual history is equally important and often overlooked. Find out if the patient is sexually active and provide information about pregnancy or sexually transmitted diseases, if needed.

If you are unsure about the patient's level of disability, shift to the mental status examination and assess simple calculations, vocabulary, memory, and abstract thinking.

See Chapter 19, Mental Status, pp. 650–663.

For patients with severe cognitive disabilities, you will have to turn to the family or caregivers for the history. Identify the person who accompanies the patient, but always show interest in the patient first. Establish rapport, make eye contact, and engage in simple conversation. Ask if the patient uses Alternative or Augmentative Communication (AAC).[26,27] As with children, avoid "talking down" or condescending behavior. The patient, family members, caregivers, or friends will notice and appreciate your respect.

Augmentative and alternative communication (AAC) includes all forms of communication (other than oral speech), such as facial expressions or gestures, use of symbols or pictures, or writing. People with severe speech or language problems may use special augmentative aids, such as picture and symbol communication boards or electronic devices.

The Patient With Personal Problems

Patients may ask you for advice about personal problems that fall outside the range of your clinical expertise. Should the patient quit a stressful job, for example, or move out of state? Instead of responding, ask what alternatives the patient has considered, related pros and cons, others who have provided advice, and what supports or resources are available. Letting the patient talk through the problems is more therapeutic than giving your own opinions.

Sexuality in the Nurse–Patient Relationship

Nurses occasionally find themselves physically attracted to their patients. Similarly, patients may make sexual overtures or exhibit flirtatious behavior toward nurses. The emotional and physical intimacy of the nurse–patient relationship may lend itself to these sexual feelings.

If you become aware of such feelings in yourself, accept them as a normal human response, and bring them to conscious level to keep them from affecting your professional behavior. Denial can increase the risk of responding inappropriately. *Any* sexual contact or romantic relationship with patients is *unethical;* keep your relationship with the patient within professional bounds, and seek help if you need it.[28]

Sometimes nurses meet patients who are seductive or make sexual advances. It is tempting to ignore this behavior hoping it will go away. Calmly but firmly, make it clear that your relationship is professional, not personal. If unwelcome overtures continue, leave the room and find a chaperone before continuing the interview. You should also reflect on your image. Has your clothing or demeanor been inappropriate? Have you been overly warm with the patient? It is your responsibility to reflect and avoid sending misleading signals.

ETHICS OF INTERVIEWING

Ethics and Professionalism

A chapter on interviewing would not be complete without mention of the ethics related to patient information. The potential power of the nurse–patient communication calls for guidance beyond one's innate sense of morality.[28] Ethics are a set of principles crafted through reflection and discussion to define what is right and wrong. Medical ethics guide professional behavior. The principle of *confidentiality* is of paramount importance in the nurse–patient relationship. The nurse is obligated to protect patient information. Simply deleting the patient's name from a story may not be adequate protection. For example, a student may tell a friend a baby was born today with club feet at ABC hospital. If only one baby was born on this day at ABC hospital, the baby can be identified.

Information may only be shared with appropriate health care team members. At the start of the interview, the patient should be told with whom the information will be shared. Do not agree to a patient's request not to reveal a piece of information with anyone before you know what the information is. Should such a request be made, tell the patient that if information revealed is harmful to self or another person, then you are obligated to share it with the appropriate person. Confidentiality is a key quality that fosters the nurse–patient relationship.

BIBLIOGRAPHY

CITATIONS

1. Lein C, Wills CE. Using patient-centered interviewing skills to manage complex patient encounters in primary care. *J Am Acad Nurse Pract*. 2007;19:215–220.

2. Hastings C. The lived experiences of the illness: making contact with the patient. In: Benne P, Wrubel J, eds. *The Primacy of Caring: Stress and Coping in Health and Illness*. Menlo Park, CA: Addison-Wesley; 1989.

3. Epstein RM. Mindful practice. *JAMA*. 1999;282(9):833–839.

4. Stokowski L. Electronic Nursing Documentation: Charting New Territory. Medscape Nurses. Available at: http://www.medscape.com/viewarticle/810573_1. 2013. Accessed August 3,2015.

5. Ventres W, Kooienga S, Vuvkovic N, et al. Physicians, patients and the electronic health record: an ethnographic analysis. *Ann Fam Med*. 2006;4(2):124–131.

6. Cerrato P. Do Your EHR Manners Turn Patients Off? Medscape Business of Medicine. Available at: http://www.medscape.com/viewarticle/809237. 2013. Accessed August 3, 2015.

7. Sheldon LK, Foust J. *Communication for Nurses: Talking with Patients*. 3rd ed. Burlington, MA: Jones and Bartlett; 2014.

8. Platt FW, Gaspar DL, Coulehan JL, et al. "Tell me about yourself": the patient-centered interview. *Ann Int Med*. 2001;134(11):1079–1085.

9. White J, Levinson W, Roter D. "Oh, by the way…:" the closing moments of the medical visit. *J Gen Intern Med*. 1994;9(1):24–28.

10. Smith RC. *Patient-Centered Interviewing: An Evidence-Based Method*. Philadelphia, PA: Lippincott Williams & Wilkins; 2002.

11. Von Korff M, Shapiro S, Burke JD, et al. Anxiety and depression in a primary care clinic. *Arch Gen Psychiatry*. 1987;44(2): 152–156.

12. Kleinman A, Eisenberg L, Good B. Culture, illness, and care: clinical lessons from anthropological and cross-cultural research. *Ann Intern Med*. 1978;88(2):251–258.

13. Lang F, Floyd MR, Beine KL. Clues to patients' explanations and concerns about their illnesses: a call for active listening. *Arch Fam Med*. 2000;9(3):222–227.

14. Brown JB, Weston W, Stewart M. Patient-centered interviewing part II: finding common ground. *Can Fam Physician*. 1989;35:153–157.

15. Coulehan JL, Block MR. *The Medical Interview: Mastering Skills for Clinical Practice*. 4th ed. Philadelphia, PA: FA Davis Company; 2001.

16. Lipkin M Jr, Putnam SM, Lazare A, et al., eds. *The Medical Interview: Clinical Care, Education, and Research*. New York, NY: Springer-Verlag; 1995.

17. Office for Civil Rights—HIPAA, U.S. Department of Health and Human Services. Available at: http://www.hhs.gov/ocr/privacy/index.html. Accessed July 28, 2015.

18. Platt FW. *Field Guide to the Difficult Patient Interview*. Philadelphia, PA: Lippincott Williams and Wilkins; 1999.

19. Kübler-Ross E. *On Death and Dying*. New York, NY: Macmillan; 1997.

20. Jacobs EA, Sadowski LS, Rathous PJ. The impact of enhanced interpreter service intervention on hospital costs and patient satisfaction. *J Gen Intern Med*. 2007;22(suppl 2):306–311.

21. Au M, Taylor EF, Gold M. *Improving Access to Language Services in Health Care*. Rockville, MD: *Agency for Healthcare Research and Quality*; http://www.ahrq.gov/research/findings/factsheets/literacy/langserv/index.html

22. USDHHS. Part 2: Verbal Communication: Working Effectively With an Interpreter. https://hclsig.thinkculturalhealth.hhs.gov/ProviderContent/section3/part2/section3-2-6.asp? Accessed July 31, 2015.

23. USDHHS: Office of Minority Health. Communication Tools: InterpretTool. pdf Available at: https://www.thinkculturalhealth.hhs.gov/Content/communication_tools.asp. Accessed August 4, 2015.

24. Hardt E, Jacobs EA, Chen A. Insights into the problems that language barriers may pose for the medical interview. *J Gen Intern Med*. 2006;21(12):1357–1358.

25. Welch J. Building a foundation for brief motivational interviewing: communication to promote health literacy and behavior change. *J Contin Educ Nurs*. 2014;45(12):566–572.

26. American Speech-Language-Hearing Association (ASHA). Augmentative and Alternative Communication (AAC). http://www.asha.org/public/speech/disorders/AAC./ Accessed July 31, 2015.

27. Hemsley B, Balandin S, Worrall L. Nursing the patient with complex communication needs: time as a barrier and a facilitator to successful communication in hospital. *J Adv Nurs*. 2012;68(1):116–126.

28. American Nurses Assoc. *Nursing Code of Ethics*. Nursebooks.org. Available at: http://nursingworld.org/DocumentVault/Ethics_1/Code-of-Ethics-for-Nurses.html. Accessed August 1, 2015.

ADDITIONAL REFERENCES

Building a Therapeutic Relationship: The Techniques of Skilled Interviewing

Ferguson LF, Ward H, Card S, et al. Putting the "patient" back into patient-centered care: An education perspective. *Nurse Educ Pract*. 2013;13(4):283.

Noordman J, van der Weijden T, van Dulmen S. Effects of video-feedback on the communication, clinical competence and motivational interviewing skills of practice nurses: a pre-test posttest control group study. *J Adv Nurs*. 2014;70(10):2272–2283.

O'Hagan S, Manias E, Elder C, et al. What counts as effective communication in nursing? Evidence from nurse educators' and clinicians' feedback on nurse interactions with simulated patients. *J Adv Nurs*. 2014;70(6):1344–1355.

Riley JB. *Communication in Nursing*. St. Louis, MO: Mosby; 2008.

Schuster PM. *Communication for Nurses: How to Prevent Harmful Events and Promote Patient Safety*. Philadelphia, PA: F.A. Davis; 2010.

Williams C, Davis C. *Therapeutic Interaction in Nursing*. Boston, MA: Jones and Bartlett; 2005.

Adapting Interviewing Techniques to Specific Situations

Americans with Disabilities Act Home Page, U.S. Department of Justice. Available at http://www.ada.gov/#Anchor-47857. Accessed July 21, 2015.

Barnett S. Cross-cultural communication with patients who use American sign language. *Fam Med*. 2002;34(5):376–382.

Iezzoni LI, O'Day BL, Killeen M, et al. Communicating about health care: observations from persons who are deaf or hard of hearing. *Ann Intern Med*. 2004;140(5):356–362.

Marcus EN. The silent epidemic—the health effects of illiteracy. *N Engl J Med*. 2006;355(4):339–341.

LEARNING OBJECTIVES

The student will:

1. Explain the four types of histories and when each is used.

2. Describe the components of a comprehensive health history.

3. Obtain a comprehensive health history from a patient.

This chapter explains how to obtain a patient health history. All history information is considered subjective data. Consider the health history as a chance for the patient to tell his or her "story."

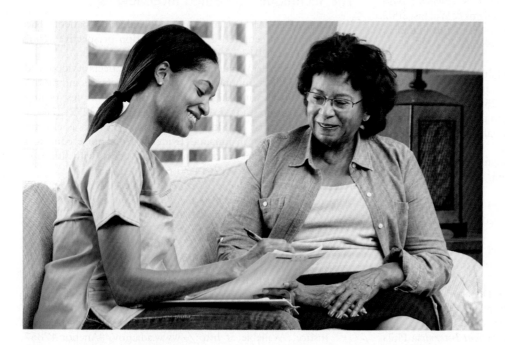

How much history to gather varies based on the purpose of the patient encounter. The admission of a new patient to a clinic, hospital, long-term care facility, or visiting nurse agency usually requires a ***comprehensive health assessment***. This history provides the nurse with a full picture of the patient's health status, as well as health promotion and risk reduction needs. The comprehensive history includes the patient's current health problems, past history, family history, a review of body systems, and health patterns. It provides a basis for assessing patient concerns, health status, risk factors, and health promotion.

A *focused or problem-oriented assessment* is appropriate in many situations, especially when the patient is known to the nurse or health care facility. For example, a patient hospitalized for surgery, who develops shortness of breath postoperatively or a college student visiting the University Health Services for a sore throat. Here the nurse focuses on gathering information mostly on the patient's current problem. The patient's symptoms, age, and this history will determine the extent of the physical examination to perform.

A *follow-up history* is a form of a focused assessment. The patient is returning to have a problem evaluated after treatment, or a second-shift nurse may be following up on a problem identified by a nurse on an earlier shift. Here the nurse gathers data to evaluate whether the treatment plan was successful.

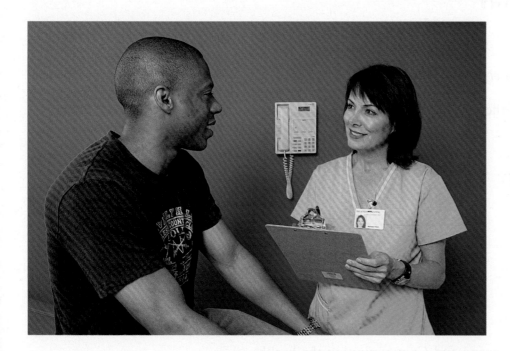

A medical emergency generates a fourth type of data collection, *the emergency history*. The data collection is focused on the patient's emergent problem with a systematic prioritization of need based on the patient's presentation. Very rapid assessment is performed in life-threatening situations, for example, assessment of circulation, airway, and breathing (CAB) when cardiac arrest is suspected.

Mastery of all the components of the comprehensive history provides proficiency and the ability to select the elements most pertinent to the patient encounter.

The Health History: Comprehensive or Focused?	
Comprehensive Assessment	**Focused Assessment**
• Is appropriate for new patients in all settings • Provides fundamental and personalized knowledge about the patient • Strengthens the nurse–patient relationship • Provides baselines for future assessments • Creates a platform for health promotion through education and counseling	• Is appropriate for established patients, especially during routine or urgent care visits • Addresses focused concerns or symptoms • Assesses symptoms restricted to a specific body system

THE COMPREHENSIVE ADULT HEALTH HISTORY

Overview

The seven components of the *Comprehensive Adult Health History* are:

- Identifying Data and Source of the History

- Chief Complaint(s)

- History of Present Illness (HPI)

- Past History

- Family History

- Review of Systems

- Health Patterns

See Chapter 23, Assessing Children: Infancy Through Adolescence for *comprehensive pediatric health histories.*

As described in Chapter 3, Interviewing and Communication the health history may not spring forth in this order. The interview is more fluid. Follow the *patient's* cues to elicit the patient's narrative of illness, provide empathy, and strengthen rapport. For the documentation, transform the patient's language and story into the seven components of the history familiar to all members of the health care team. This restructuring can organize clinical reasoning and provide a template for identification of patient problems.

Review the features of the components of the adult health history described below; then study the more detailed explanations that follow.

Overview: Components of the Adult Health History

Identifying Data	• *Identifying data*—such as age, date of birth, gender, occupation, marital or relationship status, education level, primary language spoken and read. • *Source of the history*—usually the patient, but can be a family member or friend, letter of referral, or the medical record. • If appropriate, establish *source of referral*, because a written report may be needed.
Reliability	May vary according to the patient's memory, trust, and mood. Note whether the patient or other source appears reliable when giving the history. If judged unreliable, provide reason why.
Chief Complaint(s)	The one or more symptoms or concerns causing the patient to seek care.
History of Present Illness	• Elaborates the *Chief Complaint*; describes how each symptom developed. • Includes patient's thoughts and feelings about the illness. • Pulls in relevant portions of the *Review of Systems*, called "pertinent positives and negatives" (see p. 72). • May include *medications, allergies,* and habits of *smoking* and *alcohol,* which are frequently pertinent to the present illness.
Past History	• Lists childhood Illnesses • Lists adult illnesses with dates for at least three categories: medical, surgical, and psychiatric • Includes health maintenance practices such as immunizations, screening tests, lifestyle issues, and home safety • Includes risk factors
Family History	• Outlines or diagrams age and health, or age and cause of death, of siblings, parents, grandparents, and children • Documents presence or absence of specific illnesses in family, such as hypertension, coronary artery disease, etc.
Review of Systems	• Documents presence or absence of common symptoms related to each major body system
Health Patterns	• Documents personal/social history

Initial Information

Date and Time of History

The date is always important. Be sure to document the time the history was obtained.

Identifying Data

These include age, gender, birth date, marital or relationship status, occupation, and any other biographic data appropriate to the agency. Knowledge of the patient's education level and primary language will help the nurse assess the patient's health literacy level. The *source of history* can be the patient (primary source) or a family member, friend, health care provider, or the medical record (secondary sources). Designating the *source* helps the nurse and reader assess the type of information provided and possible biases.

Health literacy is the degree to which individuals have the capacity to obtain, process, and understand basic health information and services needed to make appropriate health decisions[1]. If a formal assessment would be beneficial, there are tools that may be used to assess an individual's health literacy available from the Agency for Healthcare Research and Quality.[2]

Reliability

Document the reliability of the person providing the information. For example, "The patient is vague when describing symptoms, and details are confusing" or "The patient appears reliable." This judgment reflects the quality of the information provided by the patient and is usually made at the end of the interview.

Chief Complaint(s)

Make every attempt to quote the patient's own words. For example, "My stomach hurts and I feel awful." Sometimes patients have no specific complaints. Report their goals instead. For example, "I have come for my regular check-up" or "I've been admitted for a thorough evaluation of my heart." In the hospital setting, the chief complaint may be the same as the admitting diagnosis, but do not assume this is always so. The patient may have other concerns or problems.

History of Present Illness

This section of the history is a complete, clear, and chronologic account of the problems prompting the patient to seek care. The narrative should include the onset of the problem, the setting in which it has developed, its manifestations, and any treatments. The HPI should reveal the patient's responses to the symptoms and the effect the illness has had on daily living.

Key Elements of the History of Present Illness

- Seven attributes of each principal symptom
- Self-treatment for the symptom by the patient or family
- Past occurrences of the symptom(s)
- Pertinent positives and/or negatives from the review of systems
- Risk factors or other pertinent information related to the symptom

Seven Attributes of a Symptom

Remember the mnemonic from Chapter 2 that may help the novice history taker gather all the symptom attributes.

- **OLD CART,** or **O**nset, **L**ocation, **D**uration, **C**haracteristic Symptoms, **A**ssociated Manifestations, **R**elieving/Exacerbating Factors, and **T**reatment

1. **O**nset. When did (does) it start? Setting in which it occurs, including environmental factors, personal activities, emotional reactions, or other circumstances that may have contributed to the illness.

2. **L**ocation. Where is it? Does it radiate?

3. **D**uration. How long does it last?

4. **C**haracteristic Symptoms. What is it like? How severe is it? (For pain, ask a rating on a scale of 1 to 10.)

5. **A**ssociated Manifestations. Have you noticed anything else that accompanies it?

6. **R**elieving/Exacerbating Factors. Is there anything that makes it better or worse?

7. **T**reatment. What have you done to treat this? Was it effective?

See Chapter 2, Critical Thinking in Health Assessment, p. 13 for a more complete list of questions for each attribute.

Self-Treatment

Be sure to ask what over-the-counter (OTC) or prescribed medication or other treatments (e.g., ice packs or alternative therapies) the patient has tried to alleviate the symptoms. If the patient has already tried the typical first course of treatment and it has failed, the provider will need to consider either more advanced treatment or an alternative diagnosis. For example, if the patient complains of heartburn that was unrelieved by an antacid, the problem may be cardiac in origin and not a gastrointestinal problem.

Past Occurrences of the Symptom

The patient may have had the same or similar problems in the past. Inquire about this and ask what treatment(s) were previously used and the results.

Pertinent Positives and/or Negatives

Pertinent positives and/or negatives from the review of systems related to the chief complaint should be sought (e.g., a history of asthma in a patient with difficulty breathing). These data may help differentiate diagnoses and individualize nursing interventions.

Risk Factors or Other Pertinent Information

Risk factors or other pertinent information related to the symptom is frequently relevant, such as risk factors for coronary artery disease in a patient with chest pain, or current medications that may have side effects similar to the complaint.

Past History

Key Elements of the Past History
• Allergies
• Medications
• Childhood illnesses
• Adult Illnesses
• Health Maintenance

Allergies

Allergies to medications, foods, insects, and/or environmental factors, such as pollens should be noted. Be sure to record the specific reaction to each allergen, for example, rash, nausea, anaphylaxis, etc.

Medications

Medications, including name, dose/route, and frequency of use, are included. Also list home remedies, nonprescription (OTC) drugs, vitamins, mineral or herbal supplements, oral contraceptives, and medicines borrowed from family members or friends. If the patient is unsure, ask him or her to bring in all medications to see exactly what is taken.

Childhood Illnesses

Childhood illnesses, such as measles, rubella, mumps, whooping cough, chickenpox, rheumatic fever, scarlet fever, and polio, are included in the Past History. Also included are any chronic childhood illnesses, such as asthma.

 Concept Mastery Alert

When obtaining information from the patient about medications, it is extremely important to ask about and document all adverse effects and all allergic responses to medications that the patient reports. An adverse effect is not the same as an allergic reaction. A patient who has experienced an adverse effect may still receive the medication if the need for the medication is greater than the risk of the adverse effect. In most cases, if a patient experiences an allergic reaction to a medication, this prevents the patient from ever receiving the medication again.

Adult Illnesses

Adult Illnesses in each of the following areas:

- *Medical:* Illnesses such as diabetes, hypertension, hepatitis, asthma, or HIV; hospitalizations with reason for hospitalization

- *Surgical:* Dates, reasons for surgery, and types of operations or treatments

- *Accidents:* Type, dates, treatment, and residual disability of major accidents

- *Psychiatric:* Illness and time frame, hospitalizations, and treatments

Health Maintenance

- *Immunizations:* Ask whether the patient has received vaccines for tetanus, pertussis, diphtheria, polio, measles, mumps, rubella, influenza, varicella, hepatitis A and B, *Haemophilus influenzae* type b (Hib), HPV Meningococcal, and Pneumococcal. Include the dates of original and booster immunizations. (The Centers for Disease Control and Prevention updates vaccine recommendations yearly for different age groups. To obtain the most current recommendations, go to the website http://www.cdc.gov/vaccines/schedules/index.html.)

For patients over 50 years of age, ask if they have had the Shingles vaccine. The vaccine is recommended by the CDC for adults 60 years and older, but the vaccine has been approved by the FDA for adults 50 to 59 years of age as well.

- *Screening Tests:* Such as tuberculin tests, cholesterol tests, stool for occult blood, Pap smears, and mammograms. Include the results and the dates the tests were performed. Alternatively, screening tests may be asked about during and documented in the Review of Systems.

- *Safety Measures:* Seat belts in cars, smoke/carbon monoxide detectors, sports helmets or padding, etc.

- *Risk Factors:*

Tobacco:	Do you use or have you ever used tobacco?
	Do you smoke or chew tobacco?
	Do you use electronic cigarettes?
	At what age did you start?
	How many packs per day (ppd) do you smoke? How many ppd in the past?
Environmental Hazards:	Are you exposed to any hazards in your home or work environment?
Substance Abuse:	Do you use or have you ever used marijuana, cocaine, heroin, or other recreational drugs?
	Do you drink high-energy (*high-caffeine)* drinks? What kind and how much?
Alcohol:	How much alcohol do you drink per sitting and per week?

Alcohol and Drugs

Many nurses hesitate to ask patients about use of alcohol and drugs, whether prescribed or illegal. Misuse of alcohol or drugs often directly contributes to symptoms and the need for care and treatment. In 2013, an estimated 24.6 million Americans aged 12 or older were current illicit drug users. This estimate represents 9.4% of the population aged 12 or older. Recreational drugs include marijuana/hashish, cocaine (including crack), heroin, hallucinogens, and inhalants. Prescription medications (pain relievers, tranquilizers, stimulants, and sedatives) used nonmedically are also extremely dangerous.

In 2013, 22.9% or 60.1 million people aged 12 or older reported binge alcohol drinking in the past 30 days. Heavy drinking was reported by 6.3% of the population aged 12 or older, or 16.5 million people. Among young adults aged 18 to 25 years, the rate of binge drinking was 37.9%, and the rate of heavy drinking was 11.3%.[3]

Despite the high prevalence of substance abuse disorders they remain underdiagnosed. Because of the high incidence nurses should routinely ask about current and past use of alcohol or drugs, patterns of use, and family history.[4] Adolescents and older adults should be included in the assessment of drug or alcohol misuse.

Alcohol

Questions about alcohol and other drugs follow naturally after questions about cigarettes. "What do you like to drink?" or "Tell me about your use of alcohol" are good opening questions that avoid the easy yes or no response. Remember to assess what the patient considers alcohol—some patients do not use this term for wine or beer. Two additional questions—"Have you ever had a drinking problem?" and "When was your last drink?"—along with a drink within 24 hours are suspicious for problem drinking.[5–7] To detect problem drinking, use a well-validated short screening tool that does not take much time. The most widely used screening questions are the **CAGE** questions about **C**utting down, **A**nnoyance if criticized, **G**uilty feelings, and **E**ye-openers.

The Cage Questionnaire

Have you ever felt the need to **Cut down** on drinking?
Have you ever felt **Annoyed** by criticism of your drinking?
Have you ever felt **Guilty** about drinking?
Have you ever taken a drink first thing in the morning (**Eye-opener**) to steady your nerves or get rid of a hangover?

Adapted from Mayfield D, McLeod G, Hall P. The CAGE questionnaire: validation of a new alcoholism screening instrument. *Am J Psychiatry.* 1974;131:1121–1123.

Two or more affirmative answers to the CAGE questionnaire suggest alcohol misuse and have a sensitivity that ranges from 43% to 94% and a specificity that ranges from 70% to 96%.[4,7] If you detect misuse, you need to ask about blackouts (loss of memory about events during drinking), seizures, accidents, or injuries while drinking, job problems, conflict in personal relationships, or legal problems. Also ask specifically about drinking while driving or operating machinery.[8,9]

Illicit Drugs

As with alcohol, questions about drugs should be more focused in order to get answers that distinguish use from misuse. A good opening question is, "Have you ever used any drugs other than those required for medical reasons?" From there, either ask specifically about patterns of use (last use, how often, substances used, amount) or inquire about modes of consumption. "Have you ever injected a drug?" "Have you ever smoked or inhaled a drug?" "Have you ever taken a pill for nonmedical reasons?" As choices of drugs of abuse change, it is important to stay up to date about the most current hazards and risks from overdose.

Another approach is to adapt the CAGE questions to screening for substance abuse by adding "or drugs" to each question. Once you identify substance abuse, continue further with questions like, "Are you always able to control your use of drugs?" "Have you had any bad reactions?" "What happened … Any drug-related accidents, injuries, or arrests? Job or family problems?" and "Have you ever tried to quit? Tell me about it."

Family History

The family history is an important part of the patient history. An accurate family history can identify diseases, which the patient is at increased risk of developing. Early and routine screening as well as education on diet and lifestyle changes can be incorporated into the patient's plan of care. Patients should also be encouraged to keep their own record of diseases and causes of death in the family. Family history tools, both electronic and printed are available to assist the patient to do this.

Under *Family History,* the nurse records the age and health, or age and cause of death, of each immediate relative, including parents, grandparents, siblings, children, and grandchildren. *In addition, each of the following conditions should be reviewed with the patient to determine whether they are present or absent in the family:* hypertension, coronary artery disease, elevated cholesterol levels, stroke, diabetes, thyroid or renal disease, arthritis, tuberculosis, asthma or lung disease, headache, seizure disorder, mental illness, suicide, substance abuse, cancer and the site, genetic diseases and allergies, as well as symptoms reported by the patient. Be sure to ask if there are any other diseases not mentioned. The family history may be documented in written or electronic format per agency protocol. A

Family history tools available on the web include:

US Surgeon General, My Family Health Portrait: https://familyhistory.hhs.gov/FHH/html/index.html

Utah Health Family Tree: www.health.utah.gov/genomics

genogram is a diagram of the family history. It provides a visual record that allows the provider to quickly identify disease patterns within the family. Using a genogram while taking notes during the history, is a quick, accurate way to remember the information provided by the patient. (See figure below, for an example.)

Genogram Key

Female
Male
Unknown
Died
Patient
Gay
Lesbian
Bisexual

Children
Divorced

Transgender people:
Man to woman
Woman to man

A&W   Alive and Well
Write current diseases under each member's symbol, e.g.
HTN   Hypertension
MI   Myocardial Infarction
CVA   Cerebral Vascular Accident
CABG Coronary Artery Bypass Graft

Genogram Sample

Review of Systems

Understanding and using *Review of Systems* questions are often challenging for beginning students. Think about asking a series of questions going from "head to toe." It is helpful to prepare the patient for the questions to come by saying, "The next part of the history may feel like a hundred questions, but they are important and I want to be thorough." Most *Review of Systems* questions pertain to *symptoms,* but on occasion some nurses also include diseases like pneumonia or tuberculosis.

Start with a fairly general question as you address each of the different systems. This focuses the patient's attention and allows you to shift to more specific questions about systems that may be of concern. Examples of starting questions are "How are your ears and hearing?" "How about your lungs and breathing?" "Any trouble with your heart?" "How is your digestion?" "How about your bowels?" Note that you will vary the need for additional questions depending on the patient's age, complaints, and general state of health and your clinical judgment.

The *Review of Systems* questions may uncover problems that the patient has overlooked, particularly in areas unrelated to the *present illness*. Significant health events, such as a major prior illness or a parent's death, require full exploration. Remember that *major health events should be recorded under the Present Illness or Past History in your documentation.* Keep your technique flexible. Interviewing the patient yields various findings that you organize into formal written format only after the interview and examination are completed.

Listed below is a standard series of review-of-system questions. As you gain experience, the "yes or no" questions, placed at the end of the inter- view, will take no more than several minutes. Remember to pause after each symptom to give the patient time to respond. Do not use medical terms with the patient, for example, say "blurred vision" for diplopia.

General: Usual weight, recent weight change, any clothes that fit more tightly or loosely than before. Weakness, fatigue, or fever.

Skin: Rashes, lumps, sores, itching, dryness, changes in color; changes in hair or nails; changes in size or color of moles.

Head, Eyes, Ears, Nose, Throat (HEENT):
Head: Headache, head injury, dizziness, lightheadedness.
Eyes: Vision, glasses or contact lenses, last examination, pain, redness, excessive tearing, double or blurred vision, spots, specks, flashing lights, glaucoma, cataracts.
Ears: Hearing, tinnitus, vertigo, earaches, infection, discharge. If hearing is decreased, use or nonuse of hearing aids.
Nose and sinuses: Frequent colds; nasal stuffiness, discharge, or itch- ing; hay fever; nosebleeds; sinus trouble.
Throat (or mouth and pharynx): Condition of teeth and gums; bleed- ing gums; dentures, if any, and how they fit; last dental examina- tion; sore tongue; dry mouth; frequent sore throats; hoarseness.

Neck: "Swollen glands"; goiter; lumps, pain, or stiffness in the neck.

Breasts: Lumps, pain, or discomfort; nipple discharge; self-exam- ination practices; last examination by a health care provider; last mammogram.

Respiratory: Cough, sputum (color, quantity), hemoptysis, dyspnea, wheezing, pleurisy, TB testing. You may include asthma, bronchitis, emphysema, pneumonia, and tuberculosis.

Cardiovascular: Heart trouble, high blood pressure, rheumatic fever, heart murmurs; chest pain or discomfort; palpitations, dyspnea, orthopnea, paroxysmal nocturnal dyspnea, edema; results of past electrocardiograms or other cardiovascular tests.

Gastrointestinal: Trouble swallowing, heartburn, appetite, nausea.
Bowel movements, stool color and size, change in bowel habits, pain with defecation, rectal bleeding, black or tarry stools, hemorrhoids, constipation, diarrhea.
Abdominal pain, food intolerance, excessive belching, or passing of gas.
Jaundice, liver, or gallbladder trouble; hepatitis.

Peripheral vascular: Muscle pain with walking (intermittent claudication); leg cramps; varicose veins; past clots in the veins; swelling in calves, legs, or feet; color change in fingertips or toes during cold weather; swelling with redness or tenderness.

Urinary: Frequency of urination, polyuria, nocturia, urgency, burning or pain during urination, hematuria, urinary infections, kidney or flank pain, kidney stones, ureteral colic, suprapubic pain, incontinence; in males, reduced caliber or force of the urinary stream, hesitancy, dribbling.

Reproductive:
Male: Hernias, discharge from or sores on the penis, testicular pain or masses, scrotal pain or swelling, history of sexually transmitted diseases (STDs) and their treatments.
Sexual habits, interest, function, satisfaction, birth control methods, condom use, and problems. Concerns about HIV infection. Human Papillomavirus infection or vaccine (HPV).
Female: Age at menarche; regularity, frequency, and duration of periods; amount of bleeding; bleeding between periods or after intercourse; date of last menstrual period; dysmenorrhea.
Age at menopause, menopausal symptoms, postmenopausal bleeding.
Vaginal discharge, itching, sores, lumps, STDs and treatments. Number of pregnancies, number and type of deliveries, number of abortions (spontaneous and induced), complications of pregnancy, birth control methods. Sexual preference, interest, function, satisfaction, any problems, including dyspareunia. Concerns about HIV infection. Human papillomavirus infection or vaccine (HPV).
If the patient was born before 1971, exposure to diethylstilbestrol (DES) from maternal use during pregnancy.

Maternal DES use during pregnancy is linked to vaginal and cervical carcinoma.

Musculoskeletal: Muscle or joint pain, stiffness, arthritis, gout, backache. If present, describe location of affected joints or muscles, any swelling, redness, pain, tenderness, stiffness, weakness, or limitation of motion or activity; include timing of symptoms (e.g., morning or evening), duration, and any history of trauma. Neck or low back pain. Joint pain with systemic features such as fever, chills, rash, anorexia, weight loss, or weakness.

Psychiatric: Nervousness; tension; mood, including depression, memory change, suicide attempts.

Neurologic: Headache, dizziness, vertigo; fainting, blackouts, seizures, weakness, paralysis, numbness or loss of sensation, tingling or "pins and needles," tremors or other involuntary movements; seizures. Changes in mood, attention, or speech; changes in orientation, memory, insight, or judgment.

Hematologic: Anemia, easy bruising or bleeding, past transfusions, transfusion reactions.

Endocrine: Thyroid issues, heat or cold intolerance, excessive sweating, excessive thirst or hunger, polyuria, change in glove or shoe size.

Health Patterns

The *Health Patterns* section provides a guide for gathering personal/social history from the patient and daily living routines that may influence health and illness.

Health Pattern	Sample Questions
Self-perception–self-concept: Describes self-concept and perceptions of self (e.g., body image, feeling state, self-esteem, personal identity, and social identity)	How would a friend describe you? How do you feel about your ability to handle ___? If you could change anything about yourself, what would you change?
Value-belief: Describes patterns of values, beliefs (including spiritual), or goals that guide choices or decisions	What is your source of strength and hope? Is religion or God significant to you? Describe how.
Activity-exercise: Describes pattern of exercise, activity, leisure, and recreation	Describe your exercise routine or activities. Describe your leisure and recreation activities. Have you experienced any change in your activities due to your illness?

(continued)

Sleep-rest: Describes patterns of sleep, rest, and relaxation	At what time do you usually retire and awaken? Do you feel rested?
Nutrition: Describes pattern of food and fluid consumption	Describe a typical day's diet. Are you on any special diet?
Role-relationship: Describes pattern of role interactions and relationships. Includes roles, family functioning and problems, and work and neighborhood environment	Who lives with you? Describe the relationships you have with your family and friends. Who provides support for you? Describe your job. What is your neighborhood like? Do you feel safe?
Coping-stress-tolerance: Describes general coping pattern and its effectiveness in terms of stress tolerance	What are the current stressors in your life? What do you do to reduce stress?

SENSITIVE TOPICS THAT CALL FOR SPECIFIC APPROACHES

Nurses talk with patients about many subjects that are emotionally charged. Even seasoned clinicians are affected by societal taboos enveloping certain subjects: abuse of alcohol or drugs, sexual practices, death and dying, financial concerns, racial and ethnic bias, family interactions, domestic violence, psychiatric illnesses, physical deformities, bowel function, and others. Many of these topics trigger strong personal responses related to family, cultural, and societal value systems. Mental illness, drug use during pregnancy, and sexual practices are examples of issues that may evoke biases that can affect the patient interview. This section explores challenges to the nurse in several of these sensitive areas.

Several basic principles can help guide your response to sensitive topics:

Guidelines for Broaching Sensitive Topics

- *The single most important rule is to be nonjudgmental.* The nurse's role is to learn about the patient and help the patient achieve better health. Disapproval of behaviors or elements in the health history will only interfere with this goal.

- *Explain why you need to know certain information.* This makes patients less apprehensive. For example, say to patients, "Because sexual practices put people at risk for certain diseases, I ask all of my patients the following questions."
- Find opening questions for sensitive topics and learn the specific kinds of information needed for your assessments.
- Finally, consciously acknowledge whatever discomfort you are feeling. Denying your discomfort may lead you to avoid the topic altogether.

Look into strategies for becoming more comfortable with sensitive areas. Examples include reading about these topics in nursing, medical, and lay literature; talking to selected colleagues and teachers openly about your concerns; taking courses that help you explore your own feelings and reactions; and, ultimately, reflecting on your own life experience. Take advantage of all these resources. Whenever possible, listen to experienced nurses, and then practice similar discussions with your own patients.

The Sexual History

Asking questions about sexual behavior can be lifesaving. Sexual behaviors determine risks for pregnancy and STDs—good interviewing helps prevent or reduce these risks. Sexual practices may be directly related to the patient's symptoms and integral to both diagnosis and treatment. Many patients have questions or concerns about sexuality that they would discuss more freely if asked about sexual health. Finally, sexual dysfunction may result from use of medication or from misinformation that, if recognized, can be readily addressed.

You can introduce questions about sexual behavior at multiple points in an interview. If the chief complaint involves genitourinary symptoms, include questions about sexual health as part of "expanding and clarifying" the patient's story. You can ask these questions as part of the Review of Systems. You can bring them into discussions about Health Maintenance, along with diet, exercise, and screening tests, or as part of the lifestyle issues or important relationships covered in the Personal and Social History. Do not forget this area of inquiry just because the patient is elderly or has a disability or chronic illness.

An orienting sentence or two is often helpful: "To assess your risk for various diseases, I need to ask you some questions about your sexual health and practices" or "I routinely ask all patients about their sexual function." For more specific complaints you might state, "To figure out why you have this discharge and what we should do about it, I need to ask some questions about your sexual activity." Try to be matter-of-fact in your style; the patient will be likely to follow your lead. *Use specific language.* Refer to genitalia with explicit words such as penis or vagina and avoid phrases like "private parts." Choose words that the patient understands or explain what you mean. "By intercourse, I mean when a man inserts his penis into a woman's vagina."

See specific questions in Chapter 21, Reproductive Systems, pp. 754–756.

In general, ask about both specific sexual behaviors and satisfaction with sexual function. Here are examples of questions that help patients reveal their concerns:

- "When was the last time you had intimate physical contact with someone? Did that contact include sexual intercourse?" Using the term "sexually active" can be ambiguous. Patients have been known to reply, "No, I just lie there."

- "Do you have sex with men, women, or both?" Individuals may have sex with persons of the same gender, yet not consider themselves gay, lesbian, or bisexual. Some gay and lesbian patients have had sex with the opposite gender. Your questions should always be about the behaviors.

- "How many sexual partners have you had in the last 6 months? In the last 5 years? In your lifetime?" Again, these questions give the patient an easy opportunity to acknowledge multiple partners. Ask also about routine use of condoms. "How often do you use condoms?"

- It is important to ask all patients, "Do you have any concerns about HIV infection or AIDS?" even if no explicit risk factors are evident.

Note that these questions make no assumptions about marital status, sexual preference, or attitudes toward pregnancy or contraception. Listen to each of the patient's responses, and ask additional questions as indicated. To elicit information about sexual behaviors, you will need to ask more specific and focused questions than in other parts of the interview.

The Mental Health History

Cultural constructs of mental and physical illness vary widely, causing marked differences in acceptance and attitudes. Think how easy it is for patients to talk about diabetes and taking insulin compared with discussing schizophrenia and using psychotropic medications. Ask open-ended questions initially. "Have you ever had any problem with emotional or mental illnesses?" Then move to more specific questions such as "Have you ever visited a counselor or psychotherapist?" "Have you ever been prescribed medication for emotional issues?" "Have you or has anyone in your family ever been hospitalized for an emotional or mental health problem?"

For patients with depression or thought disorders such as schizophrenia, a careful history of their illness is in order. Depression is common worldwide but still remains underdiagnosed and undertreated, therefore routine screening is recommended. Be sensitive to reports of mood changes or symptoms such as fatigue, unusual tearfulness, appetite or weight changes, insomnia, and vague somatic complaints. Two opening screening questions are: "Over the past 2 weeks, have you felt down, depressed, or hopeless?" and "Over the past 2 weeks, have you felt little interest or pleasure in doing things?"[11] If the patient seems depressed, also ask about thoughts of suicide: "Have you ever thought about hurting yourself or ending your life?" As with chest pain, you must evaluate severity—both depression and angina are potentially lethal.

For further approaches, turn to Chapter 19, Mental Status, pp. 650–663.

Many patients with schizophrenia or other psychotic disorders can function in the community and tell you about their diagnoses, symptoms, hospitalizations, and current medications. You should investigate their symptoms and assess any effects on mood or daily activities.

Family Violence

Violence is a serious public health problem. Because of the high prevalence of physical, sexual, and emotional abuse, many authorities recommend the routine screening of all female patients for domestic violence.[12] However men can also be victims of violence. Other patients at increased risk are children and the elderly.[10,13] As with other sensitive topics, start this part of the interview with general "normalizing" questions: "Because abuse is common in many women's lives, I've begun to ask about it routinely." "Are there times in your relationships that you feel unsafe or afraid?" "Many women tell me that someone at home is hurting them in some way. Is this true for you?" "Within the last year, have you been hit, kicked, punched, or otherwise hurt by someone you know? If so, by whom?" As with other segments of the history, use a pattern that goes from general to specific, less difficult to more difficult.

Physical abuse—often not mentioned by either victim or perpetrator—should be considered in the following situations.

- If injuries are unexplained, seem inconsistent with the patient's story, are concealed by the patient, or cause embarrassment
- If the patient has delayed getting treatment for trauma
- If there is a past history of repeated injuries or "accidents"
- If the patient or person close to the patient has a history of alcohol or drug abuse
- If the partner tries to dominate the interview, will not leave the room, or seems unusually anxious or solicitous

When abuse is suspected, it is important to spend part of the encounter alone with the patient. Use the transition to the physical examination as a reason to ask the other person to leave the room. If the patient is also resistant, do not force the situation, potentially placing the victim in jeopardy. Be attuned to diagnoses that have a higher association with abuse, such as pregnancy.

Child abuse is unfortunately also common. Asking parents about their approach to discipline is a routine part of well-child care. You can also ask parents how they cope with a baby who will not stop crying or a child who misbehaves: "Most parents get upset when their baby cries (or their child has been naughty). How do you feel when your baby cries?" "What do you do when your baby won't stop crying?" "Do you have any fears that you might hurt your child?" Find out how other caregivers or companions handle these situations as well.

DOCUMENTING THE HEALTH HISTORY

Documentation of the patient's health history is frequently computerized today. The record must be accurate and thorough no matter the type of documentation system used. A sample written documentation of the history can be seen in Chapter 2, Critical Thinking in Health Assessment, pp. 20–22.

BIBLIOGRAPHY

CITATIONS

1. National Network of Libraries of Medicine. Health Literacy. August 2014. Available at: http://nnlm.gov/outreach/consumer/hlthlit.html. Accessed November 20, 2015.
2. Health Literacy Measurement Tools (Revised). November 2014. *Agency for Healthcare Research and Quality*. Rockville, MD. Available at: http://www.ahrq.gov/professionals/quality-patient-safety/quality-resources/tools/literacy/index.html. Accessed November 20, 2015.
3. Substance Abuse and Mental Health Services Administration. *Results from the 2013 National Survey on Drug Use and Health: Summary of National Findings*, NSDUH Series H-48, HHS Publication No. (SMA) 14–4863. Rockville,

MD: Substance Abuse and Mental Health Services Administration; 2014.
4. Cheal NE, McKnigh-Eily L, Weber MK. Alcohol screening and brief intervention: a clinical solution to a vital public health issue. *Am Nurse Today*. 2014;9(9):34–35.
5. Cyr MG, Wartman SA. The effectiveness of routine screening questions in the detection of alcoholism. *JAMA*. 1988;259(1):51–54.
6. Dhalla S, Kopec JA. The CAGE questionnaire for alcohol misuse: a review of reliability and validity studies. *Clin Invest Med*. 2007;30(1):33–41.
7. Alcohol Misuse: Screening and Behavioral Counseling Interventions in Primary Care. May, 2013. US Preventative Services Task Force. http://www.uspreventiveservicestaskforce.

org/Page/Document/UpdateSummaryFinal/alcohol-misuse-screening-and-behavioral-counseling-interventions-in-primary-care?ds=1&s=alcohol%20misuse. Accessed August 9, 2015.

8. Ewing JA. Detecting alcoholism: the CAGE questionnaire. *JAMA*. 1984;252(14):1905–1907.

9. National Institute on Alcohol Abuse and Alcoholism. Helping patients who drink too much. A clinician's guide. Updated 2007. Available at: http://pubs.niaaa.nih.gov/publications/Practitioner/CliniciansGuide2005/clinicians_guide.htm. Accessed August 9, 2015.

10. U.S. Preventative Services Task Force Recommendations: Intimate Partner Violence and Abuse of Elderly and Vulnerable Adults: Screening. January 2013. Accessed at: http://www.uspreventiveservicestaskforce.org/Page/Document/UpdateSummaryFinal/intimate-partner-violence-and-abuse-of-elderly-and-vulnerable-adults-screening?ds=1&s=partner%20violence. Accessed August 10, 2015.

11. Lakkis NA, Mahmassani DM. Screening instruments for depression in primary care: a concise review for clinicians. *Postgrad Med*. 2015;127(1):99–106.

12. Nelson HD, Bougatsos C, Blazina I. Screening women for intimate partner violence: a systematic review to update the U.S. Preventive Services Task Force recommendation. *Ann Intern Med*. 2012;156(11):796–808.

13. CDC Injury Prevention & Control: Division of Violence Prevention. Available at: http://www.cdc.gov/violenceprevention/index.html. Accessed August 10, 2015.

ADDITIONAL REFERENCES

Health Promotion and Counseling

Centers for Disease Control and Prevention. Vaccines andimmunizations. Available at: http://www.cdc.gov/vaccines/. Accessed August 10, 2015.

National Guideline Clearinghouse. Agency for Healthcare Research and Quality (AHRQ). Available at: http://www.ahrq.gov/clinic/. Accessed August 10, 2015.

Substance Abuse and Mental Health Services Administration. Available at: http://store.samhsa.gov/home. Accessed August 9, 2015.

Cultural and Spiritual Assessment

LEARNING OBJECTIVES

The student will:

1. Explain why culture is important in the health assessment process.

2. Define cultural competency and cultural humility.

3. Demonstrate behaviors that show sensitivity to a patient's culture during the assessment process.

4. Explain the difference between spirituality and religion.

5. Explain why the patient's spiritual needs should be assessed.

6. Use a spiritual assessment tool to assess a patient's spiritual needs.

CULTURAL ASSESSMENT

"**Cultural assessment** refers to a systematic, comprehensive examination of individuals, families, groups, and communities regarding their health-related cultural beliefs, values, and practices. Cultural assessments form the foundation for the clients' plan of care, providing valuable data for setting mutual goals, planning care, intervening, and evaluating the care."[1] Patients do not live in isolation; they are part of families, communities, ethnic groups, and cultures. To accurately assess patients' health needs, the nurse must assess patients within the context of their background. Global migration has greatly increased the challenges of providing health care to patients with health care beliefs, practices, and needs different from the health care provider.[2] Culture and ethnicity determines interpersonal communication style, as well as health beliefs, values, and practices. Culture shapes not only the patient's beliefs but also the nurse's. This chapter will discuss the importance of culture and spirituality in relation to health assessment.

There are many definitions of *culture*. Purnell defines culture as "the totality of socially transmitted behavioral patterns, arts, beliefs, values, customs, lifeways, and all other products of human work and thought characteristic of a population of people that guide their worldview and decision making."[3] In other words, *culture* is the system of shared ideas, rules, and meanings that influences how we view the world, experience it emotionally, and behave in relation to other people. It can be viewed as the "lens" through which we perceive and make sense of the world we inhabit. The meaning of culture is broader than the term *ethnicity*. An ethnic group is composed of "individuals who self-identify membership with or belong to a group with shared values, ancestry and experiences."[4] *Race*, on the other hand, is a socially constructed concept of dividing people into populations or groups on the basis of various sets of physical characteristics, usually based on genetic ancestry. Most biologists and anthropologists today do not recognize race as a biologically valid classification, in part because there is more genetic variation within groups than between them. However, research in genetics, genomics, and epigenetics has expanded dramatically and has had a profound influence on the health of people around the world. Humans are more alike than different genetically—only 0.1% of human DNA varies from another person—but these genetic variations explain why susceptibility to common diseases differs among individuals and populations. It also provides the knowledge needed to safely administer medications and counsel patients regarding the preventions and risk of disease.[3] Knowledge of a patient's genetic background is important and should be identified during the history.

Culture is not limited to ethnic or minority groups; everyone has a culture. For example, LGBT individuals, members of a religion, and teenagers may identify with the culture of their group. Likewise, individuals with disabilities, such as hearing impaired or physically impaired, recognize a connection to their culture due to the social construct. Nurses should recognize and be sensitive to the cultural needs of all patients.[5,6] The Office of Minority Health further defines culture as: "The thoughts, communications, actions, customs, beliefs, values and institutions of racial, ethnic, religious or social groups. Culture defines: how health care information is received; how rights and protections are exercised; what is considered to be a health problem; how symptoms and concerns about the problem are expressed; who should provide treatment for the problem; and what type of treatment should be given."[7] The goal of Healthy People 2020 is to reduce health disparities among ethnic or cultural groups in the United States.[8] In order to accomplish this OMH created the *National Standards for Culturally and Linguistically Appropriate Services in Health and Health Care* (the *National CLAS Standards*). The principal standard is: "Provide effective, equitable, understandable, and respectful quality care and services that are responsive to diverse cultural health beliefs and practices, preferred languages, health literacy, and other communication needs."

The National CLAS Standards: The National Standards for Culturally and Linguistically Appropriate Services in Health and Health Care

Principal Standard

1. Provide effective, equitable, understandable, and respectful quality care and services that are responsive to diverse cultural health beliefs and practices, preferred languages, health literacy, and other communication needs.

Governance, Leadership, and Workforce

2. Advance and sustain organizational governance and leadership that promotes CLAS and health equity through policy, practices, and allocated resources.
3. Recruit, promote, and support a culturally and linguistically diverse governance, leadership, and workforce that are responsive to the population in the service area.
4. Educate and train governance, leadership, and workforce in culturally and linguistically appropriate policies and practices on an ongoing basis.

Communication and Language Assistance

5. Offer language assistance to individuals who have limited English proficiency and/or other communication needs, at no cost to them, to facilitate timely access to all health care and services.
6. Inform all individuals of the availability of language assistance services clearly and in their preferred language, verbally and in writing.
7. Ensure the competence of individuals providing language assistance, recognizing that the use of untrained individuals and/or minors as interpreters should be avoided.
8. Provide easy-to-understand print and multimedia materials and signage in the languages commonly used by the populations in the service area.

Engagement, Continuous Improvement, and Accountability

9. Establish culturally and linguistically appropriate goals, policies and management accountability, and infuse them throughout the organizations' planning and operations.
10. Conduct ongoing assessments of the organization's CLAS-related activities and integrate CLAS-related measures into assessment measurement and continuous quality improvement activities.
11. Collect and maintain accurate and reliable demographic data to monitor and evaluate the impact of CLAS on health equity and outcomes and to inform service delivery.
12. Conduct regular assessments of community health assets and needs and use the results to plan and implement services that respond to the cultural and linguistic diversity of populations in the service area.
13. Partner with the community to design, implement and evaluate policies, practices and services to ensure cultural and linguistic appropriateness.

14. Create conflict- and grievance-resolution processes that are culturally and linguistically appropriate to identify, prevent, and resolve conflicts or complaints.
15. Communicate the organization's progress in implementing and sustaining CLAS to all stakeholders, constituents, and the general public.

US Department of Health and Human Services, Office of Minority Health. Think Cultural Health. Available at: https://www.thinkculturalhealth.hhs.gov/Content/clas.asp

Nursing has long recognized and practiced holistic care of the patient, and attention to culture is a part of caring for the whole patient. The nurse communicates with and cares for people of many different cultures. One does not have to be versed in every culture to provide culturally appropriate care, but one must be open and sensitive to other cultures. The term *cultural competence* recognizes the need for a set of skills necessary to care for people of different cultures. However, cultural competence must not be reduced to knowledge of a static set of traits and beliefs for particular ethnic groups that is applied to every member of the group. In reality, there are subgroups and variations within cultural groups. For example, there are many subcultures among Hispanic and Asian peoples. In addition, culture is everchanging and always being revised as group members interact with each other and the world around them.

Campinha-Bacote developed a model of cultural competence that defines culture as a process, not a state. The nurse sees herself or himself **becoming** culturally competent, not **being** culturally competent. Campinha-Bacote sees "cultural desire" as the motivation the nurse needs to "want to" and not "need to" become culturally aware, culturally knowledgeable, and culturally skillful and to seek cultural encounters. One becomes culturally competent by "genuinely seeking cultural encounters, obtaining cultural knowledge, conducting culturally-sensitive assessments and being humble to the process of cultural awareness."[9,10]

Ellis Fletcher created the concept of *cultural sensibility,* "a deliberative pro-active behavior by health care providers who examine cultural situations through thoughtful reasoning, responsiveness and discreet (attentive, considerate and observant) interactions."[11] One first identifies one's own biases, prejudices, and stereotypes about cultures, races, or ethnicity. The nurse then uses reflective thinking to analyze interactions and events in order to develop cultural awareness.

Trevalon and Murray-Garcia developed the concept of cultural humility when caring for patients from culturally diverse backgrounds. Cultural humility is defined as a "process that requires humility as individuals continually engage in self-reflection and self-critique as lifelong learners and reflective practitioners."[12] It is a process that includes "examining cultural beliefs and cultural systems of both patients and nurses to locate the points of cultural dissonance or synergy that contribute to patients' health outcomes."[13] It calls for health providers to reduce the power imbalance that exists in nurse–patient relationships and maintain mutually respectful and dynamic partnership with patients.

As you can see there is overlap among theorists, but *self-reflection* is a common denominator. Begin your self-reflection by answering the following questions.

1. Am I aware of my biases? Prejudices? Stereotypes?

2. Am I comfortable interacting with people from different cultures?

3. Do I seek out experiences with other cultures?

4. Do I seek out opportunities to learn about other cultures?

5. Do I respect the beliefs of individuals from other cultures?

6. Do I know how to access language interpreter services for patients?

Now read the following vignettes, and observe how cultural differences and unconscious bias can unwittingly lead to poor communication and disrupt the quality and outcomes of patient care.

Bias A preference or an inclination, especially one that inhibits impartial judgment, for example, the attitudes or feelings that we attach to perceived differences in other cultures.

Prejudice A disapproving or negative attitude that is not rooted in fact or accurate information.

Stereotype A uniform image of one group that is believed by another group. A fixed, over-generalized belief about a particular group or class of people.

SCENARIO 1

A 28-year-old taxi driver from Ghana who has recently moved to the United States complained to a friend about U.S. medical care. He had gone to the clinic because of fever and fatigue. He described being weighed, having his temperature taken, and having a cloth wrapped tightly, to the point of pain, around his arm. The nurse, a 36-year-old woman from Washington, D.C., had asked the patient many questions, examined him, and wanted to take blood, which the patient had refused. The patient's final comment was "… and she didn't even give me chloroquine!"—his primary reason for seeking care. The man from Ghana was expecting few questions, no examination, and treatment for malaria, which is what fever usually means in Ghana.

In this example, cross-cultural miscommunication is understandable and thus less threatening to explore. Unconscious bias leading to miscommunication, however, occurs in many clinical interactions. Consider the next scenario, which is closer to home.

SCENARIO 2

A 16-year-old high school student came to the local teen health center because of painful menstrual cramps that were interfering with concentrating at school. She was dressed in a tight top and short skirt and had multiple facial piercings. The 30-year-old provider asked the following questions: "Are you passing all of your classes? What kind of job do you want after high school? What kind of birth control do you want?" The teen felt pressured into accepting birth control pills, even though she had clearly stated she had never had intercourse and planned to postpone it until she got married. She was an honor student planning to go to college, but the nurse did not elicit these goals. The chief complaint of cramps was dismissed as minor, when the provider said, "Oh you can just take some ibuprofen. Cramps usually get better as you get older." The patient will not take the birth control pills that were prescribed, nor will she seek health care soon again. She experienced the encounter as an interrogation, therefore she failed to gain trust in her health care provider. In addition, the nurse's questions made assumptions about her life and did not show respect for her health concerns. Even though the provider pursued important psychosocial domains, the patient received ineffective health care because of conflicting cultural values and nurse bias.

In both of these cases, the failure stems from mistaken assumptions or biases. In the first case, the nurse did not consider the patient's belief about his symptoms and expectations for care. In the second case, the nurse allowed stereotypes to dictate the agenda instead of listening to the patient and respecting her as an individual. Each of us has our own cultural background and biases. These do not simply fade away as we become nurses. We must continually learn about different cultures and how to therapeutically interact with each person as an individual with varying degrees of cultural influences.

Avoid letting personal impressions about cultural groups turn into professional stereotyping rather than understanding. For example, you may have heard that Hispanic patients are more dramatic when they express pain or that Asian patients are stoic. Recognize these are stereotypes. Evaluate each patient with pain as an individual, being aware of your reaction to the patient's communication style. Work on becoming aware of your own values and biases, developing communication skills that transcend cultural differences, and building therapeutic partnerships based on respect for each patient's life experience. The framework, described in the next section, will allow you to approach each patient as a unique individual.

THE THREE DIMENSIONS OF CULTURAL HUMILITY

- *Self-awareness.* Learn about your own biases—we all have them.

- *Respectful communication.* Work to eliminate assumptions about what is "normal." Learn directly from your patients—they are the experts on their culture and illness.

- *Collaborative partnerships.* Build your patient relationships on respect and mutually acceptable plans.

Self-Awareness

Start by exploring your own cultural identity.

1. How do you describe yourself in terms of ethnicity, class, region or country of origin, religion, and political affiliation? Don't forget the characteristics that could be areas of change for an individual such as life roles, sexual orientation, gender, or physical ability.

2. What aspects of your family of origin do you identify with, and how are you different from your family of origin?

3. How do these identities influence your beliefs and behaviors?

A more challenging task is to bring our own values and biases to a conscious level. *Values* are the standards we use to measure our own and others' beliefs and behaviors. *Biases* are the attitudes or feelings that we attach to perceived differences. Being attuned to difference is normal; in fact, in the distant past, reacting to differences may have preserved life. Instinctively knowing members of one's own group is a survival skill that we may have outgrown as a society but that is still actively, if unconsciously, at work.

Feeling guilty about our biases makes it hard to recognize and acknowledge them. Start with less threatening constructs, like the way an individual relates to time, a culturally determined phenomenon. Are you always on time—a positive value in the Western culture? Or do you tend to run a little late? How do you feel about people whose habits are opposite to yours? Next time you attend a meeting or class, notice who is early, on time, or late. Is it predictable? Think about the role of physical appearance. Do you consider yourself thin, midsize, or heavy? How do you feel about your weight? What does prevailing U.S. culture teach us to value in physique? How do you feel about people who have different weights?

Respectful Communication

Given the complexity of global society, no one can possibly know the health beliefs and practices of every culture and subculture. Let your patients be the experts on their own unique cultural perspectives. Even if patients have trouble describing their values or beliefs, they can often respond to specific questions. Find out about the patient's cultural background. Review the section "Explore the Patient's Perspective" in Chapter 3, Interviewing and Communication, p. 47. for questions to use. Maintain an open, respectful, and inquiring attitude. "What did you hope to get from this visit?" If you have established rapport and trust, patients will be willing to teach you. Be aware of questions that contain assumptions. And always be ready to acknowledge your areas of ignorance or bias. "I know very little about Ghana. What would have happened at a clinic there if you had these concerns?" Or, with the second patient and with much more difficulty, "I

 Concept Mastery Alert

Before beginning a cultural assessment of a patient, the nurse must conduct a self-examination to determine any personal biases and prejudices that may exist unintentionally. This self-examination allows the nurse to become fully aware of possible unacknowledged feelings and beliefs. This is an important first step. Once this is accomplished, the nurse can gain knowledge and an awareness of the culture's health practices.

The RESPECT Model can provide a guide for cross-cultural communication.

mistakenly made assumptions about you that are not right. I apologize. Would you be willing to tell me more about yourself and your future goals?"

The RESPECT Model

What is most important in considering the effectiveness of your cross-cultural communication, whether it is verbal, nonverbal, or written, is that you remain open and maintain a sense of respect for your patients. The RESPECT Model[14] can help you remain effective and patient-centered in all of your communication with patients.

Rapport
- Connect on a social level
- See the patient's point of view
- Consciously suspend judgment
  Recognize and avoid making assumptions

Empathy
- Remember the patient has come to you for help
- Seek out and understand the patient's rationale for his/her behaviors and illness
- Verbally acknowledge and legitimize the patient's feelings

Support
- Ask about and understand the barriers to care and compliance
- Help the patient overcome barriers; Involve family members if appropriate
- Reassure the patient you are and will be available to help

Partnership
- Be flexible
- Negotiate roles when necessary
- Stress that you are working together to address health problems

Explanations
- Check often for understanding
- Use verbal clarification techniques

Cultural competence
- Respect the patient's cultural beliefs
- Understand that the patient's views of you may be defined by ethnic and cultural stereotypes
- Be aware of your own cultural biases and preconceptions
- Know your limitations in addressing health issues across cultures
- Understand your personal style and recognize when it may not be working with a given patient

Trust
- Recognize that self-disclosure may be difficult for some patients; Consciously work to establish trust

Guide to Providing Effective Communication and Language Assistance Services
www.ThinkCulturalHealth.hhs.gov

OMH
U.S. Department of
Health and Human Services
Office of Minority Health

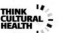

THINK
CULTURAL
HEALTH

Learning about specific cultures, especially those living in your geographic area, is valuable because it helps you provide culturally appropriate nursing care to patients from other cultures. A complete review of cultural health beliefs and practices is beyond the scope of this text. You must search out resources to expand your knowledge and this should be a lifelong learning subject. College courses, books, and conferences on culture are helpful resources. Go to movies filmed in different countries to better understand the perspective of different cultures. Learn about

Consider various barriers to health care to your patient and their family, for example, costs of appointments/medicines, lack of health insurance, distance between home and clinic/hospital, lack of a car, poor English skills, and lack of understanding of Western medical care.

the health concerns of different ethnic groups. Investigate the barriers to health care in your community. Most importantly, be open to learning from each patient. Do not assume that your impressions about a given cultural group apply to the individual before you.

On-line Self-Study Resources

The OMH under The Department of Health and Human Services sponsors *Culturally Competent Nursing Care,* an engaging e-learning program designed to help you build knowledge and skills related to cultural and linguistic competency. Available at: https://www.thinkculturalhealth. hhs.gov/Content/ContinuingEd. asp#nursing_care

National Center for Cultural Competence. Georgetown University. Promoting Cultural and Linguistic Competency provides multiple resources and tools. Available at: http://nccc. georgetown.edu/.

Collaborative Partnerships

Through continual work on self-awareness and seeing through the "lens" of others, the nurse lays the foundation for the collaborative relationship that best supports the patient's health. Communication based on trust, respect, and your willingness to reexamine assumptions allows patients to be more open to expressing views that diverge from the dominant culture. They may have strong feelings such as anger or shame. You, the nurse, must be willing to listen to and validate these feelings, and not let your own feelings of discomfort or time pressure prevent you from exploring painful areas. You must be willing to reexamine your beliefs about what is the "right approach" to clinical care in a given situation. Make every effort to be flexible and creative as you develop shared plans that reflect the patients' knowledge about their best interests, congruent with their beliefs and effective clinical care.

Transcultural Perspectives on the Health History

Culture impacts history taking in multiple ways. Knowledge of the cultural or ethnic groups in your practice region will help you better understand and interpret the patient's needs. Knowledge of categories of dissonance will help the novice recognize potential problems. Time in social conversation, use of silence, distance between the interviewer and client, eye contact, modesty, use of touch, and gestures vary by culture. A patient's nonverbal communication may confuse a novice nurse when it is different from the nurse's communication style. It can be disconcerting working with a person whose culture reverses nodding the head for "yes" and shaking the head for "no," as seen in Bulgaria. Experiencing discomfort or frustration during the history may be a clue that there is cultural dissonance. It is best to stop and clarify the situation with the patient.

Cultural and ethnic variations may be evident during the physical examination, and some of these will be noted in the text during the system examinations.

Cultural Variations in Communication Include

Time spent in social conversation before discussing the purpose of the visit.

Amount of time the patient and nurse are comfortable with silence; "no one talking."

Distance between the interviewer and client. Comfort with interpersonal space.

Eye contact—varies from none to continuous. Avoidance of eye contact is considered a sign of respect in some cultures.

Comfort with being touched: for example, shaking hands when greeting a new patient is not done in some cultures; or touch between sexes is not permissible.

Gestures while talking. Some cultures "talk with their hands," while others are very still.

Modesty, especially during examination.

THE HEALTH ASSESSMENT

Aspects of culture relevant to health assessment include[1,3]:

1. Communication and language

2. Family structure

3. Family roles and organization

4. Social networks

5. Educational background and learning style

6. Nutrition

7. Childbearing and child-rearing practices

8. High-risk behaviors

9. Health care beliefs and practices

10. Health care practitioners

11. Spirituality and religion

A full cultural assessment can be quite lengthy and take more time than the nurse has on admission. The questions in the box below will provide the nurse with basic essential information.

Cultural Assessment

Culture and Language
How would you like to be addressed?
Do you consider yourself a part of cultural group(s)?
Where were you born? Where have you lived since then? And when (during what years)?
What language do you speak at home? What other languages so you speak? What language is preferred for communicating with health care providers?
How well do you understand, speak, and read English?

Spirituality
Do you practice a particular religion? What prayers, rituals, and/or diet would you like to continue in the hospital? Would you like the priest/rabbi/imam/minister/leader to be notified?

Nutrition
What foods are preferred? When and where are meals eaten? Are special foods preferred during illness, or religious seasons (e.g., Lent or Ramadan)?

Reason for Hospitalization
What do you think caused the illness? What do you call this illness?

Family
Who belongs to the family? Who is the decision maker on health issues?

Nursing Care
What interventions would be used for this illness in your culture?
How do you feel about health care givers of a different sex or culture?

Transcultural perspectives for the health history are presented in the box on the next page. Biocultural variations in the physical examination will be noted in the body systems chapters of the textbook.

Introduction

It is generally better to begin the interview using formal titles. Ask the patient how he or she would like to be addressed. Inquire what language the patient speaks, if it is not English. Be aware that some languages have different versions; for example, Chinese may be Mandarin, Cantonese, or another dialect.

Source

Note whether an interpreter was used for the history and indicate his or her relationship to the patient and a contact phone number. See Chapter 3, Interviewing and Communication, pp. 60–61 for more information on working with an interpreter.

Reason for Seeking Care

Patients may interpret their symptoms per their cultural view, as the man from Ghana in the example. There are also *cultural-bound syndromes*, which are "illnesses" defined by a particular culture but that have no corresponding illness in Western medicine. For example, symptoms may be attributed to actions by another individual. This may be called "evil eye," or "mal ojo" in Spanish. To the patient or parent of a child, these are very real events and must be taken seriously. Referral to a healer of the patient's culture may be the best option at times. Use a question at the end of the interview, such as, "What did you hope to get from this visit?" to identify disconnects between patient and nurse or additional concerns the patient may have.

Self-Treatment

Be sure to ask what treatment the patient has used already and whether it helped. Traditional or alternative medicine remedies should be clarified.

Medications

When asking about medications, include herbal remedies and medicines from alternative health care providers. For example, Ayurvedic medicine is a system of traditional medicine native to India and practiced in other parts of the world as a form of alternative medicine.

Family and Social History

Family is important in all cultures, but definitions of family and who is included in the family may vary among cultures. In the history, note the family structure and who the decision makers are for the family, especially for health care issues.

Review of Systems

Ask about health promotion activities for each system as these may vary. One may also ask about symptoms of diseases commonly seen in the patient's ethnic or genetic background.

Adapted from Andrews MA, Boyle JS. *Transcultural Concepts in Nursing Care.* 7th ed. Philadelphia, PA: Lippincott Williams & Wilkins; 2015.

RECORDING YOUR FINDINGS

Mr. L. is a 28-year-old man, who emigrated from Ghana 4 months ago, with his family, wife M. and children, a boy 6 years and girl 4 years. He speaks and understands English well, but reports difficulty reading medical reports. He came to the clinic because he was experiencing a fever alternating with chills and is very tired, which he believes is malaria. He has had malaria twice before, while in Ghana, the last time was a month before he moved to the United States. He was treated with chloroquine pills and the malaria resolved.

SPIRITUAL ASSESSMENT

Many definitions of spirituality have been proposed. The difficulty in defining spirituality may lie in the lack of conceptual clarity of the term.[15,16] Spirituality is a dimension of culture, and it is culture-specific in how it is viewed. Nurses and researchers of Western culture have tried to separate spirituality from religion, but this may do a disservice to non-Western cultures, where spirituality rises from religious beliefs or exposure to a religious culture. An estimated 77% of the world is religious,[17] and for them religion is the basis of spirituality. Spirituality is a vital human experience shared by all humans; atheists and also nonpractitioners have a spiritual dimension. Purnell broadly define spirituality as "all behaviors that give meaning to life and provide strength to the individual."[3] Buck defines spirituality as "that most human of experiences that seeks to transcend self and find meaning and purpose through connection with others, nature and/or a Supreme Being, which may or may not involve religious structures or traditions."[15] Religion may be described as a system of beliefs or a practice of worship. The North American Nursing Diagnosis Association (NANDA) defines spirituality as "A pattern of experiencing and integrating meaning and purpose in life through connectedness with self, others, art, music, literature, nature, and/or a power greater than oneself."[18]

When an individual's sense of purpose or meaning of life is threatened, spiritual distress may result. This may be a response to illness or the loss of a relative or friend. NANDA recognizes *Spiritual Distress* and *Readiness for Enhanced Spiritual Well-being* as nursing diagnoses. Nursing care includes assessment of the patient's spiritual needs and implementation of care related to these needs. The generalist nurse is not prepared to provide intense spiritual counseling,[17] just as he or she does not provide intense nutrition counseling or physical therapy. However, the nurse may provide spiritual care by supporting the patient's practice of spirituality such as prayer or meditation; being present during unpleasant experiences; listening to the patient share fears, thoughts, or distress; providing opportunities for the patient to practice religious rituals; or referring the patient to a priest, minister, rabbi, imam, or religious leader of the patient's choice.

Spiritual Distress is "A state of suffering related to the impaired ability to experience meaning in life through connections with self, others, the world, or a superior being."[18]

Loss History

Person	Objects
Losses of Other People Death of: 1. Parent(s) 2. Spouse/Partner 3. Sibling 4. Child 5. Grandchild 6. Grandparent(s) 7. Friend 8. Relative	**Concrete Losses** • Personal Possessions • Money • Pet • Job • Stocks, Bonds • Residence
	Personal Attributes
Loss of Other People—Through: • Separation • Divorce • Geographic Move • Job Loss • Retirement • Miscarriage • Drug Abuse	**Developmental Losses** • Loss of Fertility • Loss of Mobility • Loss of Vision • Loss of Hearing • Loss of Natural Hair Color • Loss of Hair • Loss of Skin Tone
Part of Self **Loss of Self Through:** • Physical Illness • Divorce • Spouse's Death • Job Loss • Retirement • Substance Abuse • Mental Illness • Abortion • Surgery • Physical/Emotional Abuse • Sexual Abuse	**Abstract Losses** • Hopes • Dreams • Faith • Childhood • Humor • Femininity/Virility
Social Role • Loss of Job • Loss of Partner and Social Contacts • Loss of Status in Society	**Questions to Consider:** • Immediate reaction to the loss • Feelings at the time of loss • The client's age at the time of loss • What did the client remember most about the experience? • Coping Mechanisms • Support Systems • What did the client find most difficult to adjust to?

Adapted from Ginette G. Ferszt, PhD, RN, PMHCNS-BC, Professor, College of Nursing, University of Rhode Island.

The nurse approaches spiritual assessment in two tiers. Patients will not discuss deep concerns until a trusting relationship has been built with the nurse. During the first meeting, the nurse obtains a brief assessment of general information, such as the patient's religion and whether the patient would like a minister, priest, rabbi, or other religious person to be informed of the hospitalization. Does the patient have any rituals or prayers to be continued in the hospital? Nursing care schedules can be arranged to allow time for prayer during the day. Explaining to the patient that research has shown a connection between physical health and spiritual comfort will help the patient understand why questions about spirituality are being asked. The patient's diagnosis may cause fears or concerns. The nurse can ask, "Do you have any concerns or fears because of your diagnosis?" The patient may not be ready to discuss the feelings aroused by the illness. By providing an opening for discussion, the nurse communicates willingness to listen when the patient wishes to discuss spiritual concerns. Listening is an important part of being *present* with a patient. Nursing *presence* "is a holistic and reciprocal exchange between the nurse and patient that involves a sincere connection and sharing of human experience through active listening, attentiveness, intimacy and therapeutic touch, spiritual exploration, empathy, caring and compassion, and recognition of the patient's psychological, psychosocial, and physiologic needs."[19,20] Nursing presence is often what patients value most from the nurse.

Observe the patient's nonverbal cues that may indicate the patient is distressed, such as little or no affect, pitch of voice, posture, facial expression, crying, or inappropriate anger. Sitting with the patient and reflecting back to the patient what the nurse sees may encourage the patient to express concerns. "I noticed that after the doctor discussed your diagnosis you have been very quiet and appear sad. Do you have any concerns?" The key nursing action here is to *listen*, not talk. Allow the patient to talk. Use the techniques discussed in Chapter 3 to encourage the patient to express feelings and concerns.

The patient may make statements that reflect spiritual distress such as "Why did I get cancer?" "I'm a burden to my family," and "I just don't know what to do." These statements should be addressed. Again, let the patient do the talking. The nurse should not offer solutions; rather, the nurse should use the interviewing techniques to help the patient identify the problem and resources used in the past to cope with problems: "What helps you cope?" "What is your source of strength? Source of hope?" "Who are your support persons?" If more help is needed, the nurse can refer the patient to a specialist.

Stoll's guidelines for spiritual assessment provide an outline for the novice to begin assessing a patient's spiritual needs.

Stoll's Guidelines for Spiritual Assessment

Concept of God or Deity
1. Is religion or God significant to you? If yes, can you describe how?
2. Is prayer helpful to you? What happens when you pray?

3. Does a God or deity function in your personal life? If yes, can you describe how?

4. How would you describe your God or what you worship?

Sources of Hope and Strength

1. Who is the most important person to you?

2. To whom do you turn when you need help? Are they available?

3. In what ways do they help?

4. What is your source of strength and hope?

5. What helps the most when you are afraid or need special help?

Religious Practices

1. Do you feel your faith (or religion) is helpful to you? If yes, would you tell me how?

2. Are there any religious practices that are important to you?

3. Has being sick (or what has happened to you) made any difference in your practice of praying or religious practices?

4. What religious books or symbols are helpful to you?

Relation between Spiritual Beliefs and Health

1. What has bothered you most about being sick (or what is happening to you)?

2. What do you think is going to happen to you?

3. Has being sick (or what has happened to you) made any difference in your feelings about God or the practice of your faith?

4. Is there anything that is especially frightening or meaningful to you now?

From Stoll RI. Guidelines for spiritual assessment. *Am J Nurs.* 1979;79(9):1574–1577.

Incorporating cultural and spiritual assessment into one's nursing practice may seem awkward at first. Like other nursing skills, this becomes easier with practice and experience. Practice the assessments with your classmates or friends and relatives, where you may feel more comfortable. Knowledge of the patient's cultural and spiritual needs can make the difference between successful health care and poor care. You can build patient and family trust and understanding of health care in the United States; this will help ensure they follow directions and continue to seek medical care in the future.

BIBLIOGRAPHY

CITATIONS

1. Andrews MA, Boyle JS. *Transcultural Concepts in Nursing Care.* 7th ed. Philadelphia, PA: Lippincott Williams & Wilkins; 2015.

2. Douglas MK, Rosenkoetter M, Pacquiao DF, et al. Guidelines for implementing culturally competent nursing care. *J Transcult Nurs.* 2014;25(2):109–121.

3. Purnell LD. *Transcultural Health Care: A Culturally Competent Approach.* 4th ed. Philadelphia, PA: F.A. Davis; 2013.

4. Leininger MM, McFarland MR. *Transcultural Nursing: Concept Theories, Research and Practice.* 3rd ed. New York, NY: McGraw-Hill; 2002.

5. Wichinski KA. Providing culturally proficient care for transgender. *Nursing.* 2015;45:58–73.

6. Zunner BP, Grace PJ. The ethical nursing care of transgender patients. *Am J Nurs.* 2012;112(12):61–64.

7. Office of Minority Health. USDHHS. Cultural and Linguistic Competency. Available at: http://minorityhealth.hhs.gov/omh/browse.aspx?lvl=1&lvlid=6. Accessed September 1, 2015.

8. Healthy People 2020. Office of Disease Prevention and Health Promotion. Available at: http://www.healthypeople.gov/2020/about/foundation-health-measures/Disparities. Accessed September 1, 2015.

9. Campinha-Bacote J. The process of cultural competence in the delivery of healthcare services: a model of care. *J Transcult Nurs.* 2002;13(3):181–184.

10. Campinha-Bacote J. The process of cultural competence in the delivery of healthcare services, 2010. Available at: http://www.transculturalcare.net./ Accessed June 17, 2010.

11. Ellis Fletcher SN. *Cultural Sensibility in Health Care.* Indianapolis: Sigma Theta Tau International; 2015.

12. Tervalon M, Murray-Garcia J. Cultural humility versus cultural competence: a critical distinction in defining physician training outcomes in multicultural education. *J Health Care Poor Underserved.* 1998;9(2):117–125.

13. Tervalon M. Components of culture in health for medical students' education. *Acad Med.* 2003;78(6):570–576.

14. Mutha S, Allen C, Welch M. *Toward culturally competent care: A toolbox for teaching communication strategies.* San Francisco, CA: Center for Health Professions, University of California; 2002.

15. Buck HG. Spirituality: concept analysis and model development. *Holistic Nurs Pract.* 2006;20(6):288–292.

16. Sessanna L, Finnell D, Jezewski MA. Spirituality in nursing and health related literature: a concept analysis. *J Holistic Nurs.* 2007;25(4):252–262.

17. Fowler M. Come; give me a taste of Shalom. In: Pinch W, Haddad A, eds. *Nursing and Health Care Ethics: A Legacy and a Vision.* Silver Spring, MD: American Nurses Association; 2008.

18. Herdman TH, Kamitsuru S, eds. *NANDA International. Nursing Diagnoses: Definitions and Classification.* Oxford: Wiley Blackwell; 2014:2015–2017.

19. Caldeira S, Timmins F. Editorial: Time as presence and opportunity: the key to spiritual care in contemporary nursing practice. *J Clin Nurs.* 2015;24(17/18):2355.

20. Hessel JA. Presence in nursing practice: a concept analysis. *Holistic Nurs Pract.* 2009;23(5):276–281.

ADDITIONAL REFERENCES

Spiritual Care

Barnum BS. *Spirituality in Nursing: The Challenges of Complexity.* 3rd ed. New York, NY: Springer; 2011.

Biro AL. Creating conditions for good nursing by attending to the spiritual. *J Nurs Manag.* 2012;20:1002–1011.

Hodge D. Administering a two-stage spiritual assessment in healthcare settings: a necessary component of ethical and effective care. *J Nurs Manag.* 2015;23(1):27–38.

Kirkham S, Pesut B, Meyerhoff H, et al. Spiritual caregiving at the juncture of religion, culture and state. *Can J Nurs Res.* 2004;36(4):149–169.

Miner-Williams D. Putting a puzzle together: making spirituality meaningful for nursing using an evolving theoretical framework. *J Clin Nurs.* 2006;15:811–821.

Narayan MC. Culture's effects on pain assessment and management. *Am J Nurs.* 2010;110(4):38–47.

O'Brien ME. *Spirituality in Nursing: Standing on Holy Ground.* 3rd ed. Sudbury, MA: Jones and Bartlett; 2008.

Reinert KG, Campbell JD, Bandeen-Roche K, et al. Gender and race variation in the intersection of religious involvement, early trauma, and adult health. *J Nurs Scholar.* 2015;47(4):318–327.

Taylor E. *Spiritual Care: Nursing Theory, Research and Practice.* Upper Saddle River, NJ: Pearson Prentice Hall; 2002.

Culture

Beard KV, Gwanmesia E, Miranda-Diaz G. Culturally competent care: using the ESFT model in nursing. *Am J Nurs.* 2015;115(6):58–62.

Garneau AB, Pepin J. Cultural competence: a constructivist definition. *J Transcult Nurs.* 2015;26(1):9–15.

Goode TD, National Center for Cultural Competence. Georgetown University Center for Child & Human Development. University Center for Excellence in Developmental Disabilities, Education, Research & Service. Adapted Promoting Cultural Competence and Cultural Diversity for Personnel Providing Services and Supports to Children with Special Health Care Needs and their Families. June 1989 (Revised 2009). Available at: http://nccc.georgetown.edu/resources/assessments.html. Accessed August 21, 2015.

Herdman TH, Kamitsuru S, eds. *NANDA International. Nursing Diagnoses: Definitions and Classification.* Oxford: Wiley Blackwell; 2014:2015–2017.

Leininger M, McFarland M. *Culture Care Diversity and Universality: A Worldwide Nursing Theory.* 2nd ed. Boston, MA: Jones and Bartlett Publishers; 2006.

McEvoy M. Culture and spirituality as an integrated concept in pediatric care. *MCN Am J Matern/Child Nurs.* 2003;25(1):39–43.

Miller S. Cultural humility is the first step to becoming global care providers. *J Obstet Gynecol Neonatal Nurs.* 2009;38(1):92–93.

Myers VA. *What If I Say the Wrong Thing?* Chicago: ABA Publishing; 2013.

National Center for Cultural Competence. Georgetown University. Promoting Cultural and Linguistic Competency: Self-Assessment Checklist for Personnel Providing Primary Health Care Services. Available at: http://nccc.georgetown.edu/resources/assessments.html. Accessed August 21, 2015.

Office of Minority Health. The RESPECT Model. Available at: https://hclsig.thinkculturalhealth.hhs.gov/ProviderContent/Section3/Part1/Section3–1–4.asp. Accessed August 24, 2015.

Shen Z. Cultural competence models and cultural competence assessment instruments in nursing: a literature review. *J Transcult Nurs.* 2015;26(3):308.

Sherman RO. How to avoid biased thinking. *American Nurse Today.* 2015;10(3):12–14.

Spector R. *Cultural Diversity in Health and Illness.* 7th ed. Pearson Prentice Hall; 2009.

Sullivan CG. Implementing culturally competent care. *Nurs Outlook.* 2015;63(2):227–229.

Tarzian AJ. Exploring diversity and disparities: an evolving journey. In: Pinch W, Haddad A, eds. *Nursing and Health Care Ethics: A Legacy and a Vision.* Silver Spring, MD: American Nurses Association; 2008.

6 Physical Examination: Getting Started

LEARNING OBJECTIVES

The student will:

1. Describe how to individualize the physical examination approach based on the patient's needs and the environment.

2. Select an environment that enhances the accuracy of the physical examination.

3. Discuss the environmental features necessary to ensure patient safety and comfort during a physical examination.

4. Describe and use the equipment for performing a physical examination.

5. Identify safety precautions when conducting the physical examination.

6. Indicate the correct order and how to use the four cardinal techniques.

The physical examination should be performed once you understand the patient's concerns and have elicited a careful history. When learning about physical assessment, students often want to proceed directly to the examination; however, the collection of subjective information during history taking assists to focus your examination accordingly. At first, you may feel unsure of your skills and how the patient will relate to you. With practice, your skills in physical examination will grow, and you will gain confidence. Through study and repetition, the examination will soon flow more smoothly, and the attention will shift from technique and how to handle instruments to what you hear, see, and feel. Touching the patient's body will seem more natural, and you will learn to minimize discomfort to the patient. Before long, you will gain proficiency, and what once took between 1 and 2 hours will take considerably less time. You will continually hone these important relational and clinical skills throughout your practice.

The physical examination is a process to obtain objective data from the patient. The subjective data in the health history is obtained prior to the examination and will assist the nurse to navigate through a complex examination. Each body system connects to another. A finding in one system may not be an isolated finding. For example, the patient who presents with a chief complaint of blurred vision may be having vision changes because of age, an injury, a retina or macular affliction, or changes due to hyperglycemia. The purpose of the physical examination is to determine changes in a patient's health status and how to respond to a problem as well as promote healthy lifestyles and well-being. A decision to perform a comprehensive or a focused assessment is described in Chapter 4, The Health History and is made on an individual basis.

THE COMPREHENSIVE ADULT PHYSICAL EXAMINATION

Beginning the Examination: Setting the Stage

As new practitioners, the impetus is to dive in and begin the physical examination. However, as in anything worthwhile, preparation is paramount.

See Chapter 23, Assessing Children: Infancy Through Adolescence, for the comprehensive examination of infants, children, and adolescents.

See Chapter 24, Assessing Older Adults, for more details on this comprehensive examination.

Before beginning the physical examination, think through the approach to the patient, professional demeanor, and how to make the patient feel comfortable and relaxed. Review the measures that promote the patient's physical comfort and safety, making any necessary adjustments in the lighting and surrounding environment. Refer to specific accommodations for various age groups, found in Chapter 23, Assessing Older Adults and Chapter 24, Assessing Children: Infancy Through Adolescence. Remember to gather the equipment and review the patient chart, if available, prior to entering the room.

Preparing for the Physical Examination

- Reflect on your approach to the patient.
- Adjust the lighting and the environment.
- Check that the equipment is available and in working order.
- Make the patient comfortable.
- Choose the sequence of examination.

Reflect on Your Approach to the Patient

When first examining patients, feelings of insecurity are inevitable, but these will soon diminish with experience. As you enter the room, identify yourself as a nursing student. Appear calm and organized, even when you feel inexperienced. It is common to forget part of the examination, especially at first. If that occurs, simply examine that area out of sequence. It is not unusual to go back to the patient and ask to check one or two items that might have been overlooked.

Beginners will need to spend more time than experienced nurses on select portions of the examination, such as the fundoscopic examination or cardiac auscultation. To avoid alarming the patient, warn the patient ahead of time by saying, for example, "I would like to spend extra time listening to your heart and the heart sounds, but this doesn't mean I hear anything wrong."

Many patients view the physical examination with some anxiety. They feel vulnerable, physically exposed, apprehensive about possible pain, and uneasy about what the nurse may find. At the same time, they appreciate your concern about their health and respond to your attention. With these considerations in mind, the skillful nurse is thorough without wasting time, systematic but flexible, and gentle yet not afraid to cause discomfort should it be required. The skillful nurse examines each region of the body and at the same time is aware of the whole patient, notes the wince or worried glance, and shares information that calms, explains, and reassures.

As a beginner, *avoid interpreting your findings*. You are not the patient's primary caregiver, and your views may be premature or incorrect. As you grow in experience and responsibility, sharing findings will become more appropriate. If the patient has specific concerns, discuss them with your faculty. At times, you may discover abnormalities such as an ominous mass or a deep ulceration. Always avoid showing distaste, alarm, or other negative reactions. Keeping your verbal and nonverbal communication in check is paramount. If you find anything that is unusual or disturbing, always talk with your clinical instructor.

Adjust the Lighting and the Environment

Nurses practice in a variety of settings and flexibility and creativity are warranted to insure adequate lighting and a conducive environment for physical examination and patient care. Several environmental factors affect the caliber of your examination. For best results it is important to "set the stage" so that both you and the patient are comfortable. Awkward positioning for both you and the patient, impairs detection of physical findings. Take the time to adjust the bed to a convenient height (but be sure to lower it when finished), and ask the patient to move toward you, turn over or shift position whenever this makes examining selected areas of the body easier.

Good lighting and a quiet environment make a difference in what you see and hear but may be hard to arrange. Do the best you can. If a television interferes with auscultating heart sounds, politely ask the nearby patient to lower the volume and remember to thank the patient as you leave.

Tangential lighting is optimal for inspecting structures such as the jugular venous pulse, the thyroid gland, and the apical impulse of the heart. It casts light across body surfaces that shows contours, elevations, and depressions, whether moving or stationary, into sharper relief. When light is perpendicular to the surface or diffuse, shadows are reduced and subtle undulations across the surface are lost. Experiment with focused, tangential lighting across the tendons on the back of your hand; try to see the pulsations of the radial artery at your wrist.

TANGENTIAL LIGHTING

PERPENDICULAR LIGHTING

Check Your Equipment

Prior to the start of the physical examination, collect all necessary equipment and supplies and check all are in working order. For example, check the batteries in the penlight and oto/ophthalmoscope to confirm they turn on. This ensures a smooth flow during the examination and avoids having to leave the patient during the examination to search for equipment.

List of Equipment for Physical Examination

- Hand sanitizer
- Examination gloves
- Alcohol wipes

- Paper and pen, or computer
- Draw sheet or drape
- Stadiometer
- Scale
- Examination light/gooseneck lamp
- Thermometer
- Watch with a second hand
- Sphygmomanometer
- Stethoscope
- Pulse oximeter
- Doppler
- Ophthalmoscope
- Otoscope/speculums
- Nasal speculum
- Scents for testing sense of smell (e.g., mint, coffee, or alcohol swab if other scents are not available)

- Snellen chart or visual acuity card to test distant vision
- Near vision card

- Opaque card
- Penlight
- Tongue depressors
- 2 × 2-gauze pads
- Cup of water
- Ruler and flexible tape measure, preferably marked in centimeters

- Goniometer
- Scoliometer
- Reflex hammer
- Tuning forks 128 and 512 Hz
- Q-tips, paper clips, or other disposable objects for testing sense of touch
- Cotton
- Mini-mental status examination tool

Pictures and basic details are provided in the box below, with additional information in the corresponding systems chapters on how the equipment will facilitate your examination of the patient. Specific equipment is necessary for each component of the physical examination.

Explanation of Equipment and Instruments for the Physical Examination

- Stadiometer. Measures height and must be installed at the correct height and mounted to the wall to achieve accurate measurements.
- Scale. Measures weight and needs to be calibrated per institutional policy.
- Ophthalmoscope. Visualize the interior of the eye, especially the retina.

This side of the ophthalmoscope faces the patient. Letter **A** on the picture above is below and to the left of the wheel used to change the size/color of the light emitted from this side. **B** indicates the wheel used to change the diopter focus.

This side faces the nurse; the top ridge of the scope rests against the nurse's eyebrow. **B** indicates the wheel that changes the diopters and **C** indicates the indicator of diopters.

- Otoscope. Visualize the ear canal and ear drum.
- Speculum. Cone-shaped attachment, attaches to otoscope to examine ear.

- Nasal speculum. Opens the nasal passage to visualize in the nose.
- Snellen chart or visual acuity card. Tests distant vision.
- Near vision card. Tests near vision.
- Opaque card. Cover the eye not being examined.
- Penlight. Provides additional light for viewing various areas of the body and check eyes.
- Tongue depressors. Use for mouth examination.
- 2 × 2 gauze pads. Use during tongue examination.
- Examination light/gooseneck lamp. Provides additional lighting.

- Thermometer. Used for measuring temperature.

- Watch with a second hand. Times respiration and pulse rates.
- Sphygmomanometer. Measures blood pressure.
- Stethoscope with the following characteristics:
  - Stethoscopes range in length from 22–31 inches. The tubing can range from ~17–22 inches in length and should be chosen based on practitioner preference and comfort.
  - Ear tips that fit snugly and painlessly. To get this fit, choose ear tips of the proper size, align the ear pieces with the angle of the ear canals, and adjust the spring of the connecting metal band to a comfortable tightness.

- A bell and a diaphragm. The disk at the end of the stethoscope is the bell and diaphragm. The bell is the smaller, cupped side of the stethoscope and transmits lower-pitched sounds and the diaphragm is the larger, flatter side of the stethoscope and this transmits higher-pitched sounds. By rotating the disk at the end of the stethoscope you can change from the bell to the diaphragm as needed. By tapping lightly on the disk you can determine which side is open for sound transmission. If you own a stethoscope that has the bell and diaphragm on the same side then you will press firmly to use the diaphragm and barely press at all to use the bell.

- Pulse oximeter. Measures oxygen saturation.
- Doppler. Detects blood flow and pulses.
- Reflex hammer. Tests strength of a reflex.

- Tuning forks. Two-pronged with tines that form a U-shape. Tests vibration (128 Hz) and sound (512 Hz). The frequency is found on the front of the tuning fork.

128 Hz
512 Hz

- Q-tips, paper clips, or other disposable objects. Tests two-point discrimination.
- Cotton. Tests the sense of light touch.
- Q-tip or broken tongue blade. Tests the sense of sharp touch.

- Substances with distinct odors (e.g., vanilla and coffee). Test for sensory perception of smell and taste.
- Two test tubes (optional) for testing temperature sensation

Familiarity of each piece of equipment is necessary for specific techniques and will be explained in more detail in corresponding chapters.

Observe Standard and Universal Precautions

Prior to beginning the physical examination and working with patients, study the Centers for Disease Control and Prevention (CDC) guidelines to protect patients and examiners from the spread of infectious disease. These precautions can be found at the CDC website. Advisories for standard and methicillin-resistant *Staphylococcus aureus* (*MRSA*) precautions and for universal precautions are briefly summarized here.[1–7]

- *Standard and MRSA precautions:* Standard precautions are based on the principle that all blood, body fluids, secretions, excretions (except sweat), nonintact skin, and mucous membranes may contain transmissible infectious agents. These practices apply to all patients in any setting. They include hand hygiene; use of personal protective equipment (gloves, gowns, and mouth, nose, and eye protection); safe injection practices; safe handling of contaminated equipment or surfaces; respiratory hygiene and cough etiquette; patient isolation criteria; and precautions relating to equipment, toys, solid surfaces, and laundry handling. Because hand hygiene practices have been shown to reduce the transmission of multidrug resistant organisms, especially MRSA and

 Concept Mastery Alert

Gloves, which are used during patient care for numerous reasons, are essential in preventing a nurse's hands from becoming a vehicle for the transmission of organisms from one patient to another. That is, a nurse puts on gloves to care for a patient, then removes the gloves and discards them appropriately. Before entering another patient's room, the nurse performs hand hygiene. These actions disrupt the chain of infection. Gloves do not limit a nurse's exposure to body fluids and secretions. Rather, they prevent it.

vancomycin-resistant enterococcus (VRE),[2-7] the CDC hygiene recommendations are reproduced below. White coats and stethoscopes also harbor bacteria and should be cleaned frequently. Stethoscopes should be wiped before and after use with every patient.[8,9]

Centers for Disease Control: Key Recommendations for Hand Hygiene

1. Key situations where hand hygiene should be performed include:
   a. Before touching a patient, even if gloves will be worn
   b. Before exiting the patient's care area after touching the patient or the patient's immediate environment
   c. After contact with blood, body fluids or excretions, or wound dressings
   d. Prior to performing an aseptic task (e.g., placing an IV, preparing an injection)
   e. If hands will be moving from a contaminated-body site to a clean-body site during patient care
   f. After glove removal
2. Use soap and water when hands are visibly soiled (e.g., blood, body fluids), or after caring for patients with known or suspected infectious diarrhea (e.g., *Clostridium difficile,* norovirus). Otherwise, the preferred method of hand decontamination is with an alcohol-based hand rub.[10]

- *Universal precautions:* Universal precautions are a set of guidelines designed to prevent parenteral, mucous membrane, and noncontact exposures of health care workers to blood-borne pathogens, including the human immunodeficiency virus (HIV) and hepatitis B virus (HBV). Immunization with the hepatitis B vaccine for health care workers with exposure to blood is an important adjunct to universal precautions. The following fluids are considered potentially infectious: all blood and other body fluids containing visible blood, semen, and vaginal secretions; and cerebrospinal, synovial, pleural, peritoneal, pericardial, and amniotic fluids. Protective barriers include gloves, gowns, aprons, masks, and protective eyewear. All health care workers should follow the precautions for safe injections and prevention of injury from needle sticks, scalpels, and other sharp instruments and devices. Report to your health service immediately if such injury occurs.[2-4]

Make the Patient Comfortable

Patient Privacy and Comfort

Your access to the patient's body is a unique and time-honored privilege in the role of the nurse. Showing sensitivity for privacy and patient modesty must be ingrained in your professional behavior and conveys respect for the patient's vulnerability. Close nearby doors, draw the curtains in the hospital or examining room, and wash your hands thoroughly before the examination begins.

During the examination, be aware of the patient's feelings and any discomfort. Respond to the patient's facial expressions and ask "Are you okay?" or "Is this painful?" to elicit unexpressed worries or sources of pain. Adjusting the angle of the bed or examining table, rearranging the pillows, or adding blankets for warmth demonstrates that you are attentive to the patient's well-being.

Draping the Patient

You will acquire the art of *draping the patient* with the gown or draw sheet as you learn each segment of the examination in the chapters ahead.

Tips for Draping the Patient

- *Your goal is to visualize one area of the body at a time.* This preserves the patient's modesty and helps you focus on the area being examined.
- With the patient sitting, auscultate the lungs with the gown untied in back.
- For the breast examination, uncover the right breast and keep the left chest draped. Re-drape the right chest, then uncover the left chest and proceed to examine the left breast and heart.
- For the abdominal examination, only the abdomen should be exposed. Adjust the gown to cover the chest and place the sheet or drape at the inguinal area.
- To help the patient prepare for potentially awkward segments, briefly describe the plan before starting, for example, "Now I am going to move your gown so I can check the pulse in your groin area."

Courteous Clear Instructions

Make sure the instructions to the patient at each step in the examination are courteous and clear. For example, "I would like to examine your abdomen now, so please, lie down." Let the patient know if you anticipate they may experience discomfort.

Keeping the Patient Informed

As you proceed with the examination, talk with the patient so see if he or she wants to know about your findings. Is the patient curious about the lung findings or your method for assessing the liver or spleen? Tell the patient the results of the vital signs and use this as a teaching moment.

When you have completed the examination, tell the patient your general impressions and what to expect next. For hospitalized patients, make sure the patient is comfortable and safe and rearrange the immediate environment to the patient's satisfaction. To promote safety and prevent falls, be sure to lower the bed, place the side table and personal items within reach, and raise the bed rails. As you leave, clean your equipment, dispose of any waste materials, and wash your hands.

The Cardinal Techniques of Examination

Before you begin the examination, study the four cardinal techniques of examination. Plan your sequence and scope of examination and how you will position the patient.

The physical examination relies on four classic techniques: inspection, palpation, percussion, and auscultation. You will learn in later chapters about additional maneuvers that are important in amplifying physical diagnosis, such as having the patient lean forward to better detect the murmur of aortic regurgitation or balloting the patella to check for joint effusion.

These four techniques—inspection, palpation, percussion, and, finally, auscultation—will *always* be used in this order, in all systems, with the exception of the abdomen. During the abdominal examination, the pattern will be inspection, auscultation, percussion, and palpation. Auscultation follows inspection so as not to increase bowel motility with palpation.

Cardinal Techniques of Examination

• Inspection	Close observation of the details of the patient's appearance, behavior, and movement such as facial expression, mood, body build and conditioning, skin conditions such as petechiae or ecchymoses, eye movements, pharyngeal color, symmetry of thorax, height of jugular venous pulsations, abdominal contour, lower extremity edema, and gait.
• Palpation	Tactile pressure from the palmar fingers or finger pads to assess areas of skin elevation, depression, warmth, or tenderness; lymph nodes; pulses; contours and sizes of organs and masses; and crepitus in the joints. Metacarpal/phalangeal joint or ulnar surface of the hand is used to detect vibration.

• Percussion	Use of the striking or *plexor finger,* usually the third, to deliver a rapid tap or blow against the distal *pleximeter finger,* usually the distal third finger of the left hand laid against the surface of the chest or abdomen, to evoke a sound wave such as resonance or dullness from the underlying tissue or organs. This sound wave also generates a tactile vibration against the pleximeter finger.	
• Auscultation	Use of the diaphragm and bell of the stethoscope to detect the characteristics of heart, lung, and bowel sounds, including location, timing, duration, pitch, and intensity. For the heart this involves sounds from closure of the four valves, extra sounds from blood flow into the atria and ventricles, and murmurs. Auscultation also permits detection of bruits or turbulence over arterial vessels.	

Sequence of Examination

The key to a thorough and accurate physical examination is developing a systematic sequence of examination. Organize your comprehensive or focused examination around four general goals:

• Maximize the patient's comfort

• Maintain patient safety

• Avoid unnecessary changes in position

• Enhance clinical accuracy and efficiency

Patients can be nervous during physical examinations related to the examination itself or to the possible findings. As a new practitioner, you may also feel nervous. With practice, you will become more self-assured. Initially, practice in the lab with friends posing as simulated patients. This repetition will enhance your skills and this confidence will also help to allay patient's anxiety. Additionally, maintain a person's privacy by pulling the curtain, draping the person to decrease exposure and to prevent chilling. Watch patient nonverbal communication for indications of pain or uneasiness. Answer questions and talk with the patient and indicate what you plan to do and your findings.

Patient safety is paramount. This may take multiple forms, from the initial washing of hands, to moving on and off the examination table using fall prevention techniques or remembering to clean equipment, especially your stethoscope's bell and diaphragm with an alcohol swab, before and after each use.[10,11]

In general, move from "head to toe." Avoid examining the patient's feet, for example, before checking the face or mouth. You will quickly see that some segments of the examination are best assessed when the patient is sitting, such as examination of the head and neck and the thorax and lungs, whereas others are best obtained with the patient supine, such as the abdominal examination. You want to optimize the time with your patient in one position and avoid unnecessary changes in position, which may be difficult for some patients.

Frequent positional changes in a patient with shortness of breath may increase breathing patterns or a patient with joint pain may experience increased pain. Both of these examples demonstrate the importance of limiting unnecessary changes and maintaining good flow of the physical examination.

Examining From the Patient's Right Side

This book recommends examining the patient from the patient's *right side*, moving to the opposite side or foot of the bed or examining table only as necessary. This is the standard position for the physical examination and has several advantages compared with the left side: estimates of jugular venous pressure are more reliable, the palpating hand rests more comfortably on the apical impulse, the right kidney is more frequently palpable than the left, and examining tables are frequently positioned to accommodate a right-side approach.

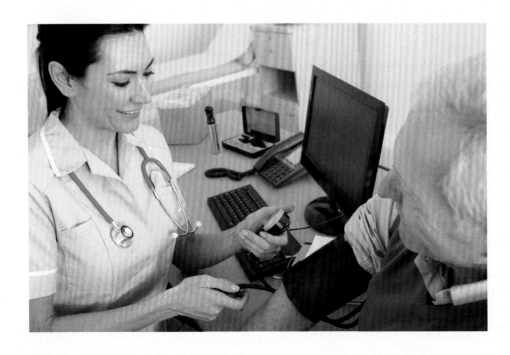

Left-handed students are encouraged to adopt right-sided positioning, even though at first it may seem awkward. It still may be easier to use the left hand for percussing or for holding instruments such as the otoscope or reflex hammer.

As you study the body systems in the upcoming chapters and review the techniques associated with each examination, you will begin to understand the components of the physical examination. Once you have learned how to examine each body system, you will methodically formulate the composition and flow of the head-to-toe physical examination. Chapter 22, Putting It All Together, has a detailed list of how to incorporate the systems with limited position changes while maintaining continuity of the examination. The culmination of the course is the ability to incorporate the skills learned and perform a head to toe physical examination, keeping in mind patient safety and comfort and thoroughness of the examination. At first, you may need notes to remind you what to look for, but over time this sequence will become habit.

BIBLIOGRAPHY

CITATIONS

1. U.S. Preventive Services Task Force. Guide to clinical preventive services 2014: recommendations of the U.S. Preventive Services Task Force. June 2014. Available at http://www.ahrq.gov/professionals/clinicians-providers/guidelines-recommendations/guide/. See also U.S. Preventive Services Task Force: Recommendations for Primary Care Practice. December 2013. Available at http://www.uspreventiveservicestaskforce.org/Page/Name/recommendations. Accessed November 11, 2015.

2. Centers for Disease Control and Prevention (CDC). Standard precautions. Guidelines for isolation precautions: preventing transmission of infectious agents in healthcare settings 2007. Updated December 2010. Available at http://www.cdc.gov/hicpac/2007IP/2007isolationPrecautions.html. Accessed November 11, 2015.

3. Centers for Disease Control and Prevention (CDC). Standard precautions. Excerpt from the guidelines for isolation precautions: preventing transmission of infectious agents in healthcare settings 2007. Updated September 2015. Available at http://www.cdc.gov/ncidod/dhqp/gl_isolation_standard.html. Accessed November 11, 2015.

4. Centers for Disease Control and Prevention. Hand hygiene in healthcare settings. Updated October 2015. Available at http://www.cdc.gov/handhygiene/. Accessed November 12, 2015.

5. Centers for Disease Control and Prevention. Bloodborne infectious diseases: HIV/AIDS, Hepatitis B, Hepatitis C. Universal precautions for the prevention for transmission of bloodborne infections, p. 66. Updated December 2011. Available at http://www.cdc.gov/niosh/topics/bbp/universal.html. Accessed November 12, 2015.

6. Centers for Disease Control and Prevention. Information about MRSA for healthcare and patients September 2013. Available at http://www.cdc.gov/mrsa/healthcare/patient/. Accessed November 11, 2015.

7. Centers for Disease Control and Prevention. Information about MRSA for healthcare personnel, September 2015. Available at http://www.cdc.gov/ncidod/dhqp/ar_mrsa_healthcareFS.html#. Accessed November 11, 2015.

8. Bearman G, Bryant K, Leekha S, et al. Healthcare personnel attire in non-operating-room settings. *Infect Control Hosp Epidemiol*. 2014;35:107–121.

9. Treakle AM, Thom KA, Furuno JP, et al. Bacterial contamination of health care workers' white coats. *Am J Infect Control*. 2009;37:101–105.

10. Centers for Disease Control and Prevention. Guide to infection prevention in outpatient settings. Minimum expectations for safe care. Updated September 2014. Available at http://www.cdc.gov/HAI/settings/outpatient/outpatient-care-guidelines.html. Accessed November 11, 2015.

11. Cronenwett L, Sherwood G, Barnsteiner J, et al. Quality and safety education. *Nsg Outlook*. 2007;55(3):122–131.

ADDITIONAL READINGS

Alexander EK. Perspective: moving students beyond an organ-based approach when teaching medical interviewing and physical examination skills. *Acad Med*. 2008;83(10):906–909.

Bremner M, Aduddell K, Bennett D, et al. The use of human patient simulators: best practices with novice nursing students. *Nurse Educ*. 2006;31(4):170–174.

Davies RH, Rees B. In praise of the physical examination: include "eyeballing" the patient. *BMJ*. 2010;340:c291.

Herrle S, Corbett E, Fagan M, et al. Bayes' theorem and physical examination: probability assessment and diagnostic decision-making. *Acad Med*. 2011;86(5):618–627.

Horner G. Genitourinary assessment: an integral part of a completer physical examination. *J Pediatr Health Care.* 2007;21(3): 162–170.

Khattab A, Rawlings B. Assessing nurse practitioner students using a modified objective structured clinical examination (OSCE). *Nurse Ed Today.* 2001;21(7):541–550.

Moosapur H, Raza M, Rambod M, et al. Conceptualization of category-oriented likelihood ration: a useful tool for clinical diagnostic reasoning. *BMC Med Educ.* 2011; 11:94.

Noon A. The cognitive processes underpinning clinical decision in triage assessment: a theoretical conundrum? *Intl Emerg Nurs.* 2014;22(1):40–46.

Numminen O, Meretoja R, IhoahoH, et al. Professional competence of practicing nurses. *J Clin Nurs.* 2013;22(10): 1411–1423.

Rushwort E. Objective structured clinical examination (OSCE): Review of literature and implications for nursing education. *Nurse Ed Today.* 2007;27(5):481–490.

Shinozaki E, Yamauchi T. Nursing competencies for physical assessment of the respiratory system in Japan. *Nurs Health Sci.* 2009;11(3):285–292.

Unsworth J, Tucker G, Hindmarsh Y. Man versus machine: the importance of manual blood pressure measurement skills amongst registered nurses. *J of Hosp Adm.* 2015;4(6): 61–67.

Vergehese A, Horwitz RI. In praise of the physical examination. *BMJ.* 339:1385–1386.

Beginning the Physical Examination: General Survey, Vital Signs, and Pain

LEARNING OBJECTIVES

The student will:

1. Identify the components of the general survey.
2. Identify appropriate subjective questions based on initial observations.
3. Demonstrate how to measure blood pressure, pulse, respiration, and temperature.
4. Discuss variations in vital signs and the possible causes.
5. Describe the different types of pain.
6. Perform and document a pain assessment using information from the health history and the physical examination.

The General Survey chapter provides an overview of the nurse's initial patient assessment prior to exploring each system in detail. The objective observation of the patient begins with the first moments of the encounter and continues throughout the history and physical examination. The nonverbal cues collected during the general survey enable the nurse to select appropriate subjective questions for the individual patient to garner more information. Many factors are assessed, such as the patient's general appearance, apparent state of health, demeanor, facial expression or affect, grooming, posture, and gait. Height and weight would also be assessed with the general survey and will be covered in detail in Chapter 8, Nutrition and Hydration.

As the assessment skills of the nurse become more attuned to individual patients, the distinguishing features of each patient are depicted so well in words that a colleague could envision the person.

Many factors contribute to the patient's makeup—genetic composition, early illnesses, socioeconomic status, culture, gender identity and expression, nutrition, degree of fitness, mood state, geographic location, and age cohort. Recall that the patient's status affects many of the characteristics you assess, including blood pressure, posture, mood and alertness, facial coloration, dentition, condition of the tongue and gingiva, color of the nail beds, and muscle bulk, to name a few.

Recapture the observations you have been making since the first moments of the interaction and refine them throughout your assessment. Does the patient hear you when greeted in the waiting room or examination room?... rise with ease?... walk easily or stiffly? If hospitalized when you first meet, what is the patient doing—sitting up and enjoying television?... lying in bed? What occupies the bedside table—a magazine?... a stack of "get well" cards?... a Bible or a Koran?... an emesis basin?... nothing at all? Each of these observations should raise one or more tentative hypotheses about the patient to consider during future assessments.

General Survey—Initial Observations

Physical Appearance and Apparent State of Health and Mood
- Overall appearance and apparent age
- Level of consciousness
- Facial features and expressions
- Demeanor and affect
- Posture
- Gait
- Motor activity
- Speech
- Skin color and lesions
- Dress and personal hygiene

The "vital signs" include blood pressure, heart rate, respiratory rate, and temperature.

Although pain is a subjective finding, in order to ensure frequent pain assessment, especially in a hospital or rehabilitation setting, pain has been labeled the "fifth vital sign." Pain assessment is commonly missed, and when pain is noted, it is often not effectively managed. Pain is a frequent motivator for people to seek health care.

Depending on the clinical setting, some might also consider oxygen saturation using a pulse oximeter, blood glucose level, or the Glasgow Coma Scale as the fifth vital sign.

GENERAL APPEARANCE

Apparent State of Health

Try to make a general judgment based on observations throughout the encounter. Support it with the significant details. Does the patient look his or her age?... appear ill?... unhappy?... fatigued?

Acutely or chronically ill, frail, or fit and robust.

Level of Consciousness

Is the patient awake, alert, and responsive to you and others in the environment? If not, promptly assess the level of consciousness. Orientation can be checked by asking about person, place, time, and situation (Chapter 19, Mental Status).

Facial Expression

Observe the facial expression at rest, during conversation, during the physical examination, and in interaction with others. Watch closely for eye contact. Is it natural?... sustained and unblinking?... quickly averted?... absent?

Are the movements of the face symmetric?... is there *ptosis*?... an uneven smile?

Check for the stare of hyperthyroidism; the immobile face of parkinsonism; the flat or sad effect of depression. Decreased eye contact may be cultural, or may suggest anxiety, fear, or sadness. Asymmetry of the face could be a stroke, palsy, or injury to the cranial nerve.

Posture, Gait, Motor Activity, and Speech

What is the patient's preferred posture? Assess the patient before calling his or her name in the waiting room. How is the patient sitting? Does the position or nonverbal communication change when you are in the room with the patient?

Patients often prefer sitting upright in left-sided heart failure and leaning forward with arms braced in chronic obstructive pulmonary disease (COPD).

Is the patient restless or quiet? How often does the patient change position? How fast/slow are the movements?

Anxious patients appear agitated and restless. Patients in pain often avoid movement.

Is there any apparent involuntary motor activity? Are some body parts immobile? Which ones?

Look for tremors, other involuntary movements, or paralysis. See Chapter 20, The Nervous System, Table 20-11, Tremors and Involuntary Movements, pp. 740–741.

Does the patient walk smoothly, with comfort, self-confidence, and balance, or is there a limp or discomfort, fear of falling, loss of balance, or any movement disorder? Does the patient use an assistive device to ambulate?... cane?... walker?... brace?

See Chapter 20, The Nervous System, Table 20-4, Abnormalities of Gait and Posture, p. 732. An impaired gait increases risk of falls.

Is the patient's speech articulate?... garbled?... rapid or slow?

Fatigue is a nonspecific symptom with many causes. It refers to a sense of weariness or loss of energy that patients describe in various ways. "I don't feel like getting up in the morning" ... "I don't have any energy"... "I just feel blah"... "I'm all done in"... "I can hardly get through the day"... "By the time I get to the office I feel as if I've done a day's work." Because fatigue is a normal response to hard work, sustained stress, or grief, try to elicit the life circumstances in which it occurs. Fatigue unrelated to such situations requires further investigation.

Fatigue is a common symptom of depression and anxiety states, but also consider infections (such as hepatitis, infectious mononucleosis, and tuberculosis); endocrine disorders (hypothyroidism, adrenal insufficiency, diabetes mellitus); heart failure; chronic disease of the lungs, kidneys, or liver; electrolyte imbalance; moderate to severe anemia; postural orthostatic tachycardia syndrome (POTS); malignancies; nutritional deficits; and medications.

Use open-ended questions to explore the attributes of the patient's fatigue, and encourage the patient to fully describe what he or she is experiencing. Important clues about etiology often emerge from a good psychosocial history, exploration of sleep patterns, and a thorough review of systems.

Weakness is different from fatigue. It denotes a demonstrable loss of muscle power and will be discussed later with other neurologic symptoms (see Chapter 20, The Nervous System, pp. 680–681).

Weakness, especially if localized in a neuroanatomic pattern, suggests possible neuropathy or myopathy.

Odors of the Body and Breath

Odors can be important diagnostic clues, such as the fruity odor of diabetes or the scent of alcohol. (For the scent of alcohol, the CAGE questions, Chapter 4, The Health History, pp. 74–75, will help you determine possible misuse.)

Breath odors of alcohol, acetone (diabetes), pulmonary infections, uremia, or liver failure

Never assume that alcohol on a patient's breath explains changes in mental status or neurologic findings.

These changes may have serious but treatable causes such as hypoglycemia, subdural hematoma, or postictal state.

Skin Color and Obvious Lesions

Inspect for any changes in skin color, scars, plaques, or nevi (see Chapter 9, The Integumentary System).

Pallor, cyanosis, jaundice, rashes, bruises, or any changes should be assessed in greater detail.

Dress, Grooming, and Personal Hygiene

How is the patient dressed? Is the clothing appropriate for the temperature and weather? Is it clean, properly buttoned, and zipped? Does it fit? How does it compare with clothing worn by people of comparable age and social group?

Excess clothing may reflect the cold intolerance of hypothyroidism; hide a skin rash or scars from self-mutilation or needle marks; mask anorexia; or signal personal lifestyle preferences.

Has the patient added additional holes on the belt to enlarge? To make smaller?

May indicate weight gain or weight loss

Take note of the patient's shoes. Are there holes or cut-outs? Or is the patient wearing slippers? Are the laces tied?

Holes or slippers may indicate gout, bunions, or other painful foot conditions. Shoes that are worn out can contribute to foot and back pain, calluses, falls, and infection. Untied laces or slippers also suggest edema.

Is the patient wearing any unusual jewelry? Are there any body piercing? Tattoos? When and where were they obtained?

Copper bracelets suggest joint pain. Piercings or tattoos may appear on any part of the body.

Note the patient's hair, fingernails, and use of make-up. They may be clues to the patient's personality, culture, self-regard, or lifestyle.

"Grown-out" hair and nail polish suggest the length of a possible illness or change in circumstances. Bitten fingernails may reflect stress. Yellowing of the index and middle finger may indicate a smoker.

Do personal hygiene and grooming seem appropriate to the patient's age, lifestyle, occupation, and socioeconomic group? These are norms that vary widely based on each individual.

Neglected appearance may appear in depression and dementia, but should be compared with the patient's norm.

Signs of Distress

- Cardiac or respiratory distress

Is there clutching the chest, pallor, diaphoresis, labored breathing, wheezing, coughing, shortness of breath, or sitting in a tripod position?

- Pain

Is there grimacing, crying, diaphoresis, holding, favoring, or protecting a body part or area of the body?

Does the patient show evidence of the problems below?

- Anxiety or depression

Are there anxious facial expressions, fidgety movements, cold moist palms, inexpressive or flat affect, poor eye contact, or psychomotor slowing? See Chapter 19, Mental Status.

THE VITAL SIGNS

Vital signs are an integral part of the assessment. These include the blood pressure, heart rate, respiratory rate, and temperature. These important measurements may be completed at the start of the physical examination. If any vital sign is not within the normal parameters, then rechecking during the cardiovascular or respiratory system examinations would be prudent.

During the assessment, check the blood pressure and the pulse. To check the pulse, the heart rate can be assessed by counting the radial pulse with your fingers, or the apical pulse with your stethoscope at the cardiac apex. Keeping contact with the patient as if still checking the pulse, count the respiratory rate without alerting the patient, as breathing patterns may unconsciously change if the patient knows breaths are being counted. The temperature may be taken in various anatomic sites, which depends on the individual patient and the equipment available. Further details on techniques for ensuring accuracy of the vital signs are provided later in the chapter.

See Chapter 14, The Cardiovascular System, Table 14-3, Variations and Abnormalities of the Apical Impulse, p. 426, and See Chapter 13, The Respiratory System, Table 13-4, Abnormalities in Rate and Rhythm of Breathing, p. 365.

BLOOD PRESSURE

Monitoring Blood Pressure

More than 80 million Americans have an elevated blood pressure. In close to half of the people with high blood pressure (46%), the condition is not well controlled.[1] Detection and management are integral in patient care. High blood pressure impacts both genders and all races of people, and the statistics are predicted to climb in upcoming years. The American Heart Association indicates the trends for hypertension in the United States continues to increase as depicted on the chart below:

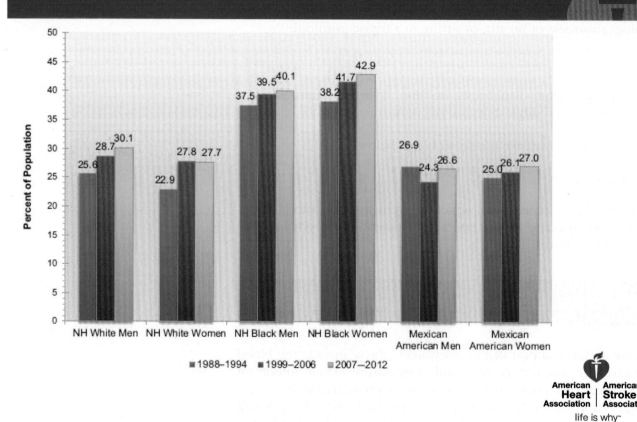

Age-Adjusted Prevalence Trends for High Blood Pressure in Adults, ≥20 years of age
(NHANES 1988–1994, 1999–2006, and 2007–2012)

Mozaffarian D, Benjamin EJ, Go AS, Arnett DK, et al; on behalf of the American Heart Association Statistics Committee and Stroke Statistics Subcommittee. Heart disease and stroke statistics—2015 update: a report from the American Heart Association. Available at https://www.heart.org/idc/groups/ahamah-public/@wcm/@sop/@smd/documents/downloadable/ucm_470707.pdf. Accessed November 20, 2015.

Screening at office visits or health fairs often detects an elevated blood pressure. Follow-up and confirmation of an elevated reading has moved into the home environment. Studies have shown that home and ambulatory blood pressure monitoring confirms more cardiovascular disease and end-organ damage than office measurements (see Chapter 14, The Cardiovascular System).[2]

Attention to accuracy of both the equipment and the technique and detail in the reading of blood pressure is crucial. Errors in blood pressure measurement can increase the risk of unnecessary treatment or misdiagnosis. Blood pressure devices may be aneroid, hybrid, or electronic, and there are international protocols for evaluating their accuracy.[3] Some offices may continue to use mercury, although these are no longer available for sale.

Self-monitoring of blood pressure by well-instructed patients using approved devices improves blood pressure control, especially when it is done two times daily at the upper arm with automatic readouts.[4,5]

Choice of Blood Pressure Cuff (Sphygmomanometer)

Take the time to choose a cuff of appropriate size for your patient's arm. Follow the guidelines listed, and advise your patients about how to choose the best cuff for home use and the need to have it re-calibrated routinely. Educate patients on the best options and make them aware that although the wrist and finger monitors are popular, they are less accurate. Patients at home need to be able to demonstrate correct technique to insure accurate readings.

Selecting the Correct Size Blood Pressure Cuff

- Width of the inflatable bladder of the cuff should be about 40% of the upper arm circumference (about 12 to 14 cm in the average adult).
- Length of the inflatable bladder should be about 80% of upper arm circumference (almost long enough to encircle the arm).
- The standard cuff is 12 × 23 cm, appropriate for arm circumferences up to 28 cm.

If the cuff is too *small* (narrow), the blood pressure will read *high*.

If the cuff is too *large* (wide), the blood pressure will read *low* on a small arm and *high* on a large arm.[6]

Technique for Measuring Blood Pressure

Before assessing the blood pressure, take several steps to make sure your measurement will be accurate. Proper technique is important and reduces the inherent variability arising from the patient or examiner, the equipment, and the procedure itself.[7,8]

Steps to Ensure Accurate Blood Pressure Measurement

- The patient should avoid smoking, exercise, or caffeine for 30 minutes before the blood pressure is measured.
- The examination room should be quiet and a comfortable temperature.
- The patient should sit quietly for at least 5 minutes in a chair, with both feet flat on the floor and legs uncrossed.
- The arm selected should be accessible and without clothing, fistulas for dialysis, scars from brachial artery that was accessed for a deep vein intravenous, or lymphedema from axillary node dissection or radiation therapy.
- Palpate the brachial artery to confirm that it has a viable pulse.
- Position the arm so that the brachial artery, at the antecubital crease, is *at heart level*—roughly level with the fourth interspace at its junction with the sternum.
- If the patient is seated, rest the arm on a table a little above the patient's waist.

If the brachial artery is *below* heart level, the blood pressure will be higher.

If the brachial artery is *higher,* the blood pressure will be lower.[8,9]

Measuring the Blood Pressure

Blood pressure is the measurement of the pressure on the walls of the blood vessels. Systole is the pressure in the arteries when the left ventricle contracts and diastole is the pressure in arteries when the heart muscle rests and refills with blood.

- **Position the cuff and the arm.**

  - The arm is at heart level.

  - Center the inflatable bladder over the brachial artery.

  - The lower border of the cuff should be about 2.5 cm above the antecubital crease.

  - Secure the cuff snugly.

  - Slightly flex the patient's arm at the elbow.

A loose cuff or a bladder that balloons outside the cuff leads to false high readings.

- **Estimate the systolic pressure and add 30 mm Hg**.

  - To determine how high to raise the cuff pressure, first estimate the systolic pressure by palpation.

  - As you feel the brachial artery with the fingers of one hand, inflate the cuff until the brachial pulse disappears.

  - Read this pressure on the manometer and *add 30 mm Hg*.

  - Deflate the cuff promptly and completely and wait 15 to 30 seconds.

  - Use of this sum as the target for subsequent inflations prevents discomfort from unnecessarily high cuff pressures. It also avoids the occasional error caused by an *auscultatory gap*—a silent interval that may be present between the systolic and the diastolic pressures.

- **Position the stethoscope over the brachial artery.**

  - Now place the bell (or diaphragm) of a stethoscope lightly over the brachial artery, taking care to make an air seal with its full rim.

  - The *Korotkoff sounds* are heard using either the bell or the diaphragm. Both sides of the stethoscope have similar results and each is reliable.[10] Each practitioner may choose a bell or diaphragm as long as they can hear the sounds clearly.

  - Do not allow the stethoscope to touch the cuff or clothing.

An unrecognized auscultatory gap may lead to serious underestimation of systolic pressure (150 instead of 200 in the example below) or overestimation of diastolic pressure.

If you find an auscultatory gap, record your findings completely (e.g., 200/98 with an auscultatory gap from 170 to 150).

An auscultatory gap is associated with arterial stiffness and atherosclerotic disease.[11]

- **Identify the systolic blood pressure.**

  - Inflate the cuff rapidly again to the previously determined estimated systolic blood pressure.

  - Deflate the cuff slowly at a rate of about 2 to 3 mm Hg per second.

  - Note the level when you hear the sounds of at least two consecutive beats. This is the *systolic* pressure.

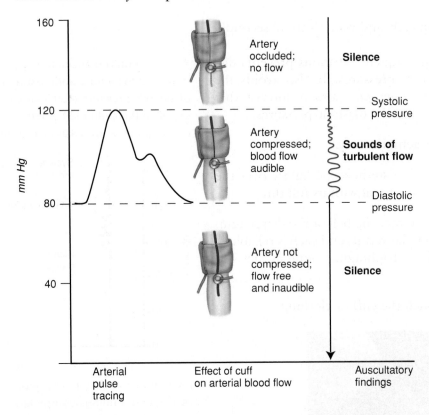

- **Identify the diastolic blood pressure.**

  - Continue to deflate the cuff slowly until the sounds become muffled and disappear.

  - To confirm the disappearance point, listen as the pressure falls another 10 to 20 mm Hg.

  - Then deflate the cuff rapidly to zero.

  - The disappearance point, which is usually only a few mm Hg below the muffling point, provides the best estimate of true *diastolic* pressure.

In some people, the muffling point and the disappearance point are farther apart. Occasionally, as in aortic regurgitation, the sounds never disappear. If the difference is 10 mm Hg or greater, record both figures (e.g., 154/80/68).

- **Average two or more readings.**

  - Read both the systolic and the diastolic levels to the nearest 2 mm Hg.[12]

  - Wait at least 2 minutes and repeat.

  - Average your readings.

  - If the first two readings differ by more than 5 mm Hg, take additional readings.

- When using an aneroid instrument, hold the dial so that it faces you directly. Avoid slow or repetitive inflations of the cuff, because the resulting venous congestion can cause false readings.

  > By making the sounds less audible, venous congestion may produce artificially low systolic and high diastolic pressures.

- **Measure blood pressure in both arms at least once.**

  - Blood pressure should be taken in both arms at least once. Normally, there may be a difference in pressure of 5 mm Hg and sometimes up to 10 mm Hg. Subsequent readings should be made on the arm with the higher pressure.

  > Pressure difference of more than 10 to 15 mm Hg occurs in subclavian steal syndrome, aortic dissection and supravalvular aortic stenosis and should be investigated.

Blood pressure cuff selection is important. Attention to cuff size is crucial to alleviate incorrect readings which can result in inaccurate treatment. If the correct cuff is not available, one should be ordered to accommodate the patient's size. Inconsistencies include:

Errors That Result in False High Readings

- Cuff too small (narrow)

- Cuff too loose or uneven

- Arm below heart level

- Arm not supported

- Inflating or deflating cuff too slowly (high diastolic)

- Deflating cuff too quickly (low systolic and high diastolic)

Errors That Result in False Low Readings

- Cuff too large (wide)

- Arm above heart level

- Repeating assessments too quickly

- Inaccurate level of inflation

- Pressing stethoscope too tightly against pulse

Classification of Normal and Abnormal Blood Pressure

The Joint National Committee on Prevention, Detection, Evaluation, and Treatment of High Blood Pressure VII Report (JNC 7) recommends using the mean of two or more properly measured seated blood pressure readings, taken on two or more office visits, for diagnosis of hypertension.[8,12] Blood pressure measurement should be verified in the contralateral arm. This report identifies four levels of systolic and diastolic hypertension, affirmed by the American Society of Hypertension in 2013.[13] Note that either component may be high. In 2014, the Joint National Committee issued the JNC 8 recommendation, "2014 Evidence-Based Guideline for the Management of High Blood Pressure in Adults" based on rigorous scientific review of clinical trial data.[14] This report focuses more narrowly on thresholds and goals for pharmacologic treatment. For patients age 18 to 60, in the general population, JNC 8 recommends treatment to lower BP at a diastolic BP of 90 or greater (strong evidence) and systolic BP of 140 or greater (expert opinion). For patients 60 years of age or older, JNC 8 recommends treatment for BP 150/90 or higher. The JNC 8 Report also recommends a higher treatment threshold than JNC 7 for patients with diabetes and chronic kidney disease (CKD), at 140/90 or higher.

There has been increased attention over the report and many groups such as the American Heart Association (AHA), the American College of Cardiology (ACC), and the Centers for Disease Control and Prevention support the JNC 7 parameters. Many are not convinced the new guidelines set by JNC 8 are appropriate and are concerned about the potential disservice to disparate groups such as the elderly, blacks, and women.

JNC 8 Blood Pressure Classification—Adults Older Than 18 Years		
Category	**Systolic (mm Hg)**	**Diastolic (mm Hg)**
Normal	<120	<80
Prehypertension	120–139	80–89
Hypertension stage 1—age ≥18 to <60; diabetes or renal disease—age ≥60	140–159; 150–159	90–99; 90–99
Hypertension stage 2	≥160	≥100

Note that the blood pressure goal for patients with hypertension, diabetes, or renal disease in the JNC 7 report was less than 130/80.

Assessment of hypertension also includes its effects on target "end organs"—the eyes, heart, brain, and kidneys. Look for hypertensive retinopathy, left ventricular hypertrophy, and neurologic deficits suggesting stroke. Renal assessment requires urinalysis and blood tests of renal function.

When the systolic and diastolic levels fall in different categories, use the higher category. For example, 170/92 mm Hg is stage 2 hypertension; 135/96 mm Hg is stage 1 hypertension. In *isolated systolic hypertension,* systolic blood pressure is 140 mm Hg or greater, and diastolic blood pressure is less than 90 mm Hg.

Treatment of isolated systolic hypertension in patients 60 years of age or older reduces mortality and complications from cardiovascular disease.[15]

Low Blood Pressure

Interpret relatively low levels of blood pressure in the light of past readings and the patient's present clinical state.

A pressure of 110/70 mm Hg would usually be normal, but could also indicate significant hypotension if past pressures have been high.

If indicated, assess *orthostatic hypotension,* common in older adults. Measure blood pressure and heart rate in two positions—*supine* after the patient is resting from 3 to 10 minutes, then within 3 minutes once the patient *stands up.* Normally, as the patient rises from the horizontal to the standing position, systolic pressure drops slightly or remains unchanged, while diastolic pressure rises slightly. Orthostatic hypotension is a drop in systolic blood pressure of at least 20 mm Hg or in diastolic blood pressure of at least 10 mm Hg within 3 minutes of standing.[16,17]

Causes of orthostatic hypotension include medications, moderate or severe blood loss, prolonged bed rest, and diseases of the autonomic nervous system.

See Chapter 24, Assessing Older Adults.

SPECIAL CIRCUMSTANCES

Weak or Inaudible Korotkoff Sounds

Consider technical problems such as erroneous placement of your stethoscope, failure to make full skin contact with the bell, or diaphragm and venous engorgement of the patient's arm from repeated inflations of the cuff. Also, consider the possibility of shock or vascular disease.

When you cannot hear any Korotkoff sounds, you may be able to estimate the systolic pressure by palpation. Alternative methods such as Doppler techniques or direct arterial pressure tracings may be necessary.

To intensify Korotkoff sounds, one of the following methods may be helpful:

- Raise the patient's arm before and while you inflate the cuff. Then lower the arm and determine the blood pressure.

- Inflate the cuff. Ask the patient to make a fist several times, and then determine the blood pressure.

Arrhythmias

Irregular rhythms produce variations in pressure and therefore unreliable measurements. Ignore the effects of an occasional premature contraction. With frequent premature contractions or atrial fibrillation, determine the average of several observations and note the measurements are approximate. Ambulatory monitoring for 2 to 24 hours is recommended.[18]

Detection of an irregularly irregular rhythm suggests *atrial fibrillation.* For all irregular patterns, obtain an ECG to identify the type of rhythm.

White Coat Hypertension

"White coat hypertension" describes hypertension in people whose blood pressure measurements are higher in the office than at home or in more relaxed settings. This phenomenon occurs in 10% to 25% of patients, especially women and anxious individuals, and may last for several visits. Try to relax the patient, including remote telehealth, and re-measure the blood pressure later in the encounter. Home monitoring has been used effectively to alleviate treatment in these individuals.

Home or ambulatory hypertension, unlike "white coat" or isolated office hypertension, signals increased risk of cardiovascular disease.[18–21]

The Obese or Very Thin Patient

For the *obese arm,* use a cuff 15 cm in width. If this cuff is too short despite a large circumference, use a thigh cuff or a very long cuff. If the arm circumference is greater than 50 cm and not amenable to use of a thigh cuff, wrap an appropriately sized cuff around the forearm, hold the forearm at heart level and feel for the radial pulse.[18] Other options include using a Doppler probe at the radial artery or an oscillometric device. For the *very thin arm,* consider using a pediatric cuff.

Using a small cuff overestimates systolic blood pressure in obese patients.[13]

The Hypertensive Patient With Systolic Blood Pressure Higher in the Arms Than the Legs

Coarctation of the aorta in children or adults generally presents with systolic hypertension, greater in the arms than the legs. Assess blood pressure in the legs and "femoral delay" at least once in every hypertensive patient.

Coarctation of the aorta arises from narrowing of the thoracic aorta, usually distal to the left subclavian artery. Compare blood pressures in the arms and legs. In normal patients, the systolic blood pressure should be 5 to 10 mm higher in the lower extremities than in the arms. Coarctation of the aorta and occlusive aortic disease are distinguished by hypertension in the upper extremities and low blood pressure in the legs and by diminished or delayed femoral pulses.[22]

- Compare blood pressures in the arms and legs.

- Compare the volume and timing of the radial and femoral pulses. Normally, volume is equal and the pulses occur simultaneously.

HEART RATE AND RHYTHM

Examine the arterial pulses, the heart rate and rhythm, and the amplitude and contour of the pulse wave.

Heart Rate

The radial pulse is commonly used to assess the heart rate. With the pads of your index and middle fingers, compress the radial artery until a maximal pulsation is detected. If the rhythm is regular and the rate seems normal, count the rate for 30 seconds and multiply by 2. If the rate is unusually fast or slow, however, count it for 60 seconds. The range of normal is 60 to 100 beats per minute.[23]

An elevated resting heart rate is associated with increased risk of cardiovascular disease and mortality.[24]

Rhythm

Begin by palpating the radial pulse. If there are any irregularities, assess the rhythm at the cardiac apex by listening with your stethoscope. Premature beats of low amplitude may not be transmitted to the peripheral pulses and the heart rate can be seriously underestimated. Is the rhythm regular or irregular? If irregular, try to identify a pattern: (1) Do early beats appear in a basically regular rhythm? (2) Does the irregularity vary consistently with respiration? (3) Is the rhythm totally irregular?

See Chapter 14, The Cardiovasuclar System, Table 14-1, Selected Heart Rate and Rhythms, p. 424.

Table 14-2, Selected Irregular Rhythms, p. 425.

If the radial pulse is irregular or the patient's condition calls for a more precise pulse rate, then an apical pulse should be assessed for 1 minute. The examiner places the stethoscope at the apex (fifth intercostal space at the midclavicular line) and auscultates the S_1 and S_2, noting the rate and rhythm. An electrocardiogram (ECG) should be checked to determine the rhythm.

Chapter 15, The Peripheral Vascular System, Table 15-5, Abnormalities of Arterial Pulse and Pressure Waves, p. 471.

RESPIRATORY RATE AND RHYTHM

Observe the *rate, rhythm, depth,* and *effort of breathing.* Count the number of respirations (one respiration includes an inspiration and an expiration) in 1 minute either by visual inspection or by subtly listening over the patient's trachea with your stethoscope during your examination of the head and neck or chest. Normally, adults take 12 to 20 breaths per minute in a quiet, regular pattern. An occasional sigh is normal. Check to see if expiration is prolonged.

See Table 13-4, Abnormalities in Rate and Rhythm of Breathing, p. 365.

Prolonged expiration is common in COPD.

TEMPERATURE

Research notes the most accurate core body temperature is the blood temperature in the pulmonary artery. However, everyday clinical practice relies on noninvasive routes such as the oral, rectal, axillary, tympanic membrane, and temporal artery measurements. Tympanic membrane and temporal artery temperatures use infrared thermometry.[25]

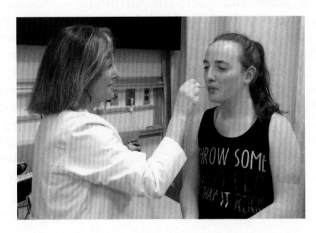

The average *oral temperature,* usually quoted at 37°C (98.6°F), fluctuates considerably. In the early morning hours, it may fall as low as 35.8°C (96.4°F), and in the late afternoon or evening; it may rise as high as 37.3°C (99.1°F).

Rectal temperatures are *higher* than oral temperatures by an average of 0.4 to 0.5°C (0.7 to 0.9°F), but this difference is also quite variable.

In contrast, *axillary temperatures* are *lower* than oral temperatures by approximately 1°F, but take 5 to 10 minutes to register and are generally considered less accurate than other measurements.

Tympanic membrane temperatures can be more variable than oral or rectal temperatures. Studies vary in methodology, but suggest that in adults, *oral and temporal artery temperatures* correlate more closely with the pulmonary artery temperature, but are about 0.5°C lower.[26,27]

Fever or pyrexia refers to an elevated body temperature. *Hyperpyrexia* refers to extreme elevation in temperature, above 41.1°C (106°F), while *hypothermia* refers to an abnormally low temperature, below 35°C (95°F) rectally.

Taking oral temperatures is not recommended when patients are unconscious, restless, or unable to close their mouths. Temperature readings may be inaccurate and thermometers may be broken by unexpected movements of the patient's jaws. Options are available—rectal, tympanic, temporal artery, or axilla—and should be chosen based on individual situations and availability.

Rapid respiratory rates tend to increase the discrepancy between oral and rectal temperatures. In these situations, rectal, tympanic, temporal, or axilla temperatures are more reliable.

Causes of fever include infection, trauma, such as surgery or crush injuries, malignancy, blood disorders such as acute hemolytic anemia, drug reactions, and immune disorders such as collagen vascular disease.

Oral Temperatures

Place the disposable cover over the probe and insert the thermometer under the tongue. Ask the patient to close both lips, and then watch closely for the digital readout. An accurate temperature recording usually takes about 10 seconds. Note that hot or cold liquids, and even smoking, can alter the temperature reading. In these situations, it is best to delay measuring the temperature for 10 to 15 minutes. Due to breakage and/or mercury exposure, glass thermometers are giving way to electronic thermometers; however, if they may still be used in homes. Glass thermometers take approximately 3 minutes to register.

The chief cause of hypothermia is exposure to cold. Other predisposing causes include reduced movement as in paralysis, interference with vasoconstriction as from sepsis or excess alcohol, starvation, hypothyroidism, or hypoglycemia. Elderly people are especially susceptible to hypothermia and also less likely to develop fever.

Rectal Temperatures

Select a rectal thermometer probe (usually red). Place the disposable cover over the probe and lubricate it. Ask the patient to lie on one side with the hip flexed and insert the thermometer about 3 to 4 cm (1.5 in) into the anal canal, in a direction pointing to the umbilicus. Wait about 10 seconds for the digital temperature recording to appear.

Tympanic Membrane Temperatures

The tympanic membrane shares the same blood supply as the hypothalamus, where temperature regulation occurs in the brain. Accurate temperature readings require access to the tympanic membrane. This is an increasingly common practice and is quick, safe, and reliable if performed properly. Make sure the external auditory canal is free of cerumen, which lowers temperature readings. Place the cover on and position the probe in the canal so that the infrared beam is aimed at the tympanic membrane. Wait 2 to 3 seconds until the digital temperature reading appears.

Temporal Artery Temperatures

A temporal artery thermometer measures the blood flow through the superficial temporal artery, which branches off the external carotid artery and lies within a millimeter of the skin surface of the forehead and behind the ear lobes. Place the probe against the center of the forehead and depress the infrared scanning button. Continue holding the button and slowly slide the probe midline across the forehead to the hairline (not down the side of the face). Move the probe from the forehead and touch behind the earlobe. Release the button and the temperature will be visible on the display.[28]

Axillary Temperatures

Place a probe cover over the electronic thermometer probe and place the thermometer in the middle of the axilla. This technique can be used with unconscious patients. It is not recommended in patients with rapid temperature changes as it lags behind rapid core changes.

Fever, Chills, and Night Sweats

Fever refers to an abnormal elevation in body temperature (see pp. 135–136 for definitions of normal). Ask about fever if patients have an acute or chronic illness. Find out whether the patient has used a thermometer to measure the temperature. Bear in mind that errors in technique can lead to unreliable information. Has the patient felt feverish or unusually hot, noted excessive sweating, or felt chilly and cold? Try to distinguish between subjective *chilliness* and a *shaking chill* with shivering throughout the body and chattering of teeth.

Feeling cold, goosebumps, and shivering accompany a rising temperature, while feeling hot and sweating accompany a falling temperature. Normally the body temperature rises during the day and falls during the night. When fever exaggerates this swing, *night sweats* may occur. Malaise, headache, and pain in the muscles and joints often accompany fever.

Fever has many causes. Focus your questions on the timing of the illness and its associated symptoms. Become familiar with patterns of infectious diseases that may affect your patient. Inquire about travel, contact with sick people, or other unusual exposures. Be sure to inquire about medications

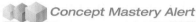
Concept Mastery Alert

The tympanic membrane temperature is the most reliable core body temperature measurement that can be done without invasive monitoring devices. The tympanic membrane is supplied by a tributary of the internal carotid artery that supplies the hypothalamus, the body's thermoregulatory center or the area where temperature regulation occurs in the brain.

Recurrent shaking chills suggest more extreme swings in temperature and systemic *bacteremia*.

Feelings of heat and sweating also accompany menopause. Night sweats occur in tuberculosis and malignancy.

because they may cause fever. In contrast, recent ingestion of aspirin, acetaminophen, corticosteroids, and nonsteroidal anti-inflammatory drugs may mask fever and affect the temperature recorded at the time of the physical examination.

ACUTE AND CHRONIC PAIN

Pain is one of the most common symptoms prompting health care. Each year, approximately 100 million Americans report persistent, chronic pain which is often under-assessed and under-treated.[29] A comprehensive approach to guide physical examination and management should be adopted in practice, as pain is a leading cause of disability and contributes significantly to health care costs.

Referred pain and visceral pain are discussed in further detail in Chapter 16, The Gastrointestinal and Renal Systems, pp. 477–478.

Assessing Acute and Chronic Pain

The International Association for the Study of Pain defines *pain* as "an unpleasant sensory and emotional experience associated with actual or potential tissue damage." The experience of pain is complex and multifactorial. Pain involves sensory, emotional, and cognitive processing but may lack a specific physical etiology.[30]

Chronic pain may be a spectrum disorder related to mental health and somatic conditions. See Chapter 19, Mental Status, pp. 648–649.

Acute pain usually is associated with a physical cause and is triggered in the nervous system to alert the body to injury, disease, or inflammation. Acute pain arises quickly and is short lived. This temporary, normal protective feature aids in preventing additional injury and resolves after treatment and healing takes place.[31]

Chronic pain is defined in several ways: pain not associated with cancer or other medical conditions that persists for more than 3 to 6 months; pain lasting more than 1 month beyond the course of an acute illness or injury; or pain recurring at intervals of months or years.[31,32] More than 40% of patients with chronic pain report that their pain is poorly controlled.[32] Pain affects more Americans than cancer, heart disease, and diabetes combined.

Adopt a multidisciplinary measurement–based approach to assessing the patient's pain, carefully listening to the patient's description of the many features of pain and contributing factors. Pain is subjective and only the patient can really tell you how severe the pain is. Use one of the multiple accepted screening tools available.[33]

Onset

When did the pain begin? How? Does it occur at a specific time of day?

Location

Ask the patient to point to the pain, because lay terms may not be specific enough to localize the site of origin. Also ask about radiation of pain.

Duration

Is it constant? Does it come and go?

Characteristic Symptoms

Assessing the severity of the pain is especially important. Use a consistent method to determine severity, based on your practice site guidelines.[34]

Three types of scales are commonly used in practice to *Assess Pain Severity:*

- *Visual Analog Scale:* a 110-mm long vertical or horizontal line, explain to the person that each line stands for a degree of pain starting at one end on the left or on top with no pain and ends with severe pain (far right or bottom). Ask the patient to point to the level of pain on the scale.[35]

- *Numeric Rating Scale:* using a scale with 0 being no pain and 10, the worst pain imaginable, a person notes their pain on the point scale.[36]

- *Verbal Pain Rating Scale:* using a scale to describe pain which includes verbalization such as: No pain–Mild–Moderate–Severe–Worst pain imaginable.

- *Combinations of pain scales include:* the Faces Pain Scale (http://wongbakerfaces.org) used for children as well as patients with language barriers or cognitive impairment[37] and the Defense & Veterans Pain Rating Scale (DVPRS) tool (below). Each of these tools has a face for a person who is happy and does not hurt at all and correlates with a 0 and progresses up the pain scale to a 10 which is unimaginable pain and hurts badly. Ask the patient to choose the face that correlates best to the pain.[38]

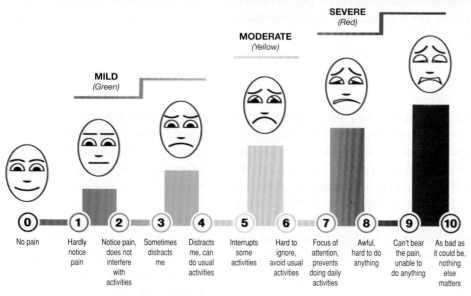

From Defense & Veterans Center for Integrative Pain Management; http://www.dvcipm.org.

Multidimensional tools like the Brief Pain Inventory and the McGill Pain Questionnaire are also available; these take longer to administer but address the effects of pain on the patient's activity level.[39]

Also ask the patient the following questions:

Describe the pain. Is it sharp? Dull? Burning?
Does it follow a particular pattern?
Is it related to an injury or a particular movement? Stressful event?

Associated Manifestations

Does anything occur when you experience the pain? Nausea? Vomiting? Headaches? Burning? Itching?

Relieving Factors

What makes the pain better? Worse?

See Chapter 3, Interviewing and Communication, p. 45.

Treatments

Be sure to ask about any treatments that the patient has tried, including medications, physical therapy, and alternative medicines. A comprehensive medication history helps to identify drugs that interact with analgesics and reduce their efficacy.

Identify any comorbid conditions such as arthritis, diabetes, HIV/AIDS, substance abuse, sickle cell disease, or psychiatric disorders. These can have significant effects on the patient's experience of pain.[40]

Chronic pain is the leading cause of disability and impaired performance at work. Inquire about the effects of pain on the patient's daily activities, mood, sleep, work, and sexual activity.

Health Disparities

Be aware of the well-documented health disparities in pain treatment and delivery of care, which range from lower use of analgesics in emergency rooms for African-American and Hispanic patients to disparities in use of analgesics for cancer, postoperative, and low back pain.[41,42] Studies show that clinician stereotypes, language barriers, and unconscious clinician biases in decision making all contribute to these disparities. Critique your own communication style, be aware of nonverbal cues, seek information and best practice standards, and improve your techniques of patient education and empowerment as first steps in ensuring uniform and effective pain management.[44]

See Institute of Medicine report, Relieving Pain in America: A Blueprint for Transforming Prevention, Care, Education, and Research.[43]

Nonverbal cues may include wincing, sweating, protectiveness of painful area, facial grimacing, or unusual posture favoring one limb or body area.

Types of Pain

Be familiar with recent advances in the scientific understanding of pain processes, described in several excellent modules for nurses available online.[31] Review the summary of types of pain in the following box to aid in your understanding of caring for patients in pain.

Types of Pain[31]	
Nociceptive or somatic pain	Pain related to tissue damage is termed *nociceptive or somatic*. Nociceptive pain can be either acute and remitting or chronic and persistent. This form of pain is mediated by the afferent A-delta and C-fibers of the sensory system that respond to noxious stimuli and is modulated by both neurotransmitters and psychological processes. Modulating neurotransmitters include endorphins, histamines, acetylcholine, and monoamines like serotonin, norepinephrine, and dopamine. These afferent nociceptors can be sensitized by inflammatory mediators.
Neuropathic pain	Pain resulting from direct injury to the peripheral or central nervous system is termed *neuropathic*. Over time, neuropathic pain may become independent of the inciting injury, become burning, lancinating, or shock-like in quality and persisting beyond healing from the initial injury. Mechanisms postulated to evoke neuropathic pain include central nervous system brain or spinal cord injury from stroke or trauma; peripheral nervous system disorders causing entrapment or pressure on spinal nerves, plexuses, or peripheral nerves; and referred pain syndromes with increased or prolonged pain responses to inciting stimuli. These triggers appear to induce changes in pain signal processing through "neuronal plasticity," leading to pain that persists beyond healing from the initial injury.[45]
Psychogenic and idiopathic pain	*Psychogenic pain* relates to the many factors that influence the patient's report of pain—psychiatric conditions like anxiety or depression, personality and coping style, cultural norms, and social support systems. *Idiopathic pain* is pain without an identifiable etiology.

Pain Management

Management of pain is complex and can be challenging. Treatment of pain requires sophisticated knowledge of nonopioid, opioid, and adjuvant analgesics and modalities of behavioral and physical therapy, which are beyond the scope of this book. More recently, health care providers have become more attentive to the care and management of patients in chronic pain. Nurses may be reluctant to administer narcotics because of fear of inducing addiction. Use of validated screening tools for opioid assessment in patients with pain and an awareness of one's own perspective in regard to pain control.[32,33]

Focus on the four A's to monitor patient outcomes:
- Analgesia
- Activities of daily living
- Adverse effects
- Aberrant drug-related behaviors

RECORDING YOUR FINDINGS

The documentation of the physical examination begins with a general description of the patient's appearance, based on the General Survey. As a novice practitioner, you may initially use sentences to describe your findings. As you progress in your practice, you will use the boxes provided in the electronic health record in conjunction with phrases in the comment boxes. The style below contains phrases appropriate for most write-ups.

Choose vivid and graphic adjectives, as if you are painting a picture in words. Avoid clichés such as "well developed" or "well nourished" or "in no acute distress," because they are nondescript and could apply to any patient. You want to convey the special features of the individual patient.

Record the vital signs taken at the time of the examination. They are preferable to those taken earlier in the day by other providers.

Recording the Physical Examination—The General Survey and Vital Signs

"Mrs. Scott, a 36-year-old healthy-appearing woman, well groomed, fit, and cheerful. Height 5'6", weight 140 lb, T 37.5°C oral, P 72 and regular, R 16 even, BP 120/80 R arm sitting, 118/76 L arm sitting."

OR

"Mr. Jones, an 82-year-old man who looks pale and chronically ill. He is alert, with eye contact but unable to speak more than two or three words at a time due to shortness of breath. He has intercostal muscle retraction when breathing and sits upright in bed. He is thin, with diffuse muscle wasting. Height 6'0", weight 157 lb, T 101.2°F tympanic, P 108 and irregular, R 32 shallow/labored, BP 160/95 R arm sitting."

Suggests exacerbation of COPD.

HEALTH PROMOTION

Temperature

Education of patients or parents on how to correctly take a temperature and the normal range is important. Review the various routes and instruments necessary and have them demonstrate the skill.

Patients should be aware of the risk factors for heatstroke, such as excessive exercise in hot, humid weather conditions; poor ventilation on hot days; decreased fluid intake; and sudden exposure to hot climates.

Patients also need to be aware of the risk factors for hypothermia when there is prolonged exposure to cold temperatures. Thermometers generally used to measure fevers will not register temperatures as low as hypothermia (core 95°F and 35°C).

Pulse

Patients taking certain cardiac medications will need to take their own pulse rate prior to taking the medication and be aware of potential side effects. They need to know at what parameters to hold the medication and when to call the health care provider. Also, patients should take a pulse rate prior to and after exercise to determine the reaction to exercise.

Teach patients how to check ONE carotid pulse by lightly placing two to three fingers on the site and counting for 1 minute. Recording the rate, rhythm, and depth is important after the assessment.

Respirations

Explain to the person assessing the respirations at home that this includes a full inspiration and a full expiration for a full minute, which is measured with a watch with a second hand. Recording the rate, rhythm, and depth is important after the assessment.

Blood Pressure

Monitoring a patient's blood pressure at home may be necessary, and it is important for the nurse to verify that it is correctly done. If a manual BP is measured, it is important to assess the environment for noise levels to ensure the reading is taken in a quiet room. Check to ensure the correct cuff size is available and the person is able to apply the cuff or has a family member who is able to correctly place the cuff. Generating a list of approved electronic instruments or sphygmomanometers for home testing is helpful, and those covered by insurance should be included. Home sphygmomanometers should be checked periodically for accuracy by simultaneously taking and comparing the readings with an office or clinic sphygmomanometer.

Everyone should be aware of his or her baseline vital signs. Notification of a health care provider of deviations is very important, especially in patients who are monitoring for a specific reason. Documentation of vital signs along with associated symptoms that occur at that time, for example, shortness of breath while walking up a flight of stairs, can be recorded in a journal or tracked using a smart phone.

BIBLIOGRAPHY

CITATIONS

1. Mozaffarian D, Benjamin EJ, Go AS, et al. On behalf of the American Heart Association Statistics Committee and Stroke Statistics Subcommittee. *Heart disease and stroke statistics—2015 update: a report from the American Heart Association.* Available at https://www.heart.org/idc/groups/ahamah-public/@wcm/@sop/@smd/documents/downloadable/ucm_470707.pdf. Accessed November 20, 2015.
2. Pickering T, Shimbo D, Haas D. Ambulatory blood-pressure monitoring. *N Engl J Med.* 2006;354:2368–2374.
3. O'Brien E, Asmar R, Beilin L, et al. European Society of Hypertension recommendations for conventional, ambulatory, and more blood pressure measurement. *J Hypertens.* 2005;21(5):821–848.
4. Ghuman N, Campbell P, White W. Role of ambulatory blood pressure recording in clinical practice. *Curr Cardiol Reports.* 2009;11(6):414–421.
5. Verberk W, Kroon A, Kessles A, et al. Home blood pressure measurement: a systematic review. *J Am Coll Cardiol.* 2005;46(5):743–751.
6. Saugel B, Dueck R, Wagner J. Measurement of blood pressure. *Best Pract Res Clin Anaesthesiol.* 2014;28(4):309–322.
7. Ogedegbe G, Pickering T. Principles and techniques of blood pressure measurement. *Cardiol Clin.* 2010;28(4):571–586.
8. McManus RJ, Mant J, Roalfe A, et al. Targets and self monitoring in hypertension: randomized controlled trial and cost effectiveness analysis. *BMJ.* 2005;331(7515):493.
9. Bakx JC, van der Wel MC, van Weel C. Self monitoring of high blood pressure. *BMJ.* 2005;331(7515):466–467.
10. Kantola I, Vesalainen R, Kangassalo K, Kariluoto A. Bell or diaphragm in the measurement of blood pressure? *J Hypertens.* 2005;23(3):499–503.
11. Cavallini MC, Roman MJ, Blank SG, et al. Association of the auscultatory gap with vascular disease in hypertensive patients. *Ann Intern Med.* 1996;124(10):877–883.
12. Pickering T, Hall J, Appel L, et al. *Recommendations for Blood Pressure Measurement in Humans: An AHA Scientific Statement From the Council on High Blood Pressure Research Professional and Public Education Subcommittee.* Available at http://www.medscape.com/viewarticle/499972_5. Accessed September 8, 2015.
13. Weber M, Schiffrin E, White W. Clinical practice guidelines for the management of hypertension in the community. *J Clin Hyperten (Greenwich).* 2014;16(1):14–26.
14. James P, Oparil S, Carter B, et al. 2014 evidence-based guideline for the management of high blood pressure in adults: report from the panel members appointed to the Eighth Joint National Committee (JNC 8). *JAMA.* 2015;311(5):507–520.
15. Yano Y, Stamler J, Garside D, et al. Isolated systolic hypertension in young and middle-aged adults and 31-year risk for cardiovascular mortality: the Chicago Heart Association Detection Project in Industry study. *J Am Coll Cardiol.* 2015;65(4):327–335.
16. Lanier J, Mote M, Clay E. Evaluation and management of orthostatic hypotension. *Am Fam Physician.* 2011;84(5):527–536.
17. Metzler M, Duerr S, Granata R, et al. Neurogenic orthostatic hypotension: pathophysiology, evaluation, and management. *J Neurol.* 2013;260(9):2212–2219.
18. Eguchi K, Pickering T, Hoshide S, et al. Ambulatory blood pressure is a better marker than clinic blood pressure in predicting cardiovascular events in patients with/without type 2 diabetes. *Am J Hypertens.* 2011;21(4):10.
19. Dawes MG, Bartlett G, Coats AJ, et al. Comparing the effects of white coat hypertension and sustained hypertension on mortality in a UK primary care setting. *Ann Fam Med.* 2008;6:390–396.
20. Pierdomenico SD, Cuccurullo F. Prognostic value of white-coat and masked hypertension diagnosed by ambulatory monitoring in initially untreated subjects: An updated meta analysis. *Am J Hypertens.* 2011;24:52–58.
21. Bancej CM, Campbell N, McKay DW, et al. Home blood pressure monitoring among Canadian adults with hypertension: Results from the 2009 Survey on Living with Chronic Diseases in Canada. *Can J Cardiol.* 2010;26:e152–e157.
22. O'Brien P, Marshall AC. Coaractation of the aorta. *Circulationc.* 2015;131:e363–e365. Available at http://circ.ahajournals.org. Accessed September 9, 2015.
23. Mason JW, Ramseth DJ, Chanter DO, et al. Electrocardiographic reference ranges derived from 79,743 ambulatory subjects. *J Electrocardiol.* 2007;40:228–234.
24. Aladin AI, Whelton SP, Al-Mallah MH, et al. Relation of resting heart rate to risk for all-cause mortality by gender after considering exercise capacity (the Henry Ford Exercise Testing Project). *Am J Cardiology.* 2014:114:1701–1706.
25. Sund-Levander M, Grodzinsky E. Time for a change to assess and evaluate body temperature in clinical practice. *Int J Nurs Pract.* 2009;15(4):241–249.
26. Bridges E, Thomas K. Noninvasive measurement of body temperature in critically ill patients. *Crit Care Nur.* 2009;29(3):94–97.
27. Washington G, Matney J. Comparison of temperature measurement devices in post anesthesia patients. *J Perianesth Nurs.* 23(1):2008;36–48.

28. Exergen Manual. Temporal artery thermometer: exergen instructions for use. Available at: www.exergen.com/medical/PDFs/tat2000cmanual.pdf. Accessed June 6, 2016.

29. Institute of Medicine Report from the Committee on Advancing Pain Research, Care, and Education. *Relieving Pain in America, A Blueprint for Transforming Prevention, Care, Education and Research.* The National Academies Press; 2011.

30. Loeser J, Treede R. The Kyoto protocol of IASP basic pain terminology. *Pain.* 2008;137:473–477.

31. American Medical Association. *Pain Management: The Online Series. Module 1. Pathophysiology of Pain and Pain Assessment.* 2010. Available at http://www.ama-cmeonline.com/pain_mgmt/. Accessed September 14, 2015.

32. Song, W, Eaton, L, Gordon D, et al. Evaluation of evidence-based nursing pain management practice. *Pain Management Nursing.* 2015;16(4):456–463.

33. Babadag B, Alparslan G, Gulec S. The relationship between pain beliefs and coping with pain of algology patients. *Pain Manag Nurs.* 2015;16(6):910–919.

34. Wells N, Pasero C, McCaffery M. *Chapter 17 Improving the Quality of Care Through Pain Assessment and Management in Patient Safety and Quality: An Evidence-Based Handbook for Nurses.* Agency for Healthcare Research and Quality; 2008.

35. Wong-Baker FACES Rating Scale: from Wong DL, Hackenberry-Eaton M, Wilson D, Winkelstein ML, Schwartz P: Wong's Essentials of Pediatric Nursing, 6/e, St. Louis, p. 1301, 2001.

36. 0–10 Numeric Pain Rating Scale: From McCaffery M, Pasero C. Pain: Clinical Manual, St. Louis, p. 16, 1999.

37. Visual Analog Scale and Verbal Pain Intensity Scale: From Pain Management: Theory and Practice, edited by RK Portenoy & RM Tanner, Oxford University Press, Inc. 1996.

38. Defense and Veterans Pain Rating Scale (DVPRS). Defense & Veterans Center for Integrative Pain Management. Available at http://www.dvcipm.org/clinical-resources/pain-rating-scale. Accessed June 9, 2016.

39. Upadhyay C, Cameron K, Murphy L, et al. Measuring pain in patients undergoing hemodialysis: a review of pain assessment tools. *Kidney J.* 2014;7(4):367–372.

40. Tsao J, Plankey M, Young M. Pain, psychological symptoms and prescription drug misuse in HIV: A literature review. *J Pain Manag.* 2012;5(2):111–118.

41. Mossey JM. Defining racial and ethnic disparities in pain management. *Clin Orthoprelated Res.* 2011;469(7):1859–1870.

42. Paulson M, Dekker AH. Disparities in pain management. *J Am Osteopath Assoc.* 2005;105(6 Suppl 3):S14–7.

43. Relieving Pain in America: A Blueprint for Transforming Prevention, Care, Education, and Research. Washington, DC: The National Academies; 2011.

44. Doorenbos A, Gordon D, Tauben D, et al. A blueprint of pain curriculum across pre-licensure health sciences programs: one NIH Pain Consortium Center of Excellence in Pain Education (CoEPE) experience. *J Pain.* 2013;14(12):1533–1538.

45. Zhang X, Bao L. The development and modulation of nociceptive circuitry. *Curr Opin Neurobiol.* 2006;16(4):460–466.

Nutrition and Hydration

LEARNING OBJECTIVES

The student will:

1. Assess the nutritional status of an individual through a nutrition history and physical examination.
2. Identify persons at risk for malnutrition or overnutrition.
3. Differentiate between normal and abnormal nutrition assessment findings.
4. Identify individuals with dehydration or overhydration.

Nutritional status is a key element of overall health. Good nutrition is important for every body system. Poor nutrition may be a problem in itself (e.g., lack of vitamin D can cause rickets), or it may exacerbate an underlying disease, such as diabetes or cardiovascular disease. Low protein reserves will impede healing (e.g., from surgery). Poor nutrition in children may delay growth and contribute to cognitive issues in school. Problems in nutrition may be the result of many factors.

Weight gain occurs when caloric intake exceeds caloric expenditure over time and typically appears as increased body fat. Hypothyroidism may cause weight gain by reducing body metabolism. Weight gain may also reflect abnormal accumulation of body fluids. When the retention of fluid is mild, the fluid may not be visible, but several pounds of fluid usually appear as edema.

Weight loss is an important symptom with many causes. Mechanisms include decreased intake of food for such reasons as anorexia, dysphagia, vomiting, diarrhea, inability to absorb nutrients from the gastrointestinal tract, increased metabolic needs, allergies to foods, problems with chewing, dislike of foods, and peer pressure. Poor food choices, inability to cook or poor cooking habits, inability to access food stores, or lack of financial resources may also cause nutrition problems. The nurse sorts through the data the patient provides to identify possible sources of problems and creates a plan of care. If the nurse finds the patient needs more testing or intense counseling, the patient should be referred to a nurse practitioner, physician, or registered dietician.

Causes of weight loss include gastrointestinal diseases; endocrine disorders (diabetes mellitus, hyperthyroidism, adrenal insufficiency); chronic infections; malignancy; chronic cardiac, pulmonary, or renal failure; depression; and anorexia nervosa (see Table 8-1, p. 166).

Severe vitamin or mineral deficiencies or lack of protein, carbohydrates, or fats will produce characteristic signs and symptoms. However, it is preferred to recognize the potential deficiency in the patient's diet before signs and symptoms occur. For example, when a patient reports lactose intolerance, the nurse should assess the diet for adequate intake of calcium and vitamin D through nonmilk foods and supplements before signs of rickets develop.

Nutritional status is assessed at most nurse–patient encounters. A general screening assessment is done during a complete health assessment. If the patient's chief complaint involves nutrition or if the general screening finds unusual results, an in-depth nutrition assessment should be done. Patients admitted to long-term care facilities and patients with problems that require good nutrition to heal, such as pressure ulcers, should be thoroughly assessed. The U.S. Department of Agriculture's (USDA's) *Choose MyPlate* website (http://www.choosemyplate.gov/) is a tool to help individuals analyze their diet and set goals for a healthier diet. The nurse can use the site with a patient to demonstrate how to perform a diet analysis and track individual progress. The ChooseMyPlate.gov website includes nutrition tips, nutrition information for various populations, print materials, interactive tools as well as links to other nutrient and physical activity information.

Two screening tools to identify individuals at risk for nutritional deficits are below.

Weight loss with relatively high food intake suggests *diabetes mellitus, hyperthyroidism,* or *malabsorption.* Also consider binge eating (bulimia) with clandestine vomiting.

Poverty, old age, social isolation, physical disability, emotional or mental impairment, lack of teeth, ill-fitting dentures, alcoholism, and drug abuse increase the likelihood of malnutrition.

For tools for assessing the older adult, see the Nutrition Screening box below and the Mini Nutritional Assessment (MNA) in Chapter 24, Assessing Older Adults, p. 948.

Nutrition Screening

Nutrition Screening Checklist

I have an illness or condition that made me change the kind and/or amount of food I eat.	Yes (2 pts)	——
I eat fewer than 2 meals per day.	Yes (3 pts)	——
I eat few fruits or vegetables, or milk products.	Yes (2 pts)	——
I have 3 or more drinks of beer, liquor, or wine almost every day.	Yes (2 pts)	——
I have tooth or mouth problems that make it hard for me to eat.	Yes (2 pts)	——
I don't always have enough money to buy the food I need.	Yes (4 pts)	——
I eat alone most of the time.	Yes (1 pt)	——
I take 3 or more different prescribed or over-the-counter drugs each day.	Yes (1 pt)	——
Without wanting to, I have lost or gained 10 lb in the last 6 months.	Yes (2 pts)	——
I am not always physically able to shop, cook, and/or feed myself.	Yes (2 pts)	——
	TOTAL	——

Instructions. Check "yes" for each condition that applies, then total the nutritional score. For total scores of 3–5 points (moderate risk) or ≥6 points (high risk), further evaluation is needed (especially for the elderly).

Source: *Nutrition Screening*—American Academy of Family Physicians. Bagley B. Editorials: Nutrition and Health. Available at http://www.aafp.org/afp/980301ap/edits.html. Accessed May 19, 2011.

Rapid Screen for Dietary Intake

	Portions Consumed by Patient	Recommended
Grains, cereals, bread group	——	6–11
Fruit group	——	2–4
Vegetable group	——	3–5
Meat/meat substitute group	——	2–3
Dairy group	——	2–3
Sugars, fats, snack foods	——	—
Soft drinks	——	—
Alcoholic beverages	——	<2

Instructions. Ask the patient for a 24-hour dietary recall (or a 2-day diet intake) before completing the form.

Source: *Rapid Screen for Dietary Intake*—Nestle M. Nutrition. In: Woolf SH, Jonas S, Lawrence RS, eds. *Health Promotion and Disease Prevention in Clinical Practice.* Baltimore: Williams & Wilkins; 1996.

Hydration status is critical to every patient's health. Under- or over-hydration may accompany disease, medical treatment, and environmental conditions. The patient can die or suffer serious complications if alterations in hydration are not recognized immediately. It is the nurse who most closely monitors the patient's hydration status. Conditions that contribute to dehydration include exposure to excessive heat, exercise in heat, decreased mobility, inability to drink (e.g. a comatose patient), medications such as diuretics, vomiting and/or diarrhea, burn injuries, and hemorrhage. Conditions that contribute to overhydration include heart failure, kidney failure, liver disease, increased sodium intake, and excess intravenous fluid.

Signs and symptoms of hydration and nutrition problems are reflected in multiple body systems, including the integumentary, respiratory, cardiovascular, peripheral vascular, gastrointestinal, and musculoskeletal systems. As you read the body system chapters, note the signs and symptoms of nutrition or hydration deficits or excess. For summaries of the signs and symptoms of nutrition and hydration disorders, see Evaluating Nutritional Disorders and Assessment of Dehydration and Overhydration.

EVALUATING NUTRITIONAL DISORDERS

This chart can help you interpret your nutritional assessment findings. Body systems are listed below with signs or symptoms and the implications for each.

Body System or Region	Sign or Symptom	Implications
General	• Weakness and fatigue • Weight loss	• Anemia or electrolyte imbalance • Decreased calorie intake, increased calorie use, or inadequate nutrient intake or absorption
Skin, hair, and nails	• Dry, flaky skin • Dry skin with poor turgor • Rough, scaly skin with bumps • Petechiae or ecchymoses • Sore that won't heal • Thinning, dry hair • Spoon-shaped, brittle, or ridged nails	• Vitamin A, vitamin B-complex, or linoleic acid deficiency • Dehydration • Vitamin A deficiency • Vitamin C or K deficiency • Protein, vitamin C, or zinc deficiency • Protein deficiency • Iron deficiency
Eyes	• Night blindness; corneal swelling, softening, or dryness; Bitot spots (gray triangular patches on the conjunctiva) • Red conjunctiva	• Vitamin A deficiency • Riboflavin deficiency
Throat and mouth	• Cracks at the corner of the mouth • Magenta tongue • Beefy, red tongue • Soft, spongy, bleeding gums • Swollen neck (goiter)	• Riboflavin or niacin deficiency • Riboflavin deficiency • Vitamin B_{12} deficiency • Vitamin C deficiency • Iodine deficiency
Cardiovascular	• Edema • Tachycardia, hypotension	• Protein deficiency • Fluid volume deficit
Gastrointestinal	• Ascites	• Protein deficiency
Musculoskeletal	• Bone pain and bow leg • Muscle wasting	• Vitamin D or calcium deficiency • Protein, carbohydrate, and fat deficiency
Neurologic	• Altered mental status • Paresthesia	• Dehydration and thiamine or vitamin B_{12} deficiency • Vitamin B_{12}, pyridoxine, or thiamine deficiency

Assessment of Dehydration and Overhydration

Dehydration: Deficient Fluid Volume
- Symptoms
  - Thirst
  - Diaphoresis
  - Vomiting/diarrhea
- Signs
  - Short-term weight loss
  - Dry mucous membranes / eyes
  - Sunken eyes
  - Decreased skin turgor
  - Fever
  - Decreased BP and pulse pressure
  - Increased Pulse rate and decreased pulse amplitude
  - Decreased urine output and increased specific gravity
  - Decrease in venous filling
  - Alteration in mental status
  - Weakness
- Contributing factors
  - Exposure to excessive heat
  - Exercise in heat
  - Decreased mobility
  - Inability to drink
  - Older age
  - Medications—diuretics
  - Burns
  - Hemorrhage
  - Vomiting/diarrhea
  - Fever

Overhydration: Excess Fluid Volume
- Signs
  - Short-term weight gain
  - Edema
  - Increased BP decreased or bounding pulse
  - Jugular vein distention
  - S3 heart sound
  - Fine crackles in lungs
  - Dyspnea
  - Alteration in mental status
  - Urine output and urine-specific gravity may be decreased or increased depending on diagnosis.
- Contributing factors
  - Heart failure
  - Kidney failure
  - Liver disease
  - Increased sodium intake
  - IV fluid overload

THE HEALTH HISTORY

In the general assessment the nurse assesses nutrition during the Review of Systems (ROS) and Health Patterns. Under the ROS the patient is asked about weight changes, fatigue, allergies, and problems in the gastrointestinal system, which may signal nutrition problems. Under Health Patterns the patient's nutrition and exercise patterns are elicited. These may also help the nurse identify a patient problem with nutrition (see Chapter 4, The Health History, pp. 79-80).

Common or Concerning Symptoms

- Changes in weight, usually unintended
- Anorexia
- Changes in the senses of taste or smell
- Difficulty chewing or swallowing

Changes in Weight

Changes in weight result from changes in body tissues or body fluid.

Rapid changes in weight over a few days suggest an increase or decrease in body fluids, not tissues.

Begin with broad open-ended questions, such as "Tell me about your weight gain (loss)." Use the "OLD CART" mnemonic to ask follow-up questions.

Onset: When did you notice the change in your weight? When do you think it began?

Location: Is the weight gain (loss) distributed over your whole body or in a particular area?

Weight gain or swelling in the lower legs may indicate water retention due to cardiac or peripheral vascular disease, not a nutrition problem.

Duration: Has the gain (loss) been consistent? In spurts? Have you alternated between gaining and losing weight?

Characteristic Symptoms: How much weight have you gained (lost)? How does your weight compare to a year (6 months) ago? Have you experienced increased hunger (or anorexia) during this time? Do you have difficulty chewing? Has your sense of smell changed? Taste?

Associated Manifestations: Do you tire easily? Do you often feel cold? Is your skin drier than usual? Are your ankles swollen? Have you noticed a change in the fit of your clothes? Have you changed your diet during this time? Have you changed your exercise routines or patterns of living? Who cooks for you? Who shops for you? Any change in your teeth? Dentures?

Relieving Factors: Has anything helped you lose (gain) weight?

Treatment: Have you tried any diets or supplements to lose (gain) weight?

Follow-up on other symptoms in a similar fashion.

Be sure to ask the patient about food allergies or intolerances, such as lactose intolerance. Ask about chronic illnesses in the patient and family, as these may be related to the nutrition problems.

If an in-depth nutrition assessment is needed, a nutrition history form is helpful. One such form is given below.

Nutrition History	
Assessment Area	**Sample Questions**
Food pattern	How many meals/snacks do you eat a day? Which is the biggest meal? How many meals do you eat outside the home? Where are they eaten? Are you on any special diet or fad diet? Do you use food supplements, e.g. protein shakes? If yes, which ones?
Personal food preferences	Are any foods particularly liked or disliked? Are there any foods you feel are harmful or beneficial? Do you have any cultural or religious preferences?
Food preparation	Who does the cooking? How are the foods prepared? What type of oil is used for frying (saturated or unsaturated)? What spices or condiments are commonly used?
Finances	Is there enough money for food? Would you eat any differently if more money was available for food? Do you use any supplementary financial program?
Accessibility	Who does the shopping? When? Where? How close is your preferred grocery store? Is there transportation to the market?
Patient health	Do you have any trouble with chewing or digesting food? How often do you have a bowel movement? Do you take any nutritional supplements or vitamins? What type? How much? Do you have any food allergies or food intolerances? What medications do you take? Dose? How often? Do you drink alcohol? What type? How much? Per day? Per week? Do you smoke? How many packs per day?

	Please rate your stress level on a scale of 1–10. (1 being low stress and 10 being extremely stressed.) Does the stress affect your appetite?
	Have you ever been tested for anemia or had your cholesterol level tested? Results?
	Are you happy with your health?
	Do you have an eating disorder? Heart disease? Osteoporosis? Diabetes? Obesity? or Gastrointestinal (GI) disorder?
Exercise pattern	Describe your exercise on a typical day (or week).
Body image	Are you satisfied with your weight?
	What would you change about your body, if you could?
Family health	Is there any heart disease, osteoporosis, diabetes, obesity, or GI disorders in the family?
Family dietary patterns	Does anyone in the family eat a special diet?
	Does the family eat meals together? How often?
	Is mealtime a social time?

In addition to the nutrition history, the nurse should collect a sample food intake record. The nurse can ask the patient for a 24-hour recall of food and beverage intake. This is efficient if the patient can accurately remember the types and quantities of foods and beverages. If time allows, the patient can be given a sheet to record a 2-day diet intake or a weekly diary. The nurse can help the patient analyze the record at a later appointment, or if hospitalized or in a long-term care facility use the patient intake record.

PHYSICAL EXAMINATION

Signs of poor nutrition may occur in any body system. Usually by the time a sign appears the condition is fairly severe. See the chart on Evaluating Nutritional Disorders (p. 149).

The nurse looks for signs of nutritional problems and hydration problems during the general head-to-toe physical examination. For example, assessment of the skin for nutritional deficits begins with the general survey and continues as one moves through the examination from head to toe. When a full patient examination is not necessary, the nurse can systematically look for signs of nutrition or hydration problems.

General Survey

Begin the physical examination with the patient's *height and weight* and vital signs. Note the patient's *body frame*. Is it small, medium, or large?

The head

The neck

The shoulder

Center of gravity

The sacral area

The hip joint

The knee

The ankle

The patient's *body mass index* (BMI) can be calculated from the height and weight. See p. 157 for how to calculate the BMI.

The proportion of weight to height can indicate whether the patient is over- or underweight. Note that individuals with large muscle mass may have a falsely high calculated BMI. This must be taken into account before assuming the patient is obese or overweight.

Height Measurement

1. Have the patient remove shoes and hat.

Have patient undo hair styles or remove hair pieces or ornaments that add height, if possible.

2. Use a stadiometer attached to the wall.

3. The patient should stand facing away from the wall with a straight back and the heels, hips, shoulders, and occiput aligned.

4. The patient's head, back, buttocks, and heels should be against the wall.

5. Record the patient's height.

6. Children younger than 2 years who cannot stand up should have their body length measured supine on a length measuring board. Chapter 23, Assessing Children, p. 822.

Weight Measurement

The balance beam scale is frequently used in health care agencies for patients who can stand up. Digital scales are used for infants and patients who cannot stand up and need chair or bed scales. Read the instructions for such scales.

Weight can vary during the day. If serial weights are needed, the patient should be weighed at the same time in the morning, on the same scale, and in the same clothing. In the hospital this is often the hospital gown.

For the balance beam scale:

1. First zero the balance beam.
   a. Be sure the movable weights are at zero.
   b. If necessary, move the counter weights until the pointer is balanced in the middle at zero.

1. Have the patient remove shoes and outer clothing for a one-time weight.

2. The patient should step on the scale facing the balance beam.

3. Slide the large weight forward first. When the pointer is overbalanced downward, slide the large weight back to the previous notch.

4. Slide the small weight forward until the beam is balanced.

5. Read and document weight.

Individuals who have problems concerning weight, such as an eating disorder, may prefer to face away from the measurement beam.

Skin, Hair, and Nails

Thoroughly inspect the skin for dryness, flaking, cracking, or sores that will not heal. Assess skin color and turgor. Inspect the hair for texture, thinning, and loss of color. Check the nails for shape and brittleness.

A pale color in fair-skinned patients or pale palms and mucous membranes in dark-skinned patients may indicate anemia.

Turgor recoil greater than 3 seconds may indicate dehydration.

Vitamin deficiencies may cause changes in skin, hair, and nails. See the chart, Evaluating Nutritional Disorders (p. 149).

Head, Ears, Eyes, Nose, and Throat (HEENT)

Inspect for dark circles under the eyes.

Allergies may cause circles.

Inspect the mucous membranes for dryness, color, and intactness. Note cracking at the corners of the mouth, bleeding gums, and changes in tongue color. Look for an enlarged thyroid gland.

Dry membranes and sunken eyes indicate dehydration. Pale membranes may indicate anemia. Bleeding gums, cracking, and color changes may indicate vitamin deficiencies.

An enlarged thyroid may indicate lack of iodine or thyroid malfunction.

Respiratory

Assess lung sounds for adventitious sounds.

Fine crackles may indicate fluid overload in cardiac failure or pulmonary edema.

Cardiovascular and Peripheral Vascular

Measure blood pressure and pulse rate and amplitude. Assess peripheral vein filling.

Tachycardia, a weak pulse and decreased blood pressure can indicate dehydration, while a increased jugular venous distension and increased blood pressure may mean overhydration. Flat veins with hands or feet dependent may indicate dehydration; full veins when hands and feet elevated may indicate overhydration.

Inspect arms and legs for edema, petechiae, and ecchymoses.

Petechiae and ecchymoses may be due to a lack of vitamin C or K. Edema may be secondary to a protein deficiency, fluid retention in cardiac failure or venous stasis in peripheral vascular disease.

Gastrointestinal

Observe for distension and ascites.

Abdominal distention and ascites may be due to protein deficiency liver disease and low albumin.

Measure waist circumference. Place the tape measure over bare skin just above the hip bones. Have the patient take a breath and measure the waist after exhalation.

The waist circumference indicates central body fat. Waist circumference greater than 40 in in men and greater than 35 in in women is related to an increased risk for cardiovascular disease.[1]

Musculoskeletal

Note muscle wasting or flaccidity, bone pain, and bowing of tibia. Measure arm circumference.

Muscle wasting and flaccidity may be secondary to protein deficiency. Lack of vitamin D can cause bone pain and bowing of the legs.

Neurologic

Note changes in mental status, irritability, inability to concentrate, or paresthesias.

Dehydration and lack of vitamins may cause these symptoms.

Calculate the BMI

Use the patient's measurements of height and weight to calculate the *body mass index,* or *BMI.* Body fat consists primarily of adipose in the form of triglycerides and is stored in subcutaneous, interabdominal, and intramuscular fat deposits that are difficult to measure directly. The BMI incorporates estimated but more accurate measures of body fat than weight alone. Note that BMI criteria for overweight and obesity are not rigid points but guidelines for estimating increasing risks to patient health and well-being from both excess and low weight. For older adults, there is a disproportionate risk for undernutrition.

BMI standards are derived from two surveys: the National Health Examination Survey, consisting of three survey cycles between 1960 and 1970, and the National Health and Nutrition Examination Survey, conducted over three cycles between the 1970s and the 1990s.

There are several ways to obtain the BMI, as shown in the accompanying table. Choose the method most suited to your practice. The National

BMI Calculation Set up

1. Use the Body Mass Index table on p. 158.
   a. Find the patient's height in inches in the first column.
   b. Move across the height row to the column with the patient's weight in pounds
   c. Follow the weight column up to the BMI number.
2. Use the "BMI calculator" from NIH at https://www.nhlbi.nih.gov/health/educational/lose_wt/BMI/bmicalc.htm
3. Calculate the BMI using one of the following formulas.

Unit of Measure	Method of Calculation
Weight in *pounds,* height in *inches*	$BMI = \dfrac{Weight (Pound)}{Height^2 (Inches^2)} \times 703$ Example: Weight = 150 lbs, Height = 5'5" (65") Calculation: $[150 \div (65)^2] \times 703 = 24.96$
Weight in *kilograms,* height in *meters*	$BMI = \dfrac{Weight (Kilogram)}{Height^2 (Meters^2)}$ Example: Weight = 68 kg, Height = 165 cm (1.65 m) Calculation: $68 \div (1.65)^2 = 24.98$

Conversion formulas: 2.2 lbs = 1 kg; 1.0 inch = 2.54 cm; 100 cm = 1 meter.

Source: CDC. Division of Nutrition, Physical Activity and Obesity. About BMI. Available at http://www.cdc.gov/healthyweight/assessing/bmi/adult_bmi/#Interpreted. Accessed February 15, 2016.

Institutes of Health and the National Heart, Lung, and Blood Institute caution that people who are very muscular, for example, body builders may have a high BMI but still be healthy.[2] Likewise, the BMI for people with low muscle mass and reduced nutrition may appear inappropriately "normal."

Body Mass Index Table

BMI	Normal								Overweight								Obese				
	19	20	21	22	23	24	25	26	27	28	29	30	31	32	33	34	35	36	37	38	39
Height (inches)	Body Weight (pounds)																				
58	91	96	100	105	110	115	119	124	129	134	138	143	148	153	158	162	167	172	177	181	186
59	94	99	104	109	114	119	124	128	133	138	143	148	153	158	163	168	173	178	183	188	193
60	97	102	107	112	118	123	128	133	138	143	148	153	158	163	168	174	179	184	189	194	199
61	100	106	111	116	122	127	132	137	143	148	153	158	164	169	174	180	185	190	195	201	206
62	104	109	115	120	126	131	136	142	147	153	158	164	169	175	180	186	191	196	202	207	213
63	107	113	118	124	130	135	141	146	152	158	163	169	175	180	186	191	197	203	208	214	220
64	110	116	122	128	134	140	145	151	157	163	169	174	180	186	192	197	204	209	215	221	227
65	114	120	126	132	138	144	150	156	162	168	174	180	186	192	198	204	210	216	222	228	234
66	118	124	130	136	142	148	155	161	167	173	179	186	192	198	204	210	216	223	229	235	241
67	121	127	134	140	146	153	159	166	172	178	185	191	198	204	211	217	223	230	236	242	249
68	125	131	138	144	151	158	164	171	177	184	190	197	203	210	216	223	230	236	243	249	256
69	128	135	142	149	155	162	169	176	182	189	196	203	209	216	223	230	236	243	250	257	263
70	132	139	146	153	160	167	174	181	188	195	202	209	216	222	229	236	243	250	257	264	271
71	136	143	150	157	165	172	179	186	193	200	208	215	222	229	236	243	250	257	265	272	279
72	140	147	154	162	169	177	184	191	199	206	213	221	228	235	242	250	258	265	272	279	287
73	144	151	159	166	174	182	189	197	204	212	219	227	235	242	250	257	265	272	280	288	295
74	148	155	163	171	179	186	194	202	210	218	225	233	241	249	256	264	272	280	287	295	303
75	152	160	168	176	184	192	200	208	216	224	232	240	248	256	264	272	279	287	295	303	311
76	156	164	172	180	189	197	205	213	221	230	238	246	254	263	271	279	287	295	304	312	320

Source: Adapted from National Institutes of Health and National Heart, Lung, and Blood Institute: Clinical Guidelines on the Identification, Evaluation and Treatment of Overweight and Obesity in Adults: The Evidence Report. June 1998. Available at: http://www.nhlbi.nih.gov/health/educational/lose_wt/BMI/bmi_tbl.htm. Accessed May 11, 2016.

If the BMI is 35 or higher, measure the patient's *waist circumference*. With the patient standing, measure the waist just above the hip bones. The patient may have excess body fat if the waist measures:

- ≥35 inches for women

- ≥40 inches for men

HEALTH PROMOTION AND COUNSELING

Important Topics for Health Promotion and Counseling

- Optimal weight, nutrition, and diet
- Exercise
- Hydration

Optimal Weight, Nutrition, and Diet

Fewer than half of U.S. adults maintain a healthy weight, with a BMI between 18.5 and 24.9. Obesity has increased in every segment of the U.S. population, regardless of age, gender, ethnicity, or socioeconomic status. Review the alarming statistics about the rising prevalence of obesity nationally and worldwide in the table below.[3–5]

See Table 8-2 (p. 167).

Obesity at a Glance

- According to the National Health and Nutrition Examination Surveys (NHANES) (2009–2010), nearly 69% of U.S. adults are overweight or obese (BMI ≥25), including 71% of men, 66% of women; overall, about 35% of U.S. adults are obese.[6]
- 31.8% of U.S. children and adolescents (2–19 years) are obese or overweight.[6]
- Health disparities: the prevalence of being overweight or obese varies by ethnic and socioeconomic groups.[7]
- Overweight and obesity increase risk of heart disease, numerous types of cancers, type 2 diabetes, stroke, arthritis, sleep apnea, infertility, and depression.
- More than 80% of people with type 2 diabetes[8] and 20% of people with hypertension or elevated cholesterol are overweight or obese.
- Obesity is increasing worldwide: although being poor in the world's poorest countries is associated with underweight and malnutrition, being poor in a middle-income country adopting a Western lifestyle is associated with increased risk of obesity.[9]
- Only 65% of obese U.S. adults report that health care professionals have told them they were overweight. Less than half report being advised to lose weight.[10]

To promote optimal patient weight and nutrition, adopt the four-step approach outlined below. Even reducing weight by 5% to 10% can improve blood pressure, lipid levels, and glucose tolerance and reduce the risk of diabetes or hypertension.

Four Steps to Promote Optimal Weight and Nutrition

- Measure BMI and waist circumference; identify risk of overweight and obesity.
- Assess dietary intake.
- Assess the patient's motivation to change.
- Provide counseling about nutrition and exercise.

See Table 8-3 (p. 168).

Take advantage of the resources available for patient assessment and counseling summarized in the following sections. Review the role of weight in the growing prevalence of *metabolic syndrome* in Chapter 14, The Cardiovascular System.

See Table 8-2 (p. 167).

Step 1: Measure the BMI and Assess Risk Factors

Classify the BMI according to the national guidelines in the following table. If the BMI is *above 25,* assess the patient for *additional risk factors* for heart disease and other obesity-related diseases: hypertension, high low-density lipoprotein (LDL) cholesterol, low high-density lipoprotein (HDL) cholesterol, high triglycerides, high blood glucose, family history of premature heart disease, physical inactivity, and smoking. Patients with a BMI over 25 and two or more risk factors should pursue weight loss, especially if the waist circumference is elevated.

Adults with a BMI greater than 25, men with waist circumferences greater than 40 in, and women with waist circumferences greater than 35 in are at increased risk for heart disease and obesity-related diseases.

Measuring the waist-to-hip ratio (waist circumference divided by hip circumference) may be a better risk predictor for individuals older than 75 years. Ratios greater than 0.95 in men and greater than 0.85 in women are considered elevated.

Classification of Overweight and Obesity by BMI

	Obesity Class	BMI (kg/m^2)
Underweight		<18.5
Normal		18.5–24.9
Overweight		25.0–29.9
Obesity	I	30.0–34.9
	II	35.0–39.9
Extreme obesity	III	≥40

Source: National Institutes of Health and National Heart, Lung, and Blood Institute: Clinical Guidelines on the Identification, Evaluation, and Treatment of Overweight and Obesity in Adults: The Evidence Report. NIH Publication 98–4083. June 1998. Available at http://www.nhlbi.nih.gov/guidelines/obesity/ob_gdlns.pdf. Accessed September 16, 2015.

Step 2: Assess Dietary Intake

Obtain a nutrition history (see pp. 152–153) and a diet intake record. Analyze the patient's intake record. The USDS's *Choose MyPlate* site online is an excellent resource to help you analyze the patient's intake record.

Step 3: Assess the Patient's Motivation to Change

Assess the patient's readiness to make the lifestyle changes that promote weight loss. Prochaska's model of change helps the nurse tailor interventions to the patient's stage of readiness. See Table 8-3, p. 168.

Step 4: Provide Counseling about Nutrition and Exercise

Advising patients about diet and weight loss is important, especially in light of the many, often contradictory dieting options in the popular press. The following three resources provide excellent guidelines for counseling your patients:

- USPS Task Force. Final Recommendation Statement: Obesity in Adults: Screening and Management, June 2012. Available at http://www.uspreventiveservicestaskforce.org/Page/Document/Recommendation StatementFinal/obesity-in-adults-screening-and-management. Accessed February 14, 2016.

- U.S. Department of Health and Human Services and U.S. Department of Agriculture. Dietary Guidelines for Americans 2015–2020. Available at http://www.cnpp.usda.gov/2015–2020-dietary-guidelines-americans. Accessed February 14, 2016.

- USDA Choose MyPlate. Weight Management. Available at http://www.choosemyplate.gov/weight-management-calories. Accessed February 14, 2016.

Diet recommendations hinge on assessment of the patient's motivation and readiness to lose weight and individual risk factors. The *The Evidence*

 Concept Mastery Alert

When completing a nutritional history, the nurse needs to be alert for findings that may suggest anorexia nervosa. Patients with anorexia nervosa are preoccupied with controlling their environment so that they limit the number of calories ingested and perform exercise to lose even those limited calories. They have a low body mass index and other physical symptoms related to starvation. This is in contrast to patients with bulimia nervosa, who may be of normal weight or even overweight and are preoccupied with eating and often engage in binge eating followed by purging.

Report on Managing Overweight and Obesity in Adults[1] recommend the following general guidelines:

- A 10% weight reduction over 6 months, or a decrease of 500 to 1000 kcal/day, for overweight and obese adults.

- A weight loss goal of ½ to 1 lb per week because more rapid weight loss does not lead to better results at 1 year.[11]

These guidelines recommend low-calorie diets of 1200 to 1500 kcal per day for women and 1500 to 1700 kcal per day for men. Interventions that combine nutrition education, diet, and exercise (see Moderate and Vigorous Exercise table on p. 164) with behavioral therapy are most likely to succeed. The *Clinical Guidelines* cite evidence supporting the role of moderate physical activity in weight loss and weight loss maintenance programs: it enhances and may assist with maintenance of weight; it increases cardiorespiratory fitness; and it may decrease abdominal fat.

If the BMI falls *below 18.5*, be concerned about eating disorders, or other medical conditions. These conditions are summarized in Table 8-1 (p. 166).

Once you have assessed food intake, nutritional status, and motivation to adopt healthy eating behaviors or lose weight, give patients the "recommendations for healthy eating patterns" of the Dietary Guidelines for Americans 2015–2020, as summarized and adapted below.

Recommendations for Healthy Eating Patterns[12]

- Consume a variety of foods within and among the basic food groups while staying within calorie requirements.
- A healthy diet includes:
  - A variety of vegetables from all subgroups—dark green, red and orange, legumes (beans and peas), starchy, and other
  - Fruits, especially whole fruits
  - Grains, at least half of which are whole grains
  - Fat-free or low-fat dairy, including milk, yogurt, cheese, and/or fortified soy beverages
  - A variety of protein foods, including seafood, lean meats and poultry, eggs, legumes (beans and peas), and nuts, seeds, and soy products
  - Oils, monosaturated or unsaturated
- Limit saturated fats and *trans* fats, and added sugars.
- Limit sodium to 2,300 mg per day for children >14 years and older.
- If you drink alcoholic beverages, do so in moderation: one drink per day for women and two drinks per day for men.
- Maintain moderate physical activity for at least 30 minutes each day, for example, walking 3 to 4 miles per hour.

Assess adolescent females and women of childbearing age for adequate intake of iron and folic acid. Assist adults older than 50 years to identify foods rich in vitamin B_{12} and calcium. Advise older adults and those with dark skin or low exposure to sunlight to increase intake of vitamin D.

See Table 8-4 (p. 169).

Blood Pressure and Diet

With respect to blood pressure, there is reliable evidence that regular and frequent exercise, decreased sodium intake, increased potassium intake, and maintenance of a healthy weight reduce the risk for developing hypertension as well as lower blood pressure in adults who are already hypertensive. Explain to patients that most dietary sodium comes from salt (sodium chloride). The recommended daily allowance (RDA) of sodium is less than 2,300 mg, approximately 1 teaspoon, per day. However, individuals with hypertension, diabetes or chronic kidney disease, age of 51 years or older, or African-American ethnic heritage should consume no more than 1,500 mg sodium per day.[13] Patients need to read food labels closely, especially the Nutrition Facts panel. Low-sodium foods are those with sodium listed at less than 5% of the RDA of 2,400 mg or less. For nutritional interventions to reduce the risk for cardiac disease, refer to Chapter 14, The Cardiovascular System, pp. 421–422.

See Table 8-5 (p. 169).

Exercise

Fitness is a key component of both weight control and weight loss. Adults should do at least 2 hours and 30 minutes each week of aerobic physical activity at a moderate level OR 1 hour and 15 minutes each week of aerobic physical activity at a vigorous level—An example of moderate intensity activity is walking briskly, 3 miles in an hour or faster.[14] However, research has discovered that if a middle-aged or older woman with a normal body mass index wants to maintain her weight over an extended period, she must engage in the equivalent of 60 minutes per day of physical activity at a moderate intensity. Overweight women must restrict their caloric intake in addition to exercise to achieve weight loss.[15]

Patients can increase exercise by such simple measures as parking farther away from their place of work or using stairs instead of elevators. A safe goal for weight loss is ½ to 2 lb per week.

Moderate and Vigorous Exercise

A 154-lb man (5′10″) will use up about the number of calories listed doing each activity below. **Those who weigh more will use more calories, and those who weigh less will use fewer.** The calorie values listed include both calories used by the activity and calories used for normal body functioning.

	Approximate Calories Used by a 154-lb Man	
	In 1 hour	**In 30 minutes**
Moderate Physical Activities:		
Hiking	370	185
Light gardening/yard work	330	165
Dancing	330	165
Golf (walking and carrying clubs)	330	165
Bicycling (<10 miles per hour)	290	145
Walking (3½ miles per hour)	280	140
Weight training (general light workout)	220	110
Stretching	180	90
Vigorous Physical Activities:		
Running/jogging (5 miles per hour)	590	295
Bicycling (more than 10 miles per hour)	590	295
Swimming (slow freestyle laps)	510	255
Aerobics	480	240
Walking (4½ miles per hour)	460	230
Heavy yard work (chopping wood)	440	220
Weight lifting (vigorous effort)	440	220
Basketball (vigorous)	440	220

Source: U.S. Department of Agriculture: Inside the Pyramid—Calories Used. Available at http://www.choosemyplate.gov/physical-activity-calories-burn. Accessed September 30, 2015.

Hydration

According to the Report of the Dietary Guidelines Advisory Committee on the Dietary Guidelines for Americans, "In order to prevent dehydration, water must be consumed daily. Healthy individuals who have routine access to fluids and who are not exposed to heat stress consume adequate water to meet their needs." Purposeful drinking may be warranted for individuals who are exposed to heat stress or who perform sustained vigorous physical activity in extreme heat. Current guidelines recommend athletes use their thirst as a guide to regulate their intake of fluids, because purposeful over drinking of water or low-sodium sports drinks can lead to hyponatremia.[16] The older adult is at increased risk of morbidity and mortality from dehydration. In view of the ongoing obesity epidemic, individuals are encouraged to drink water and other fluids with few or no calories.

"Based on an extensive review of evidence, an Institute of Medicine (IOM) panel in 2004 concluded that the combination of thirst and usual drinking behavior, especially the consumption of fluids with meals, is sufficient to maintain normal hydration. However, because water needs vary considerably and because there is no evidence of chronic dehydration in the general population, a minimum intake of water cannot be set."[17]

Individuals with limited ability to obtain fluids for themselves, such as persons with disabilities, older adults in nursing homes, or persons confined to a bed, are at increased risk for dehydration. These patients' hydration status should be assessed at least daily and appropriate fluids provided.

TABLE
8-1

Eating Disorders and Excessively Low BMI

In the United States an estimated 5 to 10 million women and 1 million men suffer from eating disorders. These severe disturbances of eating behavior are often difficult to detect, especially in teens wearing baggy clothes or in individuals who binge and then induce vomiting or evacuation. Be familiar with the two principal eating disorders, anorexia nervosa and bulimia nervosa. Both conditions are characterized by distorted perceptions of body image and weight. Early detection is important, because prognosis improves when treatment occurs in the early stages of these disorders.

Clinical Features

Anorexia Nervosa

- Refusal to maintain minimally normal body weight (or BMI above 17.5)
- Afraid of appearing fat
- Frequently starving but in denial; lacking insight
- Often brought in by family members
- Initial symptoms may be failure to make expected weight gains in childhood or adolescence, amenorrhea in women, loss of libido or potency in men
- Associated with depressive symptoms such as depressed mood, irritability, social withdrawal, insomnia, decreased libido
- Additional features supporting diagnosis: self-induced vomiting or purging, excessive exercise, use of appetite suppressants and/or diuretics
- Biologic complications
  - *Gynecological:* amenorrhea
  - *Endocrine:* hypercortisolemia, hypoglycemia, osteoporosis, euthyroid hypothyroxinemia
  - *Cardiovascular disorders:* bradycardia, hypotension, arrhythmias, cardiomyopathy
  - *Metabolic disorders:* hypokalemia, hypochloremic metabolic alkalosis, increased BUN, edema
  - *Other:* dry skin, dental caries, delayed gastric emptying, constipation, anemia, osteoporosis

Bulimia Nervosa

- Repeated binge eating followed by self-induced vomiting; misuse of laxatives, diuretics, or other medications; fasting; or excessive exercise
- Often with normal weight
- Overeating at least twice a week during 3-month period; large amounts of food consumed in short period (~2 hours)
- Preoccupation with eating; craving and compulsion to eat; lack of control over eating; alternating with periods of starvation
- Dread of fatness but may be obese
- Subtypes of
  - *Purging:* bulimic episodes accompanied by self-induced vomiting or use of laxatives, diuretics, or enemas
  - *Nonpurging:* bulimic episodes accompanied by compensatory behavior such as fasting, exercise, but without purging
- Biologic complications

See changes listed for anorexia nervosa, especially weakness, fatigue, mild cognitive disorder; also erosion of dental enamel, parotid gland swelling, pancreatitis, mild neuropathies, seizures, hypokalemia, hypochloremic metabolic acidosis, hypomagnesemia

Sources: Hudson JI, Hiripi E, Pope HG Jr, Kessler RC. The prevalence and correlates of eating disorders in the National Comorbidity Survey Replication. *Biol Psychiatry.* 2007;61(3):348; World Health Organization. *The ICD-10 Classification of Mental and Behavioral Disorders: Diagnostic Criteria for Research.* Geneva: World Health Organization; 1993; American Psychiatric Association. *DSM-5: Diagnostic and Statistical Manual of Mental Disorders.* 5th ed. Washington, DC: American Psychiatric Association; 2013; Andersen AE. Eating disorders: In: Sadock BJ, Sadock VA, Ruiz P, eds. *Kaplan and Sadock's Comprehensive Textbook of Psychiatry.* 9th ed. New York: Wolters Kluwer; Lippincott Williams & Wilkins; 2009.

TABLE

8-2

Obesity-Related Risk Factors and Diseases

Cardiovascular
- Hypertension
- Congestive heart failure
- Cor pulmonale
- Varicose veins
- Pulmonary embolism
- Coronary artery disease

Endocrine
- The metabolic syndrome
- Type 2 diabetes
- Dyslipidemia
- Polycystic ovarian syndrome/androgenicity
- Amenorrhea/infertility/menstrual disorders

Gastrointestinal
- Gastroesophageal reflux disease (GERD)
- Nonalcoholic fatty liver disease (NAFLD)
- Cholelithiasis
- Hernias
- Cancer: colon, pancreas, esophagus, liver

Genitourinary
- Urinary stress incontinence
- Obesity-related glomerulopathy
- Hypogonadism (male)
- Cancer: breast, cervical, ovarian, uterine pregnancy complications
- Nephrolithiasis, chronic renal disease

Integument
- Striae distensae (stretch marks)
- Status pigmentation of legs
- Lymphedema
- Cellulitis
- Intertrigo, carbuncles
- Acanthosis nigricans/skin tags

Musculoskeletal
- Hyperuricemia and gout
- Immobility
- Osteoarthritis (knees, hips)
- Low back pain

Neurologic
- Stroke
- Idiopathic intracranial hypertension
- Meralgia paresthetica

Psychological
- Depression/low self-esteem
- Body image disturbance
- Social stigmatization

Respiratory
- Dyspnea
- Obstructive sleep apnea
- Hypoventilation syndrome
- Hypoventilation syndrome/pickwickian syndrome
- Pulmonary embolism
- Asthma

Source: Kushner RF. *Roadmaps for Clinical Practice: Case Studies in Disease Prevention and Health Promotion—Assessment and Management of Adult Obesity: A Primer for Physicians.* Chicago, IL: American Medical Association; 2003.

TABLE 8-3

Obesity: Stages of Change Model and Assessing Readiness

Stage	Characteristic	Patient Verbal Cue	Appropriate Intervention	Sample Dialogue
Precontemplation	Unaware of problem, no interest in change	"I'm not really interested in weight loss. It's not a problem."	Provide information about health risks and benefits of weight loss	"Would you like to read some information about the health aspects of obesity?"
Contemplation	Aware of problem, beginning to think of changing	"I know I need to lose weight, but with all that's going on in my life right now, I'm not sure I can."	Help resolve ambivalence; discuss barriers	"Let's look at the benefits of weight loss, as well as what you may need to change."
Preparation	Realizes benefits of making changes and thinking about how to change	"I have to lose weight, and I'm planning to do that."	Teach behavior modification; provide education	"Let's take a closer look at how you can reduce some of the calories you eat and how to increase your activity during the day."
Action	Actively taking steps toward change	"I'm doing my best. This is harder than I thought."	Provide support and guidance, with a focus on the long term	"It's terrific that you're working so hard. What problems have you had so far? How have you solved them?"
Maintenance	Initial treatment goals reached	"I've learned a lot through this process."	Relapse control	"What situations continue to tempt you to overeat? What can be helpful for the next time you face such a situation?"

Sources: American Medical Association. Roadmaps for Clinical Practice—Case Studies in Disease Prevention and Health Promotion—Assessment and Management of Adult Obesity: A Primer for Physicians. Communication and Counseling Strategies. Booklet 8. Chicago, November 2003. Adapted from Prochaska JO, DiClemente CC. Toward a comprehensive model of change. In: Miller WR, ed. *Treating Addictive Behaviors*. New York: Plenum; 1986:3–27.

TABLE 8-4 Nutrition Counseling: Sources of Nutrients

Nutrient	Food Source
Calcium	Dairy foods such as yogurt, milk, and natural cheeses Breakfast cereal, fruit juice with calcium supplements Dark green leafy vegetables such as collards, turnip, and mustard greens; kale; bok choy sardines
Iron	Clams, mussels, oysters, sardines, anchovies Lean meat, dark turkey meat Iron-fortified cereals Spinach, peas, lentils, turnip greens, artichokes Enriched and whole-grain bread Dried prunes and raisins
Folate	Cooked dried beans and peas Oranges, orange juice Dark-green leafy vegetables; spinach, mustard greens Liver Black-eyed peas, lentils, okra, chick peas, peanuts Folate fortified cereals
Vitamin D	Vitamin D–fortified milk, orange juice, and cereals Cod liver oil; swordfish, salmon, herring, mackerel, tuna, trout Egg yolk Mushrooms

Source: Adapted from U.S. Department of Health and Human Services and U.S. Department of Agriculture. *2015–2020 Dietary Guidelines for Americans.* 8th ed.. December 2015. Available at http://health.gov/dietaryguidelines/2015/guidelines/; Choose MyPlate.gov. Available at http://www.choosemyplate.gov/index.html. Accessed September 30, 2015; Office of Dietary Supplements, National Institutes of Health. *Dietary Supplement Fact Sheets: Calcium; Vitamin D.* Available at http://ods.od.nih.gov/factsheets/list-all/. Accessed September 30, 2015.

TABLE 8-5 Patients With Hypertension: Recommended Changes in Diet

Dietary Change	Food Source
Increase foods high in potassium	Baked white or sweet potatoes, cooked greens such as spinach Bananas, plantains, many dried fruits, orange juice
Decrease foods high in sodium	Canned foods (soups, tuna fish) Pretzels, potato chips, pickles, olives Many processed foods (frozen dinners, ketchup, mustard) Batter-fried foods Table salt, including for cooking

Source: Adapted from U.S. Department of Health and Human Services and U.S. Department of Agriculture. *2015–2020 Dietary Guidelines for Americans.* 8th ed. December 2015. Available at http://health.gov/dietaryguidelines/2015/guidelines/

BIBLIOGRAPHY

CITATIONS

1. National Heart Lung, and Blood Institute (NHLBI). Managing Overweight and Obesity in Adults: Systematic Evidence Review from the Obesity Expert Panel: The Evidence Report. April 2014. Available at http://www.nhlbi.nih.gov/health-pro/guidelines/in-develop/obesity-evidence-review. Accessed February 14, 2016.

2. National Institutes of Health and National Heart, Lung, and Blood Institute. Calculate Body Mass Index. Available at http://www.nhlbi.nih.gov/health/educational/wecan/healthy-weight-basics/body-mass-index.htm. Accessed October 2, 2015.

3. Go AS, Mozaffarian D, Roger VL, et al. Heart disease and stroke statistics—2014 update: a report from the American Heart Association. *Circulation*. 2014;129(3):e28–e292.

4. Ogden CL, Carroll MD, Kit BK, et al. Prevalence of childhood and adult obesity in the United States, 2011–2012. *JAMA*. 2014;311(8):806–814.

5. May AL, Freedman D, Sherry B, et al. Obesity—United States, 1999–2010. *MMWR Surveill Summ*. 2013;62(Suppl 3):120–128.

6. NHLBI. Why Obesity Is a Health Problem. Available at http://www.nhlbi.nih.gov/health/educational/wecan/healthy-weight-basics/obesity.htm. Accessed October 2, 2015.

7. CDC. Division of Nutrition, Physical Activity, and Obesity. Overweight and Obesity. Available at http://www.cdc.gov/obesity/data/index.html. Accessed February 18, 2016.

8. CDC. Diabetes Public Health Resource: Age-Adjusted Percentage of Adults Aged 18 Years or Older with Diagnosed Diabetes Who Were Overweight, United States, 1994–2010. Available at http://www.cdc.gov/diabetes/statistics/comp/fig7_overweight.htm. Accessed October 2, 2015.

9. Ng M, Fleming T, Robinson M, et al. Global, regional, and national prevalence of overweight and obesity in children and adults during 1980–2013: a systematic analysis for the Global Burden of Disease Study 2013. *Lancet*. 2014;384(9945):766–781.

10. Schauer GL, Halperin AC, Mancl LA, et al. Health professional advice for smoking and weight in adults with and without diabetes: findings from BRFSS. *J Behav Med*. 2013;36:10.

11. CDC. Division of Nutrition, Physical Activity, and Obesity. Losing weight: What is a healthy weight loss? Available at www.cdc.gov.healthyweight/losing_weight/index.html. Accessed May 4, 2016.

12. U.S. Department of Health and Human Services and U.S. Department of Agriculture. Dietary Guidelines for Americans 2015–2020. Available at http://www.cnpp.usda.gov/2015–2020-dietary-guidelines-americans. February 13, 2016.

13. Center for Disease Control and Prevention. CDC Features: Most Americans Should Consume Less Sodium (1,500 mg./Day or Less). Available at http://www.cdc.gov/salt/index.htm. Accessed September 30, 2015.

14. ChooseMyPlate Physical Activity. Available at http://www.choosemyplate.gov/physical-activity-amount. Accessed September 30, 2015.

15. Lee I-M, Djoussé L, Sesso HD, et al. Physical activity and weight gain prevention. *JAMA*. 2010;303(12):1173–1179.

16. Hew-Butler T, Rosner MH, Fowkes-Godek S, et al. Statement of the Third International Exercise-Associated Hyponatremia Consensus Development Conference, Carlsbad, California, 2015. *Clin J Sport Med*. 2015;25:303–320.

17. Report of the Dietary Guidelines Advisory Committee on the Dietary Guidelines for Americans, Part D, Section 6: Sodium, Potassium, and Water 2010. Available at http://origin.www.cnpp.usda.gov/Publications/DietaryGuidelines/2010/DGAC/Report/D-6-SodiumPotassiumWater.pdf. Accessed October 2, 2015.

ADDITIONAL REFERENCES

Budd GM, Peterson JA. The obesity epidemic, Part 1: Understanding the origins. *Am J Nurs*. 2014;114(12):40–45.

Budd GM, Peterson JA. The obesity epidemic, Part 2: Nursing assessment and intervention. *Am J Nurs*. 2015;115(1):38–46.

Freitag E, Edgecombe G, Baldwin I, et al. Determination of body weight and height measurement for critically ill patients admitted to the intensive care unit: A quality improvement project. *Aust Crit Care*. 2010;23:197—207.

Gaffney KF, Kitsantas P, Brito A, et al. Baby Steps in the Prevention of Childhood Obesity: IOM Guidelines for Pediatric Practice. *J Pediatr Nurs*. 2014;29(2):108–113.

Malone SK, Lipman TH. The Significance of Abdominal Obesity in Youth. *J Pediatr Nurs*. 2014;29(5):489–490.

U.S. Preventative Services Task Force. Final Recommendation Statement: *Obesity in Adults: Screening and Management*. June 2012. Available at http://www.uspreventiveservicestaskforce.org/Page/Document/RecommendationStatementFinal/obesity-in-adults-screening-and-management. Accessed February 13, 2016.

UNIT 2 Body Systems

The Integumentary System

The student will:

1. Identify the structures of the skin, nails, and hair.
2. Explain the functions of the integumentary system.
3. Identify risk factors for pressure ulcers.
4. Identify risk factors for skin cancer.
5. Obtain an accurate history of the integumentary system.
6. Appropriately prepare and position the patient for the integumentary examination.
7. Describe the equipment necessary to perform an integumentary examination.
8. Correctly perform an integumentary examination.
9. Accurately describe primary, secondary, and vascular lesions.
10. Discuss risk reduction and health promotion strategies to reduce skin cancer.

Intact and functioning skin is essential for the life and health of the patient. The skin is the largest and heaviest organ of the body, accounting for approximately 16% of body weight and covering an area of roughly 1.2 to 2.3 m^2.

Nursing assessment of the integumentary system is frequently superficial, unless the patient has a significant problem, such as third-degree burns. A thorough integumentary assessment requires time; turning heavy, unconscious, or uncooperative patients in order to perform the assessment may be difficult during a busy shift. For the nurse, assessment of the skin is much more than discovering skin lesions or diseases. Examination of the skin can reveal signs of systemic diseases, medication side effects, dehydration, overhydration, or physical abuse; allow early identification of potentially cancerous lesions and risk factors for pressure ulcer formation; and identify the need for hygiene and health promotion education.

ANATOMY AND PHYSIOLOGY

The skin keeps the body in homeostasis despite daily assaults from the environment. The skin

1. **provides a barrier** protecting the body from

   a. injury secondary to mechanical, chemical, thermal, and ultraviolet (UV) light sources.

   b. penetration by microorganisms.

   c. loss of water and electrolytes, thereby preventing dehydration.

2. **regulates body temperature** by allowing heat dissipation through sweat glands and heat storage through subcutaneous insulation.

3. **synthesizes vitamin D** from cholesterol by the action of UV light.

4. **allows sensory perception** via end sensory organs for touch, pain, temperature, and pressure.

5. **provides nonverbal communication,** such as posture, facial movements, or vasomotor responses such as blushing.

6. **provides identity** through skin color and facial features.

7. **allows wound repair** through cell replacement of surface injuries.

8. **allows excretion of metabolic wastes,** such as electrolytes, minerals, sugar, or uric acid.

Hair, nails, and sebaceous and sweat glands are considered appendages of the skin. The skin and its appendages undergo many changes during aging. Turn to Chapter 24, Assessing Older Adults (pp. 930–931), to review normal and abnormal changes of the skin with aging.

Skin

The skin contains three layers: the epidermis, the dermis, and the subcutaneous tissues.

The most superficial layer, the *epidermis,* is thin, devoid of blood vessels, and itself divided into two layers: an outer horny layer of dead keratinized cells and

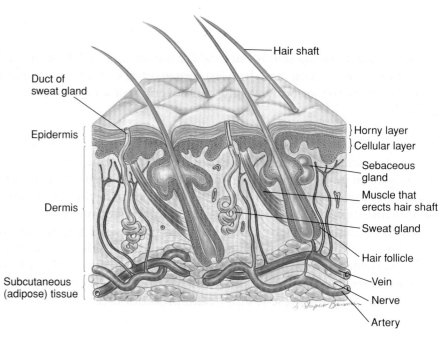

Labels: Hair shaft, Duct of sweat gland, Epidermis, Horny layer, Cellular layer, Sebaceous gland, Muscle that erects hair shaft, Dermis, Sweat gland, Hair follicle, Vein, Subcutaneous (adipose) tissue, Nerve, Artery

an inner cellular layer where both melanin and keratin are formed. Migration from the inner layer to the top layer takes approximately 1 month.

The epidermis depends on the underlying *dermis* for its nutrition. The dermis is well supplied with blood. It contains connective tissue, sebaceous glands, sweat glands, and hair follicles. It merges below with *subcutaneous,* or *adipose tissue,* also known as fat.

The color of healthy skin depends primarily on four pigments: melanin, carotene, oxyhemoglobin, and deoxyhemoglobin. The amount of *melanin,* the brownish pigment of the skin, is genetically determined and is increased by exposure to sunlight. *Carotene* is a golden yellow pigment that exists in subcutaneous fat and in heavily keratinized areas such as the palms and soles.

Another yellow color in the skin may be jaundice, due to deposition of bilirubin in the skin. Liver disease, biliary duct obstruction, or increased destruction of red blood cells increases serum bilirubin, which is then deposited in the skin. Jaundice is easiest to observe in the sclera, nails, palms, and soles. See Chapter 16, The Gastrointestinal and Renal Systems, for further discussion of jaundice.

Hemoglobin, which circulates in the red cells and carries most of the oxygen of the blood, exists in two forms. *Oxyhemoglobin,* a bright red pigment, predominates in the arteries and capillaries. An increase in blood flow through the arteries to the capillaries causes a reddening of the skin (e.g., with blushing), whereas the opposite change usually produces pallor. The skin of light-colored people is normally redder on the palms, soles, face, neck, and upper chest.

As blood passes through the capillary bed, oxyhemoglobin loses its oxygen to the tissues and changes to *deoxyhemoglobin*—a darker and somewhat bluer pigment. An increased concentration of deoxyhemoglobin in cutaneous blood vessels gives the skin a bluish cast known as *cyanosis.*

Cyanosis is of two kinds. If the oxygen level in the arterial blood is low, cyanosis is *central* and indicates decreased oxygenation in the patient. If the oxygen level is normal, cyanosis is *peripheral.* Peripheral cyanosis occurs when cutaneous blood flow decreases and slows, and tissues extract more oxygen than usual from the blood. Peripheral cyanosis may be a response to anxiety or a cold environment.

Skin color is also affected by the scattering of light reflected back through the cloudy superficial layers of the skin or vessel walls. This scattering makes the color look more blue and less red. The bluish color of a subcutaneous vein results from this effect; it appears much bluer than the venous blood obtained on venipuncture.

Hair

Adults have two types of hair: *vellus hair,* which is short, fine, inconspicuous, and relatively unpigmented; and *terminal hair,* which is coarser, thicker, more conspicuous, and usually pigmented. Scalp hair and eyebrows are examples of terminal hair.

Nails

Nails protect the distal ends of the fingers and toes. The firm, rectangular, and usually curving *nail plate* gets its pink color from the vascular *nail bed* to which the plate is firmly attached. Note the white moon, or *lunula*, and the white free edge of the nail plate. Roughly one fourth of the nail plate (the *nail root*) is covered by the proximal nail fold. The *cuticle* extends from the fold and, functioning as a seal, protects the space between the fold and the plate from external moisture. *Lateral nail folds* cover the sides of the nail plate. Note that the angle between the proximal nail fold and nail plate is normally less than 180 degrees.

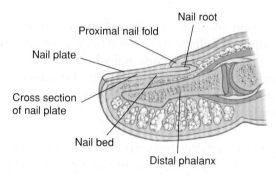

Fingernails grow approximately 0.1 mm daily; toenails grow more slowly.

Sebaceous Glands and Sweat Glands

Sebaceous glands produce sebum, a fatty substance secreted onto the skin surface through the hair follicles. These glands are present on all skin surfaces except the palms and soles. The sebum lubricates hair and skin and reduces water loss through the skin.

Sweat glands are of two types: eccrine and apocrine. The *eccrine glands* are widely distributed, open directly onto the skin surface, and by their sweat production help to control body temperature. In contrast, the *apocrine glands* are found chiefly in the axillary and genital regions, usually open into hair follicles, and are stimulated by emotional stress. Bacterial decomposition of apocrine sweat is responsible for adult body odor.

THE HEALTH HISTORY

The purpose of the integumentary history is to identify the following:

Diseases of the skin
Systemic diseases that have skin manifestations
Physical abuse
Risk for pressure ulcer formation
Risk for skin cancer
Need for health promotion education regarding the skin

Common or Concerning Symptoms	
Rash	Lesions
Nonhealing lesions	Bruising (ecchymosis)
Moles	Hair loss
Growths	Nail changes

The patient with an integumentary issue will frequently state the problem when asked the purpose of the visit. The nurse can use the OLD CART mnemonic to ask follow-up questions in order to obtain a full description of the condition. For example, if the patient reports a rash, ask:

Onset: When did it start?
   Have you started any new medications or changed existing medications?
   Have you been out of the country recently?
   Have you ever had similar symptoms in the past?
Location: Where is it located?
   Has it changed size or spread to another part of your body?
Duration: How long have you had the rash?
   Does it come and go?
Characteristic symptoms: Describe your rash.
   What did it first look like?
   Has it changed?
Associated manifestations: Does it itch?
   Is there any discharge?
Relieving/exacerbating factors: Have you used or done anything that seems to make it better? Does anything make it worse?
Treatment: Have you put anything on it to treat it?

If the patient does not offer a specific complaint, be sure to ask about each of the symptoms above. Start with broad open-ended questions:

"Have you noticed any changes in your skin? Your hair? Your nails?"
"Have you had any rashes? Sores? Lumps? Itching?"

Even subtle changes in moles or skin lesions may indicate cancerous changes and need follow-up. Ask, "Have you noticed any moles you are concerned about or that have changed at all?" "Any new moles?" If the patient reports such moles, ask how they have changed and pursue any personal or family history of melanoma or skin cancer.

Many contagious diseases present with skin rashes, for example, rubeola, rubella, and varicella.

Past History

Do you have any skin diseases such as melanoma, eczema, or psoriasis?
Do you have diabetes or peripheral vascular disease?
Do you have any allergies or food sensitivities?
Have you ever had a severe sunburn? How many second-degree sunburns have you experienced?

Have you ever been on corticosteroid medications for more than 2 weeks?
What prescribed or over-the-counter medications do you take?
What immunizations have you had?

Family History

Do any family members have the same or similar symptoms?
Has anyone in your family had melanoma, eczema, or psoriasis or skin biopsies?
Does anyone in your family have allergies?

Lifestyle and Personal Habits

Describe your bathing and shampooing routines. Have you changed product brands recently?
Do you wear false nails or wigs?
Do you go to a nail salon or gym?
How much sun exposure do you receive daily?
How often do you use sunscreen? What SPF value of sunscreen do you use?
Do you perform skin self-examinations? How often?
Are you exposed to any chemicals or radiation at home or work?
What are your hobbies?
Describe a typical day's diet.

PHYSICAL EXAMINATION

Equipment for Examination	
Good lighting	Magnifying glass
Ruler or measuring tape	Gloves

The examination of the skin, hair, and nails begins with the General Survey and continues throughout the physical examination. Make sure the patient wears a gown that allows close inspection of all anterior and posterior skin surfaces. A sheet can be used to maintain privacy and cover the parts of the body not being examined. Wash your hands and explain the examination to the patient.

Inspect the entire skin surface in good light, preferably natural light or artificial light that resembles it. Correlate your findings with observations of the mucous membranes, especially when assessing skin color, because diseases may appear in both areas. Techniques for examining these membranes are described in Chapter 11, The Eyes, and Chapter 12, Ears, Nose, Mouth and Throat.

To sharpen your observations, turn to the tables at the end of the chapter to better identify skin colors and patterns and types of lesions that you may encounter during the examination.

Patients at risk for skin cancer, may not request a skin examination, so the general physical examination is an important opportunity to look for melanomas and other skin cancers, especially in hard to see areas such as the back and posterior legs.

Artificial light often distorts colors and masks jaundice.

Skin

Inspect and palpate the skin. Note these characteristics:

Color. Skin color will vary according to genetic background and may have fair, olive, tan, brown, or golden hues. Color change may be general, affecting all the skin or localized, confined to an area, for example, the right forearm. Patients may notice a change in their skin color before the nurse does. Ask about it.

Look for increased pigmentation (brownness), loss of pigmentation, or redness of the skin. Is it generalized or local? If local, indicate its location.

See Table 9-1, Skin Color Changes, p. 193.

Assess for cyanosis or pallor. Look for the red color of oxyhemoglobin versus the pallor in its absence. These are best observed where the horny layer of the epidermis is thinnest and causes the least scatter: the fingernails, the lips, and the mucous membranes, particularly those of the mouth and the palpebral conjunctiva. In dark-skinned people, inspecting the palms and soles may also be useful.

Pallor results from decreased redness in *anemia* and decreased blood flow, as occurs in fainting or arterial insufficiency.

Central cyanosis is best identified in the lips, oral mucosa, and tongue. The lips, however, may turn blue in the cold, and melanin in the lips may simulate cyanosis in darker-skinned people.

Causes of *central cyanosis* include advanced lung disease, congenital heart disease, and hemoglobinopathies.

Cyanosis of the nails, hands, and feet may be central or peripheral in origin. Anxiety or a cold examining room may cause peripheral cyanosis.

Cyanosis in *congestive heart failure* is usually peripheral, reflecting decreased blood flow, but in *pulmonary edema*, it may also be central. *Venous obstruction* may cause peripheral cyanosis.

Look for the yellow color of jaundice in the sclera. Do not confuse a normal scleral yellow pigmentation in dark-skinned individuals with jaundice. Rather, observe the hard palate with a bright light for jaundice. Jaundice may also appear in the palpebral conjunctiva, lips, hard palate, undersurface of the tongue, tympanic membrane, and skin. Pressing the skin over a bony prominence and observing the color when your finger is removed will accentuate the yellow hue.

Jaundice suggests liver disease or excessive hemolysis of red blood cells.

For the yellow color that accompanies high levels of carotene, look at the palms, soles, and face.

Carotenemia. See Table 9-1, Skin Color Changes, p. 193.

Moisture. Note excessive dryness, sweating, and oiliness. Skin should be dry to touch without flaking or cracking. Perspiration may appear on the face, hands, axillae, or skin folds in response to a warm environment; increased metabolic activity, such as fever or exercise; and anxiety or pain. Excessive dryness, often accompanied by flaking, or excessive sweating (diaphoresis) may indicate a problem. Carefully inspect skin folds where moisture may cause skin breakdown.

Dryness in hypothyroidism; oiliness in acne. Dry skin with parched cracked lips, dry mucous membranes, and lack of tears indicate dehydration.

Temperature. Use the backs of your hands to make this assessment. In addition to identifying generalized warmth or coolness of the skin, note the temperature of any areas with increased pigmentation or erythema.

Generalized warmth in fever, *hyperthyroidism;* coolness in *hypothyroidism.* Local warmth of inflammation or cellulitis.

Texture. Note the roughness or smoothness of the skin. Normal skin feels smooth and firm with an even surface.

Roughness in *hypothyroidism;* velvety texture in *hyperthyroidism.*

Mobility and Turgor. Lift a fold of skin below the clavicle, the forearm, or on the abdomen and note the ease with which it lifts up (mobility) and the speed with which it returns into place (turgor). Normally the skin promptly returns into place.

Do not test turgor on the dorsal surface of the hand in the older adult, this will result in a false-positive finding due to loss of subcutaneous tissue.

Decreased mobility in edema, *scleroderma;* decreased turgor in dehydration.

Edema. The presence of excess fluid in the interstitial spaces is edema. It may be localized due to an injury or may be the result of a systemic problem (e.g., heart failure). Systemic edema most often occurs in the dependent portions of the body, the feet, legs, and sacral area. The skin appears puffy and feels tight. Mobility is decreased and cyanosis or jaundice in the skin is obscured.

Edema may be pitting or nonpitting. In pitting edema the interstitial water is mobile and can be translocated with the pressure exerted by a finger. A "pit" or depression is left for 5 to 30 seconds. The degree of pitting is measured on a 1 to 4 scale.

See Chapter 15, The Peripheral Vascular System and Lymphatic System, for a further discussion of edema.

Scale	Depression
1+	2 mm
2+	4 mm
3+	6 mm
4+	8 mm

Nonpitting edema reflects a condition in which serum proteins have accumulated in the interstitial space with the water and coagulated. This is frequently seen with local infection or trauma and is called brawny edema.

Lesions. Inspect the skin for lesions. A lesion is a circumscribed pathologic alteration of the skin. Lesions may be classified as primary (*initial lesions*), secondary (*lesions that arise from primary lesions*) and vascular lesions. Document the following characteristics of any lesion(s).

See Table 9-4, Primary Skin Lesions, pp. 196–198.

Table 9-5, Secondary Skin Lesions, p. 199.

Table 9-6, Secondary Skin Lesions—Depressed, p. 200.

Table 9-7, Acne Vulgaris—Primary and Secondary Lesions, p. 201.

Table 9-8, Vascular and Purpuric Lesions of the Skin, p. 202.

(a) ***Color.*** Is the color uniform or variegated?

- Use "skin-colored" to describe a lesion that is the same shade as the patient's skin.

- For red lesions or rashes, blanch the lesion by pressing it firmly with your finger or a glass slide to see if the redness temporarily blanches then refills.

Blanching lesions are *erythematous* and suggest inflammation.

(b) ***Size.*** Measure with a ruler in millimeters or centimeters. For oval lesions, measure in the long axis then perpendicular to the axis.

(c) ***Elevation.*** Flat, *cannot palpate the lesion with eyes closed.* Raised, or pedunculated (attached to a stalk, e.g., a skin tag).

(d) ***Number.*** Can be solitary, multiple, or if multiple, how many. Also consider estimating the total number of the type of lesion you are describing.

(e) ***Texture.*** Palpate the lesion to see if it is smooth, fleshy, verrucous or warty, or scaling (keratotic).

Scaling can be greasy, like *seborrheic dermatitis* or *seborrheic keratoses,* dry and fine like *tinea pedis,* or hard and keratotic like *actinic keratoses* or *squamous cell carcinoma.*

(f) ***Type of skin lesions*** (e.g., macules, papules, vesicles, nevi).

(g) ***Shape and Pattern.*** Are they round, oval, linear, clustered, annular (in a ring), arciform (in an arc), bulls-eye, geographic, or serpiginous (serpent- or worm-like)? Are they dermatomal, covering a skin band that corresponds to a sensory nerve root (*dermatome*). See Chapter 20, The Nervous System, pp. 701–703.

Vesicles in a unilateral dermatomal pattern are typical of herpes zoster. See Table 9-3, Skin Lesions—Patterns and Shapes, p. 195.

(h) ***Anatomic location and distribution*** over the body. Are they generalized or localized? Do they, for example, involve the exposed surfaces, the intertriginous or skin-fold areas, extensor or flexor areas, or acral (peripheral) areas? Do they involve areas exposed to specific allergens or irritants, such as wrist bands, rings, or industrial chemicals?

Many skin diseases have typical distributions. *Acne* affects the face, upper chest, and back; *psoriasis,* the knees and elbows (among other areas); and *Candida* infections, the intertriginous areas. See Table 9-2, Skin Lesions—Anatomic Location and Distribution, p. 194.

Evaluating the Patient With Decreased Mobility

People with decreased mobility or who are hospitalized, especially when they are emaciated, elderly, or neurologically impaired, are particularly susceptible to skin damage and ulceration. *Pressure sores* result when sustained compression obliterates arteriolar and capillary blood flow to the skin. Sores may also result from the shearing forces created by bodily movements. When a person slides down in bed from a partially sitting position or is dragged rather than lifted up from a supine position, for example, the movements may distort the soft tissues of the buttocks and close off the arteries and arterioles. Friction and moisture further increase the risk.

Assess every patient by carefully inspecting the skin that overlies the sacrum, buttocks, greater trochanters, knees, and heels. Roll the patient onto one side to see the sacrum and buttocks. Inspect the skin folds where moisture promotes maceration and skin breakdown.

It is easier to prevent pressure ulcers than heal them. Every patient with decreased mobility and all hospitalized patients should be assessed for the risk factors that lead to pressure ulcers. The risk factors may then be mitigated to prevent pressure ulcers. The Braden Scale is a simple effective tool that evaluates levels of risk for ulcer development in the patient. With its high reliability, predictive validity, and ease of use, the Braden Scale can be used to assess patients as often as every shift if needed.[1,2] Six factors are rated using a matrix scoring system: sensory perception, moisture, activity, mobility, nutrition, and friction and shear. A lower score indicates that the patient has a lower functional level and is at higher risk for ulcer formation. Levels of risk for developing pressure ulcers are rated according to the following scores:

- 19 to 23: not at risk

- 15 to 18: mild risk

- 13 to 14: moderate risk

- 10 to 12: high risk

- 9 or lower: very high risk

See pp. 184–185 for Braden Scale.

Concept Mastery Alert

Improved patient outcomes related to pressure ulcers is crucial. If a patient develops a pressure ulcer but it does not show signs of healing, the nurse must first evaluate the client's current outcomes and the current measures being used to determine which measures are effective and which are ineffective. Then the nurse needs to revise the patient's plan of care, modifying or adjusting the ineffective measures to meet the patient's needs and thus improve the patient's outcome.

See Table 9-12, Pressure Ulcers, p. 206.

Local redness of the skin warns of impending necrosis, although some deep pressure sores develop without antecedent redness. Ulcers may be seen.

Hair

Inspect and palpate the hair. Note its quantity, distribution, and texture.

Alopecia refers to hair loss—diffuse, patchy, or total. Sparse hair is seen in *hypothyroidism;* fine, silky hair in *hyperthyroidism.* See Table 9-13, Hair Loss, p. 207.

The color of hair depends on the amount of melanin present and varies from pale blond to black. Graying occurs with aging and may begin in the 20s. Texture varies from silky fine to coarse and thick, straight to varying degrees of curly. As people age, hair tends to feel coarser and drier. However, if such changes occur over a few weeks or months, it may indicate a systemic disease or poor nutrition.

The amount of hair tends to decrease with aging in both men and women. Male pattern baldness is considered a normal change. See Table 9-13, Hair Loss, p. 207.

Inspect the scalp for lesions, flaking, and parasites by separating the hair at 1-inch to 2-inch intervals with your fingers or a swab.

Inspect the body, axillae, and pubic hair for amount and distribution as well as parasites. Loss of hair on the legs may indicate peripheral artery disease, while changes in pubic or axilla hair may indicate hormonal problems.

Nails

Inspect and palpate the fingernails and toenails. Note their color and shape and any lesions. Nails should be pink with white lunulae; smooth and firm in texture; rounded in shape with a 160-degree angle between the nail base and skin; and firmly attached to the nail bed. Longitudinal bands of pigment may be seen in the nails of people who have darker skin.

See Table 9-14, pp. 208–209.

Normal angle 160 degrees

Swollen, springy, floating

Angle greater than 160 degrees

Normal angle

Clubbing

Braden Scale for Predicting Pressure Sore Risk

Patient's Name _____   Evaluator's Name _____   Date of Assessment _____

	1	2	3	4
SENSORY PERCEPTION Ability to respond meaningfully to pressure-related discomfort	**1. Completely Limited** Unresponsive (does not moan, flinch, or grasp) to painful stimuli, due to diminished level of consciousness or sedation OR limited ability to feel pain over most of body.	**2. Very Limited** Responds only to painful stimuli. Cannot communicate discomfort except by moaning or restlessness OR has a sensory impairment which limits the ability to feel pain or discomfort over half of body.	**3. Slightly Limited** Responds to verbal commands, but cannot always communicate discomfort of the need to be turned. OR has some sensory impairment which limits ability to feel pain or discomfort in 1 or 2 extremities.	**4. No Impairment** Responds to verbal commands. Has no sensory deficit which would limit ability to feel or voice pain or discomfort.
MOISTURE Degree to which skin is exposed to moisture	**1. Constantly Moist** Skin is kept moist almost constantly by perspiration, urine, etc. Dampness is detected every time patient is moved or turned.	**2. Very Moist** Skin is often, but not always moist. Linen must be changed at least once a shift.	**3. Occasionally Moist** Skin is occasionally moist, requiring an extra linen change approximately once a day.	**4. Rarely Moist** Skin is usually dry. Linen only requires changing at routine intervals.
ACTIVITY Degree of physical activity	**1. Bedfast** Confined to bed.	**2. Chairfast** Ability to walk severely limited or nonexistent. Cannot bear own weight and/or must be assisted into chair or wheelchair.	**3. Walks Occasionally** Walks occasionally during day, but for very short distances, with or without assistance. Spends majority of each shift in bed or chair.	**4. Walks Frequently** Walks outside room at least twice a day and inside room at least once every 2 hours during waking hours.
MOBILITY Ability to change and control body position	**1. Completely Immobile** Does not make even slight changes in body or extremity position without assistance.	**2. Very Limited** Makes occasional slight changes in body or extremity position but unable to make frequent or significant changes independently.	**3. Slightly Limited** Makes frequent though slight changes in body or extremity position independently.	**4. No Limitation** Makes major and frequent changes in position without assistance.

	1. Very Poor	2. Probably Inadequate	3. Adequate	4. Excellent
NUTRITION Usual food intake pattern	Never eats a complete meal. Rarely eats more than half of any food offered. Eats 2 servings or less of protein (meat or dairy products) per day. Takes fluids poorly. Does not take a liquid dietary supplement OR Is NPO and/or maintained on clear liquids or IVs for more than 5 days.	Rarely eats a complete meal and generally eats only about half of any food offered. Protein intake includes only 3 servings of meat or dairy products per day. Occasionally will take a dietary supplement. OR Receives less than optimum amount of liquid diet or tube feeding.	Eats over half of most meals. Eats a total of 4 servings of protein (meat, dairy products) per day. Occasionally will refuse a meal, but will usually take a supplement when offered OR Is on a tube feeding or TPN regimen which probably meets most nutritional needs.	Eats most of every meal. Never refuses a meal. Usually eats a total of 4 or more servings of meat and dairy products. Occasionally eats between meals. Does not require supplementation.
	1. Problem	2. Potential Problem	3. No Apparent Problem	
FRICTION AND SHEAR	Requires moderate to maximum assistance in moving. Complete lifting without sliding against sheets is impossible. Frequently slides down in bed or chair, requiring frequent repositioning with maximum assistance. Spasticity, contractures, or agitation leads to almost constant friction.	Moves feebly or requires minimum assistance. During a move skin probably slides to some extent against sheets, chair, restraints, or other devices. Maintains relatively good position in chair or bed most of the time but occasionally slides down.	Moves in bed and in chair independently and has sufficient muscle strength to lift up completely during move. Maintains good position in bed or chair.	

Total Score _____

RECORDING YOUR FINDINGS

Note that initially you may use sentences to describe your findings; later you will use phrases. The style below contains phrases appropriate for most write-ups.

Recording the Physical Examination—The Skin

"Color pink. Skin warm and moist. Nails without clubbing or cyanosis. No suspicious nevi. No rash, petechiae, or ecchymoses."

OR

"Marked facial pallor, with circumoral cyanosis. Palms cold and moist. Cyanosis in nailbeds of fingers and toes. One raised blue-black nevus, 1 × 2 cm, with irregular border on right forearm. No rash."

Suggests central cyanosis and possible melanoma

OR

"Facial ruddiness. Skin icteric. 3 spider angiomas over anterior torso. Palmar erythema. Single pearly papule with depressed center and telangi-ectasias, 1 × 1 cm, on posterior neck above collarline. No suspicious nevi. Nails with clubbing but no cyanosis."

Suggests possible liver disease and basal cell carcinoma

HEALTH PROMOTION AND COUNSELING

Important Topics for Health Promotion and Counseling

* Skin cancer prevention
* Risk factors for skin cancers
* Avoidance of excessive sun exposure and artificial tanning lamps
* Use of sunscreen

Nurses play an important role in educating patients about early detection of suspicious moles, protective measures for skin care, and the hazards of excessive sun exposure. Skin cancers are the most common cancers in the United States.[3] They are caused by a combination of genetic predisposition and ultraviolet radiation exposure. Fair-skinned individuals are at highest risk.

Almost all skin cancers are of three types:

* *Basal cell carcinoma,* arising in the lowest, or basal, level of the epidermis, accounts for most of skin cancers. These cancers arise in sun-exposed areas, usually on the head and neck. They are pearly white and translucent, tend to grow slowly, and rarely metastasize.

* *Squamous cell carcinoma,* arise in the upper layer of the epidermis. These cancers are often crusted and scaly with a red, inflamed or ulcerated appearance; they can metastasize.

* *Melanoma,* arising from the pigment-producing melanocytes in the epidermis that give the skin its color, is the most lethal type, due to its high rate of metastasis and high rate of mortality at advanced stages,

See Table 9-9, Skin Tumors, p. 203 and Table 9-10, Benign and Malignant Nevi, p. 204.

causing over 70% of skin cancer deaths.[4] The incidence of melanoma has more than doubled in the past three decades, the most rapid increase of any cancer.[5] Melanoma is now the fifth most frequently diagnosed cancer in men and the seventh most frequently diagnosed in women. In the United States in 2014, the estimated lifetime risk was 1 in 48 for whites (2%), 1 in 200 for Hispanics, and 1 in 1,000 for African Americans.[6]

Risk Factors for Melanoma

Educate patients about *risk factors for melanoma*. Early detection of melanoma, when 3 mm or less, significantly improves prognosis.

Risk Factors for Melanoma[7-9]

- Personal or family history of previous melanoma
- Atypical or dysplastic moles (moles that change in size or color)
- Male gender
- 50 or more common moles
- Red or light hair
- Light eye or skin color, especially skin that freckles or burns easily
- Actinic keratoses, solar lentigines (acquired brown macules on sun-exposed areas)
- Ultraviolet radiation from heavy sun exposure, sunlamps, or tanning booths
- Severe blistering sunburns, especially in childhood
- Immunosuppression from HIV or chemotherapy

The *Melanoma Risk Assessment Tool* developed by the National Cancer Institute, available at http://www.cancer.gov/melanomarisktool/ can be used to help patients assess their risk for melanoma. It assesses an individual's 5-year risk of developing melanoma based on geographic location, gender, race, age, history of blistering sunburns, complexion, number and size of moles, freckling, and sun damage.[7]

Preventing Skin Cancer

Avoiding Ultraviolet Radiation and Tanning Beds

Increasing lifetime sun exposure correlates directly with increasing risk of skin cancer. Intermittent sun exposure appears to be more harmful than chronic exposure.[10] The best defense against skin cancers is to avoid ultraviolet radiation exposure by limiting time in the sun, avoiding mid-day sun, using sunscreen, and wearing sun-protective clothing with long sleeves and hats with wide brims.

Advise patients to avoid indoor tanning, especially children, teens, and young adults. Use of indoor tanning beds, especially before age 35, increases risk of melanoma by as much as 75%.

In 2009, the International Agency for Research on Cancer classified ultra-violet-emitting tanning devices as "carcinogenic to humans."[11] Options for tanning include self-tanning products or sprays in conjunction with sunscreen.

Regular Use of Sunscreen Prevents Skin Cancer

There are many myths about sunscreen. A landmark study in 2011 demonstrated that the regular use of sunscreen decreases the incidence of melanoma.[12] Advise patients to use at least Sun Protective Factor (SPF) 30 and broad spectrum protection. For water exposure, patients should use water-resistant sunscreens.

Free information about protection and proper use of sunscreen are available from the American Academy of Dermatology and the Skin Cancer Foundation.[9,13]

Skin Cancer Screening

Clinician Screening

Although the U.S. Preventive Services Task Force found insufficient evidence (Grade I) to recommend routine skin cancer screening by primary care physicians, the Task Force does advise clinicians to "remain alert for skin lesions with malignant features" during routine physical examinations and references the ABCDE criteria.[14–17] The American Cancer Society and the American Academy of Dermatology recommend *full body examinations* for patients over age 50 or at high risk, since melanoma can appear in any location.[18] High-risk patients are those with a personal or family history of multiple or dysplastic nevi or previous melanoma. Both new and changing nevi should be closely examined, since at least half of melanomas newly arise from isolated melanocytes rather than pre-existing nevi. Also take advantage of "opportunistic screening" when assessing other body systems, such as the respiratory system, or when bathing a patient.

Patient Screening

Instructions for the Skin Self-Examination

The American Academy of Dermatology recommends regular self-examination of the skin using the following techniques. Instruct patients with risk factors for skin cancer and melanoma, especially those with a history of high sun exposure, prior or family history of melanoma and 50 or more moles or more than 5 to 10 atypical moles, to perform regular self-skin examinations. The patient will need a full-length mirror, a hand-held mirror, and a well-lit room that provides privacy. Teach the patient the **ABCDE-EFG** method for assessing moles, and show the patient the photos of benign and malignant nevi in Table 9-10, Benign and Malignant Nevi, p. 204.

Approximately half of melanomas are initially detected by patients or their partners.

Patient Instructions for the Skin Self-Examination

Examine your body front and back in the mirror, then right and left sides with arms raised.

Bend elbows and look carefully at forearms, upper underarms, and palms.

Look at the backs of your legs and feet, the spaces between your toes, and the sole.

Examine the back of your neck and scalp with a hand mirror. Part hair for a closer look.

Finally, check your back and buttocks with a hand mirror.

Source: Adapted from American Academy of Dermatology. Detect Skin Cancer. Available at https://www.aad.org/spot-skin-cancer/learn-about-skin-cancer/detect-skin-cancer. Accessed October 29, 2015.

Inspecting Moles

Patients and clinicians who find moles should apply the ***ABCDE-EFG method*** to screen for melanoma. Sensitivity ranges from 43% to 97%, and specificity from 36% to 100%.[19] Any suspicious mole or skin lesion should be referred to a dermatologist for follow-up. Patients who examine their skin regularly are more likely to have thinner melanomas if detected. See Table 9-10, Benign and Malignant Nevi, p. 204.

ABCDEs for Early Recognition of Possible Melanoma

- **A** for asymmetry of one side of mole compared to the other
- **B** for irregular borders, especially ragged, notched, or blurred
- **C** for variation or change in color, especially blue or black
- **D** for diameter ≥6 mm or different from others, especially if changing, itching, or bleeding
- **E** for evolving or changing rapidly in size, symptoms, or morphology (the most sensitive criterion. This history may prompt biopsy of a benign-appearing lesion.)

Some have suggested adding EFG to help detect aggressive nodular melanomas because they are often:

- **E** for **E**levated
- **F** for **F**irm to palpation
- **G** for **G**rowing progressively over several weeks

TABLE
9-1

Skin Color Changes–General

Changes in Pigmentation

Cyanosis

Cyanosis is the somewhat bluish color that is visible in these toenails and toes. Compare this color with the normally pink fingernails and fingers of the same patient. Impaired venous return in the leg caused this example of peripheral cyanosis. Cyanosis, especially when slight, may be hard to distinguish from normal skin color.

Erythema

Red hue, increased blood flow, seen here as the "slapped cheeks" of *erythema infectiosum* ("fifth disease").

Carotenemia

The yellowish palm of carotenemia is compared with a normally pink palm, sometimes a subtle finding. Unlike jaundice, carotenemia does not affect the sclera, which remains white. The cause is a diet high in carrots and other yellow vegetables or fruits. Carotenemia is not harmful but indicates the need for assessing dietary intake.

Jaundice

Jaundice makes the skin diffusely yellow. Contrast this patient's skin color with the examiner's hand. Jaundice is seen most easily and reliably in the sclera, as shown here. It may also be visible in mucous membranes. Causes include *liver disease* and *hemolysis of red blood cells*.

Sources of photos: *Tinea Versicolor*—Ostler HB, Mailbach HI, Hoke AW, et al. *Diseases of the Eye and Skin: A Color Atlas*. Philadelphia, PA: Lippincott Williams & Wilkins; 2004; *Vitiligo, Erythema*—Goodheart HP. *Goodheart's Photoguide of Common Skin Disorders: Diagnosis and Management*. 2nd ed. Philadelphia, PA: Lippincott Williams & Wilkins; 2003.

Skin Color Changes—Local

Café-Au-Lait Spot
A slightly but uniformly pigmented macule or patch with a somewhat irregular border, usually 0.5–1.5 cm in diameter; benign. Six or more such spots, each with a diameter of >1.5 cm, however, suggest neurofibromatosis. (The small, darker macules are unrelated.)

Vitiligo
In vitiligo, depigmented macules appear on the face, hands, feet, extensor surfaces, and other regions and may coalesce into extensive areas that lack melanin. The brown pigment is normal skin color; the pale areas are vitiligo. The condition may be hereditary. These changes may be distressing to the patient.

Tinea Versicolor
Common superficial fungal infection of the skin, causing hypopigmented, slightly scaly macules on the trunk, neck, and upper arms (short-sleeved shirt distribution). They are easier to see in darker skin and in some are more obvious after tanning. In lighter skin, macules may look reddish or tan instead of pale.

Acanthosis Nigricans
A skin condition characterized by areas of dark, velvety discoloration in body folds and creases. The affected skin can become thickened. Most often, seen in the armpits, groin and neck. Frequently associated with obesity and diabetes.

TABLE
9-2

Skin Lesions—Anatomic Location and Distribution

Document the anatomic location of lesions and their distribution, e.g., discrete round red macule on dorsum of foot, scattered brown papules across upper posterior chest.

Herald lesion

Red oval papules across anterior and posterior chest.

Silvery scaly patches, on the extensor surfaces.

Example: Pityriasis Rosea.

Example: Psoriasis

Tan, flat, scaly lesions anterior and posterior chest.

Silvery scaly patches mainly on flexor surfaces.

Example: Tinea Versicolor.

Example: Atopic Eczema.

Source: Hall JC. *Sauer's Manual of Skin Diseases*. 8th ed. Philadelphia, PA: Lippincott Williams & Wilkins; 2000; Photos from Goodheart HP. *Goodheart's Photoguide of Common Skin Disorders: Diagnosis and Management*. 2nd ed. Philadelphia, PA: Lippincott Williams & Wilkins; 2003.

TABLE
9-3

Skin Lesions—Patterns and Shapes

Linear lesions appear as a straight line.

Example: Linear epidermal nevus

Geographic areas of one color, with variably scalloped borders interface with another color.

Example: Mycosis fungoides

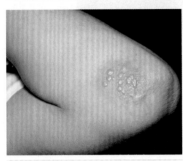

Clustered lesions are grouped

Example: Herpes simplex

Serpiginous lesions appear to creep from one part to another. The margin has a wavy or serpentine border

Example: Tinea corporis

Annular, arciform have a circular shape.

Example: Annular lesion of tinea faciale (ringworm)

Confluent lesions are lesions that run together.

Example: Small-vessel vasculitis

Target lesions have a bulls-eye appearance.

Example: Lyme disease

Zosteriform lesions follow a nerve dermatome. See Dermatome maps, Chapter 20, The Nervous System, pp. 701–703.

Example: Herpes zoster (shingles)

Sources of photos: *Linear Epidermal Nevus, Herpes Simplex, Tinea Faciale*—Goodheart HP. *Goodheart's Photoguide of Common Skin Disorders: Diagnosis and Management*. 2nd ed. Philadelphia, PA: Lippincott Williams & Wilkins, 2003; *Mycosis Fungoides, Tinea Corporis*—Hall JC. *Sauer's Manual of Skin Diseases*. 8th ed. Philadelphia, PA: Lippincott Williams & Wilkins, 2000; *Herpes zoster*—Hall JC. *Sauer's Manual of Skin Diseases*. 9th ed. Philadelphia, PA: Lippincott Williams & Wilkins, 2006; *Small-vessel vasculitis*—Marder VJ, Aird WC, Bennett JS, Schulman S, White GC II. *Hemostasis and Thrombosis*. 6th ed. Philadelphia, PA: Wolters Kluwer | Lippincott Williams & Wilkins, 2012; *Lyme disease*—Engleberg NC, Dermody T, DiRita V. *Schaechter's Mechanisms of Microbial Disease*. 5th ed. Wolters Kluwer | Lippincott Williams & Wilkins; 2012.

TABLE
9-4

Primary Skin Lesions (*initial presentation*)

Flat Lesions: Nonpalpable lesions with local changes in skin color
Macule—Less than 1.0 cm

Example: Vitiligo

Example: Hemangioma

Patch—1.0 cm or larger

Example: Café-au-lait spot

Palpable Elevated Lesions and Solid Masses

Plaque—Elevated superficial lesion 1.0 cm or larger, often formed by coalescence of papules

Example: Psoriasis

Example: Psoriasis

Papule—Less than 1.0 cm

Example: Psoriasis

Nodule—Marble-like lesion larger than 0.5 cm, often deeper and firmer than a papule

Example: Dermatofibroma

Cyst—Nodule filled with expressible material, either liquid or semisolid

Example: Epidermal Inclusion Cyst

Wheal—A somewhat irregular, often reddish or deeper brown on patients with dark complexions, superficial area of localized skin edema

Example: Urticaria

Palpable Elevated Fluid-Filled, Round or Oval Lesions (blisters)

Vesicle—Less than 1.0 cm; filled with serous fluid

Example: Herpes Simplex

Bulla—1.0 cm or larger; filled with serous fluid

Example: Insect Bite

(table continues on page 198)

TABLE
9-4

Primary Skin Lesions
(*initial presentation*) (continued)

Pustule—Filled with pus

Example: Acne

Example: Small Pox

Burrow—A minute, slightly raised tunnel in the epidermis, commonly found on the finger webs and on the sides of the fingers. It looks like a short (5–15 mm), linear or curved gray line and may end in a tiny vesicle. Skin lesions include small papules, pustules, lichenified areas, and excoriations. With a magnifying lens, look for the *burrow* of the mite that causes scabies.

Example: Scabies

Sources of photos: *Hemangioma, Café-au-Lait Spot, Psoriasis* [bottom], *Dermatofibroma, Herpes Simplex*—Hall JC. *Sauer's Manual of Skin Diseases*. 9th ed. Philadelphia, PA: Lippincott Williams & Wilkins, 2006; *Vitiligo, Psoriasis* [top], *Epidermal Inclusion Cyst, Urticaria, Insect Bite, Acne, Scabies*—Goodheart HP. *Goodheart's Photoguide of Common Skin Disorders: Diagnosis and Management*. 2nd ed. Philadelphia, PA: Lippincott Williams & Wilkins; 2003; *Small Pox*—Ostler, HB, Mailbach HI, Hoke AW, et al. *Diseases of the Eye and Skin: A Color Atlas*. Philadelphia, PA: Lippincott Williams & Wilkins; 2004.

TABLE
9-5

Secondary Skin Lesions Arise From Primary Lesions (seen in overtreatment, excess scratching, infection of primary lesions)

Scales—Flakes of dead exfoliated epidermis. Color may be white, gray or silvery. Texture may be fine or thick.

Example: Ichthyosis Vulgaris

Example: Dry Skin

Crust—The dried residue of skin exudates such as serum, pus, or blood; can be red-brown, orange, or yellow.

Example: Impetigo

Lichenification—Visible and palpable thickening of the epidermis and roughening of the skin with increased visibility of the normal skin furrows (often from chronic rubbing)

Example: Neurodermatitis

Scars—Flat connective tissue left after an injury or disease heals. Can be red or purple initially; older scars can fade to silver or white.

Example: Hypertrophic Scar From Steroid Injections

Keloid—Hypertrophic scarring that extends beyond the borders of the initiating injury

A

B

Example: Keloid A—shoulder   B—earlobe

Sources of photos: *Lichenification*—Hall JC. *Sauer's Manual of Skin Diseases.* 9th ed. Philadelphia, PA: Lippincott Williams & Wilkins; 2006; *Ichthyosis, Dry Skin, Hypertrophic Scar, Keloids*—Goodheart HP. *Goodheart's Photoguide of Common Skin Disorders: Diagnosis and Management.* 2nd ed. Philadelphia, PA: Lippincott Williams & Wilkins; 2003.

TABLE
9-6

Secondary Skin Lesions—Depressed

Erosion—Nonscarring wearing away of the superficial epidermis; surface is moist but does not bleed

Example: Aphthous stomatitis, moist area after the rupture of a vesicle, as in chickenpox

Excoriation—Linear or punctate erosions caused by scratching

Example: Cat scratches

Fissure—A linear crack in the skin, often resulting from excessive dryness

Example: Athlete's foot

Ulcer—A deeper loss of epidermis and dermis; may bleed and scar

Example: Stasis ulcer of venous insufficiency, syphilitic chancre

Sources of photos: *Erosion, Excoriation, Fissure*—Goodheart HP. *Goodheart's Photoguide of Common Skin Disorders: Diagnosis and Management.* 2nd ed. Philadelphia, PA: Lippincott Williams & Wilkins; 2003; *Ulcer*—Hall JC. *Sauer's Manual of Skin Diseases.* 8th ed. Philadelphia, PA: Lippincott Williams & Wilkins; 2000.

TABLE
9-7

Acne Vulgaris—Primary and Secondary Lesions

Acne vulgaris is the most common cutaneous disorder in the United States, affecting more than 85% of adolescents.[20] Acne is a disorder of the pilosebaceous follicle that involves proliferation of the keratinocytes at the opening of the follicle; increased production of sebum, stimulated by androgens, which combines with keratinocytes to plug the follicular opening; growth of *Propionibacterium acnes,* an anaerobic diphtheroid normally found on the skin; and inflammation from bacterial activity and release of free fatty acids and enzymes from activated neutrophils.[20] Cosmetics, humidity, heavy sweating, and stress are contributing factors.

Lesions appear in areas with the greatest number of sebaceous glands, namely, the face, neck, chest, upper back, and upper arms. They may be primary, secondary, or mixed.

Primary Lesions

Mild Acne

Open and closed comedones, occasional papules

Moderate Acne

Comedones, papules, pustules

Severe Cystic Acne

Secondary Lesions

Acne With Pitting and Scars

Sources of photos: Goodheart HP. *Goodheart's Photoguide of Common Skin Disorders: Diagnosis and Management.* 2nd ed. Philadelphia, PA: Lippincott Williams & Wilkins; 2003.

TABLE
9-8

Vascular and Purpuric Lesions of the Skin

Vascular Lesions		
Spider Angioma[a]	**Spider Vein**[a]	**Cherry Angioma**
Color and Size Fiery red. From very small to 2 cm	Bluish. Size variable, from very small to several inches	Bright or ruby red; may become brownish with age. 1–3 mm
Shape Central body, sometimes raised, surrounded by erythema and radiating legs	Variable. May resemble a spider or be linear, irregular, cascading	Round, flat or sometimes raised, may be surrounded by a pale halo
Pulsatility and Effect of Pressure Often seen in center of the spider, when pressure with a glass slide is applied. Pressure on the body causes blanching of the spider.	Absent. Pressure over the center does not cause blanching, but diffuse pressure blanches the veins	Absent. May show partial blanching, especially if pressure applied with edge of a pinpoint
Distribution Face, neck, arms, and upper trunk; almost never below the waist	Most often on the legs, near veins; also on the anterior chest	Trunk; also extremities
Significance Usually normal; solitary or few. If numerous in telangiectatic mats, may indicate liver disease. Also seen in pregnancy, vitamin B deficiency.	Often accompanies increased pressure in the superficial veins, as in varicose veins	None; increases in size and numbers with aging

Purpuric Lesions	
Petechia/Purpura	**Ecchymosis**
Color and Size Deep red or reddish purple. Petechia, 1–3 mm; purpura, larger	Purple or purplish blue, fading to green, yellow, and brown with time. Variable size, larger than petechiae, >3 mm
Shape Rounded, sometimes irregular; flat	Rounded, oval, or irregular; may have a central subcutaneous flat nodule (a hematoma)
Pulsatility and Effect of Pressure Absent. No effect from pressure	Absent. No effect from pressure
Distribution Variable	Variable
Significance Blood outside the vessels; If on dorsal forearms, is usually *actinic purpura* from chronic sun exposure. May indicate a bleeding disorder or, if petechiae, emboli to skin; palpable purpura in *vasculitis*	Blood outside the vessels; often secondary to bruising or trauma; also seen in bleeding disorders

[a]These are telangiectasias, or dilated small vessels that look red or bluish.
Sources of photos: *Spider Angioma*—Marks R. *Skin Disease in Old Age*. Philadelphia, PA: JB Lippincott; 1987; *Petechia/Purpura*—Kelley WN. *Textbook of Internal Medicine*. Philadelphia, PA: JB Lippincott; 1989.

TABLE
9-9

Skin Tumors

Actinic Keratosis

Superficial, flattened papules covered by a dry scale. Often multiple; can be round or irregular; pink, tan, or grayish. Appear on sun-exposed skin of older, fair-skinned people. Though benign, 1 of every 1,000 per year develops into squamous cell carcinoma (suggested by rapid growth, induration, redness at the base, and ulceration). Keratoses on face and hand, typical locations, are shown.

Seborrheic Keratosis

Common, benign, yellowish to brown raised lesions that feel slightly greasy and velvety or warty and have a "stuck on" appearance. Typically multiple and symmetrically distributed on the trunk of older people, but may also appear on the face and elsewhere. In black people, often younger women, may appear as small, deeply pigmented papules on the cheeks and temples (dermatosis papulosa nigra).

Basal Cell Carcinoma

A basal cell carcinoma, though malignant, grows slowly and seldom metastasizes. It is most common in fair-skinned adults 40 years or older, and usually appears on the face. An initial translucent nodule spreads, leaving a depressed center and a firm, elevated border. Telangiectatic vessels are often visible.

Squamous Cell Carcinoma

Usually appears on sun-exposed skin of fair-skinned adults older than 60 years. May develop in an actinic keratosis. Usually grows more quickly than a basal cell carcinoma, is firmer, and looks redder. The face and the back of the hand are often affected, as shown here.

Sources of photos: *Basal Cell Carcinoma*—Rapini R. *Squamous Cell Carcinoma, Actinic Keratosis, Seborrheic Keratosis*—Hall JC. *Sauer's Manual of Skin Diseases.* 9th ed. Philadelphia, PA: Lippincott, Williams & Wilkins; 2006.

TABLE
9-10

Benign and Malignant Nevi

Benign Nevus

The *benign nevus,* or common mole, usually appears in the first few decades. Several nevi may arise at the same time, but their appearance usually remains unchanged. Note the following typical features and contrast them with those of atypical nevi and melanoma:

- Round or oval shape
- Sharply defined borders
- Uniform color, especially tan or brown
- Diameter <6 mm
- Flat or raised surface

Changes in these features raise the specter of *atypical (dysplastic) nevi,* or melanoma. Atypical nevi are varied in color but often dark and larger than 6 mm, with irregular borders that fade into the surrounding skin. Look for atypical nevi primarily on the trunk. They may number more than 50 to 100.

A

Malignant Melanoma

Learn the ***ABCDE-EFG*** of melanoma from these reference standard photographs from the American Cancer Society:

- **A***symmetry* (Fig. A)
- Irregular **B***orders,* especially notching (Fig. B)
- Variation in **C***olor,* especially mixtures of black, blue, and red (Figs. B, C)
- **D***iameter* >6 mm (Fig. C)
- **E***volving,* a mole changing in size, shape or color.
- **E** for **E**levated
- **F** for **F**irm to palpation
- **G** for **G**rowing progressively over several weeks

Review *melanoma risk factors* such as intense year-round sun exposure, blistering sunburns in childhood, fair skin that freckles or burns easily (especially if blond or red hair), family history of melanoma, and nevi that are changing or atypical, especially if the patient is older than 50 years. Changing nevi may have new swelling or redness beyond the border, scaling, oozing, or bleeding, or sensations such as itching, burning, or pain.

On darker skin, look for melanomas under the nails, on the hands, or on the soles of the feet.

B

C

Source: Courtesy of American Cancer Society; American Academy of Dermatology.

TABLE
9-11

Diseases and Related Skin Conditions[21]

Addison disease	Hyperpigmentation of skin and mucous membranes
Chronic renal disease	Pallor, xerosis, pruritus, hyperpigmentation, uremic frost, metastatic calcification in the skin, calciphylaxis, "half and half" nails, hemodialysis-related skin disease
Cushing disease	Striae, skin atrophy, purpura, ecchymoses, telangiectasias, acne, moon facies, buffalo hump, hypertrichosis
Diabetes	Diabetic dermopathy, acanthosis nigricans, neuropathic ulcers, peripheral vascular disease
Disseminated intravascular coagulation	Skin necrosis, petechiae, ecchymoses, hemorrhagic bullae, purpura fulminans
Dyslipidemias	Xanthomas (tendon, eruptive, and tuberous), xanthelasma (may occur in healthy people)
Hypothyroidism	Dry, rough, and pale skin; coarse and brittle hair; myxedema; alopecia (lateral third of the eyebrows to diffuse); skin cool to touch; thin and brittle nails
Hyperthyroidism	Warm, moist, soft, and velvety skin; thin and fine hair; alopecia; vitiligo; pretibial myxedema (in Graves disease); hyperpigmentation (local or generalized)
Kawasaki disease	Mucosal erythema (lips, tongue, and pharynx), strawberry tongue, cherry red lips, polymorphous rash (primarily on trunk), erythema of palms and soles with later desquamation of fingertips
Liver disease	*Jaundice, spider angiomas* and other telangiectasias, palmar erythema, *Terry nails,* pruritus, purpura, caput medusae
Meningococcemia	Pink macules and papules, *petechiae,* hemorrhagic petechiae, hemorrhagic bullae, purpura fulminans
Peripheral vascular disease	Dry, scaly, shiny atrophic skin; dystrophic, brittle toenails; cool skin; hairless shins; ulcers; pallor; cyanosis; gangrene
Pregnancy (physiologic changes)	Melasma, increased pigmentation of areolae, linea nigra, palmar erythema, varicose veins, striae, *spider angiomas,* hirsutism, pyogenic granuloma
Systemic lupus erythematosus	Photosensitivity, malar (butterfly) rash, discoid rash, alopecia, vasculitis, oral ulcers, Raynaud phenomenon
Thrombocytopenic purpura	*Petechiae, ecchymoses*
Viral exanthems	
Coxsackie A (hand, foot, and mouth)	Oral ulcers; macules, papules, and vesicles on hands, feet, and buttocks
Erythema infectiosum (fifth disease)	Erythema of cheeks ("slapped cheeks") followed by erythematous, pruritic, reticulated (net-like) rash that starts on trunk and proximal extremities (rash worsens with sun, fever, and temperature changes)
Roseola infantum (HSV 6)	Erythematous, maculopapular, discrete rash (often fever present) that begins on head and spreads to involve trunk and extremities, petechiae on soft palate
Rubella (German measles)	Erythematous, maculopapular, discrete rash (often fever present) that begins on head and spreads to involve trunk and extremities, petechiae on soft palate
Rubeola (measles)	Erythematous, maculopapular rash that begins on head and spreads to involve trunk and extremities (lesions become confluent on face and trunk, but are discrete on extremities), Koplik spots on buccal mucosa
Varicella (chickenpox)	Generalized, pruritic, vesicular (vesicles on an erythematous base, "dewdrop on a rose petal") rash begins on trunk and spreads peripherally, lesions appear in crops and are in different stages of healing
Herpes zoster (shingles)	Pruritic, vesicular rash (vesicles on an erythematous base) in a dermatomal distribution

Source: Hall JC. *Sauer's Manual of Skin Diseases.* 9th ed. Philadelphia, PA: Lippincott Williams & Wilkins; 2006.

TABLE
9-12

Pressure Ulcers

Pressure (*decubitus*) ulcers usually develop over bony prominences subject to unrelieved pressure, resulting in ischemic damage to underlying tissue. Prevention is important: inspect the skin thoroughly for *early warning signs of erythema that blanches with pressure,* especially in patients with risk factors.

Pressure ulcers form most commonly over the sacrum, ischial tuberosities, greater trochanters, and heels. A commonly applied staging system, based on depth of destroyed tissue, is illustrated below. Note that necrosis or eschar must be débrided before ulcers can be staged. Ulcers whose base is covered with eschar or sloughing tissue are "unstageable." Ulcers may not progress sequentially through the four stages.[22]

Inspect ulcers for signs of infection (drainage, odor, cellulitis, or necrosis). Fever, chills, and pain suggest underlying **osteomyelitis**. Address the patient's overall health, including *comorbid conditions* such as vascular disease, diabetes, immune deficiencies, collagen vascular disease, malignancy, psychosis, or depression; nutritional status; pain and level of analgesia; risk for recurrence; psychosocial factors such as learning ability, social supports, and lifestyle; and evidence of polypharmacy, overmedication, or abuse of alcohol, tobacco, or illicit drugs.[23]

Risk Factors for Pressure Ulcers

- Decreased mobility, especially if accompanied by increased pressure or movement causing friction or shear stress
- Decreased sensation, from brain or spinal cord lesions or peripheral nerve disease

- Decreased blood flow from hypotension or microvascular disease such as diabetes or atherosclerosis
- Fecal or urinary incontinence
- Presence of fracture
- Poor nutritional status or low albumin

| | Stage I | Stage II | Stage III | Stage IV |

Epidermis —
Dermis —
Fat —
Muscle —
Bone —

Stage I

Pressure-related alteration of intact skin, with changes in temperature (warmth or coolness), consistency (firm or boggy), sensation (pain or itching), or color (red, blue, or purple on darker skin; red on lighter skin)

Stage II

Partial-thickness skin loss or ulceration involving the epidermis, dermis, or both

Stage III

Full-thickness skin loss, with damage to or necrosis of subcutaneous tissue that may extend to, but not through, underlying muscle

Stage IV

Full-thickness skin loss, with destruction, tissue necrosis, or damage to underlying muscle, bone, or supporting structures

Source: National Pressure Ulcer Advisory Panel, Reston, VA.

TABLE
9-13 Hair Loss

Alopecia Areata

Clearly demarcated round or oval patches of hair loss, usually affecting young adults and children. There is no visible scaling or inflammation.

Trichotillomania

Hair loss from pulling, plucking, or twisting hair. Hair shafts are broken and of varying lengths. More common in children, often in settings of family or psychosocial stress.

Tinea Capitis ("Ringworm")

Round scaling patches of alopecia. Hairs are broken off close to the surface of the scalp. Usually caused by fungal infection from *tinea tonsurans*. Mimics seborrheic dermatitis.

Sources of photos: *Alopecia Areata [left], Trichotillomania [left]*—Hall JC. *Sauer's Manual of Skin Diseases*. 9th ed. Philadelphia, PA: Lippincott Williams & Wilkins; 2006; *Alopecia Areata [right], Tinea Capitis*—Goodheart HP. *Goodheart's Photoguide of Common Skin Disorders: Diagnosis and Management*. 2nd ed. Philadelphia, PA: Lippincott Williams & Wilkins; 2003; *Trichotillomania [right]*—Ostler HB, Mailbach HI, Hoke AW, et al. *Diseases of the Eye and Skin: A Color Atlas*. Philadelphia, PA: Lippincott Williams & Wilkins; 2004.

TABLE
9-14

Findings in or Near the Nails

Paronychia

A superficial infection of the proximal and lateral nail folds adjacent to the nail plate. The nail folds are often red, swollen, and tender. Represents the most common infection of the hand, usually from *Staphylococcus aureus* or *Streptococcus* species, and may spread until it completely surrounds the nail plate. Creates a felon if it extends into the pulp space of the finger. Arises from local trauma due to nail biting, manicuring, or frequent hand immersion in water.

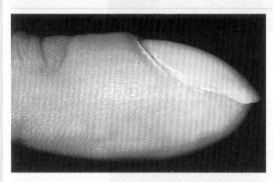

Clubbing of the Fingers

Clinically a bulbous swelling of the soft tissue at the nail base, with loss of the normal angle between the nail and the proximal nail fold. The angle increases to 180 degrees or more, and the nail bed feels spongy or floating. The mechanism is still unknown but involves vasodilatation with increased blood flow to the distal portion of the digits and changes in connective tissue, possibly from hypoxia, changes in innervation, genetics, or a platelet-derived growth factor from fragments of platelet clumps. Seen in congenital heart disease, interstitial lung disease and lung cancer, inflammatory bowel diseases, and malignancies.[24]

Onycholysis

A painless separation of the whitened opaque nail plate from the pinker translucent nail bed. Starts distally and progresses proximally, enlarging the free edge of the nail. Local causes include trauma from excess manicuring, psoriasis, fungal infection, and allergic reactions to nail cosmetics. Systemic causes include diabetes, anemia, photosensitive drug reactions, hyperthyroidism, peripheral ischemia, bronchiectasis, and syphilis.

Terry Nails

Nail plate turns white with a ground-glass appearance, a distal band of reddish brown, and obliteration of the lunula. Commonly affects all fingers, although may appear in only one finger. Seen in liver disease, usually cirrhosis, congestive heart failure, and diabetes. May arise from decreased vascularity and increased connective tissue in nail bed.

Sources of photos: *Clubbing of the Fingers, Paronychia, Onycholysis, Terry Nails*—Habif TP. *Clinical Dermatology: A Color Guide to Diagnosis and Therapy*. 2nd ed. St. Louis: CV Mosby; 1990; *White Spots, Transverse White Lines, Psoriasis, Beau Lines*—Sams WM Jr, Lynch PJ. *Principles and Practice of Dermatology*. New York, NY: Churchill Livingstone; 1990.

White Spots *(Leukonychia)*

Trauma to the nails is commonly followed by nonuniform white spots that grow slowly out with the nail. Spots in the pattern illustrated are typical of overly vigorous and repeated manicuring. The curves in this example resemble the curve of the cuticle and proximal nail fold.

Transverse White Bands *(Mees Lines)*

Curving transverse white bands that cross the nail parallel to the lunula. Arising from the disrupted matrix of the proximal nail, they vary in width and move distally as the nail grows out. Seen in arsenic poisoning, heart failure, Hodgkin disease, chemotherapy, carbon monoxide poisoning, and leprosy.[25]

Transverse Linear Depressions *(Beau Lines)*

Transverse depressions of the nail plates, usually bilateral, resulting from temporary disruption of proximal nail growth from systemic illness. As with Mees lines, timing of the illness may be estimated by measuring the distance from the line to the nail bed (nails grow approximately 1 mm every 6–10 days). Seen in severe illness, trauma, and cold exposure if Raynaud disease is present.[25,26]

Pitting

Punctate depressions of the nail plate caused by defective layering of the superficial nail plate by the proximal nail matrix. Usually associated with psoriasis but also seen in Reiter syndrome, sarcoidosis, alopecia areata, and localized atopic or chemical dermatitis.[25]

Sources of photos: *Clubbing of the Fingers, Paronychia, Onycholysis, Terry Nails*—Habif TP. *Clinical Dermatology: A Color Guide to Diagnosis and Therapy.* 2nd ed. St. Louis: CV Mosby; 1990; *White Spots, Transverse White Lines, Psoriasis, Beau Lines*—Sams WM Jr, Lynch PJ. *Principles and Practice of Dermatology.* New York: Churchill Livingstone; 1990.

BIBLIOGRAPHY

CITATIONS

1. Bergstrom N, Braden BJ. Predictive validity of the Braden Scale among Black and White subjects. *Nsg Res.* 2002;51(6): 398–403.

2. Siegel V. Exploring the role of the nurse in skin cancer prevention. *Dermatology Nursing.* 2010;4(12):18–22.

3. American Academy of Dermatologists. For the public: Free Resources. Treatable beatable with early detection. Available at https://www.aad.org/spot-skin-cancer/free-resources. Accessed October 29, 2015.

4. Siegel R, Desantis C, Jemal A. Cancer statistics. *CA Cancer J Clin.* 2015;65:5–29.

5. Howlader N, Noone AM, Krapcho M, et al. *SEER Cancer Statistics Review, 1975–2011.* Bethesda, MD: National Cancer Institute; 2014.

6. American Cancer Society. Key statistics about Melanoma Skin Cancer. Available at http://www.cancer.org/cancer/skincancer-melanoma/detailedguide/melanoma-skin-cancer-key-statistics. Accessed October 29, 2015.

7. American Cancer Society. Melanoma Risk Tool. Available at http://www.cancer.gov/melanomarisktool/. Accessed June 2, 2016.

8. Naeyaert JM, Broches L. Dysplastic nevi. *N Engl J Med.* 2003;349(23):2233–2240.

9. Division of Cancer Prevention and Control. Centers for Disease Control and Prevention. What are the risk factors for skin cancer? Available at http://www.cdc.gov/cancer/skin/basic_info/risk_factors.htm. Accessed June 2, 2016.

10. National Cancer Institute. Genetics of Skin Cancer (PDQ®). Melanoma. Available at http://www.cancer.gov/cancertopics/pdq/genetics/skin/HealthProfessional/page4. October 29, 2015.

11. El Ghissassi F, Baan R, Straif K, et al.; WHO International Agency for Research on Cancer Monograph Working Group. A review of human carcinogens—part D: radiation. *Lancet Oncol.* 2009;10:751–752.

12. Green AC, Williams GM, Logan V, et al. Reduced melanoma after regular sunscreen use: randomized trial follow-up. *J Clin Oncol.* 2011;29:257–263.

13. Skin Cancer Foundation. Sun protection. Available at http://www.skincancer.org/prevention/sun-protection. Accessed October 19, 2015.

14. U.S. Preventive Services Task Force. Screening for skin cancer. Recommendation statement. *Ann Intern Med.* 2009;150:188. Available at http://www.uspreventiveservicestaskforce.org/Page/Topic/recommendation-summary/skin-cancer-screening?ds=1&s=. Accessed October 19, 2015.

15. Wolff T, Tai E, Miller T. Screening for skin cancer: an update of the evidence for the U.S. Preventive Services Task Force. *Ann Intern Med.* 2009;150:194. Available at http://www.ncbi.nlm.nih.gov/books/NBK34051./. Accessed October 19,2015.

16. American Cancer Society. Skin cancer Prevention and Early Detection, 2010. Available at http://www.cancer.org/cancer/skincancer/index. Accessed October 19, 2015.

17. American Academy of Dermatology. What to look for: ABCDEs of Melanoma. Available at https://www.aad.org/public/spot-skin-cancer/learn-about-skin-cancer/detect/what-to-look-for. Accessed June 2, 2016.

18. American Academy of Dermatology. Skin cancer. Available at https://www.aad.org/media-resources/stats-and-facts/conditions/skin-cancer. Accessed October 19, 2015.

19. Abbasi NR, Shaw HM, Rigel DS, et al. Early diagnosis of cutaneous melanoma: revisiting the ABCD criteria. *JAMA.* 2004;292:2771–2776.

20. American Academy of Dermatology. American Academy of Dermatology issues new guidelines of care for acne treatment. Available at https://www.aad.org/media/news-releases/acne-guidelines. Accessed June 2, 2016.

21. Hall JC. Sauer's Manual of Skin Diseases. 9th ed. Philadelphia, PA: Lippincott Williams & Wilkins; 2006.

22. National Pressure Ulcer Advisory Panel. Prevention and Treatment of Pressure Ulcers: Clinical Practice Guidelines. Washington, DC: National Pressure Ulcer Advisory Panel; 2009. Available at http://www.npuap.org/resources/educational-and-clinical-resources/prevention-and-treatment-of-pressure-ulcers-clinical-practice-guideline/. Accessed June 2, 2016.

23. Patton RM. Is Diagnosis of Pressure Ulcers within an RN's Scope of Practice? *American Nurse Today.* 2005;5(1):20.

24. Spicknall KE, Zirwas MJ, English JC 3rd. Clubbing: an update on diagnosis, differential diagnosis, pathophysiology, and clinical relevance. *J Am Acad Dermatol.* 2005;52(6): 1020–1028.

25. Fawcett RS, Hart TM, Lindford S, et al. Nail abnormalities: clues to systemic diseases. *Am Fam Phys.* 2004;69(6): 1418–1425.

26. Hanford RR, Cobb MW, Banner NT. Unilateral Beau's lines associated with a fractured and immobilized wrist. *Cutis.* 1995;56(5):263–264.

ADDITIONAL READINGS

Anderson J, Langemo D, Hanson D, et al. Wound & skin care. What you can learn from a comprehensive skin assessment. *Nursing.* 2007;37(4):65–66.

Barr J. Nursing assessment of the integumentary system. *Ostomy Wound Manag.* 2006;52(6):20–22.

Habif TP. *Clinical Dermatology: A Color Guide to Diagnosis and Therapy.* 6th ed. New York, NY: Mosby; 2016.

Hess C. Performing a skin assessment. *Adv Skin Wound Care.* 2008;21(8):392.

Johannsen L. Skin assessment. *Dermatol Nurs.* 2005;17(2): 165–166.

Joint Commission on Accreditation of Healthcare Organizations. Assessing a patients' risk for pressure ulcers: compliance tips for national patient safety goal 14. *Joint Commission Perspectives on Patient Safety.* 2008;8(10):9–11.

Massey D. The value and role of skin and nail assessment in the critically ill. *Nurs Crit Care.* 2006;11(2):80–85.

Miller AJ, Mihm MC. Melanoma. *N Engl J Med.* 2006;355(1):51–65.

Scanlon E, Stubbs N. Pressure ulcer risk assessment in patients with darkly pigmented skin. *Professional Nurse.* 2004;19(6):339–341.

Schon MP, Henning-Boehncke W. Psoriasis. *N Engl J Med.* 2005;352(18):1899–1912.

Warner-Maron, I. The Risk of Risk Assessment: Pressure Ulcer Assessment and the Braden Scale. *Anna Long Term Care,* 2015;23:5 - May 2015, http://www.annalsoflongtermcare.com/article/risk-risk-assessment-pressure-ulcer-assessment-and-braden-scale. Accessed October 15, 2015.

10 The Head and Neck

LEARNING OBJECTIVES

The student will:

1. Identify the basic structures and function of the head and neck and the purpose of each.

2. Collect an accurate health history of the head and neck.

3. State questions used during the assessment of a patient with a headache.

4. Perform the physical examination techniques to evaluate the head and neck.

5. Document the physical examination results.

6. Identify the measures for prevention of traumatic brain injury.

The head and neck contains the cranium, face, sensory organs, neck, thyroid gland, and lymph nodes. This chapter is an overview of the head/cranium. Each of these sequential areas will be addressed with additional anatomical detail followed by the assessment, including an example of subjective health history questions and objective physical examination techniques in upcoming chapters.

THE HEAD

Anatomy and Physiology of the Head

The head is the upper portion of the body consisting of the skull and face. Regions of the head take their names from the underlying bones of the skull: the frontal, parietal, temporal, and occipital areas. Knowing this anatomy helps locate and describe physical findings. The face is the anterior portion of the head and encompasses the sensory organs, which are the focus of upcoming Chapter 11, The Eyes, and Chapter 12, Ears, Nose, Mouth, and Throat. Additional systems coincide with the head and neck and are addressed in future chapters, including cranial nerves in Chapter 20, The Nervous System, cervical vertebrae in Chapter 18, The Musculoskeletal System, and the blood supply to the head and neck in Chapter 15, The Peripheral Vascular System and Lymphatic System.

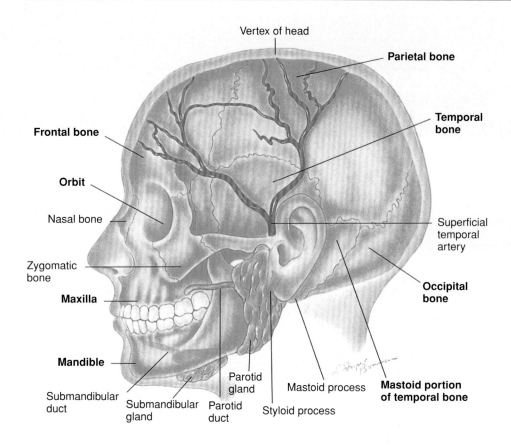

Vertex of head

Parietal bone

Frontal bone

Temporal bone

Orbit

Nasal bone

Superficial temporal artery

Zygomatic bone

Maxilla

Occipital bone

Mandible

Parotid gland

Submandibular duct

Submandibular gland

Parotid duct

Styloid process

Mastoid process

Mastoid portion of temporal bone

THE HEALTH HISTORY

Common or Concerning Symptoms of the Head

- Headache
- Head injury
- Head or neck surgery
- Traumatic brain injury

Headache

Headache is one of the most common complaints in clinical practice, with a prevalence of 47% of the adult population experiencing symptoms in the past year.[1,2] Although there are varying types, degrees, and causes, headaches are a global issue that knows no boundaries and impacts people of all ages, races, socioeconomic status, and locations.

Tension headaches are the most common headache, although many individuals self-treat this type of headache. Migraine headaches are by far the most frequent cause of headaches seen in office practice, as migraines are often the most debilitating, lasting up to 3 days. Every headache warrants careful evaluation for life-threatening causes such as meningitis,

See Table 10-1, Primary Headaches, p. 229, and Table 10-2, Secondary Headaches, pp. 230–231.

subdural or intracranial hemorrhage, or tumor. It is important to elicit a full description of the headache and all seven attributes of the patient's pain (see p. 45). Is the headache one-sided or bilateral? Severe with sudden onset? Steady or throbbing? Continuous or intermittent (comes and goes)?

Look for "red flags" that raise suspicion of worrisome secondary causes: recent onset (less than 6 months); onset after 50 years of age; acute onset like a "thunderclap," or "the worst headache of my life"; markedly elevated blood pressure; presence of rash or signs of infection; presence of cancer, HIV, or pregnancy; vomiting; recent head trauma; or persisting neurologic deficits.

The history is critical in determining the focus of the physical examination. Using "OLD CART," ask the patient specifically about symptoms related to each system.

The opening questions are:

"Have you experienced unusually severe headaches?"
"Have you experienced unusually frequent headaches?"

If the patient noticed unusually severe or frequent headaches, then further assessment is helpful.

Onset: When did you first notice the headache?

Location: Where do you feel the headache? Can you point to the area(s)?
Duration: How long has this been going on?
   Did the headache begin suddenly (in a few minutes or less than an hour) or gradually (over a few hours or days)?
   Is it temporary or constant?
   When does the pain begin (morning, evening)? Does it wake you at night?
   How long do the headaches last?
   Are they recurring?
   Is there a pattern?
Characteristic symptoms: Describe what it feels like (throbbing, hammering, squeezing).
   Describe the pain on a scale of 1 to 10 with 1 being minimal pain and 10 being the worst pain you ever felt.

Primary headaches have no identifiable underlying cause. *Secondary headaches* arise from other conditions—some of these may endanger the patient's life.[3]

The most important attributes are the headaches' severity and chronologic patterns. If a headache is severe and of sudden onset, consider subarachnoid hemorrhage, meningitis, or stroke.

Migraine and *tension headaches* are episodic and tend to peak over several hours. New and persisting, progressively severe headaches raise concerns of *tumor, abscess,* or *mass.*

Unilateral headache is seen in *migraine and cluster headaches.*[1,3] Tension headaches often arise in the temporal areas; cluster headaches may be retroorbital.

Associated manifestations: Do you notice any other symptoms when this occurs? Blurred vision? Nausea? Vomiting? Dizziness?

Nausea and vomiting are common with *migraine* but also occur with *brain tumors* and *subarachnoid hemorrhage.*

What happened prior to the headache? Did anything precipitate the pain?

Is there a prodrome of unusual feelings such as euphoria, craving for food, fatigue, or dizziness? Is there an aura with neurologic symptoms, such as change in vision or numbness or weakness in an arm or leg?

Approximately 60% to 70% of patients with migraine have a prodrome prior to onset; 20% experience an aura, including photophobia, scintillating scotomata, or reversible visual and sensory symptoms.

What brings the headache on (specific foods or drinks, exercise, stress, work, environment, menstruation)?

Is there a history of overuse of analgesics (e.g., NSAIDS), ergotamine, or triptans?

Consider medication overuse in patients with chronic daily headache taking symptomatic medications more than 2 days a week.[1,3]

Do you have a family or personal history of headaches?

Family history may be positive in patients with migraines.

Did you experience a head injury or brain trauma in the past? When?

Relieving Factors: What have you tried to make the headache go away? (e.g., Sleep? Dark room? Cool compresses? Relaxation techniques?)

Ask whether coughing, sneezing, or changing the position of the head has any effect (better, worse, or none) on the headache. Such maneuvers may increase pain from a brain tumor and acute sinusitis.

What has worked the best? What has not worked at all?

Does anything make it worse?

How have the headaches affected your daily life and activities?

Treatment:

Has anyone treated you for headaches in the past? (e.g., physician, nurse practitioner, holistic practitioner, herbalist, acupuncturist, or massage therapist).

If yes, what type of headache was diagnosed?

Have you used any medication? If yes, then the name of the medication, dosage, and effect?

Traumatic Brain Injury

Traumatic brain injury (TBI) is a blow to the head or a piercing head injury that interferes with the function of the brain. Not all injuries to the head result in a TBI, and those that do occur span from mild to severe. Mild cases involve a slight change in mental status or consciousness and severe is an extended change postinjury. The severe cases account for approximately 30% of all deaths related to injuries.[4,5]

Have you experienced head trauma or brain injury in the past?
Onset: When did this occur? Can you describe what happened?
Do you remember when you hurt your head?
Precipitating Factors: What happened to cause the TBI? (e.g., Absence of protective equipment or helmet? Environmental)?
Location: Can you show me where you hurt your head?
Duration: Did you lose consciousness? If yes, for how long? Did you fall first or lose consciousness first?
Characteristic symptoms: Did you experience any symptoms prior to the head injury (headache, shortness of breath, chest pain, numbness, or tingling)?
Do you have any medical issues (cardiac history, diabetes, seizures)?
Associated manifestations: Do you experience vision changes; nausea or vomiting; attention span deficits; dizziness, confusion, drainage from the ears, nose, eyes, or mouth; tremors; seizures; or gait changes?
Relieving factors/strategies: Prevention of further injury (pp. 227–228)

THE NECK

Anatomy and Physiology of the Neck

For descriptive purposes, divide each side of the neck into two triangles bounded by the sternocleidomastoid muscle. Visualize the borders of the two triangles as follows:

- For the *anterior triangle:* the mandible above, the sternocleidomastoid laterally, and the midline of the neck medially

- For the *posterior triangle:* the sternocleidomastoid muscle, the trapezius, and the clavicle. Note that a portion of the omohyoid muscle crosses the lower portion of this triangle and can be mistaken for a lymph node or mass.

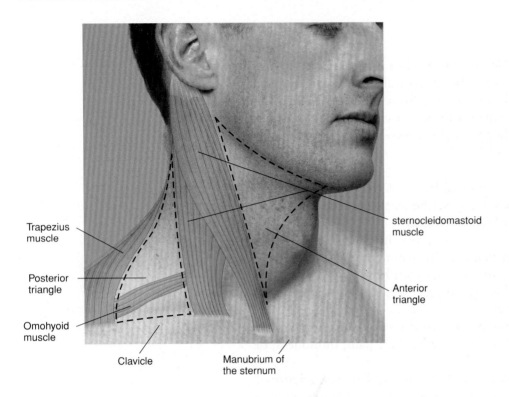

Trapezius muscle

Posterior triangle

Omohyoid muscle

Clavicle

Manubrium of the sternum

sternocleidomastoid muscle

Anterior triangle

Great Vessels

Under the sternocleidomastoids run the great vessels of the neck: the *carotid artery* and the *internal jugular vein*. The *external jugular vein* passes diagonally over the surface of the sternocleidomastoid and may be helpful when trying to identify the jugular venous pressure (see pp. 385–387).

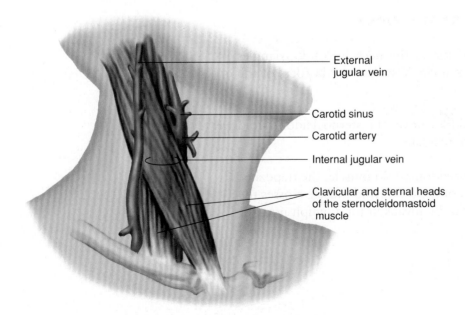

External jugular vein

Carotid sinus

Carotid artery

Internal jugular vein

Clavicular and sternal heads of the sternocleidomastoid muscle

Midline Structures and Thyroid Gland

Now identify the following midline structures: (1) the mobile *hyoid bone* just below the mandible, (2) the *thyroid cartilage*, readily identified by the notch on its superior edge, (3) the *cricoid cartilage*, (4) the *tracheal rings*, and (5) the *thyroid gland*.

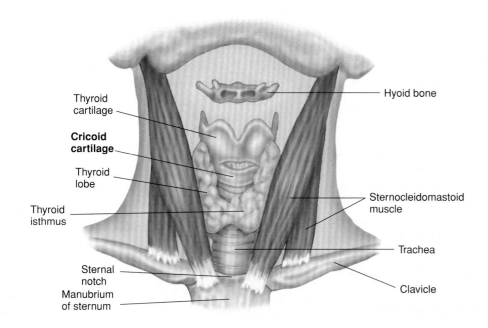

The isthmus of the thyroid gland lies across the trachea below the cricoid cartilage. The lateral lobes of this gland curve posteriorly around the sides of the trachea and the esophagus. Except in the midline, the thyroid gland is covered by thin strap-like muscles. Of these, only the sternocleidomastoids are visible. Women have larger and more easily palpable glands than men.

Lymph Nodes

The lymphatic system is a part of the immune system. Its function is to detect and eliminate foreign substances. One part of the lymph system is in the head and neck. The nurse needs to be aware of the drainage pattern.

Knowledge of the lymphatic system is important to a thorough assessment: whenever a malignant or inflammatory lesion is observed, look for involvement of the regional lymph nodes that drain it; whenever a node is

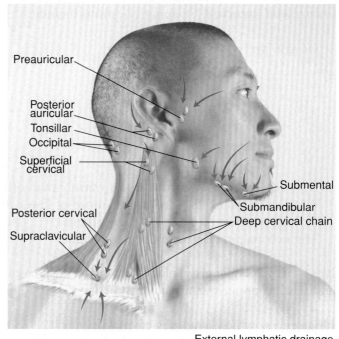

enlarged or tender, look for a source such as infection in the area that it drains.

Common or Concerning Symptoms of the Neck

- Swollen lymph nodes or neck lumps
- Enlarged thyroid gland
- Hoarseness

Ask, "Have you noticed any swollen 'glands' or lumps in your neck?" because patients are more familiar with the lay terms than with "*lymph nodes.*"

Enlarged tender lymph nodes commonly accompany pharyngitis.

O*nset:* When did you first notice the lump?

L*ocation:* Where is the lump? Is there more than one lump?

D*uration:* How long have you had the lump?

C*haracteristic symptoms:* Has the lump changed (size, tenderness, drainage, shape, consistency)?

A*ssociated manifestations:* Do you have difficulty swallowing? Have you had any recent infections? Trauma? Radiation? Surgery? History of smoking? Drinking alcohol? Chewing tobacco?

R*elieving factors:* Does anything make the lump smaller? Less tender? Have you tried compresses at the site?

T*reatment:* Have you been to a health care provider?

Assess thyroid function and ask about any evidence of an enlarged thyroid gland or goiter. To evaluate thyroid function, ask about **temperature intolerance and sweating**. Opening questions include:

With *goiter,* thyroid function may be increased, decreased, or normal.

Do you prefer hot or cold weather?

Intolerance to cold, preference for warm clothing and many blankets, and decreased sweating suggest hypothyroidism; the opposite symptoms, palpitations, and involuntary weight loss suggest *hyperthyroidism* (p. 235).

Do you dress more warmly or less warmly than other people?
What about blankets—do you use more or fewer than others at home?
Do you perspire more or less than others?
Any new palpitations or change in weight?

Note that as people grow older, they sweat less, have less tolerance for cold, and tend to prefer warmer environments.

Hoarseness, which is addressed in Chapter 12, Ears, Nose, Mouth, and Throat will frequently arise from the larynx. However, hypothyroidism can cause chronic hoarseness.

PHYSICAL EXAMINATION

Equipment

- Tangential light
- Cup of water
- Stethoscope

Abnormalities covered by the hair are easily missed, so ask if the patient has noticed anything different or any changes with the scalp or hair. Ask the patient to remove any hair pieces, hair adornments, scarves, or rubber bands. Take into consideration individual cultural practices and personal preferences when examining patients.

The Hair

Note its quantity, distribution, texture, and pattern of loss, if any. You may see loose flakes of dandruff.

Fine hair accompanies *hyperthyroidism;* coarse hair is found with *hypothyroidism.*

Tiny white ovoid granules that adhere to hairs may be nits (eggs of lice).

The Scalp

Part the hair in several places and look for scaliness, lumps, nevi, or other lesions.

Redness and scaling may indicate *seborrheic dermatitis, psoriasis;* soft lumps of *pilar cysts;* or pigmented nevi.

The Skull

Observe the general size and contour of the skull. Note any deformities, depressions, lumps, or tenderness. Learn to recognize the irregularities in a normal skull, such as those near the suture lines between the parietal and occipital bones.

Macrocephaly is an anomaly characterized by a large head in proportion to the body and an underdeveloped brain. The circumference of the head is more than two standard deviations above average for the person's age and sex.

Microcephaly is an anomaly characterized by a small head in proportion to the body and an underdeveloped brain. The circumference of the head is more than two standard deviations below average for the person's age and sex.

The Face

Note the patient's facial expression and contours. Observe for asymmetry, involuntary movements, edema, and masses.

See Table 10-3, Selected Facies, (p. 232).

The Skin

Observe the skin, noting its color, pigmentation, texture, thickness, hair distribution, and any lesions.

Acne is found in many adolescents. *Hirsutism* (excessive facial hair) occurs in some women with *polycystic ovary syndrome.*

The Neck

Observe the skin, noting its color, pigmentation, texture, thickness, hair distribution, and any lesions. *Inspect the neck,* noting its symmetry and any masses or scars. Look for enlargement of the parotid or submandibular glands, and note any visible lymph nodes.

A scar of past thyroid surgery is often a clue to under-reported thyroid disease.

The Lymph Nodes

Palpate the lymph nodes. Using the pads of your index and middle fingers, move the skin over the underlying tissues in each area in a circular motion. The patient should be relaxed, with neck flexed slightly forward and, if needed, slightly toward the side being examined. You can usually examine both sides at once. For the submental node, however, it is helpful to feel with one hand behind the mandible.

Feel in sequence for the following nodes:

1. *Preauricular*—in front of the ear

2. *Posterior auricular*—superficial to the mastoid process

3. *Occipital*—at the base of the skull posteriorly

4. *Tonsillar*—at the angle of the mandible

A "tonsillar node" that pulsates is really the carotid artery. A small, hard, tender "tonsillar node" high and deep between the mandible and the sternocleidomastoid is probably a styloid process.

5. *Submandibular*—midway between the angle and the tip of the mandible. These nodes are usually smaller and smoother than the lobulated submandibular gland against which they lie.

6. *Submental*—in the midline a few centimeters behind the tip of the mandible

7. *Superficial cervical*—superficial to the sternocleidomastoid

8. *Posterior cervical*—along the anterior edge of the trapezius

9. *Deep cervical chain*—deep to the sternocleidomastoid and often inaccessible to examination. Hook your thumb and fingers around either side of the sternocleidomastoid muscle to find them.

10. *Supraclavicular*—deep in the angle formed by the clavicle and the sternocleidomastoid

Enlargement of a supraclavicular node, especially on the left, suggests possible metastasis from a thoracic or an abdominal malignancy.

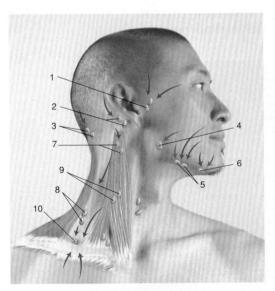

→ External lymphatic drainage
→ Internal lymphatic drainage
(e.g., from mouth and throat)

Begin palpation using the pads of the index and third fingers, and palpate the *preauricular nodes* with a gentle rotary motion. Then examine the *posterior auricular* and *occipital* lymph nodes and follow sequentially to *tonsillar,* then *submandibular.* The *submental* is palpated with one hand.

The last lymph nodes in the neck to be palpated are the *superficial cervical* and the *deep cervical chains,* located anterior and superficial to the sternocleidomastoid. Then palpate the *posterior cervical chain* along the trapezius (anterior edge) and along the sternocleidomastoid (posterior edge). Flex the patient's neck slightly forward toward the side being examined. Examine the *supraclavicular* nodes in the angle between the clavicle and the sternocleidomastoid.

Most lymph nodes cannot be palpated. When a node is detected on palpation, note its size, shape, delimitation (discrete or matted together), mobility, consistency, and any tenderness. Small, mobile, discrete, nontender nodes, sometimes termed "shotty," can frequently be found, especially in children.

Tender nodes suggest inflammation; hard or fixed nodes suggest malignancy.

Enlarged or tender nodes, if unexplained, call for (1) reexamination of the regions they drain and (2) careful assessment of lymph nodes elsewhere so that you can distinguish between regional and generalized lymphadenopathy.

Diffuse lymphadenopathy raises the suspicion of HIV or AIDS.

Occasionally you may mistake a band of muscle or an artery for a lymph node. You should be able to roll a node in two directions: up and down, and side to side. Neither a muscle nor an artery will pass this test.

The Trachea and the Thyroid Gland

To orient yourself to the neck, identify the thyroid and cricoid cartilages and the trachea below them.

- *Inspect the trachea* for any deviation from its usual midline position. Then *feel for any deviation*. Place your finger along one side of the trachea and note the space between it and the sternocleidomastoid. Compare it with the other side. The spaces should be symmetric.

  Masses in the neck may push the trachea to one side. Tracheal deviation may also signify important problems in the thorax, such as a mediastinal mass, atelectasis, or a large pneumothorax (see Table 13-7, pp. 367–368).

- *Inspect the neck for the thyroid gland.* Tip the patient's head back a bit. Using tangential lighting directed downward from the tip of the patient's chin, *inspect the region below the cricoid cartilage* for the gland. The lower shadowed border of each thyroid gland shown here is outlined by arrows.

  The lower border of this large thyroid gland is outlined by tangential lighting. *Goiter* is a general term for an enlarged thyroid gland.[5,6]

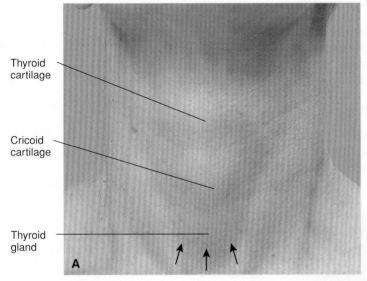

Thyroid cartilage

Cricoid cartilage

Thyroid gland

A

B

AT REST

Ask the patient to sip some water and to extend the neck again and swallow. Watch for upward movement of the thyroid gland, noting its contour and symmetry. The thyroid cartilage, the cricoid cartilage, and the thyroid gland all rise with swallowing and then fall to their resting positions.

With swallowing, the lower border of this large gland rises and looks less symmetric.

SWALLOWING

Assessment of the thyroid can be done by an anterior or posterior approach. As your skills develop, you will determine which approach is best for you; however, until you become familiar with this examination, check your visual observations with your fingers from in front of the patient and then palpate from the posterior.

Palpating the thyroid gland may seem difficult at first. Use the cues from visual inspection. Find your landmarks—the notched thyroid cartilage and the cricoid cartilage below it. Locate the *thyroid isthmus,* usually overlying the second, third, and fourth tracheal rings.

Adopt good technique, and follow the steps listed which can be used for both the anterior and posterior approach. With experience you will become more adept. The thyroid gland is usually easier to feel in a long slender neck than in a short stocky one. In shorter necks, added extension of the neck may help. In some people, however, the thyroid gland is partially or wholly substernal and not amenable to physical examination.

Steps for Palpating the Thyroid Gland

- Ask the patient to flex the neck slightly forward to relax the sterno-cleidomastoid muscles.
- Place the fingers of both hands on the patient's neck so that your index fingers are just below the cricoid cartilage.
- Ask the patient to sip and swallow water as before. Feel for the thyroid isthmus rising up under your finger pads. It is often but not always palpable.
- The lobes are somewhat harder to feel than the isthmus, so practice, Cardiovascular System is needed. The anterior surface of a lateral lobe is approximately the size of the distal phalanx of the thumb and feels somewhat rubbery.
- Note the *size, shape,* and *consistency* of the gland and identify any *nodules* or *tenderness*.
- If the thyroid gland is enlarged, listen over the lateral lobes with a stethoscope to detect a *bruit*, a sound similar to a cardiac murmur but of noncardiac origin.

Although physical characteristics of the thyroid gland, such as size, shape, and consistency, are diagnostically important, assessment of thyroid function depends on symptoms, signs elsewhere in the body, and laboratory tests.[7] See Table 10-4, Thyroid Enlargement and Function, (p. 233).

Soft consistency in *Graves disease;* firm in *Hashimoto thyroiditis,* malignancy. Benign and malignant nodules,[8,9] tenderness in thyroiditis.

A localized systolic or continuous bruit may be heard in *hyperthyroidism.*

The Carotid Arteries and Jugular Veins

Defer a detailed examination of these vessels until the patient lies down for the cardiovascular examination. Jugular venous distention may be visible in the sitting position, however, and should not be overlooked. You should also be alert to unusually prominent arterial pulsations. See Chapter 14, The Cardiovascular System for further discussion.

RECORDING YOUR FINDINGS

Recording the Physical Examination—The Head and Neck

Head—The skull is normocephalic/atraumatic (NC/AT). Hair straight, brown, and soft.
Neck—Trachea midline. Neck supple; thyroid isthmus palpable, lobes nonpalpable.
Lymph Nodes—No head or neck adenopathy.
OR
Head—The skull is normocephalic/atraumatic. Frontal balding; thin, brown hair.
Neck—Trachea midline. Neck supple; thyroid isthmus midline, lobes palpable but not enlarged.
Lymph Nodes—R submandibular and R occipital lymph palpated, 1×1 cm, rubbery, nontender and mobile.

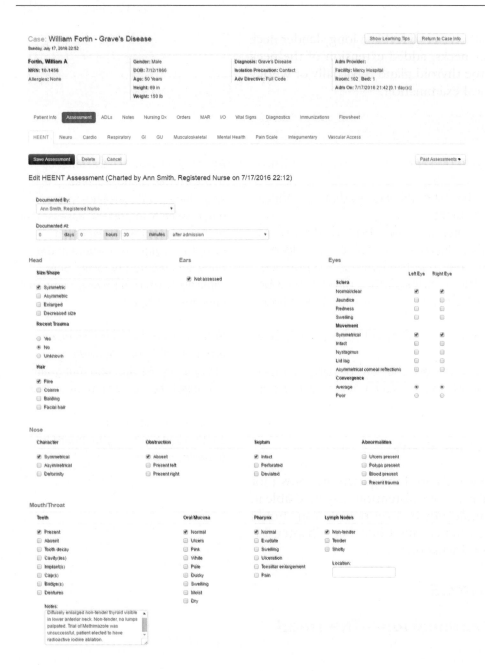

Case: William Fortin - Grave's Disease
Sunday, July 17, 2016 22:52

Fortin, William A	Gender: Male	Diagnosis: Grave's Disease	Adm Provider:
MRN: 10-1456	DOB: 7/12/1966	Isolation Precaution: Contact	Facility: Mercy Hospital
Allergies: None	Age: 50 Years	Adv Directive: Full Code	Room: 102 Bed: 1
	Height: 69 in		Adm On: 7/17/2016 21:42 [0.1 day(s)]
	Weight: 150 lb		

Show Learning Tips   Return to Case Info

Patient Info   **Assessment**   ADLs   Notes   Nursing Dx   Orders   MAR   I/O   Vital Signs   Diagnostics   Immunizations   Flowsheet

HEENT   Neuro   Cardio   Respiratory   GI   GU   Musculoskeletal   Mental Health   Pain Scale   Integumentary   Vascular Access

Save Assessment   Delete   Cancel   Past Assessments ▼

Edit HEENT Assessment (Charted by Ann Smith, Registered Nurse on 7/17/2016 22:12)

Documented By:
Ann Smith, Registered Nurse   ▼

Documented At:
| 0 | days | 0 | hours | 30 | minutes | after admission | ▼ |

Head

Size/Shape
☑ Symmetric
☐ Asymmetric
☐ Enlarged
☐ Decreased size

Recent Trauma
○ Yes
◉ No
○ Unknown

Hair
☑ Fine
☐ Coarse
☐ Balding
☐ Facial hair

Ears
☑ Not assessed

Eyes

	Left Eye	Right Eye
Sclera		
Normal/clear	☑	☑
Jaundice	☐	☐
Redness	☐	☐
Swelling	☐	☐
Movement		
Symmetrical	☑	☑
Intact	☐	☐
Nystagmus	☐	☐
Lid lag	☐	☐
Asymmetrical corneal reflections	☐	☐
Convergence		
Average	◉	◉
Poor	○	○

Nose

Character
☑ Symmetrical
☐ Asymmetrical
☐ Deformity

Obstruction
☑ Absent
☐ Present left
☐ Present right

Septum
☑ Intact
☐ Perforated
☐ Deviated

Abnormalities
☐ Ulcers present
☐ Polyps present
☐ Blood present
☐ Recent trauma

Mouth/Throat

Teeth
☑ Present
☐ Absent
☐ Tooth decay
☐ Cavity(ies)
☐ Implant(s)
☐ Cap(s)
☐ Bridge(s)
☐ Dentures

Oral Mucosa
☑ Normal
☐ Ulcers
☐ Pink
☐ White
☐ Pale
☐ Dusky
☐ Swelling
☐ Moist
☐ Dry

Pharynx
☑ Normal
☐ Exudate
☐ Swelling
☐ Ulceration
☐ Tonsillar enlargement
☐ Pain

Lymph Nodes
☑ Non-tender
☐ Tender
☐ Shotty

Location:
[   ]

Notes:
Diffusely enlarged non-tender thyroid visible in lower anterior neck. Non-tender, no lumps palpated. Trial of Methimazole was unsuccessful, patient elected to have radioactive iodine ablation.

HEALTH PROMOTION AND COUNSELING
Important Topics
Prevention of Traumatic Brain Injury

The Centers for Disease Control and Prevention note that 40% of all TBIs are caused by falls, which is the overall leading cause of TBIs in the United States. The two age groups affected significantly are children from birth to 14 years old and adults over the age of 65 years old. The statistics for the 0- to 14-year-old age group reveal that 55% of TBIs are caused by falls; the numbers increase to 81% for adults over 65 years of age. The second leading cause of TBIs is unintentional blunt trauma and the third is motor vehicle crashes.[4]

The leading causes of TBI are falls, being hit or struck by an object, and motor vehicle accidents. Teaching patients about prevention of head injuries is paramount.

To decrease the likelihood of falls, suggest the following:

- Install safety features in the home such as grab bars in the bathroom and nonslip mats in the bathtub.

- Avoid the use of throw rugs.

- Remove extension cords from high-traffic areas.

- Use rails on stairs.

- Wear nonslip, well-fitting shoes.

- Install gates on stairs.

- Install window guards.

- Do not use walkers for babies.

- Review medication lists with the health care provider to assess for side effects such as fainting or dizziness, which could lead to falls.

To prevent head injuries in motor vehicle accidents, recommend the following:

- Always use seat belts.

- Ensure small children are using car seats or booster seats appropriate for their size and weight.

- Small children should sit in the back seat especially if the car has a passenger airbag.

Traumatic brain injury (TBI) is a leading cause of death and disability in infants and children. Infants and young children have a malleable, thin skull with sutures that have not fused and a comparatively large head with weak neck muscles, which increase the risk of injury.[5]

- Never drive under the influence of alcohol or drugs, including over-the-counter medications that cause drowsiness.

- Use hands-free phones and never text when driving.

- Wear a helmet when riding motorcycles, all-terrain vehicles, motorized scooters, bicycles, horses, or snowmobiles.

Adolescents are more likely to sustain a TBI from a fall, blunt trauma (e.g., sports-related injury) or a motor vehicle accident. There has been increased research on the prevention and care of TBIs.

To avert injuries from being hit by an object, recommend the following:

- Wear helmets when participating in risky activities, such as skiing, snowboarding, skating, batting, and contact sports.

- Place heavy objects on shelves at eye level or lower.

- Avoid dangerous situations or fights.

- Lock firearms and bullets in a separate area.

Safety and prevention are ongoing, and every possible situation is not addressed here. This is an awareness issue that each individual needs to account for in his or her own surroundings. Community health nurses can be instrumental in home assessments. They are able to assist individuals, families, and communities in identifying potential risks and remediations.

Lifting the Burden: The Global Campaign to reduce the burden of headache
HEADS UP: Education initiative of the CDC to protect children and teens from concussions and other brain injuries
http://www.cdc.gov/headsup/about/index.html
SAFE KIDS Worldwide: Global organization aimed at keeping kids safe
http://www.safekids.org
Think First: National Injury Prevention Organization
http://www.thinkfirst.org
Brain Injury Association of America
http://www.biausa.org
"Help Seniors Live Better, Longer: Prevent Brain Injury": CDC program to raise awareness or TBI prevention, recognition, and response in older adults
http://www.cdc.gov/traumaticbraininjury/seniors.html

TABLE 10-1 Primary Headaches[10-15]

Headaches are classified as *primary*, without underlying pathology, or *secondary*, with a serious underlying cause often warranting urgent attention. Secondary headaches are more likely to occur after age 50 years with a sudden severe onset and should be ruled out before making the diagnosis of a primary headache.[16] About 90% of headaches are primary headaches and fall into four categories: tension, migraine, cluster, and chronic daily headache. The features of tension, migraine, and cluster headaches are highlighted below. *Chronic daily headache* is not a diagnosis, but a category containing pre-existing headaches that have been transformed into more pronounced forms of migraines, chronic tension-type headaches, and medication-overuse headaches and last more than 15 days a month for more than 3 months.[17] Risk factors include obesity; more than one headache a week; caffeine ingestion; use of headache medications >10 days a month, such as analgesics, ergots, and triptans; and sleep and mood disorders.

	Tension	Migraines	Cluster
Process	Process unclear—possibly heightened CNS pain sensitivity. Involves pericranial muscle tenderness; etiology also unclear	Neuronal dysfunction, possibly of brainstem origin, involving low serotonin level, spreading cortical depression and trigeminovascular activation; types: with aura, without aura, variants	Process unclear—possibly hypothalamic then trigeminoautonomic activation
Lifetime Prevalence	Most common headache (40%); prevalence about 50%	10% of headaches; prevalence 18% of U.S. adults; affects ~15% of women, 6% of men	<1%, more common in men.
Location	Usually bilateral; may be generalized or localized to the back of the head and upper neck or to the frontotemporal area	Unilateral in ~70%; bifrontal or global in ~30%	Unilateral, usually behind or around the eye or temple
Quality and Severity	Steady; pressing or tightening; nonthrobbing pain; mild to moderate intensity	Throbbing or aching, pain, moderate to severe in intensity; preceded by an aura in up to 30%	Sharp, continuous, intense; severe in intensity
Timing			
Onset	Gradual	Fairly rapid, reaching a peak in 1–2 hours	Abrupt; peaks within minutes
Duration	30 minutes–7 days	4–72 hours	15 minutes to 3 hours
Course	Episodic; may be chronic	Recurrent—usually monthly, but weekly in ~10%; peak incidence early to mid-adolescence	Episodic, clustered in time, with several each day for 4–8 weeks and then relief for 6–12 months
Associated Symptoms	Sometimes photophobia, phonophobia; scalp tenderness; nausea absent	Prodrome: nausea, vomiting, photophobia, phonophobia; aura in 30%; either visual (flickering, zig-zagging lines), or motor (paresthesias of hand, arm, or face, or language dysfunction)	Unilateral autonomic symptoms: lacrimation, rhinorrhea, miosis, ptosis, eyelid edema, conjunctival infection
Triggers/ Factors That Aggravate or Provoke	Sustained muscle tension, as in driving or typing; stress; sleep disturbances	Alcohol, certain foods, or stress may provoke; also menses, high altitude; aggravated by noise and bright light	During attack, sensitivity to alcohol may increase
Factors That Relieve	Possibly massage, relaxation	Quiet, dark room; sleep; sometimes transient relief from pressure on the involved artery	

Sources: Headache Classification Committee of the International Headache Society (IHS). The International Classification of Headache Disorders, 3rd edition (beta version). *Cephalalgia.* 2013;33:629; Lipton RB, Bigal ME, Steiner TJ, et al. Classification of primary headaches. *Neurology.* 2004;63:427; Sun-Edelstein C, Bigal ME, Rappoport AM. Chronic migraine and medication overuse headache: clarifying the current International Headache Society classification criteria. *Cephalalgia.* 2009;29:445; Lipton RB, Stewart WF, Seymour D, et al. Prevalence and burden of migraine in the United States: data from the American Migraine Study II. *Headache.* 2001;41:646; Fumal A, Schoenen J. Tension-type headache: current research and clinical management. *Lancet Neurol.* 2008;7:70; Nesbitt AD, Goadsby PJ. Cluster headache. *BMJ.* 2012;344:e2407.

TABLE 10-2 Secondary Headaches and Cranial Neuralgias[18-23]

Type	Process	Location	Quality and Severity
Secondary Headaches			
Analgesic Rebound	Withdrawal of medication	Previous headache pattern	Variable
Headaches from Eye Disorders			
Errors of Refraction (farsightedness and astigmatism, but not nearsightedness)	Probably the sustained contraction of the extraocular muscles, and possibly of the frontal, temporal, and occipital muscles	Around and over the eyes; may radiate to the occipital area	Steady, aching, dull
Acute Glaucoma	Sudden increase in intraocular pressure (see p. 264)	Pain in and around one eye	Steady, aching, often severe
Headache from Sinusitis	Mucosal inflammation of the paranasal sinuses	Usually frontal sinuses above the eyes or over the maxillary sinus	Aching or throbbing, severity variable; consider possible migraine
Meningitis	Viral or bacterial infection of the meninges surrounding the brain and spinal cord	Generalized	Steady or throbbing, very severe
Subarachnoid Hemorrhage— "Thunderclap Headache"	Bleeding from a ruptured cerebral saccular aneurysm; rarely from AV malformation, mycotic aneurysm	Generalized	Very severe, "the worst of my life"
Brain Tumor	Mass lesion causing displacement of or traction on pain-sensitive arteries and veins or pressure on nerves	Variable, including lobes of brain, cerebellum, barinstem	Aching, steady, dull pain worse on awakening the better after several hours
Giant Cell (Temporal) Arteritis	Transmural lymphocytic vasculitis often involving multinucleated giant cells that disrupts the internal elastic lamina of large-caliber arteries	Localized near the involved artery, most often the temporal artery in those > age 50, women > men (2:1 ratio)	Throbbing, generalized, persistent; often severe
Postconcussion Headache	Follows mild acceleration–deceleration traumatic brain injury; may involve axonal, cerebrovascular autoregulatory, neurochemical injury	Often but not always localized to the injured area	Dull, aching, constant; may have features of tension and migraine headaches
Cranial Neuralgias			
Trigeminal Neuralgia (CN V)	Vascular compression of CN V, usually near entry to pons leading to focal demyelination, aberrant discharge; 10% with causative intracranial lesion	Cheek, jaws, lips, or gums; trigeminal nerve divisions 2 and 3 > 1	Shock-like, stabbing, burning; severe

Note: Blanks appear in this table when the categories are not applicable or not usually helpful in assessing the problem.

Sources: Headache Classification Committee of the International Headache Society (IHS). The International Classification of Headache Disorders, 3rd ed. (beta version). *Cephalalgia.* 2013;33:629; Schwedt TJ, Matharu MS, Dodick DW. Thunderclap headache. *Lancet Neurol.* 2006;5:621; Van de Beek D, de Gans J, Spanjaard L, et al. Clinical features and prognostic factors in adults with bacterial meningitis. *N Engl J Med.* 2004;351:1849; Salvarini C, Cantini F, Hunder GG. Polymyalgia rheumatica and giant cell arteritis. *Lancet.* 2008;372:234; Smetana GW, Shmerling RH. Does this patient have temporal arteritis? *JAMA.* 2002;287:92; Ropper AH, Gorson KC. Clinical practice. Concussion. *N Engl J Med.* 2007;356:166. American College of Physicians. Neurology—MKSAP 16. Philadelphia, PA; 2012.

Timing			Associated Symptoms	Factors That Aggravate or Provoke	Factors That Relieve
Onset	Duration	Course			
Variable	Depends on prior headache pattern	Depends on frequency of "mini-withdrawals"	Depends on prior headache pattern	Fever, carbon monoxide, hypoxia, withdrawal of caffeine, other headache triggers	Depends on cause
Gradual	Variable	Variable	Eye fatigue, "sandy" sensations in eyes, redness of conjunctiva	Prolonged use of the eyes, particularly for close work	Rest of the eyes
Often rapid	Variable, may depend on treatment	Variable, may depend on treatment	Blurred vision, nausea, and vomiting; halos around lights, reddening of eye	Sometimes provoked by mydriatic drops	
Variable	Often daily several hours at a time, persisting until treatment	Often daily in a repetitive pattern	Local tenderness, nasal congestion, discharge, and fever	May be aggravated by coughing, sneezing, or jarring the head	Nasal decongestants, antibiotics
Fairly rapid, usually <24 hours; may be sudden onset	Variable, usually days	Viral: usually <1 week; bacterial: persistent until treatment	Fever, stiff neck, photophobia, change in mental status		Immediate antibiotics until diagnosis of if bacterial or viral
Sudden onset; can be less than a minute	Variable, usually days	Varies according to presenting severity and level of consciousness; worst if initial coma	Nausea, vomiting, loss of consciousness, neck pain. Possible prior neck symptoms from "sentinel leaks"	Rebleeding, ↑ intracranial pressure, cerebral edema	Subspecialty treatments
Variable	Often brief; depends on location and rate of growth	Intermittent but may progress in intensity over a period of days	Seizures, hemiparesis, field cuts, personality changes. Also nausea, vomiting, vision change, gait change	May be aggravated by coughing, sneezing, or sudden movements of the head	Subspecialty treatments
Gradual or rapid	Variable	Recurrent or persistent over weeks to months	Tenderness over temporal artery, adjacent scalp; fever (in ~50%), fatigue, weight loss; new headache (~60%), jaw claudication (~50%), visual loss or blindness (~15–20%), polymyalgia rheumatica (~50%)	Movement of neck and shoulders	Often sterioids
Within 7 days of the injury up to 3 months	Weeks to up to a year	Tends to diminish over time	Drowsiness, poor concentration, confusion, memory loss, blurred vision, dizziness, irritability, restlessness, fatigue	Mental and physical exertion, straining, stooping, emotional excitement, alcohol	Rest; medication
Abrupt, paroxysmal	Each jab lasts seconds but recurs at intervals of seconds or minutes	May recur daily for weeks to months then resolve; can be chronic progressive	Exhaustion from recurrent pain	Touching certain areas of the lower face or mouth; chewing, talking, brushing teeth	Medication; neurovascular decompression

TABLE
10-3

Selected Facies

Facial Swelling

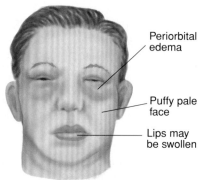

Periorbital edema

Puffy pale face

Lips may be swollen

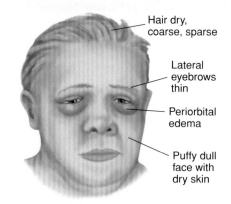

Hair dry, coarse, sparse

Lateral eyebrows thin

Periorbital edema

Puffy dull face with dry skin

Red cheeks

Hirsutism

Moon face

Cushing Syndrome
The increased adrenal cortisol production of Cushing syndrome produces a round or "moon" face with red cheeks. Excessive hair growth may be present in the mustache and sideburn areas and on the chin.

Nephrotic Syndrome
The face is edematous and often pale. Swelling usually appears first around the eyes and in the morning. The eyes may become slitlike when edema is severe.

Myxedema
The patient with severe hypothyroidism *(myxedema)* has a dull, puffy facies. The edema, often pronounced around the eyes, does not pit with pressure. The hair and eyebrows are dry, coarse, and thinned. The skin is dry.

Other Facies

Swelling

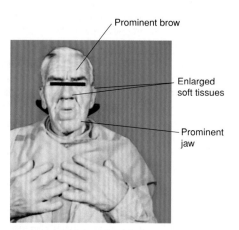

Prominent brow

Enlarged soft tissues

Prominent jaw

Stare

Decreasd mobility

Parotid Gland Enlargement
Chronic bilateral asymptomatic parotid gland enlargement may be associated with obesity, diabetes, cirrhosis, and other conditions. Note the swellings anterior to the ear lobes and above the angles of the jaw. Gradual unilateral enlargement suggests neoplasm. Acute enlargement is seen in mumps.

Acromegaly
The increased growth hormone of acromegaly produces enlargement of both bone and soft tissues. The head is elongated, with bony prominence of the forehead, nose, and lower jaw. Soft tissues of the nose, lips, and ears also enlarge. The facial features appear generally coarsened.

Parkinson Disease
Decreased facial mobility blunts expression. A mask-like face may result, with decreased blinking and a characteristic stare. Since the neck and upper trunk tend to flex forward, the patient seems to peer upward toward the observer. Facial skin becomes oily, and drooling may occur.

TABLE 10-4 — Thyroid Enlargement and Function

Diffuse Enlargement. Includes the isthmus and lateral lobes; there are no discretely palpable nodules. Causes include Graves disease, Hashimoto thyroiditis, and endemic goiter.

Single Nodule. May be a cyst, a benign tumor, or one nodule within a multinodular gland. It raises the question of malignancy. Risk factors are prior irradiation, hardness, rapid growth, fixation to surrounding tissues, enlarged cervical nodes, and occurrence in males.[8]

Multinodular Goiter. An enlarged thyroid gland with two or more nodules suggests a metabolic rather than a neoplastic process. Positive family history and continuing nodular enlargement are additional risk factors for malignancy.

TABLE 10-5 — Symptoms and Signs of Thyroid Dysfunction[7,22–26]

	Hyperthyroidism	Hypothyroidism
Symptoms	Nervousness	Fatigue, lethargy
	Weight loss despite increased appetite	Modest weight gain with anorexia
	Excessive sweating and heat intolerance	Dry, coarse skin and cold intolerance
	Palpitations	Swelling of face, hands, and legs
	Frequent bowel movements	Constipation
	Muscular weakness of the proximal type and tremor	Weakness, muscle cramps, arthralgias, paresthesias, impaired memory and hearing
Signs	Warm, smooth, moist skin	Dry, coarse, cool skin, sometimes yellowish from carotene, with nonpitting edema and loss of hair
	With Graves disease, eye signs such as stare, lid lag, and exophthalmos	Periorbital puffiness
	Increased systolic and decreased diastolic blood pressures	Decreased systolic and increased diastolic blood pressures
	Tachycardia or atrial fibrillation	Bradycardia and, in late stages, hypothermia
	Hyperdynamic cardiac pulsations with an accentuated S1	Intensity of heart sounds sometimes decreased
	Tremor and proximal muscle weakness	Impaired memory, mixed hearing loss, somnolence, peripheral neuropathy, carpal tunnel syndrome

BIBLIOGRAPHY

CITATIONS

1. World Health Organization. Atlas of Headache Disorders and Resources in the World 2011. Geneva: WHO; 2011.
2. World Health Organization. Headache Disorders. Available at: http://www.who.int/mediacentre/factsheets/fs277/en. Accessed June 10, 2015.
3. Zwart JA, Dyb G, Hagen K, et al. Analgesic use: a predictor of chronic pain and medication overuse: the Head-HUNT Study. *Neurology.* 2003;61:160–164.
4. Centers for Disease Control. Injury Prevention and Control: Traumatic Brain Injury. Available at: http://www.cdc.gov/traumaticbraininjury/get_the_facts.html. Accessed November 15, 2015.
5. Centers for Disease Control. Injury Prevention and Control: Traumatic Brain Injury in the United States Fact Sheet. Division of Unintentional Injury Prevention, June 2015. Available at: http://www.cdc.gov/TraumaticBrainInjury/factsheets_reports.html. Accessed November 15, 2015.
6. Lesnik DJ, O'Leary MA, Noordzij JP, et al. Surgical management of benign diseases of the thyroid gland. In: *Diseases of the Thyroid and Parathyroid Glands. Practical Guide.* Warszawa: MediPage;2013:83.
7. Syrenicz A, Koziołek M, Ciechanowicz K, et al. New insights into the diagnosis of nodular goiter. *Thyroid Res.* 2014;7:6.
8. Hegedus L. The thyroid nodule. *N Engl J Med.* 2004; 351(17):1764–1771.
9. Castro MR, Gharib H. Controversies in the management of thyroid nodules. *Ann Intern Med.* 2005;142(11):926–931.
10. Headache Classification Committee of the International Headache Society (IHS). The International Classification of Headache Disorders, 3rd edition (beta version). *Cephalalgia.* 2013;33:629.
11. Lipton RB, Bigal ME, Steiner TJ, et al. Classification of primary headaches. *Neurology.* 2004;63:427.
12. Sun-Edelstein C, Bigal ME, Rappoport AM. Chronic migraine and medication overuse headache: clarifying the current International Headache Society classification criteria. *Cephalalgia.* 2009;29:445.
13. Lipton RB, Stewart WF, Seymour D, et al. Prevalence and burden of migraine in the United States: data from the American Migraine Study II. *Headache.* 2001;41:646.
14. Fumal A, Schoenen J. Tension-type headache: current research and clinical management. *Lancet Neuro.* 2008;7:70.
15. Nesbitt AD, Goadsby PJ. Cluster headache. *BMJ.* 2012;344:e2407.
16. Schwedt TJ, Matharu MS, Dodick DW. Thunderclap headache. *Lancet Neurol.* 2016;5:621.
17. Van de Beek D, de Gans J, Spanjaard L, et al. Clinical features and prognostic factors in adults with bacterial meningitis. N *Engl J Med.* 2014;351:1849.
18. Salvarini C, Cantini F, Hunder GG. Polymyalgia rheumatica and giant cell arteritis. *Lancet.* 2008;372:234.
19. Smetana GW, Shmerling RH. Does this patient have temporal arteritis? *JAMA.* 2002;287:92.
20. Ropper AH, Gorson KC. Clinical practice. Concussion. *N Engl J Med.* 2007;356:166.
21. American College of Physicians. Neurology – MKSAP 16. Philadelphia, PA; 2012.
22. Nakamura H, Hirokawa M, Ota H, et al. Is an increase in thyroid nodule volume a risk factor for malignancy? *Thyroid.* 2015;804–811.
23. Williams S. Holistic management of thyroid dysfunction: The nurse's role. *Altern. Complement. Ther.* 2004;384–388.
24. Olson B. Facets of thyroid disease in women: Four case reports. *J. Wom. Health.* 2009;85–91.
25. Terris DJ, Snyder S, Carneiro-Pla D, et al. American Thyroid Association Statement on Outpatient Thyroidectomy for the American Thyroid Association Surgical Affairs Committee Writing Task Force. *Thyroid.* 2013;1193–1202.
26. Garber JR, Cobin RH, Gharib H, et al. Clinical practice guidelines for hypothyroidism in adults: cosponsored by the American Association of Clinical Endocrinologists and the American Thyroid Association. *Thyroid.* 2012;1200–1235.

ADDITIONAL REFERENCES

The Head

Bacorro WR, Sy Ortin TT, Suarez CG, et al. Validation of the MD Anderson symptom inventory-head-and-neck-filipino (MDASI-HN-F): clinical utility of symptom screening among patients with head-and-neck cancer. *BMJ Support Palliative Care.* 2015.

Bendtsen L. Treatment guidelines: implications for community-based headache treatment. *Int J Clin Pract Suppl.* 2015; (182):13–16.

Cady RK, Dodick DW, Levine HL, et al. Sinus headache: a neurology, otolaryngology, allergy, and primary care consensus on diagnosis and treatment. *Mayo Clin Proc.* 2005;80(7): 908–916.

Dowson A. The burden of headache: global and regional prevalence of headache and its impact. *Int J Clin Pract Suppl.* 2015;(182):3–7.

Faul M, Xu L, Wald MM, et al. *Traumatic Brain Injury in the United States: Emergency Department Visits, Hospitalizations and Deaths 2002–2006.* Atlanta, GA: Centers for Disease Control and Prevention, National Center for Injury Prevention and Control; 2010.

Franges EZ. When a headache is really a brain tumor. *Nurse Pract.* 2006;31(4):47–51.

Langlois JA, Rutland-Brown W, Thomas KE. *Traumatic Brain Injury in the United States: Emergency Department Visits, Hospitalizations, and Deaths.* Atlanta, GA: Centers for Disease Control and Prevention, National Center for Injury Prevention and Control; 2006.

Lipton RB, Bigal ME, Steiner TJ, et al. Classification of primary headaches. *Neurology.* 2004;63(3):427–435.

Paemeleire K, Bahra A, Evers S, et al. Medication-overuse headache in patients with cluster headache. *Neurology.* 2006; 67(1):109–113.

Straus SE, Thorpe KE, Holroyd-Leduc J. How do I perform a lumbar puncture and analyze the results to diagnose bacterial meningitis? *JAMA.* 2006;296(16):2012–2022.

Van Gijn J, Kerr RS, Rinkel GJ. Subarachnoid haemorrhage. *Lancet.* 2007;369(9558):306–318.

BIBLIOGRAPHY

Wong TY, Klein R, Sharrett AR, et al. Retinal arteriolar diameter and risk for hypertension. *Ann Intern Med*. 2004;140(4):248–255.

The Neck

Bliss SJ, Flanders SA, Saint S. A pain in the neck. *N Engl J Med*. 2004;350(10):1037–1042.

Dorshimer GW, Kelly M. Cervical pain in the athlete: common conditions and treatment. *Prim Care*. 2005;32(1):231–243.

Henry PH, Long DL. Enlargement of the lymph nodes and spleen. In: Kasper DL, Fauci AS, Longo DL, et al., eds. *Harrison's Principles of Internal Medicine*. 16th ed. New York, NY: McGraw-Hill; 2005:343–348.

Jiang Y, Zhu XD, Qu S, et al. Guidelines for squamous cell carcinoma of the head and neck: A systematic assessment of quality. *Ear Nose Throat J*. 2015;94:4–5.

Maguire T. Community-based headache management. *Int J Clin Pract Suppl*. 2015;(182):17–20.

Prisco MK. Evaluating neck masses. *Nurse Pract*. 2000;25(4):30–32, 35–36.

Schwetschenau E, Kelley DJ. The adult neck mass. *Am Fam Phys*. 2003;67(6):1190, 1192, 1195.

Silberstein S, Lipton R, Dodick D. *Wolff's Headache and Other Head Pain*. New York, NY: Oxford University Press; 2008.

Shaughnessy, Lynn D. *Radio Frequency Identification*.
Des Kapstar. 2005, Pupdf. AS: Power. DS., et. al. *Leadership and Motivation in Nursing Alliances*. 16th ed. New York: McGraw Hill. 2006. 435-443.

LEARNING OBJECTIVES

The student will:

1. Identify the components and function of the eye.

2. Collect an accurate health history of the eye.

3. Describe the physical examination techniques performed to evaluate the eye.

4. Demonstrate how to use the ophthalmoscope.

5. Identify the measures for prevention or early detection of eye disease, infections, or vision loss.

6. Perform a complete eye examination.

7. Document a complete eye assessment using information from·the health history and physical examination.

ANATOMY AND PHYSIOLOGY

The eye is the sensory organ of vision and has many critical components, including the cranial nerves. During the assessment various signs and symptoms signal changes in the eyes. The nurse's role is to detect these changes and work with the health care team to prevent injury or loss of vision.

Eye Structures

The structures of the eye are identified on this page. Note that the upper eyelid covers a portion of the iris but does not touch the pupil. The opening between the eyelids is called the *palpebral fissure*. The white sclera may look somewhat darker at its periphery. The *conjunctiva* is a clear mucous membrane with two easily visible components. The *bulbar conjunctiva,* also known as the sclera covers most of the anterior eyeball, adhering loosely to the

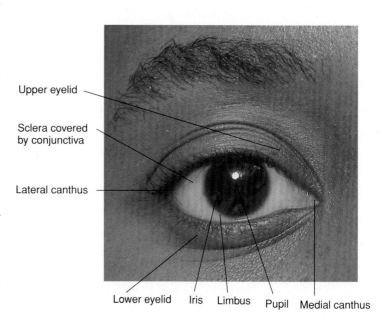

Upper eyelid

Sclera covered by conjunctiva

Lateral canthus

Lower eyelid   Iris   Limbus   Pupil   Medial canthus

underlying tissue. The *palpebral conjunctiva* lines the eyelids. The two parts of the conjunctiva merge in a folded recess that permits movement of the eyeball.

Palpebral - relates to the eyelids.

Within the eyelids lie firm strips of connective tissue called *tarsal plates*. Each plate contains a parallel row of *meibomian glands*, which open on the lid margin. The *levator palpebrae*, the muscle that raises the upper eyelid, is innervated by the oculomotor nerve, cranial nerve (CN) III. Smooth muscle, innervated by the sympathetic nervous system, also contributes to lid elevation.

A film of tear fluid protects the conjunctiva and cornea from drying, inhibits microbial growth, and gives a smooth optical surface to the cornea. This fluid comes from the meibomian glands, conjunctival glands, and lacrimal gland. The *lacrimal gland* lies mostly within the bony orbit, above and lateral to the eyeball. The tear fluid spreads across the eye and drains medially through two tiny holes called *lacrimal puncta*. The tears then pass into the *lacrimal sac* and into the nose through the *nasolacrimal duct*. You can easily find a *punctum* atop the small elevation of the lower lid medially. The lacrimal sac rests in a small depression inside the bony orbit and is not visible.

The eyeball is a spherical structure that focuses light on the neurosensory elements within the retina. The muscles of the iris control pupillary size, constricting in bright light and dilating in the dark. Muscles of the *ciliary body* control the thickness of the lens, allowing the eye to focus on near or distant objects.

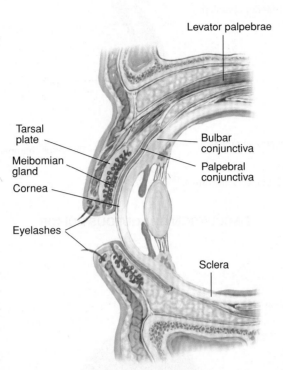

SAGITTAL SECTION OF ANTERIOR EYE WITH LIDS CLOSED

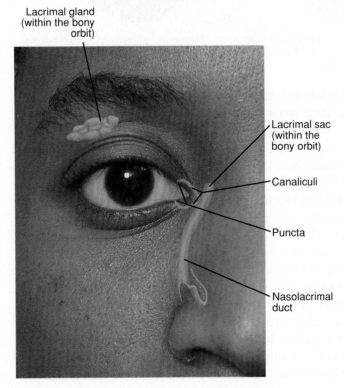

Vitreous humor is the clear gel that fills the space between the lens and the retina. The aqueous humor is a clear liquid that fills the anterior and posterior chambers of the eye, circulating between the cornea and the lens. Aqueous humor is produced by the *ciliary body,* circulates from the posterior chamber through the pupil into the anterior chamber, and drains out through the *canal of Schlemm.* This circulatory system helps to control the pressure inside the eye.

CIRCULATION OF AQUEOUS HUMOR

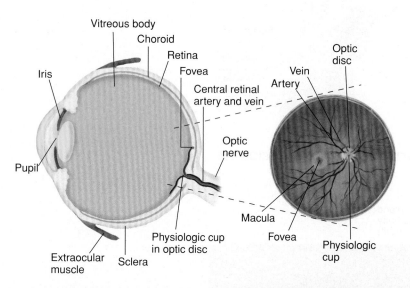

CROSS SECTION OF THE RIGHT EYE SHOWING A PORTION OF THE FUNDUS COMMONLY SEEN WITH THE OPHTHALMOSCOPE

The posterior part of the eye seen through an ophthalmoscope is often called the *fundus* of the eye. Structures here include the retina, choroid, fovea, macula, optic disc, and retinal vessels. The entire fundus is not visible at once and as the ophthalmoscope is adjusted sections of the eye appear. The optic nerve with its retinal vessels enters the eyeball posteriorly. You can find it with an ophthalmoscope at the *optic disc.* When looking into the eye with the ophthalmoscope, it is best to locate the optic disc medially and use this as your landmark. Note the margins of the disc and then locate the arteries and veins. Lateral and slightly inferior to the disc, there is a small depression in the retinal surface that marks the point of central vision. Around it is a darkened circular area called the *fovea.* The roughly circular *macula* (named for a microscopic yellow spot) surrounds the fovea but has no discernible margins. It is unusual to see the normal *vitreous body,* a transparent mass of gelatinous material that fills the eyeball behind the lens. It helps to maintain the shape of the eye.

Visual Fields

A *visual field* is the entire area seen by an eye when it looks at a central point. Fields are typically diagrammed on circles from the **patient's** point of view. The center of the circle represents the focus of gaze. The circumference is 90 degrees from the line of gaze. Each visual field, shown by the white areas below, is divided into quadrants. Note the fields extend farthest on the temporal sides. Visual fields are normally limited by the brows above, the cheeks below, and the nose medially. A lack of retinal receptors at the optic disc produces an oval blind spot in the normal field of each eye, 15 degrees temporal to the line of gaze.

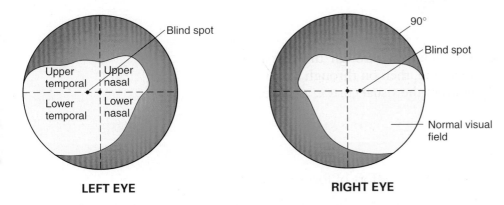

LEFT EYE   **RIGHT EYE**

When a person is using both eyes, the two visual fields overlap in an area of binocular vision. Laterally, vision is monocular.

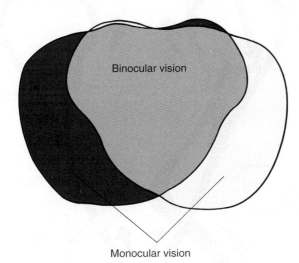

Visual Pathways

To see an image, light reflected from the image must pass through the pupil and be focused on photoreceptors in the retina. The image projected there is upside down and reversed right to left. An image from the upper nasal visual field thus strikes the lower temporal quadrant of the retina.

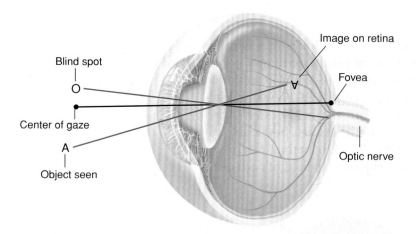

Nerve impulses, stimulated by light, are conducted through the retina, optic nerve (CN II), and optic tract on each side, then on through a curving tract called the *optic radiation*. This ends in the visual cortex, a part of the occipital lobe.

Pupillary Reactions

Pupillary size changes in response to light and to the effort of focusing on a near object.

The Light Reaction

A light beam shining onto one retina causes pupillary constriction both in that eye, termed the *direct reaction* to light, and in the contralateral (opposite) eye, the *consensual reaction* to light. The initial sensory pathways are similar to those described for vision: retina, optic nerve (CN II), and optic tract which diverges in the midbrain. Impulses back to the constrictor muscles are transmitted through the oculomotor nerve, CN III, to the constrictor muscles of the iris of each eye are transmitted through the oculomotor nerve, CN III.

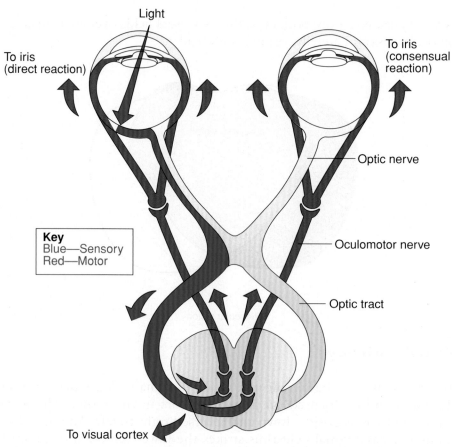

PATHWAYS OF THE LIGHT REACTION

The Near Reaction

The near reaction occurs when a person shifts gaze from a far object to a near one and the pupils constrict. This response, like the light reaction, is mediated by the oculomotor nerve (CN III). At the same time as the *pupillary constriction*, but not a part of it, are (1) *convergence* of the eyes, a medial rectus movement; and (2) *accommodation*, an increased convexity of the lenses caused by contraction of the ciliary muscles. In accommodation, the change in shape of the lenses brings near objects into focus but is not visible to the examiner.

Autonomic Nerve Supply to the Eyes

Fibers traveling in the oculomotor nerve (CN III) and producing pupillary constriction are part of the parasympathetic nervous system. The iris is also supplied by sympathetic fibers. When these are stimulated, the pupil dilates, and the upper eyelid rises a little, as if from fear. The sympathetic pathway starts in the hypothalamus and passes down through the brainstem and cervical cord into the neck. From there, it follows the carotid artery or its branches into the orbit. A lesion anywhere along this pathway may impair sympathetic effects that dilate the pupil.

Extraocular Movements

The coordinated action of six muscles: the four rectus (superior, lateral, medial, and inferior) and two oblique (inferior and superior), control the eye. To test the function of each muscle and the nerve that supplies it, ask the patient to move the eye in the direction controlled by that muscle. There are six *cardinal directions*, indicated by the lines on the figure on the next page. When a person looks down and to the right, for example, the right inferior rectus (CN III) is principally responsible for moving the right eye, whereas the left superior oblique (CN IV) is principally responsible for moving the left. If one of these

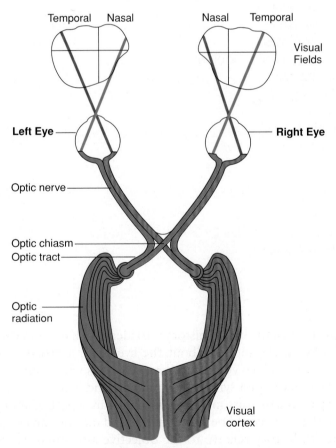

VISUAL PATHWAYS FROM THE RETINA TO THE VISUAL CORTEX

muscles is paralyzed, the eye will deviate from its normal position in that direction of gaze and the eyes will no longer appear conjugate, or parallel.

Superior rectus (III)

Lateral rectus (VI)

Inferior rectus (III)

Inferior oblique (III)

Medial rectus (III)

Superior oblique (IV)

Superior rectus (III)

Lateral rectus (VI)

Inferior rectus (III)

CARDINAL DIRECTIONS OF GAZE

THE HEALTH HISTORY

Common or Concerning Symptoms

- Changes in vision:
  - Hyperopia
  - Presbyopia
  - Myopia
  - Scotomas
- Double vision or diplopia
- Strabismus
- Blurring
- Redness
- Itching
- Discharge
- Pain
- Tearing
- Edema
- Lesions
- Visual disturbances
- Photophobia

A scotoma is an area of lost or depressed vision within the visual field and is surrounded by an area of normal vision.

Photophobia or light sensitivity is usually from excess light entering the eye, which may overexcite the photoreceptors in the retina.

The purpose of the health history is to identify changes in the eyes. The nurse should begin the inquiry about the eyes with a broad, open-ended question such as: "Have you noticed any changes with your eyes?" The patient may have developed symptoms gradually and learned to live with changes. Older patients may assume vision changes are a part of aging. They may not realize that they could be seeing better and may not answer the questions in the health history relative to the objective assessment revelations. Further investigation is crucial and more in-depth questioning should be pursued. For example: "Is your vision as good now as previously?"

If changes in vision are revealed then continue:

Is the **difficulty** during close work or at distances?

Difficulty with close work suggests hyperopia (farsightedness) or presbyopia (aging vision) with distances, myopia (nearsightedness).

Is there **blurred** vision? If yes, is the onset sudden or gradual? If sudden and unilateral, is the visual loss painless or painful? Is the blurring of the entire field of vision or only parts of it?

If sudden visual loss is unilateral and *painless,* consider vitreous hemorrhage from diabetes or trauma, macular degeneration, retinal detachment, retinal vein occlusion, or central retinal artery occlusion.

If *painful,* consider causes in the cornea and anterior chamber such as corneal ulcer, uveitis, traumatic hyphema, and acute-angle closure glaucoma.[1,2] Optic neuritis from multiple sclerosis may also be painful.[3] Immediate referral may be warranted.
If *bilateral and painless,* medications that change refraction such as cholinergics, anticholinergics, and steroids may contribute. If bilateral and painful, consider chemical or radiation exposures. If the onset of bilateral visual loss is gradual, this usually arises from *cataracts* or *macular degeneration.*[4]

If the visual field defect is partial, is it central, peripheral, or only on one side?

Slow central loss in nuclear cataract (p. 268), *macular degeneration*[4]; peripheral loss in advanced *open-angle glaucoma* (p. 264); one-sided loss in *hemianopsia* and *quadrantic defects* (p. 248).

Do lights **flash** across the field of vision?

Flashing lights with new vitreous floaters suggest detachment of vitreous from retina. Prompt eye consultation is indicated.[5]

Do **floaters** accompany this symptom?

Does it feel like a curtain is falling?

Are there **specks** in the vision or areas where you are unable to see scotomas? If so, do they move in the visual field with shifts of gaze or are they fixed?

Moving specks or strands suggest vitreous floaters; fixed defects suggest lesions in the retina or visual pathways.

Do you have double vision (diplopia)?

Are the images side by side (horizontal diplopia) or on top of each other (vertical diplopia)? Does this persist with one eye closed? Which eye is affected?

One kind of horizontal diplopia is physiologic. Hold one finger upright approximately 6 inches in front of your face, a second at arm's length. When you focus on either finger, the image of the other is double. A patient who notices this phenomenon can be reassured. Diplopia in adults may arise from a lesion in the brainstem or cerebellum, or from weakness or paralysis of one or more extraocular muscles, as in horizontal diplopia from palsy of cranial nerve CN III or VI, or vertical diplopia from palsy of CN III or IV. Diplopia in one eye, with the other closed, suggests a problem in the cornea or lens.

Do you experience:
  Redness?

Red painless eye is seen in allergies, subconjunctival hemorrhage; red eye with gritty sensation in viral conjunctivitis. Red painful eye is seen in hyphema, episcleritis, acute-angle closure glaucoma, herpes keratitis, foreign body, fungal keratitis, and sarcoid uveitis.[6] See Table 11-1, p. 264.

Infection or allergic reaction

  Excessive tearing?
  Discharge?
  Crusting?
Do you have or have you ever had lesions or growths on your eyelids or eyes?
Are your eyes painful or uncomfortable when you are in the sun or well-lit places?

Photophobia

Eye History

Do you have any past history of eye problems or eye disease?
Do you have a history of:
   Premature birth?
   Trauma or injury to the eye?
   Eye surgery? Related to injury, congenital causes, or cosmetic
      reasons?
   Eye infections?
   Strabismus?
   Amblyopia?
   Cataracts?
   Glaucoma?
   Diabetes?
   Retinal detachment?
   Macular degeneration?
   Blindness?
When was your last eye examination? Test for color blindness?
Do you wear glasses or contact lenses? Hard or soft lenses?
When did you begin to wear them?
Are they corrective or cosmetic?
How do you care for your contacts?
Do you share contacts?
How long are the contacts in your eye? Day hours? Night hours?

Family History

Do you have a family history of congenital eye diseases, cataracts, glaucoma, macular degeneration, or diabetes?

Lifestyle Habits

   Do you smoke?
   Do you wear sunglasses?
   Do you use goggles or protective eyewear? When?
   Are you on any medications/drugs that dry out the eye?

PHYSICAL EXAMINATION

Preparation of the Patient

Preparation of the patient and the environment is crucial to obtain correct findings during the eye examination. If the Snellen chart is located outside the examination room, then this portion of the examination should be completed prior to changing into a patient gown. The area should be well lit and free of distractions. The remainder of the examination will be in a quiet, well-lit room with all necessary equipment in the room.

The components of the eye examination include:

Vision tests: distal, near, and peripheral

Inspection of the eye, eyebrows, lids, conjunctiva and sclera, cornea, lens, iris, and pupils

Inspection and palpation of the lacrimal apparatus

Extraocular movements: assessment of cardinal fields, convergence, corneal light test, cover–uncover test

Inspection of the fundi including the optic disc and cup, retina, and retinal vessels

Equipment for Examination

Eye Chart (e.g., Snellen or "E" chart)
Near Vision Card (e.g., Rosenbaum or Jaegar)
Index card or opaque covering
Penlight
Ophthalmoscope

Vision Tests

Visual Acuity Tests

Eyesight is evaluated using visual acuity tests. Various tests are available to use, including the Snellen chart, the "E" chart, and the Near Vision Chart.

Snellen Test

To test the acuity of central vision and the patient's ability to see at a distance, use a well-lit Snellen eye chart. The chart has the largest letter on the top line and the smallest letters on the bottom row. Position the patient 20 feet from the wall chart. Patients who wear glasses or contact lenses, other than for reading, should wear them for the examination. Ask the patient to cover one eye with an index card (to prevent peeking through the fingers) and to read the smallest line of print possible. Coaxing to attempt the next line may improve performance. A patient who cannot read the largest letter, on the top line, should be positioned closer to the chart; note the intervening distance. Identify the smallest line of print the patient can identify more than half the letters. Record the visual acuity designated at the side of this line and note the number of letters missed, in addition note if glasses or contacts were worn. Test each eye separately and note any misread letters, squinting, or apprehension. During examination of the second eye, the patient can be asked to read the lines backward or right to left to insure the letter series is not memorized.

Documentation: right eye 20/30, left eye 20/30 (–2), with contacts.

Visual acuity is expressed as two numbers (e.g., 20/30): the numerator (top number) indicates the distance of the patient from the chart and this

Referral to an ophthalmologist should be made if vision is worse than 20/30.

number should always be 20 unless the patient moved closer for testing, and the denominator (bottom number) is the distance at which a normal eye can read the line of letters.

Normal vision is 20/20.

Better than normal vision is when the denominator or second number is smaller than the numerator or top number. For example, 20/15 vision is when a person can see from 20 feet what the normal eye can see from 15 feet.

Legally blind is 20/200. Vision of 20/200 means that at 20 feet the patient can read print that a person with normal vision could read at 200 feet.

The **"E" chart** is used for testing children's vision or people who are unable to read. It is similar to the Snellen chart as there are rows with the letter, E facing different positions. The top row is the largest and the bottom row has the smallest. The person being tested is asked to point to the direction the E is facing. Charts with the letter "C" or pictures are also available for testing.

The larger the second number, the worse the vision. "20/40 corrected" means the patient could read the 40 line with glasses (a correction).

Myopia (nearsightedness) causes focusing problems for distance vision.[7]

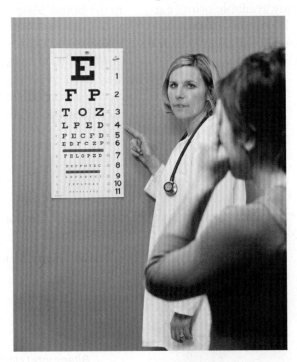

Near Vision

NEAR TEST. Test near vision with a special hand-held card (e.g., Jaeger) held 14 inches away from the eyes. The test identifies the need for reading glasses or bifocals. The card contains paragraphs and the print gradually gets smaller. The patient is asked to read the smallest paragraph possible. Both eyes are tested at the same time without corrective lenses. Generally, this test is done after the age of 40 as near vision begins to decrease.

When scoring the near test, the numerator is 14, as the card is held 14 inches away from the eyes.

Normal near vision is 14/14

Reduced near vision is when the denominator, or second number, is larger than 14. For example, 14/20 near vision is when a person has to hold the card at 14 inches when others with normal near vision can read at 20 inches.

A Jaegar number is another way for near vision to be rated. The J number delineates the text size read. The Jaegar (J) number goes up as the print size goes up. The higher number correlates with decreased near vision.

J1 is the smallest line on the chart = 20/15
J2 = 20/20
J12 = 20/100

Presbyopia (farsightedness) is the impaired near vision found in middle-aged and older people caused by the loss of elasticity of the lens of the eye. Often the patient sees better when the card is farther away.

If there are not any charts, screen visual acuity with any available print (e.g., newspaper) held at 14 inches away from the eyes. If patients cannot read even the largest letters, test their ability to count your upraised fingers and distinguish light (such as your flashlight) from dark.

In the United States, a person is usually considered legally blind when vision in the better eye, corrected by glasses, is 20/200 or less. Legal blindness also results from a constricted field of vision: 20 degrees or less in the better eye.

Peripheral Vision

Peripheral Visual Fields by Confrontation

SCREENING. **Visual fields** are tested to assess peripheral vision. Confrontation is a comparison between the patient and the nurse, provided the nurse has intact peripheral vision, to determine any areas of deficit. Screening starts in the temporal fields because most defects involve these areas. Imagine the patient's visual fields projected onto a glass bowl that encircles the front of the patient's head.

1. Stand about 2 feet away

2. Ask the patient to look with both eyes into your eyes

Field defects that are all or partly temporal include:

Homonymous Hemianopsia

Bitemporal Hemianopsia

Quadratic Defects

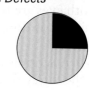

3. Spread your arms apart, just behind and lateral to the patient's head

4. Instruct the patient to point to your wiggling fingers as soon as they are seen

5. Coming from both sides, slowly move the wiggling fingers of both your hands along the imaginary bowl toward the center until the patient points to them

6. Repeat this pattern in the upper and lower temporal quadrants. Usually a person sees both sets of fingers at the same time. If so, the fields are usually normal.

Review these patterns in Table 11-2, Visual Field Defects, p. 265.

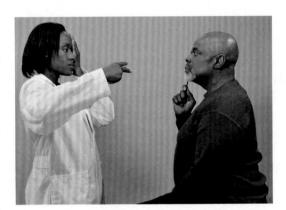

FURTHER TESTING. If you find a defect, try to establish its boundaries. Test one eye at a time. Repeat this at several levels to define the border.

1. Stand/sit at eye level, approximately 2 feet away from the patient

2. Testing one eye at a time, ask the patient to cover one eye with a card

3. With the other eye, the patient looks directly at you

4. Cover your own eye, directly across from the eye the patient has covered

5. Starting midline above the head, slowly move your wiggling finger from the periphery noting where the patient first responds by saying "now" when they see the finger

6. Repeat this in several directions/sides and levels to define the border. The person should be seeing the wiggling fingers at the same time you do

7. Repeat the steps with the opposite eye.

Field defects that are all or partly temporal include:

Review these patterns in Table 11-2, Visual Field Defects, p. 265.

Hemianopsia is when the patient is unable to see in half of the visual field and is generally on one side. This can occur after a cerebrovascular accident or stroke. The patient is unable to distinguish objects to the side of the visual midline. The loss is contralateral, which is on the opposite side of the brain lesion.

A left *homonymous hemianopsia* may thus be established.

Note: The visual field screening test works with all fields except the temporal field. For this field, start the examination with the wiggling finger behind the patient. In this instance, the examiner will see the finger at all times.

A temporal defect in the visual field of one eye suggests a nasal defect in the other eye. To test this hypothesis, examine the other eye in a similar way, again moving from the anticipated defect toward the better vision.

Small visual field defects and enlarged blind spots require a finer stimulus. Using a small red object such as a red-headed matchstick or the red eraser on a pencil, test one eye at a time. As the patient looks into your eye directly opposite, move the object about in the visual field. The normal blind spot (due to the location of the macula) can be found 15 degrees temporal to the line of gaze—the small red object disappears. (Find your own blind spots for practice.)

An enlarged blind spot occurs in conditions affecting the optic nerve such as *glaucoma, optic neuritis,* and *papilledema.*[2]

External Eye

Position and Alignment of the Eyes

Stand in front of the patient and survey the eyes for position and alignment. If one or both eyes seem to protrude, assess them from above.

Inward or outward deviation of the eyes; abnormal protrusion in Graves disease or ocular tumors

Eyebrows

Inspect the eyebrows, noting their quantity and distribution and any scaliness of the underlying skin.

Scaliness occurs in seborrheic dermatitis; lateral sparseness in hypothyroidism

Eyelids

Note the position of the lids in relation to the eyeballs. Inspect for the following:

See Table 11-3, Variations and Abnormalities of the Eyelids, p. 266.

- Width of the palpebral fissures—open area between the upper and lower eyelids

Upslanting palpebral fissures are visible in Down syndrome

- Edema of the lids

- Color of the lids

Red inflamed lid margins occur in *blepharitis,* often with crusting

- Lesions

- Condition and direction of the eyelashes

- Adequacy with which the eyelids close. Look for this especially when the eyes are unusually prominent, when there is facial paralysis, or when the patient is unconscious.

See entropion and ectropion, Table 11-3, Variations and Abnormalities of the Eyelids, p. 266.

Failure of the eyelids to close exposes the corneas to serious damage.

Lacrimal Apparatus

Briefly inspect the regions of the lacrimal gland and lacrimal sac for swelling.

See Table 11-4, Lumps and Swellings in and Around the Eyes, p. 267.

Look for excessive tearing, dryness, or crusting of the eyes. Assessment of dryness may require special testing by an ophthalmologist. To test for naso-lacrimal duct obstruction, see p. 259.

Excessive tearing may be from increased production or impaired drainage of tears. In the first group, causes include conjunctival inflammation and corneal irritation; in the second, ectropion (p. 266) and nasolacrimal duct obstruction.

Conjunctiva and Sclera

Ask the patient to look up as you depress both lower lids with your thumbs, exposing the sclera and conjunctiva. Inspect the sclera and palpebral conjunctiva for color, and note the vascular pattern against the white scleral background. Look for any nodules or swelling.

A yellow sclera indicates jaundice.

If you need a fuller view of the eye, rest your thumb and finger on the bones of the cheek and brow, respectively, and spread the lids.

Ask the patient to look to each side and down. This technique gives you a good view of the sclera and bulbar conjunctiva, but not of the palpebral conjunctiva of the upper lid. For this purpose, you need to evert the lid (see p. 260).

The local redness below is from nodular episcleritis, often self-limiting in younger adults; also seen in rheumatoid arthritis and system lupus erythematosus (SLE).

For comparisons, see Table 11-1, Red Eyes, p. 264.

Cornea and Lens

With oblique lighting, inspect the cornea of each eye for opacities and note any opacities in the lens that may be visible through the pupil.

See Table 11-5, Opacities of the Cornea and Lens, p. 265.

Iris

At the same time, inspect each iris. The markings should be clearly defined. With your light shining directly from the temporal side, look for a crescentic shadow on the medial side of the iris. Because the iris is normally fairly flat and forms a relatively open angle with the cornea, this lighting casts no shadow. There are variations in the color of the iris. Many Asians, Hispanics, or African Americans have brown eyes and many of European or Scandinavian origins have lighter eye color.

Occasionally the iris bows abnormally far forward, forming a very narrow angle with the cornea. The light then casts a crescentic shadow.

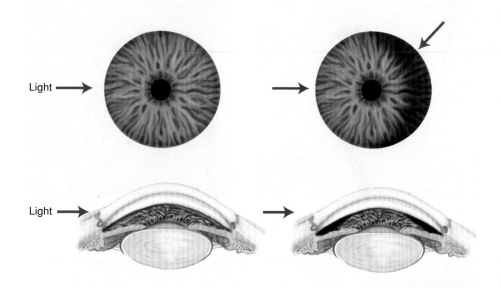

Light →

Light →

This narrow angle increases the risk for acute *narrow-angle glaucoma*—a sudden increase in intraocular pressure when drainage of the aqueous humor is blocked.

In *open-angle glaucoma*—the common form of glaucoma—the normal spatial relation between iris and cornea is preserved and the iris is fully lit.

Pupils

In dim light, inspect the *size, shape,* and *symmetry* of each pupil. Measure the pupils with a guide such as a card or a flashlight with black circles of various sizes to facilitate measurement. Document the pupil size and note if the pupil is large (>5 mm), small (<3 mm), or unequal.

Miosis refers to constriction of the pupils, *mydriasis* to dilation.

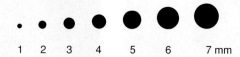

1   2   3   4   5   6   7 mm

Anisocoria is a difference in pupil size. This can normally be found in 1 in 5 people. Pupillary diameter inequality is generally <0.5 mm, however, it can be up to 1 mm. If pupillary reactions are normal, anisocoria is considered benign. If the change in pupil size is sudden and does not resolve or

Compare benign anisocoria with Horner syndrome, oculomotor nerve paralysis, and tonic pupil. See Table 11-6, Pupillary Abnormalities, p. 269.

is in combination with additional symptoms, follow-up with a health care provider is warranted.[8]

LIGHT REACTION. Test the *pupillary reaction to light*. Ask the patient to look into the distance, and shine a bright light obliquely into each pupil in turn. Both the distant gaze and the oblique lighting help to prevent a near reaction. Look for:

• The *direct reaction* (pupillary constriction in the same eye)

• The *consensual reaction* (pupillary constriction in the opposite eye)

Always darken the room and use a bright light before deciding that a light reaction is absent or abnormal.

NEAR REACTION. If the reaction to light is impaired or questionable, test the *near reaction* in dim and normal room light. Testing one eye at a time makes it easier to concentrate on pupillary responses, without the distraction of extraocular movement. Hold your finger or pencil about 10 cm from the patient's eye. Ask the patient to look alternately at it and into the distance directly behind it. Watch for pupillary constriction with near effort and convergence of the eyes.

Testing the near reaction is helpful in diagnosing Argyll Robertson and tonic (Adie) pupils (see p. 269).

Extraocular Muscles

1. *Test the six extraocular movements (EOMs).* Ask the patient to follow your finger or pencil as you sweep through the six cardinal directions of gaze. Making a wide "H" in the air, lead the patient's gaze:

   a. to the patient's extreme right

   b. to the right and upward

   c. down on the right

   d. without pausing in the middle, to the extreme left

   e. to the left and upward

   f. down on the left.

1

4

2

5

3

6

Deviations in movements can signal a brain tumor or injury. The change depends on the location of the lesion or injury. In paralysis of the CN VI, illustrated below, the eyes are conjugate in right lateral gaze but not in left lateral gaze.

LOOKING RIGHT

LOOKING LEFT

Pause during upward and lateral gaze to detect *nystagmus*. Move your finger or pencil at approximately 12 to 18 inches from the patient. Because middle-aged or older adults may have difficulty focusing on near objects, make this distance greater. Patients should maintain the head midline however, some patients move their heads to follow your finger. If necessary, hold the head in the proper midline position.

If you suspect lid lag or hyperthyroidism, ask the patient to follow your finger again as you move it slowly from up to down in the midline. The lid should overlap the iris slightly throughout this movement as depicted in the photo.

Note the rim of sclera from *proptosis*, an abnormal protrusion of the eyeball in *hyperthyroidism*, leading to a characteristic "stare" on frontal gaze.

2. Assess the extraocular movements, looking for:

- The normal *conjugate movements* of the eyes in each direction. Detect any deviation from normal or dysconjugate gaze.

See Table 11-7, Dysconjugate Gaze, p. 270.

- *Nystagmus,* a fine rhythmic oscillation of the eyes. A few beats of nystagmus on extreme lateral gaze are normal. If you see it, bring your finger in to within the field of binocular vision and look again. Nystagmus occurs normally when a person watches a rapidly moving object such as a passing train.

Sustained nystagmus within the binocular field of gaze is seen with various causes, including impairment of vision in early life, disorders of the labyrinth and the cerebellar system and drug toxicity. See Chapter 20, p. 665.

- *Lid lag* as the eyes move from up to down.

In lid lag of *hyperthyroidism,* a rim of sclera is visible above the iris with downward gaze.

3. *Test for convergence.* Ask the patient to follow your finger or pencil as you move it in toward the bridge of the nose. The converging eyes normally follow the object to within 5 to 8 cm of the nose.

Poor convergence in *hyperthyroidism*

CONVERGENCE

4. *Corneal light reflex.* Standing 2 feet in front of the patient, shine a light into the patient's eyes and ask the patient to look at it. *Inspect the reflections in the corneas.* They should be visible slightly nasal to the center of the pupils.

Asymmetry of the corneal reflections indicates a deviation from normal ocular alignment. A temporal light reflection on one cornea, for example, indicates a nasal deviation of that eye. See Table 11-7, Dysconjugate Gaze, p. 270.

5. A *cover–uncover test* may reveal a slight or latent muscle imbalance not otherwise seen (see p. 270).

Ophthalmoscopic Examination

The nurse would examine the patient's eyes *without dilating the pupils*. The view is therefore limited to the posterior structures of the retina. To see more peripheral structures, to evaluate the macula well, or to investigate unexplained visual loss, ophthalmologists dilate the pupils with mydriatic drops unless this is contraindicated.

Aperture

Indicator of diopters

Lens disc

On/off

Contraindications for mydriatic drops include (1) head injury and coma, in which continuing observations of pupillary reactions are essential, and (2) any suspicion of narrow-angle glaucoma.

At first, using the ophthalmoscope may seem awkward, and it may be difficult to visualize the fundus. With patience and practice of proper technique, the fundus will come into view, and the ability to assess important structures such as the optic disc and the retinal vessels becomes easier.

The optic disc's yellowish orange to creamy pink oval or round structure may fill the field of gaze or even exceed it. Of interest, the ophthalmoscope magnifies the normal retina about 15 times and the normal iris about 4 times. The optic disc actually measures about 1.5 mm. Follow the next steps for this important segment of the physical examination.

Steps for Examining the Optic Disc

To begin using the ophthalmoscope for assessment, the nurse needs to be aware of how it functions as there are different types. Familiarize yourself with the dials and know how to turn it on. Initially, the scope needs to be set on:

- The brightest light necessary to visualize the retina and blood vessels

- The white light (ignore the other colors)

- The circle (ignore the slits and crosses)

- "0" diopters

If the nurse wears glasses or contacts they can remain on for the examination. If the patient wears glasses they should be removed, although contacts may remain in.

Room lighting should be decreased or turned off without making the room too dark.

Explain to the patient that the ophthalmoscope light will be bright and the importance of focusing on a specific point so the eyes do not wander during the examination. Choose a point on the wall over your shoulder that the patient should stare at (you might pick a curtain or determine a spot on the wall behind you). The patient should continue to look in that direction even if you step in the line of view.

Positioning

When looking into the patient's right eye the nurse holds the scope with the right hand and uses the right eye; when looking into the patient's left eye the nurse holds the scope with the left hand and uses the left eye. Try to keep your other eye open during the examination. Using the nondominant hand and eye will take practice. It is important to master this, as it decreases the likelihood of the nurse's nose touching the patient's nose. In addition, the hand not holding the scope can brace the thumb and forefinger on the patient's eyebrow to determine the proximity to the patient and to assist with opening the patient's eye if it tends to close.

The Examination

The nurse will shine the light into the patient's eye from 6 inches away and at a 15-degree angle and will be able to see the red reflex. Follow this into the eye, resting the ophthalmoscope on your eyebrow and standing about 1.5 to 2 inches away from the patient. (It is important to get close to the patient as you will have a wider field of view.) Here the optic disc, arteries, and veins are visible. If you are unable to visualize the optic disc and vessels, keep your head still and move the diopter dial (which your index finger has been resting on) either way. If the disc becomes clearer keep turning the dial; if it becomes blurry then turn the dial in the opposite direction.

Steps for Examining the Optic Disc and the Retina

The Optic Disc
- Initially the red reflex comes into view; the nurse needs to be able to look through the red reflex to visualize the arteries and veins.
- Follow the blood vessels as they get wider. Follow the vessels medially toward the nose and look for the round yellowish orange structure described earlier as the optic disc.

EXAMINER AT 15-DEGREE ANGLE FROM PATIENT'S LINE OF VISION, ELICITING RED REFLEX

- Now, *bring the optic disc into sharp focus* by adjusting the lens of your ophthalmoscope. If both you and the patient have no refractive errors, the retina should be in focus at 0 diopters. If structures are blurred, rotate the lens disc until you find the sharpest focus.
- For example, if the patient is myopic (nearsighted), rotate the lens disc counterclockwise to the minus diopters (red); in a hyperopic (farsighted) patient, move the disc clockwise to the plus diopters (black). You can correct your own refractive error in the same way.
- *Inspect the optic disc.* Note the following features:
  - *The sharpness or clarity of the disc outline.* The nasal portion of the disc margin may be somewhat blurred, a normal finding.
  - *The color of the disc,* normally yellowish orange to creamy pink. White or pigmented crescents may ring the disc, a normal finding.
  - *The size of the central physiologic cup,* if present. It is usually yellowish white. The horizontal diameter is usually less than half the horizontal diameter of the disc.
  - *The comparative symmetry* of the eyes and findings in the fundi.

Detecting Papilledema. *Papilledema* describes swelling of the optic disc and anterior bulging of the physiologic cup. Increased intracranial pressure is transmitted to the optic nerve, causing edema of the optic nerve. Papilledema often signals serious disorders of the brain, such as meningitis, subarachnoid hemorrhage, trauma, and mass lesions, so searching for this important disorder is a priority during all your fundu-scopic examinations.

The Retina—Arteries, Veins, Fovea, and Macula
- *Inspect the retina,* including arteries and veins as they extend to the periphery, arteriovenous crossings, the fovea, and the macula. Distinguish arteries from veins based on the features listed below. Darker retinas correlate with darker irises. Those with light retinas tend to have better night vision however are more sensitive to bright light.[10]
- *Follow the vessels peripherally in each of four directions,* noting their relative sizes and the character of the arterio-venous crossings.
- Identify any lesions of the surrounding *retina* and note their size, shape, color, and distribution. As you search the retina, *move your head and instrument as a unit,* using the patient's pupil as an imaginary fulcrum. At first, you may repeatedly lose your view of the retina because your light falls out of the pupil. You will improve with practice.
- Lesions of the retina can be measured in terms of "disc diameters" from the optic disc.

Sequence of inspection from disc to macula

LEFT EYE

In a *refractive error,* light rays from a distance do not focus on the retina. In *myopia,* they focus anterior to it; in *hyperopia,* posterior to it. Retinal structures in a myopic eye look larger than normal.[9]

See Table 11-8, Normal Variations of the Optic Disc, p. 271 and Table 11-9, Abnormalities of the Optic Disk, p. 272.

An enlarged cup suggests chronic open-angle glaucoma.

PAPILLEDEMA

See Table 11-10, Ocular Fundi: Normal and Hypertensive Retinopathy, p. 275.

See Table 11-10, Ocular Fundi: Normal and Hypertensive Retinopathy, p. 273, Table 11-11, Ocular Fundi: Diabetic Retinopathy, p. 274, and Table 11-12, Retinal Arteries and Arteriovenous Crossings: Normal and Hypertensive, p. 275.

COTTON-WOOL PATCHES
Note the irregular patches between 11 and 12 o'clock, 1 to 2 disc diameters from the disc. Each measures about one-half by one-half disc diameters.

- Inspect the *fovea and surrounding macula*. Direct your light beam laterally or by asking the patient to look directly into the light. Except in older people, the tiny bright reflection at the center of the fovea helps to orient you. Shimmering light reflections in the macular area are common in young people.

Macular degeneration is an important cause of poor central vision in the elderly. Types include *dry atrophic* (more common but less severe) and *wet exudative*, or neovascular. Undigested cellular debris, called *drusen*, may be hard and sharply defined, as seen below, or soft and confluent with altered pigmentation.

Photo from Tasman W, Jaeger E, eds. *The Wills Eye Hospital Atlas of Clinical Ophthalmology*. 2nd ed. Philadelphia, PA: Lippincott Williams & Wilkins; 2001.

- *Inspect the anterior structures*. Look for opacities in the *vitreous* or *lens* by rotating the lens disc progressively to diopters of around +10 or +12. This technique allows you to focus on the more anterior structures in the eye. Vitreous floaters may be seen as dark specks or strands between the fundus and the lens. Cataracts are densities in the lens (see p. 268).

	Arteries	Veins
Color	Light red	Dark red
Size	Smaller (⅔ to ¾ the diameter of veins)	Larger
Light reflex (*reflection*)	Bright	Inconspicuous or absent

SPECIAL TECHNIQUES

For Nasolacrimal Duct Obstruction

This test helps identify the cause of excessive tearing. Ask the patient to look up. Press on the lower lid close to the medial canthus, just inside the rim of the bony orbit—this compresses the lacrimal sac. Look for fluid regurgitated out of the puncta into the eye. Avoid this test if the area is inflamed and tender.

Discharge of mucopurulent fluid from the puncta suggests an obstructed nasolacrimal duct.

(AF) For Inspection of the Upper Palpebral Conjunctiva

Adequate examination of the eye in search of a foreign body requires eversion of the upper eyelid. Follow these steps:

- Instruct the patient to look down. Have the patient to relax the eyes—with reassurance and gentle, assured, and deliberate movements. Raise the upper eyelid slightly so that the eyelashes protrude, and then grasp the upper eyelashes and pull them gently down and forward.

- Place a small stick such as an applicator or a tongue blade at least 1 cm above the lid margin (and therefore at the upper border of the tarsal plate). Push down on the stick as you raise the edge of the lid, thus everting the eyelid or turning it "inside out." Do not press on the eyeball itself.

- Secure the upper lashes against the eyebrow and inspect the palpebral conjunctiva. After your inspection, grasp the upper eyelashes and pull them gently forward. Ask the patient to look up. The eyelid will return to its normal position.

This view allows you to see the upper palpebral conjunctiva and look for a foreign body that might be lodged there.

RECORDING THE PHYSICAL EXAMINATION—
THE EYE

Case: Amy Smith
Thursday, July 28, 2016 17:19

Show Learning Tips   Return to Case Info

Smith, Amy	Gender: Female	Diagnosis: Cataract	Adm Provider:
MRN: 11-6354	DOB: 1/21/1944	Isolation Precaution: Standard	Facility: North County Clinic
Allergies: None	Age: 72 Years	Adv Directive: Full Code	Room: 10 Bed: 1
	Height:		Adm On: 7/28/2016 16:59 [0 day(s)]
	Weight:		

Patient Info   Assessment   ADLs   Notes   Nursing Dx   Orders   MAR   I/O   Vital Signs   Diagnostics   Immunizations   Flowsheet

HEENT   Neuro   Cardio   Respiratory   GI   GU   Musculoskeletal   Mental Health   Pain Scale   Integumentary   Vascular Access

Save Assessment   Delete   Cancel   Past Assessments ▾

Edit HEENT Assessment (Charted by Sarah Linkletter, Registered Nurse on 7/28/2016 17:29)

Documented By:
Sarah Linkletter, Registered Nurse   ▾

Documented At:
0   days   0   hours   30   minutes   after admission   ▾

Additional Notes

Pt. complains of cloudy vision, which has become steadily worse over last 6 mo. She now sees halos around light and can no longer drive at night. Reports right eye is worse than left.

Head

Size/Shape

☑ Symmetric
☐ Asymmetric
☐ Enlarged
☐ Decreased size

Recent Trauma

○ Yes
◉ No
○ Unknown

Hair

☑ Fine
☐ Coarse
☐ Balding
☐ Facial hair

Ears

☐ Not assessed

	Left Ear	Right Ear
Pain	☐	☐
Drainage	☐	☐
Hearing		
Intact	☑	☑
Impaired	☐	☐
Hearing device present	☐	☐
Interior		
Normal	☑	☑
Redness	☐	☐
Cerumen present	☐	☐
Swollen	☐	☐

Eyes

	Left Eye	Right Eye
Sclera		
Normal/clear	☑	☑
Jaundice	☐	☐
Redness	☐	☐
Swelling	☐	☐
Movement		
Symmetrical	☑	☑
Intact	☐	☐
Nystagmus	☐	☐
Lid lag	☐	☐
Asymmetrical corneal reflections	☐	☐
Convergence		
Average	◉	◉
Poor	○	○

Nose

Character

☑ Symmetrical
☐ Asymmetrical
☐ Deformity

Obstruction

☐ Absent
☐ Present left
☐ Present right

Septum

☑ Intact
☐ Perforated
☐ Deviated

Abnormalities

☐ Ulcers present
☐ Polyps present
☐ Blood present
☐ Recent trauma

Mouth/Throat

Teeth

☑ Present
☐ Absent
☐ Tooth decay
☐ Cavity(ies)
☐ Implant(s)
☐ Cap(s)
☐ Bridge(s)
☐ Dentures

Oral Mucosa

☑ Normal
☐ Ulcers
☐ Pink
☐ White
☐ Pale
☐ Dusky
☐ Swelling
☐ Moist
☐ Dry

Pharynx

☑ Normal
☐ Exudate
☐ Swelling
☐ Ulceration
☐ Tonsillar enlargement
☐ Pain

Lymph Nodes

☑ Non-tender
☐ Tender
☐ Shotty

Location:

Notes:

visual acuity: R eye 20/200, L eye 20/50 with glasses,
lenses: gray BL(R fully covered, L 1/2 covered),
red reflex absent in R eye)

Eyes: near vision—14/14, distal vision—20/20 bilaterally, peripheral vision—visual fields full by confrontation. EOMs intact. No nystagmus. No deviations on cover–uncover test. Convergence to 7 cm.

Thick and equal hair distribution on brows and lids. Lids tan and without lesions. Palpebral fissures equal bilaterally. No edema or ptosis. Lacrimal apparatus nontender, moist without tearing or crusting. Conjunctiva pink and sclera white bilaterally. No opacities in cornea or lens bilaterally. PERRLA. Disc yellowish orange with sharp margins. No hemorrhages or exudates. No arteriolar narrowing.

OR

Eyes: near vision—14/14, distal vision 20/50 right, 20/40 left with glasses, peripheral vision—visual fields full by confrontation. EOMs intact. No nystagmus. Cover-uncover test-no deviations. Convergence to 7 cm.

Thin hair distribution on brows and lids. Lids with light greenish, sticky substance matting the lashes. Lacrimal apparatus tender with light greenish drainage bilaterally. Negative lesions. Palpebral fissures equal bilaterally. Minimal edema bilaterally and L ptosis. Conjunctiva reddish and sclera white and cloudy bilaterally. No opacities in cornea or lens bilaterally. PERRLA. Disc yellowish orange with sharp margins. No hemorrhages or exudates. No arteriolar narrowing.

> PERRLA-pupils equal, round, and reactive to light and accommodation

HEALTH PROMOTION, DISEASE PREVENTION, AND EDUCATION

Important Topics

- Vision screening
- Eye protection
- Care of contact lenses

Vision is a critical sense for experiencing the world around us, and an area of importance for health promotion and disease prevention. Education by nurses is vital in maintaining vision and a healthy outlook for clients.

Vision Screening

Changes in vision shift with age. Young children may have changes and the U.S. Preventive Task Force (USPSTF) recommends vision screening for all children at least once between the ages of 3 and 5 years old to detect amblyopia or its risk factors. Amblyopia, also known as "lazy eye," affects approximately 2% to 4% or preschool children. This loss of vision is due to an alteration in neural pathways in the developing brain which in turn decreases use of the affected eye.

> Failure to correct amblyopia during early childhood can result in poor vision for life.

Strabismus is eye misalignment; these are found most frequently in infants and children up to 5 years old. Screening tests for detecting strabismus and amblyopia include simple inspection, the cover–uncover test, corneal light reflex, and visual acuity tests.[11]

The most common visual change in school-age children, adolescents, and young adults is refractive errors. Most school-age children are screened in school, and young adults present to their health care provider when they have changes in vision or are tested for driving examinations, employment, or physicals. The Snellen vision chart is used for the screening examination.

As aging occurs, cataracts, macular degeneration, and glaucoma become more prevalent.[12] These disorders reduce awareness of the social and physical environment and contribute to falls and injuries. To improve detection of visual defects, test visual acuity with a Snellen chart or Near Vision card. Examine the lens and fundi for clouding of the lens (*cataracts*); mottling of the *macula;* variations in the retinal pigmentation; subretinal hemorrhage or exudate (*macular degeneration*); and change in size and color of the optic cup or visual field defects (*glaucoma*).[5]

Eye Protection

Eye injuries and trauma can occur in the home, during recreational activities, and in the place of employment. Protective eyewear should be used when there is a chance of injury to the eye. Eye injury can result from numerous causes, for example, chemical splashes from cleaning supplies, metal shards or rocks flying when mowing the lawn, sports (e.g., lacrosse) injuries, body fluids entering the eye—the list is endless.[13,14] The activities and environment in which people work and play should be assessed and precautions taken to avoid eye injury and promote healthy habits. Emergency eye care education is important for individuals to react when something enters the eye such as chemicals or a blunt object or when there is a cut around the eye.[15,16] Additional education includes avoidance of direct sunlight and use of sunglasses to protect the eyes from ultraviolet radiation and individuals working with chemicals should be taught how to use devices to flush eyes and/or skin if they come in contact with chemicals.

Care of Contact Lenses

Infections can occur and injure the eye if contact lenses are not taken care of properly. Patients should remember to wash their hands when inserting or removing lenses, to wear and remove them as prescribed by the health care provider, and to keep them clean and not share contacts. If patients are using solutions, they should discard unused portions at the expiration date. Contact lens wearers may become too familiar with the routine and may need reminders that putting anything into the eye, including contacts, may cause damage if not done correctly. Contact lenses should be inspected by a lens specialist once a year for scratches or damage that can injure the eye.

TABLE 11-1

Red Eyes[7]

	Conjunctivitis	**Subconjunctival Hemorrhage**
Pattern of Redness	Conjunctival injection: diffuse dilatation of conjunctival vessels with redness that tends to be maximal peripherally	Leakage of blood outside of the vessels, producing a homogeneous, sharply demarcated, red area that fades over days to yellow and then disappears
Pain	Mild discomfort rather than pain	Absent
Vision	Not affected except for temporary mild blurring due to discharge	Not affected
Ocular Discharge	Watery, mucoid, or mucopurulent	Absent
Pupil	Not affected	Not affected
Cornea	Clear	Clear
Significance	Bacterial, viral, and other infections; allergy; irritation	Often none. May result from trauma, bleeding disorders, or a sudden increase in venous pressure, as from cough

	Corneal Injury or Infection	**Acute Iritis**	**Glaucoma**
Pattern of Redness	Ciliary injection: dilation of deeper vessels that are visible as radiating vessels or a reddish violet flush around the limbus. Ciliary injection is an important sign of these three conditions but may not be apparent. The eye may be diffusely red instead. Other clues of these more serious disorders are pain, decreased vision, unequal pupils, and a less than perfectly clear cornea.		
Pain	Moderate to severe, superficial	Moderate, aching, deep	Severe, aching, deep
Vision	Usually decreased	Decreased	Decreased
Ocular Discharge	Watery or purulent	Absent	Absent
Pupil	Not affected unless iritis develops	May be small and, with time, irregular	Dilated, fixed
Cornea	Changes depending on cause	Clear or slightly clouded	Steamy, cloudy
Significance	Abrasions, and other injuries; viral and bacterial infections	Associated with many ocular and systemic disorders	Acute increase in intraocular pressure—an emergency

TABLE
11-2

Visual Field Defects

Visual Field Defects

1. Horizontal Defect. Occlusion of a branch of the central retinal artery may cause a horizontal (altitudinal) defect. Ischemia of the optic nerve also can produce a similar defect.

1

2. Blind Right Eye (right optic nerve). A lesion of the optic nerve, and of course of the eye itself, produces unilateral blindness.

2

3. Bitemporal Hemianopsia (optic chiasm). A lesion at the optic chiasm may involve only fibers crossing over to the opposite side. Since these fibers originate in the nasal half of each retina, visual loss involves the temporal half of each field.

3

4. Left Homonymous Hemianopsia (right optic tract). A lesion of the optic tract interrupts fibers originating on the same side of both eyes. Visual loss in the eyes is therefore similar (homonymous) and involves half of each field (hemianopsia).

4

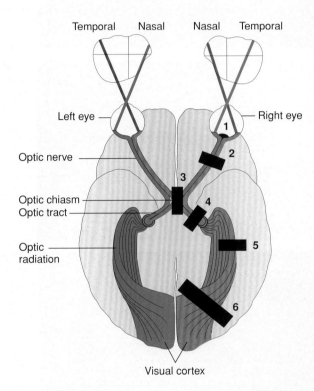

5. Homonymous Left Superior Quadrantic Defect (right optic radiation, partial). A partial lesion of the optic radiation in the temporal lobe may involve only a portion of the nerve fibers, producing, for example, a homonymous quadrantic defect.

5

6. Left Homonymous Hemianopsia (right optic radiation). A complete interruption of fibers in the optic radiation produces a visual defect similar to that produced by a lesion of the optic tract.

6

TABLE 11-3

Variations and Abnormalities of the Eyelids

Ptosis

Ptosis is a drooping of the upper lid. Causes include myasthenia gravis, damage to the oculomotor nerve, and damage to the sympathetic nerve supply (*Horner syndrome*). A weakened muscle, relaxed tissues, and the weight of herniated fat may cause senile ptosis. Ptosis may also be congenital.

Entropion

Entropion, more common in the elderly, is an inward turning of the lid margin. The lower lashes, which are often invisible when turned inward, irritate the conjunctiva and lower cornea. Asking the patient to squeeze the lids together and then open them may reveal an entropion that is not obvious.

Ectropion

In ectropion the margin of the lower lid is turned outward, exposing the palpebral conjunctiva. When the punctum of the lower lid turns outward, the eye no longer drains satisfactorily, and tearing occurs. Ectropion is more common in the elderly.

Lid Retraction and Exophthalmos

A wide-eyed stare suggests retracted eyelids. Note the rim of sclera between the upper lid and the iris. Retracted lids and a lid lag (p. 254) are often due to hyperthyroidism.

In exophthalmos the eyeball protrudes forward. When bilateral, it suggests the infiltrative ophthalmopathy of Graves hyperthyroidism. Edema of the eyelids and conjunctival injection may be associated. Unilateral exophthalmos is seen in Graves disease or a tumor or inflammation in the orbit.

Source of photos: *Ptosis, Ectropion, Entropion*—Tasman W, Jaeger E, eds. *The Wills Eye Hospital Atlas of Clinical Ophthalmology.* 2nd ed. Philadelphia, PA: Lippincott Williams & Wilkins; 2001.

TABLE 11-4	Lumps and Swellings in and Around the Eyes

Pinguecula

A harmless yellowish triangular nodule in the bulbar conjunctiva on either side of the iris. Appears frequently with aging, first on the nasal and then on the temporal side.

Episcleritis

A localized ocular redness from inflammation of the episcleral vessels. Vessels appear pink and are movable over the scleral surface. May be nodular, as shown, or may show only redness and dilated vessels.

Sty (Hordeolum)

A painful, tender red infection in a gland at the margin of the eyelid.

Chalazion

A subacute nontender and usually painless nodule involving a meibomian gland. May become acutely inflamed but, unlike a sty, usually points inside the lid rather than on the lid margin.

Xanthelasma

Slightly raised, yellowish, well-circumscribed plaques that appear along the nasal portions of one or both eyelids. May accompany lipid disorders.

Inflammation of the Lacrimal Sac (Dacryocystitis)

A swelling between the lower eyelid and nose. An *acute* inflammation (illustrated) is painful, red, and tender. *Chronic* inflammation is associated with obstruction of the nasolacrimal duct. Tearing is prominent, and pressure on the sac produces regurgitation of material through the puncta of the eyelids.

Source of photos: Tasman W, Jaeger E, eds. *The Wills Eye Hospital Atlas of Clinical Ophthalmology.* 2nd ed. Philadelphia, PA: Lippincott Williams & Wilkins; 2001.

TABLE

11-5

Opacities of the Cornea and Lens

Corneal Arcus. A thin grayish white arc or circle not quite at the edge of the cornea. Accompanies normal aging but also seen in younger people, especially African Americans. In young people, suggests possible hyperlipoproteinemia. Usually benign.

Corneal Scar. A superficial grayish white opacity in the cornea, secondary to an old injury or to inflammation. Size and shape are variable. Do not confuse with the opaque lens of a cataract, visible on a deeper plane and only through the pupil.

Pterygium. A triangular thickening of the bulbar conjunctiva that grows slowly across the outer surface of the cornea, usually from the nasal side. Reddening may occur. May interfere with vision as it encroaches on the pupil.

Cataracts. Opacities of the lenses visible through the pupil; most common in old age.

Nuclear cataract. A nuclear cataract looks gray when seen by a flashlight. If the pupil is widely dilated, the gray opacity is surrounded by a black rim.

Peripheral cataract. Produces spoke-like shadows that point inward—gray against black, as seen with a flashlight, or black against red with an ophthalmoscope. A dilated pupil, as shown here, facilitates this observation.

TABLE
11-6

Pupillary Abnormalities

Unequal Pupils (*Anisocoria*)—When anisocoria is greater in bright light than in dim light, the larger pupil cannot constrict properly. Causes include blunt trauma to the eye, open-angle glaucoma (p. 264), and impaired parasympathetic nerve supply to the iris, as in tonic pupil, oculomotor nerve paralysis, brain injury, or brain tumors. When anisocoria is greater in dim light, the smaller pupil cannot dilate properly, as in Horner syndrome, caused by an interruption of the sympathetic nerve supply. See also Table 20-9, Pupils in Comatose Patients, p. 738.

Tonic Pupil (*Adie Pupil*). Pupil is large, regular, and usually unilateral. Reaction to light is severely reduced and slowed, or even absent. Near reaction, although very slow, is present. Slow accommodation causes blurred vision. Deep tendon reflexes are often decreased.

Oculomotor Nerve (CN III) Paralysis. The dilated pupil is fixed to light and near effort. Ptosis of the upper eyelid and lateral deviation of the eye are almost always present.

Horner Syndrome. The affected pupil, though small, reacts briskly to light and near effort. Ptosis of the eyelid is present, perhaps with loss of sweating on the forehead. In congenital Horner syndrome, the involved iris is lighter in color than its fellow (*heterochromia*).

Small, Irregular Pupils. Small, irregular pupils that accommodate but do not react to light indicate *Argyll Robertson pupils*. Seen in central nervous system syphilis.

Equal Pupils and One Blind Eye. Unilateral blindness does not cause anisocoria as long as the sympathetic and parasympathetic innervation to both irises is normal. A light directed into the seeing eye produces a direct reaction in that eye and a consensual reaction in the blind eye. A light directed into the blind eye, however, causes no response in either eye.

Blind eye

Light

Blind eye

Light

TABLE
11-7

Dysconjugate Gaze

There are a variety of gaze abnormality patterns that give nurses clues about developmental disorders and cranial nerve abnormalities.

Developmental Disorders

Developmental dysconjugate gaze is caused by an imbalance in ocular muscle tone. This imbalance has many causes, may be hereditary, and usually appears in early childhood. These gaze deviations are classified according to direction:

Esotropia (Inward Deviation)   *Exotropia (Outward Deviation)*

Cover–Uncover Test

A cover–uncover test may be helpful. Here is what you would see in the right monocular esotropia illustrated above.

Corneal reflections are asymmetric.

COVER

The right eye moves outward to fix on the light. (The left eye is not seen but moves inward to the same degree.)

UNCOVER

The left eye moves outward to fix on the light. The right eye deviates inward again.

Disorders of Cranial Nerves

New onset of dysconjugate gaze in adult life is usually the result of cranial nerve injuries, lesions, or abnormalities from such causes as trauma, multiple sclerosis, syphilis, and others.

A Left Cranial Nerve VI Paralysis

LOOKING TO THE RIGHT

Eyes are conjugate.

LOOKING STRAIGHT AHEAD

Esotropia appears

LOOKING TO THE LEFT

Esotropia is maximum

A Left Cranial Nerve IV Paralysis

LOOKING DOWN AND TO THE RIGHT

The left eye cannot look down when turned inward. Deviation is maximum in this direction.

A Left Cranial Nerve III Paralysis

LOOKING STRAIGHT AHEAD

The eye is pulled outward by action of the 6th nerve. Upward, downward, and inward movements are impaired or lost. Ptosis and pupillary dilation may be associated.

TABLE
11-8

Normal Variations of the Optic Disc

Physiologic Cupping

Central cup

Temporal cup

The physiologic cup is a small whitish depression in the optic disc, from which the retinal vessels appear to emerge. Although sometimes absent, the cup is usually visible either centrally or toward the temporal side of the disc. Grayish spots are often seen at its base.

Rings and Crescents

Medullated Nerve Fibers

Rings and crescents are often seen around the optic disc. These are developmental variations in which you can glimpse either white sclera, black retinal pigment, or both, especially along the temporal border of the disc. Rings and crescents are not part of the disc itself and should not be included in your estimates of disc diameters.

Medullated nerve fibers are a much less common but dramatic finding. Appearing as irregular white patches with feathered margins, they obscure the disc edge and retinal vessels. They have no pathologic significance.

TABLE

11-9

Abnormalities of the Optic Disc

	Process	Appearance
Normal		
	Tiny disc vessels give normal color to the disc.	Color yellowish orange to creamy pink Disc vessels tiny Disc margins sharp (except perhaps nasally) The physiologic cup is located centrally or somewhat temporally. It may be conspicuous or absent. Its diameter from side to side is usually less than half that of the disc.
Papilledema		
	Venous stasis leads to engorgement and swelling	Color pink, hyperemic Often with loss of venous pulsations Disc vessels more visible, more numerous, curve over the borders of the disc Disc swollen with margins blurred The physiologic cup is not visible.
Glaucomatous Cupping		
	Increased pressure within the eye leads to increased cupping (backward depression of the disc) and atrophy. The base of the enlarged cup is pale	The physiologic cup is enlarged, occupying more than half of the disc's diameter, at times extending to the edge of the disc. Retinal vessels sink in and under it, and may be displaced nasally.
Optic Atrophy		
	Death of optic nerve fibers leads to loss of the tiny disc vessels.	Color white Tiny disc vessels absent

Sources of photos for *Normal*—Tasman W, Jaeger E, eds. *The Wills Eye Hospital Atlas of Clinical Ophthalmology.* 2nd ed. Philadelphia, PA: Lippincott Williams & Wilkins; 2001; *Papilledema, Glaucomatous Cupping, Optic Atrophy*—Courtesy of Ken Freedman, MD.

TABLE 11-10

Ocular Fundi: Normal and Hypertensive Retinopathy[7]

Normal Fundus of a Fair-Skinned Person

Inspect the optic disc. Follow the major vessels in four directions, noting their relative sizes and any arteriovenous crossings—both normal here. Inspect the macular area. The slightly darker fovea is just discernible; no light reflex is visible in this subject. Look for any lesions in the retina. Note the striped, or tessellated, character of the fundus, especially in the lower field, that comes from normal underlying choroidal vessels.

Normal Fundus of a Dark-Skinned Person

Again, inspect the disc, vessels, macula, and retina. The ring around the fovea is a normal light reflection. The color of the fundus has a grayish brown, almost purplish cast, which comes from pigment in the retina and the choroid that characteristically obscures the choroidal vessels; no tessellation is visible. The fundus of a light-skinned person with brunette coloring is redder.

Hypertensive Retinopathy[13]

Marked arteriolar-venous crossing changes are seen, especially along the inferior vessels. Copper wiring of the arterioles is present. A cotton-wool spot is seen just superior to the disc. Incidental disc drusen are also present but are unrelated to hypertension.

Hypertensive Retinopathy With Macular Star

Punctate exudates are readily visible: some are scattered; others radiate from the fovea to form a macular star. Note the two small, soft exudates about 1 disc diameter from the disc. Find the flame-shaped hemorrhages sweeping toward 7 o'clock and 8 o'clock; a few more may be seen toward 10 o'clock. These fundi show changes typical of accelerated (malignant) hypertension and are often accompanied by a papilledema (p. 258).

Source of photos: *Hypertensive Retinopathy, Hypertensive Retinopathy With Macular Star*—Tasman W, Jaeger E, eds. *The Wills Eye Hospital Atlas of Clinical Ophthalmology.* 2nd ed. Philadelphia, PA: Lippincott Williams & Wilkins; 2001.

TABLE

11-11
Ocular Fundi: Diabetic Retinopathy[16]

Diabetic Retinopathy

Study carefully the fundi in the series of photographs below. They represent a national standard used by ophthalmologists to assess diabetic retinopathy.

Nonproliferative Retinopathy, Moderately Severe
Note tiny red dots or microaneurysms. Note also the ring of hard exudates (white spots) located superotemporally. Retinal thickening or edema in the area of the hard exudates can impair visual acuity if it extends into the center of the macula (detection requires specialized stereoscopic examination).

Nonproliferative Retinopathy, Severe
In the superior temporal quadrant, note the large retinal hemorrhage between two cotton-wool patches, beading of the retinal vein just above them, and tiny tortuous retinal vessels above the superior temporal artery.

Proliferative Retinopathy, With Neovascularization
Note new preretinal vessels arising on the disc and extending across the disc margins. Visual acuity is still normal, but the risk for visual loss is high (photocoagulation reduces this risk by >50%).

Proliferative Retinopathy, Advanced
This is the same eye, but 2 years later and without treatment. Neovascularization has increased, now with fibrous proliferations, distortion of the macula, and reduced visual acuity.

Source of photos: *Nonproliferative Retinopathy, Moderately Severe; Proliferative Retinopathy, With Neovascularization; Nonproliferative Retinopathy, Severe; Proliferative Retinopathy, Advanced*—Early Treatment Diabetic Retinopathy Study Research Group. Courtesy of MF Davis, MD, University of Wisconsin, Madison.

TABLE
11-12

Retinal Arteries and Arteriovenous Crossings: Normal and Hypertensive

Normal Retinal Artery and Arteriovenous (A-V) Crossing

- Arterial wall (invisible)
- Column of blood
- Light reflex

The normal arterial wall is transparent. Only the column of blood within it can usually be seen. The normal light reflex is *narrow—about one fourth the diameter of the blood column.* Because the arterial wall is transparent, a vein crossing beneath the artery can be seen right up to the column of blood on either side.

- Vein
- Arterial wall
- Artery

Retinal Arteries in Hypertension

- Focal narrowing
- Narrowed column of blood
- Narrowed light reflex

In hypertension, the arteries may show areas of focal or generalized narrowing. The light reflex is also narrowed. The arterial wall thickens and becomes less transparent.

Copper Wiring

Sometimes the arteries, especially those close to the disc, become full and somewhat tortuous and develop an increased light reflex with a bright coppery luster.

Silver Wiring

Occasionally a portion of a narrowed artery develops such an opaque wall that no blood is visible within it. It is then called a silver wire artery.

Arteriovenous Crossing

When the arterial walls lose their transparency, changes appear in the arteriovenous crossings. Decreased transparency of the retina probably also contributes to the first two changes shown below.

CONCEALMENT OR A-V NICKING

Nicking. The vein appears to stop abruptly on either side of the artery.

TAPERING AND BANKING

Tapering. The vein appears to taper down on either side of the artery.

BANKING

Banking. The vein is twisted on the distal side of the artery and forms a dark, wide knuckle.

BIBLIOGRAPHY

CITATIONS

1. Mantravadi A, Vadhar H. Glaucoma. *Prim Care*. 2015;42(3): 437–449.

2. Ervin AM, Boland MV, Myrowitz E, et al. *Screening for glaucoma: Comparative effectiveness*. Agency for Healthcare Research and Quality (US): Report: 12-EHC037-EF, 2012.

3. Bennett JL, Nickerson M, Costello F, et al. Re-evaluating the treatment of acute optic neuritis. *J Neurol Neurosurg Psychiatry*. 2015;86(7):799–808.

4. Randolph SA. Age-related macular degeneration. *Workplace Health Saf*. 2014;62(8):352.

5. Lin KW, Hollis EM. Screening for impaired visual acuity in older adults. *Am Fam Physician*. 2011;83(2):185–186.

6. Klein BE, Klein R. Projected prevalences of age-related eye diseases. *Invest Ophthalmol Vis Sci*. 2013;54(14):14–17.

7. Smith MJ, Walline JJ. Controlling myopia progression in children and adolescents. *Adolesc Health Med Ther*. 2015;6:133–140.

8. Rucker JC. Pupillary and eyelid abnormalities. In: Daroff RB, Fenichel GM, Jankovic J, et al., eds. *Bradley's Neurology in Clinical Practice*. 6th ed. Philadelphia, PA: Saunders Elsevier; 2012: Chapter 16.

9. Wen G, Tarczy-Hornoch K, McKean-Cowdin R, et al. Prevalence of myopia, hyperopia, and astigmatism in non-Hispanic white and Asian children: Multi-ethnic Pediatric Eye Disease Study. *Ophthalmology*. 2013;120(10):2109–2116.

10. Andrews MA, Boyle JS. *Transcultural Concepts in Nursing Care*. 7th ed. Philadelphia, PA: Lippincott Williams & Wilkins; 2015.

11. U.S. Preventive Services Task Force. Vision screening for children 1 to 5 years of age: US Preventive Services Task Force Recommendation Statement. *Pediatrics*. 2011;127:340–346.

12. Katlinowski MA. "Eye" dentifying vision impairment in the geriatric patient. *Geriatric Nursing*. 2008;29:125–132.

13. Lincoln AE, Caswell AV, Almquist JL, et al. Effectiveness of the women's lacrosse protective eyewear mandate in the reduction of eye injuries. *Am J Sports Med*. 2012;40(3):611–614.

14. Kriz PK, Comstock RD, Zurakowski D, et al. Effectiveness of protective eyewear in reducing eye injuries among high school field hockey players. *Pediatrics*. 2012;130(6):1069–1075.

15. Chen AJ, Chan JJ, Linakis JG, et al. Age and consumer product-related eye injuries in the United States. *R I Med J*. 2014;97(1):44–48.

16. Ehlers JP, Shah CP, Chirag P, et al., eds. *The Wills Eye Manual: Office and Emergency Room Diagnosis and Treatment of Eye Disease*. Philadelphia, PA: Lippincott Williams & Wilkins; 2008.

CHAPTER 12

Ears, Nose, Mouth, and Throat

The student will:

1. Identify the structures and function of the ear, nose, mouth, and throat.

2. Obtain an accurate health history of the ear, nose, mouth, and throat.

3. Describe the physical examination techniques to evaluate the ear, nose, mouth, and throat.

4. Demonstrate how to use the otoscope.

5. Identify the measures for prevention or early detection of ear, sinus, and throat infections; hearing loss; change in balance; and maintenance of oral health.

6. Perform a complete ear, nose, mouth, and throat examination.

7. Document a complete ear, nose, mouth, and throat assessment utilizing information from the health history and the physical examination.

The ear is the sensory organ of hearing. Critical functions of the ear are hearing and balance. During the assessment there are various signs and symptoms that signal changes in the ears. The nurse's role is to detect changes and work with the health care team to prevent infections, loss of hearing, or loss of balance.

The nose is the sensory organ of smell. The nurse assesses changes in the sense of smell as well as changes in breathing patterns and signs of sinus infections.

The mouth and throat are the first part of the digestive system and the nurse assesses for changes in taste, eating patterns, and oral hygiene. Voice quality is also assessed. In all components of the system, the nurse assesses the patient for deviations from normal and teaches preventative practices to maintain these sensory organs.

THE EAR

Anatomy and Physiology

The ear has three compartments: the external ear, the middle ear, and the inner ear.

The External Ear

The *external ear* is composed of the pinna (auricle) and the external ear canal. The pinna consists chiefly of cartilage covered by skin and has a firm elastic consistency. Its prominent curved outer ridge is the *helix*. Parallel and anterior to the helix is another curved prominence, the *antihelix*. Inferiorly is the fleshy projection of the earlobe, or *lobule*. The ear canal opens behind the *tragus*, a triangular nodular area pointing backward over the entrance to the canal.

The function of the pinna is to gather sound waves and funnel them down the ear canal to assist in localization of sound.

The *external ear canal* or the *external acoustic meatus* curves inward and is made up of cartilage and bone. Cartilage surrounds the outer two thirds. The skin in this area is hairy and contains glands that produce cerumen (wax). The inner third of the canal is surrounded by bone and lined by thin, hairless skin. Pressure on this latter area causes pain—a point to remember when you examine the ear.

Behind the ear and below the ear canal is the mastoid part of the temporal bone. The lowest portion of this bone, the *mastoid process*, is palpable behind the lobule.

At the end of the ear canal, lies the *tympanic membrane (TM)*. The TM is a thin, semitransparent membrane that divides the external and middle ear.

The Middle Ear

The *middle ear* or *tympanic cavity* extends from the TM to the oval window. The middle ear is an air-filled cavity that transmits sound by way of three tiny bones or the *ossicles*: the *malleus* (hammer), the *incus* (anvil), and the *stapes* (stirrup). The ossicles transform sound vibrations into mechanical waves for the inner ear. The proximal end of the *Eustachian tube* connects the middle ear to the nasopharynx.

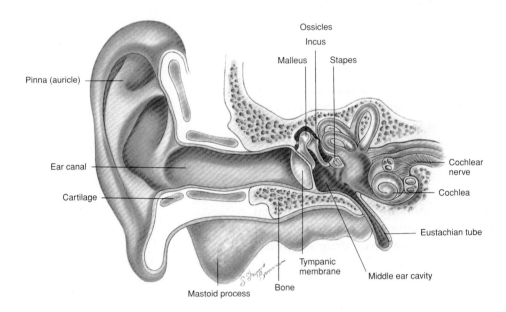

The *malleus* is one of the three ossicles and is attached to the medial TM. The *handle* and the *short process* of the malleus are the two chief landmarks of the TM. From the *umbo,* where the eardrum meets the tip of the malleus, a light reflection called the *cone of light* fans downward and anteriorly. Above the short process lies a small portion of the eardrum called the *pars flaccida*. The remainder of the TM is the *pars tensa*. Anterior and posterior malleolar folds, which extend obliquely upward from the short process, separate the pars flaccida from the pars tensa but are usually invisible unless the eardrum is retracted. A second ossicle, the *incus* can sometimes be seen through the drum and the third ossicle, the *stapes* is not visible.

The Inner Ear

The inner ear includes the *cochlea,* the *semicircular canals,* and the distal end of the *auditory nerve,* which is also known as *the vestibulocochlear nerve,* or *CN VIII.,* Movements of the stapes vibrate the perilymph in the labyrinth of the semicircular canals and the hair cells and endolymph in the ducts of the cochlea, producing electrical nerve impulses transmitted by the auditory nerve to the brain. The inner ear functions to conduct sound to the central nervous system and to assist with balance.

Much of the middle ear and all of the inner ear are inaccessible to direct examination. Some inferences concerning their condition can be made, however, by testing auditory function.

Hearing Pathways

The first part of the hearing pathway, from the external ear through the middle ear, is known as the *conductive* phase. The second part of the pathway, involving the cochlea and the cochlear nerve, is called the *sensorineural* phase.

Hearing disorders of the external and middle ear cause *conductive hearing loss*. External ear causes include cerumen impaction, *otitis externa*, trauma, *squamous cell carcinoma*, and benign bony growths such as *exostoses* or *osteomas*. Middle ear disorders include *otitis media*, congenital conditions, cholesteatomas and otosclerosis, tumors, and perforation of the TM.

Disorders of the inner ear cause *sensorineural hearing loss* from congenital and hereditary conditions, *presbycusis*, viral infections such as *rubella* and *cytomegalovirus*, *Ménière disease*, noise exposure, ototoxic drug exposure, and *acoustic neuroma*.[1]

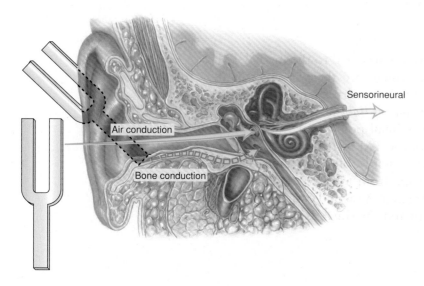

Air conduction describes the normal first phase in the hearing pathway. An alternate pathway, known as *bone conduction*, bypasses the external and middle ear and is used for testing purposes. A vibrating tuning fork, placed on the head, sets the bone of the skull into vibration and stimulates the cochlea directly. In a person with intact hearing, air conduction is more sensitive than bone conduction.

Equilibrium

The labyrinth within the inner ear senses the position and movements of the head and helps to maintain balance.

THE HEALTH HISTORY

Common or Concerning Symptoms of the Ears

- Hearing loss
- Earache
- Discharge
- Tinnitus
- Vertigo

The purpose of the nursing health history of the ears is to detect changes in the patient's hearing, ears, and balance. The opening questions are:

"How is your hearing?"
"Have you had any trouble with your ears?"

If the patient has noticed a hearing change then further assessment utilizing the mnemonic "OLD CART" is helpful.

Hearing Loss

O*nset:* When did you first notice the change in your ears/hearing?
L*ocation:* Does it involve the left ear, right ear, or both ears?
D*uration:* How long has this been going on? Did it start suddenly or gradually? Is it temporary or constant?
C*haracteristic Symptoms:* Do you notice any other symptoms when this occurs?
 Have you put anything in your ear (e.g., food, dislodged pencil eraser)?
 Has anything ever crawled/flown in your ear (e.g., bugs)?
 Do you clean your ears with cotton swabs?
 Does the inside of your ear ever feel itchy? If so, what do you do when this occurs?
 Do you scratch the inside of your ear? With what?
A*ssociated Manifestations:* Does anything else seem to be going on at the same time? Nausea? Dizziness?
 What happened prior to the hearing loss? Did anything occur before or cause the loss?
R*elieving Factors:* Does anything make it better?
T*reatment:* Have you seen anyone for this?

Do you have a history of *hearing loss?*

Hearing loss may also be congenital, from single gene mutations.[2]

Try to distinguish *conductive loss,* which results from problems in the external or middle ear, from *sensorineural loss,* which are problems in the inner ear, the cochlear nerve, or its central connections in the brain. People with sensorineural loss have particular trouble understanding speech, often complaining that others mumble; noisy environments make hearing worse. In conductive loss, noisy environments may help. Two questions may be helpful: Does the patient have difficulty understanding others or avoid noisy areas? Does a noisy environment make a difference in the ability of the person to hear?

Symptoms associated with hearing loss, such as earache or vertigo, help when assessing likely causes. In addition, inquire specifically about medications that might affect hearing and ask about sustained exposure to loud noise.

Medications that affect hearing include aminoglycosides, aspirin, nonsteroidal anti-inflammatory drugs (NSAIDs), quinine, and furosemide.

Earache

Complaints of an *earache,* or *pain in the ear,* are especially common. Ask about associated fever, sore throat, cough, or concurrent upper respiratory infection (URI). If any of these symptoms occur, there is an increased chance of an ear infection.

Otalgia is also known as ear pain. There are two types of otalgia. Primary otalgia occurs within or around the ear such as *otitis externa, otitis media, mastoiditis, or auricular infections.* Referred otalgia originates in another anatomic structure such as in the mouth, throat, or neck.[3,4]

Do you have frequent earaches?
  Onset: When did the last earache occur? How often do you have earaches?
  Location: Which ear was affected?
  Duration: How long did it last?
  Characteristic Symptoms: Did you have any other symptoms?
  Associated Manifestations: What additional symptoms were occurring or what might have occurred prior to the earache?
    Did you or anyone around you have a cold? fevers? chills?
    When was the last time you were swimming? Took a bath? Went in a hot tub? Did you go underwater?
  Relieving Factors: What relieves the pain?
  Treatment: Has this been treated previously? Currently?

Discharge

Ask about *discharge* or *otorrhea* from the ear, especially if associated with an earache or trauma.

Cerumen (wax) is normally found in the ear. The earwax tends to be yellowish to dark brown in color and a sticky consistency. In East Asians or Native Americans it is usually drier and whitish to gray in color.[5] Generally the cerumen falls out of the ear on its own or is removed with washing, however, it can build up and block the ear canal. Wax blockage is one of the most common causes of hearing loss.

Have you noticed any discharge?
When did you first notice the discharge?
In which ear?
Describe the discharge.
Color?
Consistency?
Amount?
Constant or intermittent drainage?
Does anything stop the discharge? Has it gotten worse or better?
Are you noting any other symptoms?
Sore throat?
Cough?
Respiratory infection?
Fever?
Dizziness?
Headaches?
Does anything make it better?

Discharge from the ear, if associated with an earache or trauma, is cause for additional assessment. A*cute otitis externa* and *acute or chronic otitis media* with perforation usually present with a yellow-green or purulent discharge. Generally the ear is painful and once a "pop" is felt, drainage occurs and the pain will resolve.

Tinnitus

Tinnitus is a perceived sound that has no external stimulus and commonly is heard as musical ringing or a rushing or roaring noise. It can involve one or both ears. Tinnitus may accompany hearing loss and often remains unexplained. Occasionally, popping sounds originate in the temporomandibular joint, or sounds from the neck vessels may be audible.

Tinnitus is a common symptom, increasing in frequency with age. When associated with hearing loss and vertigo, it is suggestive of Ménière disease.

Do you have ringing (tinnitus) in your ear?
When did this begin?
Is it in the left ear, right ear, or both ears?
Is this temporary or constant?
Do you notice any other symptoms when this occurs?

Vertigo

Vertigo refers to the perception that the patient or the environment is rotating or spinning. These sensations point primarily to a problem in the labyrinths of the inner ear, peripheral lesions of cranial nerve CN VIII, or lesions in its central pathways or nuclei in the brain.

See Table 12-1, Dizziness and Vertigo, p. 310.

Vertigo is a challenging symptom. Patients differ widely in what they mean by the word "dizzy." "Are there times when you feel dizzy?" is an appropriate first question, but patients often find it difficult to be more specific. Ask "Do you feel unsteady, as if you are going to fall or black out?" or "Do you feel the room is spinning or tilting (vertigo)?" Elicit information while clarifying exactly what the patient means. You may need to offer the patient several choices of wording. Ask if the patient feels pulled to the ground or off to one side, and if the dizziness is related to a change in body position. Pursue any associated feelings of clamminess or flushing, nausea, or vomiting. Check which

Feeling unsteady, lightheaded, or "dizzy in the legs" sometimes suggests a cardiovascular etiology.

A feeling of being pulled suggests true vertigo from an inner ear problem or a central or peripheral lesion of CN VIII.

medications the patient is taking and if any may be contributing to this feeling.

Do you have vertigo (dizziness)?
When did this begin?
Is this temporary or constant?
How long does it last?
What other symptoms do you experience at this time?
How does it affect your daily life?
What makes it feel better? Or go away?
What activities of daily living are impacted due to the vertigo (e.g., avoiding steps or driving a car)?
When was the last ear examination?
What were the results?
Was any further testing necessary?

Past History

Congenital hearing loss
Removal of cerumen
"Swimmer's ear"
Ear surgery
Trauma or injury to your ear(s)
Infection
Exposure to hazardous noise levels (work, home, war)
History of syphilis, rubella, meningitis

Family History

Hearing loss
Allergies
Smoking or exposure to cigarette smoke

Lifestyle Habits

Are you exposed to loud noises?
What is your occupation? Hobbies (e.g., hunting)?
Do you attend concerts? Bars? Loud places?
Do you use headphones or earbuds to listen to music?
How often? On what volume level?
Do you use lawn mower? Power tools? Firearms?
Do you live near a busy road or train tracks?
Have you ever used ear plugs/protectors? Currently?
Have you ever used hearing aid(s)? Which ear? Currently? At all times?
Have you used medications or drugs that interfere with how you hear or cause dizziness? Any medications that cause ototoxicity (e.g., large doses of antibiotics infused rapidly)?

THE NOSE AND PARANASAL SINUSES

Anatomy and Physiology

The nose has four primary functions:

1. Inspiration and expiration

2. Filtration, warmth, and moisturization of the air exchanged

3. Sensation of smell

4. Resonance of speech.

Terms used to describe the external anatomy of the nose are depicted for review.

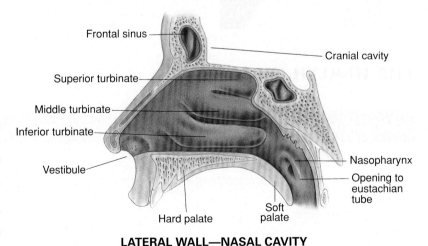

Approximately the upper third of the nose is supported by bone, the lower two thirds by cartilage. Air enters the nasal cavity through the *anterior naris* on either side, passes into the wider area known as the *vestibule,* and on through the narrow nasal passage to the nasopharynx.

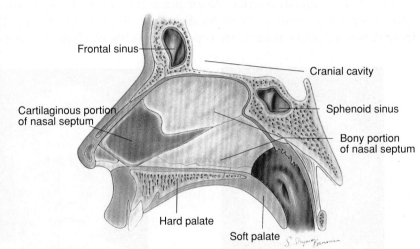

MEDIAL WALL—LEFT NASAL CAVITY (MUCOSA REMOVED)

The medial wall of each nasal cavity is formed by the *nasal septum,* which, like the external nose, is supported by both bone and cartilage. It is covered by a mucous membrane well supplied with blood. The vestibule, unlike the rest of the nasal cavity, is lined with hair-bearing skin, not mucosa.

Laterally, the anatomy is more complex. Curving bony structures, the *turbinates,* covered by a highly vascular mucous membrane protrude into the nasal cavity. Below each turbinate is a groove, or meatus, each named according to the turbinate above it. The nasolacrimal duct drains into the inferior meatus and most of the paranasal sinus drains into the middle meatus. Their openings are not usually visible.

LATERAL WALL—NASAL CAVITY

The additional surface area provided by the turbinates and the overlying mucosa aids the nasal cavities in their principal functions: cleansing, humidification, and temperature control of inspired air.

CROSS SECTION OF NASAL CAVITY-ANTERIOR VIEW

The *paranasal sinuses* are air-filled cavities within the bones of the skull. Like the nasal cavities into which they drain, they are lined with mucous membranes. The paranasal sinuses are air filled and make the skull lighter and add to speech resonance. Their locations are diagrammed below. Only the frontal and maxillary sinuses are readily accessible to clinical examination.

THE HEALTH HISTORY

Common or Concerning Symptoms of the Nose and Sinuses

* Rhinorrhea—drainage
* Congestion—difficulty breathing through the nose
* Epistaxis—bleeding
* Change in sense of smell
* Pain

The purpose of the nursing health history of the nose and sinus is to detect changes in the patient's breathing, sense of smell, nose, and sinuses. The opening questions are:

"How is your breathing?"
"Have you noticed any changes with your nose or sinuses?

Rhinorrhea refers to drainage from the nose and is often associated with *nasal congestion,* a sense of stuffiness or obstruction. These symptoms are frequently accompanied by sneezing, watery eyes, and throat discomfort, and also by itching in the eyes, nose, and throat.[6]

Causes include *viral infections, allergic rhinitis* ("hay fever"), and *vasomotor rhinitis.* Itching favors an allergic cause.

Assess the chronology of the illness. Do symptoms last for a week or so, especially when common colds and related syndromes are prevalent, or does it occur seasonally when pollens are in the air? Is it associated with specific environmental triggers? What remedies has the patient used? How well do they work? Length of time used?

Environmental triggers or seasonal association suggest *allergic rhinitis.*

Excessive use of decongestants can worsen symptoms, causing *rhinitis medicamentosa.*

Rhinorrhea

Have you noticed a runny nose (rhinorrhea) or discharge?
   Onset: When did you first notice the runny nose?
      Does it occur when pollen is in the air? When you are exposed to others with colds?
      What brings the runny nose (rhinorrhea) on? Are you at a certain place when it occurs? Does it occur at a certain time?
   Location: In which side does it occur? Both?
   Duration: How long does it last? A day? A week? A season?
      Does it interfere with sleep? Work? Activities of daily living?
   Characteristic Symptoms: Describe the runny nose (rhinorrhea).
      What color is the discharge?
      Consistency?
      Amount?
      Is it constant? or Does it come and go?
   Associated Manifestations: Have you noticed any other symptoms?
      Sore throat?
      Cough?
      Cold?
      Fever?
      Headache?
      Tenderness over the sinuses?
   Relieving Factors/**T**reatment: Does anything stop the runny nose (rhinorrhea)? Has it gotten worse or better? Does anything make it better? What remedies have worked? For how long? How well do they work?

Congestion

Did symptoms appear after a URI? Is there pain on bending forward or a maxillary toothache? Fever or local headache? Tenderness over the sinuses?

Together these suggest *acute bacterial sinusitis.* Sensitivity and specificity are highest for symptoms appearing after a URI (~90% and ~80%).[7,8]

Inquire about drugs that might cause stuffiness.

Examples are oral contraceptives, cocaine, and alcohol

Is the patient's nasal congestion limited to one side? If so, you may be dealing with a different problem that requires careful physical examination.

Consider a deviated nasal septum, foreign body, or tumor.

How long have you noticed the congestion on one side?
Have you injured your nose?
Do you remember putting anything in your nose?
Have you had surgery on your nose?
Do you have a history of polyps? Family history?
What medications are you currently taking?

Oral contraceptives, reserpine, guanethidine, and alcohol may cause stuffiness.

Epistaxis means bleeding from the nose. The blood usually originates from the nose itself, but may come from a paranasal sinus or the nasopharynx. The history can be quite graphic. However, in patients who are lying down or have bleeding that originates in posterior structures, blood may pass into the throat instead of out the nostrils. You must identify the source of the bleeding carefully—is it from the nose, or has it been coughed up or vomited? Assess the site of bleeding, its severity, and associated symptoms. Carefully differentiate epistaxis from *hemoptysis* or *hematemesis,* because each has different causes. Is it a recurrent problem? Has there been easy bruising or bleeding elsewhere in the body?

Local causes of epistaxis include trauma (especially nose picking), inflammation, drying and crusting of the nasal mucosa, tumors, and foreign bodies.

Bleeding disorders may contribute to epistaxis.

Epistaxis

O*nset:* When did you first notice the bloody nose (epistaxis)?
  What caused the bloody nose? (injury, dry room, an object?)
L*ocation:* In which side does it occur? Both?
D*uration:* How long does it last? How often do the nosebleeds occur?
C*haracteristic Symptoms:* Describe the nosebleeds.
  What color is the blood? Bright red? Black? Dark red-brown?
  Consistency?
  Amount?
  Constant or intermittent drainage?

Associated Manifestations: Have you noticed any other symptoms?
    Injury to the nose?
    Recent surgery—nose or adenoids?
    Inflammation?
    Drying of the mucous membrane?
Relieving Factors/Treatment: What makes the bleeding stop? Is it difficult to stop?
    Are taking any nasal steroid medications? e.g., Flonase

> Assess if the patient is on anticoagulation therapy or aspirin, which interfere with clotting. Nasal sprays, if overused, can contribute to the rebound effect, causing inflammation and congestion.

Change in Sense of Smell

Onset: When did you first notice the change in sense of smell? What triggered this?
    Was there any illness prior to the change in smell? Injury?
Location: In which side did the change of smell occur? Both?
Duration: Is it constant or intermittent?
Characteristic Symptoms: Are there any smells you can detect? Which ones?
Associated Manifestations: Have you noticed any other symptoms?
Relieving Factors/Treatment: Does anything relieve this or is it permanent?

Past History

Sinus infections
Upper Respiratory Infections (URI)
Allergies
Trauma or injury
Nasal or sinus surgery
Polyps
Dental history

Family History

Allergies
Asthma

Lifestyle Habits

Air quality: at home and work, how often filters are changed, age of home and work or school site, rugs
Pets: What kind? How many? Are they in the house or outside? Do they sleep in bed with the patient?
Alcohol: What kind? How much?
Tobacco use: What kind? How often? How many?
Recreational drugs: What kind? Route? How often?

> Snorting cocaine can perforate the nasal mucous membrane. Frequent use can cause chronic rhinitis.

MOUTH AND PHARYNX

Anatomy and Physiology

The *lips* are muscular folds that surround the entrance to the mouth. When opened, the gums (gingiva) and teeth are visible. Note the scalloped shape of the *gingival margins* and the pointed *interdental papillae*.

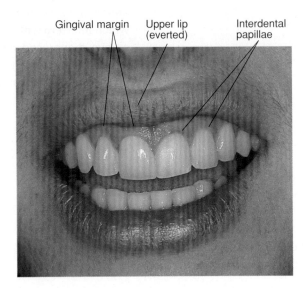

The *gingiva* is firmly attached to the teeth and to the maxilla and mandible. In lighter-skinned people, the gingiva is pale or coral pink. In darker-skinned people, it may be diffusely or partly brown, as shown in the picture. A midline mucosal fold, called a *labial frenulum,* connects each lip with the gingiva. A shallow *gingival sulcus* between the gum's thin margin and each tooth is not readily visible (but is probed and measured by dentists). Adjacent to the gingiva is the *alveolar mucosa,* which merges with the *labial mucosa* of the lip.

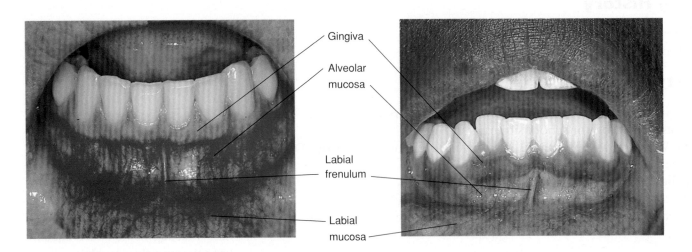

Each tooth, composed chiefly of *dentin*, lies rooted in a bony socket with only its enamel-covered crown exposed. Small blood vessels and nerves enter the tooth through its apex and pass into the pulp canal and pulp chamber.

Note the terms designating the 32 adult teeth, 16 in the upper and 16 in the lower jaw.

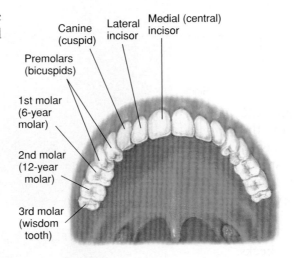

The dorsum of the *tongue* is covered with papillae, giving it a rough surface. Some of these papillae look like red dots, which contrast with the thin white coat that often covers the tongue. The undersurface of the tongue has no papillae. Note the midline *lingual frenulum* that connects the tongue to the floor of the mouth and the *ducts of the submandibular gland* (Wharton ducts) that pass forward and medially. They open on papillae that lie on each side of the lingual frenulum. The paired sublingual salivary glands lie just under the floor of the mouth mucosa.

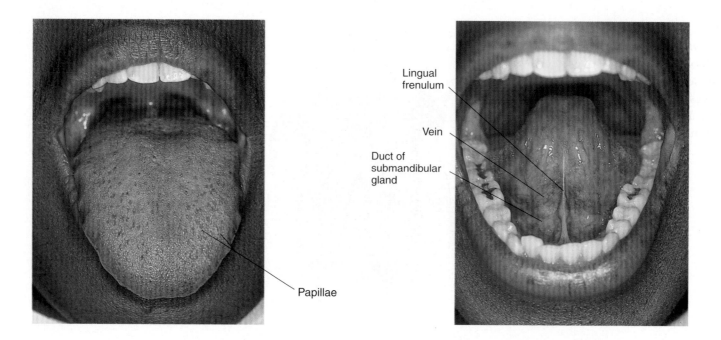

Papillae

Lingual frenulum

Vein

Duct of submandibular gland

Above and behind the tongue rises an arch formed by the *anterior* and *posterior pillars,* the *soft palate,* and the *uvula.* A meshwork of small blood vessels may web the soft palate. The *posterior pharynx* is visible in the recess behind the soft palate and tongue.

In the adjacent photograph, note the right tonsil protruding from the hollowed *tonsillar fossa,* or cavity, between the anterior and posterior pillars. In adults, tonsils are often small or absent, as in the empty left tonsillar fossa here.

The *buccal mucosa* lines the cheeks. Each *parotid duct,* sometimes termed the *Stensen duct,* opens onto the buccal mucosa near the upper second molar. Its location is frequently marked by its own small papilla.

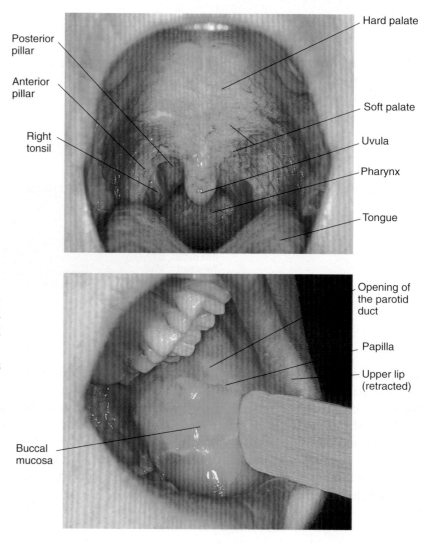

Posterior pillar

Anterior pillar

Right tonsil

Hard palate

Soft palate

Uvula

Pharynx

Tongue

Opening of the parotid duct

Papilla

Upper lip (retracted)

Buccal mucosa

THE HEALTH HISTORY

- Sore throat
- Hoarseness
- Lesions
- Sore tongue
- Bleeding gums
- Toothache
- Dysphagia

The purpose of the nursing health history of the mouth and throat is to detect changes in skin integrity, speech, or swallowing, infection, or illness.

The opening questions are:

Have you noticed any changes in your mouth or throat?
Have you had any difficulty eating? Swallowing?

Sore throat is a frequent complaint, usually associated with acute upper respiratory symptoms.

Fever, pharyngeal exudates, and anterior lymphadenopathy, especially in the absence of cough, suggest streptococcal pharyngitis, or strep throat (p. 317).[9,10]

Hoarseness refers to an altered quality of the voice, often described as husky, rough, or harsh. The pitch may be lower than before. Hoarseness usually arises from inflammation or infection of the larynx but may also develop as laryngeal lesions which press on the laryngeal nerves.[11]

Ask the patient about smoking or inhalation of other irritants, alcohol use, acid reflux, voice use, environmental allergies, and any associated symptoms. Differentiate if the problem is acute or chronic.

Acute hoarseness might be caused by voice overuse or acute viral laryngitis.

Is the problem chronic, lasting more than 2 weeks? Is there prolonged tobacco or alcohol use, cough or hemoptysis, weight loss, or unilateral throat pain?

If hoarseness lasts over 2 weeks, refer for laryngoscopy and consider causes such as *hypothyroidism*, reflux, vocal cord nodules, head and neck cancers, thyroid masses, and neurologic disorders like *Parkinson disease, amyotrophic lateral sclerosis,* or *myasthenia gravis.*

Do you experience hoarseness? If the answer is affirmative then continue the assessment.

Onset: When did the hoarseness begin? How often do you have hoarseness?

Location: Where in the throat do you feel this?

Duration: How long did it last?

Characteristic Symptoms: Did you have any other symptoms?

Associated Manifestations: What additional symptoms have occurred or what might have preceded the hoarseness?

Did you or anyone around you have a cold? Cough?

Did you overuse your voice?

Were you in a situation in which you needed to raise your voice or scream (e.g., concert, crowded area, jack hammers)?

Do you smoke? If yes, what, how many per day, and since when?

Are you around others who smoke?

Relieving Factors: What relieves the hoarseness?

Treatment: Has this been treated previously? Currently?

Additional questions for the mouth assessment would include:

A *sore tongue* may result from local lesions as well as systemic illness.

Aphthous ulcers (p. 302); sore smooth tongue of nutritional deficiency (p. 323)

How long have you had the sore tongue? Describe it?

Bleeding from the gums is a common symptom, especially when brushing teeth. What type of toothbrush is used? Hard or soft? Ask about local lesions and any tendency to bleed or bruise elsewhere.

Bleeding gums are most often caused by *gingivitis* (p. 320).

Do you have *bleeding gums?*
When did this begin?
Where is the bleeding?
Is this temporary or constant?
Do you notice any other symptoms when this occurs?
Tell me about the *toothache*.
When was the last dental examination?
What were the results?
Were any further visits necessary?
Do you have difficulty swallowing (dysphagia)?
When did this begin?
What brought it on?
Is this temporary or constant?
What other symptoms do you experience at this time?
How does it affect your daily life?
What makes it feel better or go away?
How has this changed what you eat? How has it changed who you eat with?

Do you have a history of lesions in your mouth?
    When did you first notice the lesions?
    Where are the lesions located? Are there any others?
    Describe the lesions.
        Size?
        Shape?
        Color?
        Discharge?
        Pain?
        Relationship to other lesions?
Have you noticed any other symptoms?
    Itching?
    Cough?
    Cold (respiratory infection)?
    Fever?
    Dizziness?
    Headaches?
Does anything make it better?

Past History

Sore throat
Loss of voice
Dental, mouth, or throat surgery
Trauma or injury to teeth, mouth, or throat
History of infections
Oral cancer
Sexually transmitted infection (STI)

Family History

Allergies
Smoking or exposure to smoke
Stroke
Tuberculosis

Lifestyle Habits

How many times a day do you brush your teeth?
Do you floss? How often?
Do you use tobacco? Cigarettes, cigars, a pipe, or chewing tobacco?
   How many/much per day? When did you start?
Do you smoke marijuana? Crack? Inhale any other product?
Do you drink alcohol? What? How many ounces per day?
What is your occupation?
Do you use dental dams?

PHYSICAL EXAMINATION OF THE EAR

Equipment for the Examination Includes

- Tuning fork (512 Hz preferred for hearing assessment)
- Otoscope
- Speculum
- Tongue blade
- Gloves
- Penlight

The Pinna (Auricle)

Inspect the pinna and surrounding tissue for deformities, lumps, or skin lesions.

Concept Mastery Alert

Ear pain is a common complaint with otitis externa and otitis media. Although the symptoms of both are quite similar, there are two significant differences. First, the nurse needs to evaluate pain on movement of the pinna and tragus. A positive finding is closely associated with otitis externa. Additionally, the nurse needs to evaluate for a history of exposure to water. Typically, one of the causes of otitis externa is frequent submersion of the ear in water, as would happen with a recent vacation to the beach or swimming.

See Table 12-2, Lumps on or Near the Ear (p. 311).

If ear pain, discharge, or inflammation is present, move the pinna up and down, press the tragus, and press firmly just behind the ear.

Movement of the pinna and tragus (the "tug test") is painful in acute *otitis externa* (inflammation of the ear canal), but not in *otitis media* (inflammation of the middle ear). Tenderness behind the ear occurs in *otitis media*.

Ear Canal and Drum

To see the ear canal and drum, use an otoscope with the brightest light and the largest ear speculum that inserts easily into the canal. Position the patient's head so that you can see comfortably through the otoscope. To straighten the ear canal, grasp the pinna firmly but gently and pull it upward, backward, and slightly away from the head.

Hold the otoscope handle between your thumb and fingers and brace your hand against the patient's head. Your hand and instrument can then follow unexpected movements by the patient.

Insert the speculum gently into the ear canal, directing it somewhat down and forward and through the hairs, if any, toward the eardrum.

Nontender nodular swellings covered by normal skin deep in the ear canals suggest *exostoses.* These are nonmalignant overgrowths, which may obscure the drum.

Inspect the ear canal, noting any discharge, foreign bodies, redness of the skin, or swelling. Cerumen, which varies in color and consistency from yellow and flaky to brown and sticky or even to dark and hard, may wholly or partly obscure your view.

In acute otitis externa, shown below, the canal is often swollen, narrowed, moist, pale, and tender. It may be reddened.

In *chronic otitis externa,* the skin of the canal is often thickened, red, and itchy.

RIGHT EARDRUM

Inspect the eardrum, noting its color and contour. The cone of light—usually easy to see—helps to orient you. The examiner is unable to visualize the entire eardrum at once but finds a landmark such as the cone of light and follows upward to see the handle of the malleus.

Identify the *handle of the malleus,* noting its position, and inspect the *short process of the malleus.*

Red bulging drum of acute purulent otitis media[12]; amber drum of a serous effusion. See Table 12-3, Abnormalities of the Eardrum (pp. 312–313).

An unusually prominent short process and a prominent handle that looks more horizontal suggest a retracted drum.

Gently move the speculum so that you can see as much of the drum as possible, including the *pars flaccida* superiorly and the margins of the *pars tensa.* Look for any perforations. The anterior and inferior margins of the drum may be obscured by the curving wall of the ear canal.

An advanced practitioner may evaluate the mobility of the eardrum with a pneumatic otoscope.

A serous effusion, a thickened drum, or purulent otitis media may decrease mobility. Note with a perforation, there will be no mobility.

Testing Auditory Acuity

A patient who reports difficulty hearing during the subjective questioning is twice as likely to have a hearing deficit; for patients who report normal hearing the likelihood of moderate to severe hearing impairment is only 0.13.[13]

The *whispered voice test* is a reliable screening test for hearing loss if the examiner uses a standard method of testing and exhales before whispering. Sensitivity is 90% to 100% and specificity 70% to 87%.[13–15] This test detects significant hearing loss of greater than 30 dB. A formal hearing test is still the gold standard.

Whispered Voice Test for Auditory Acuity[20]

- The patient sits and you stand 2 ft behind, so the patient is unable to read your lips.
- Test 1 ear at a time, starting with the better hearing ear.
- Using 1 finger, occlude the nontest ear and slightly rub the tragus in a circular motion preventing sound to transfer to the nontest ear.
- Exhale a full breath before whispering to ensure a quiet voice.
- Whisper a sequence with three numbers/letters, such as 2-K-5. Use a different combination for the other ear.
- Interpretation:
  - *Normal:* Patient repeats initial sequence correctly.
  - *Normal:* Patient responds incorrectly, so test a second time with a different number/letter combination; patient repeats at least three out of the possible six numbers and letters correctly.
  - *Abnormal:* Four of the six possible numbers and letters are incorrect. Conduct further testing by audiometry. (The Weber and Rinne tests are less accurate.)[13]

Testing for Conductive Versus Neurosensory Hearing Loss: Tuning Fork Tests

If hearing is diminished and a person has not passed the whisper voice test, try to distinguish between *conductive and sensorineural hearing loss.* You need a quiet room and a *512 Hertz (Hz)* tuning fork. These frequencies fall within the range of human speech (500 Hz to 3,000 Hz)—functionally the most important range. Tuning forks with lower pitches may lead to overestimating bone conduction and can also be felt as vibration. Set the fork into light vibration by briskly stroking it between the thumb and index finger or by tapping it on your forearm.

In unilateral *conductive hearing loss*, sound is heard in (lateralized to) the impaired ear. Etiologies include acute otitis media, otosclerosis, perforation of the eardrum, and obstruction of the ear canal (e.g., cerumen). See Table 12-4, Patterns of Hearing Loss, p. 314.

- *Test for lateralization (Weber test).* Place the base of the lightly vibrating tuning fork firmly on top of the patient's head or on the midforehead.

  - Ask where the patient hears the sound: on one or both sides? Normally the vibration is heard in the midline or equally in both ears. If nothing is heard, try again, pressing the fork more firmly on the head.

In unilateral *sensorineural hearing loss*, sound is heard in the good ear.

  - Restrict this test to patients with unilateral hearing loss since patients with normal hearing may lateralize, and patients with bilateral conductive or sensorineural deficits will not lateralize.

- *Compare air conduction (AC) and bone conduction (BC) (Rinne test).* Place the base of a lightly vibrating tuning fork on the mastoid bone, behind the ear and level with the canal. When the patient can no longer hear the sound, quickly place the fork close to the ear canal and ask the patient if a vibration is heard. Here the "U" of the fork should face forward, which maximizes sound transmission for the patient. Normally the sound is heard longer through air than through bone (AC > BC).

In *conductive hearing loss*, sound is heard through bone as long as or longer than it is through air (BC = AC or BC > AC). In *sensorineural hearing loss*, sound is heard longer through air (AC > BC).

PHYSICAL EXAMINATION OF THE NOSE

> ## Equipment for Examination Includes
>
> - Penlight
> - Otoscope
> - Nasal speculum or largest speculum available
> - Gloves

Inspect the anterior and inferior surfaces of the nose. Gentle pressure on the tip of the nose with your thumb usually widens the nostrils. Use a penlight or otoscope light for a partial view of each nasal *vestibule*. If the nasal tip is tender, be gentle and manipulate the nose as little as possible.

Note any asymmetry or deformity of the nose.

Test for nasal obstruction, if indicated, by pressing on each ala nasi in turn and asking the patient to breathe in.

Tenderness of the nasal tip or alae suggests local infection such as a furuncle, especially if there is a small erythematous and/or swollen area.

Vestibule

 Inspect the inside of the nose with a nasal speculum or with an otoscope and the largest ear speculum available. Tilt the patient's head back slightly and insert the speculum gently into the vestibule of each nostril, avoiding contact with the sensitive nasal septum. Hold the otoscope handle to one side to avoid the patient's chin and improve your mobility. By directing the speculum posteriorly, then upward in small steps, try to see the inferior and middle turbinates, the nasal septum, and the narrow nasal passage between them. Some asymmetry of the two sides is normal.

Deviation of the lower septum is common and may be easily visible, as illustrated in the previous photo. Deviation seldom obstructs air flow.

Middle turbinate

Nasal passage

Septum

Inferior turbinate

Observe the nasal mucosa, the nasal septum, and any abnormalities.

- The *nasal mucosa* that covers the septum and turbinates. Note its color and any swelling, bleeding, or exudate. If exudate is present, note its character: clear, mucopurulent, or purulent. The nasal mucosa is normally somewhat redder than the oral mucosa.

- The *nasal septum*. Note any deviation, inflammation, or perforation of the septum. The lower anterior portion of the septum (where the patient's finger can reach) is a common source of epistaxis (nosebleed).

- Any *abnormalities* such as ulcers or polyps.

In *viral rhinitis* the mucosa is reddened and swollen; in *allergic rhinitis* it may be pale, bluish, or red.

Fresh blood or crusting may be seen. Causes of septal perforation include trauma, surgery, and the intranasal use of cocaine or amphetamines, which can also cause septal ulceration.

Nasal polyps are pale, semitranslucent sacs of inflamed tissue that can obstruct the airway.

Inspection of the nasal cavity through the anterior naris is usually limited to the vestibule, the anterior portion of the septum, and the lower and middle turbinates. Examination with a nasopharyngeal mirror is required for detection of posterior abnormalities. This technique is used by otorhinolaryngologists (ear, nose, and throat [ENT] specialists).

Dispose of all nasal and ear specula after use. (Check the policies of your institution.)

Palpate for sinus tenderness. Press up on the *frontal sinuses* from under the bony brows, avoiding pressure on the eyes. Then press up on the *maxillary sinuses.*

Local tenderness, together with symptoms such as facial pain, pressure or fullness, purulent nasal discharge, nasal obstructions, and smell disorder, especially when present for more than 7 days, suggest *acute bacterial rhinosinusitis* involving the frontal or maxillary sinuses.[16–19]

PHYSICAL EXAMINATION OF THE MOUTH AND THROAT

Equipment for Examination Includes

- Penlight
- Tongue blade
- Gloves
- Gauze pad

Assess the teeth and teeth hygiene. Take note if the teeth are real or if the patient wears dentures. Offer a paper towel and ask the patient to remove the dentures so that you can see the underlying mucosa. If you detect any suspicious ulcers or nodules, put on a glove and palpate any lesions, noting any thickening or infiltration of the tissues that might suggest malignancy.

Bright red edematous mucosa underneath a denture suggests *denture stomatitis* (denture sore mouth). There may be ulcers or papillary granulation tissue.

Inspect the following:

The Lips

Observe their color and moisture, and note any lumps, ulcers, cracking, or scaliness.

Assess for central cyanosis or pallor from anemia. See Table 12-5, Abnormalities of the Lips (pp. 315–316).

The Oral Mucosa

Look into the patient's mouth with a good light and the help of a tongue depressor. Inspect the oral mucosa for color, ulcers, white patches, and nodules.

Leukoedema is a grayish, blue-white coloring on the buccal mucosa. This is present in 68% to 90% of individuals with darker skin and in 43% of lighter-skinned individuals. This can develop where the upper and lower teeth meet and is irritated from sucking or chewing.[20]

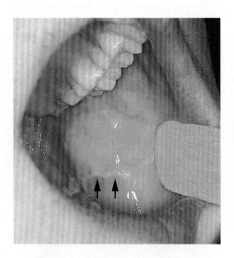

This patient has an aphthous ulcer (or canker sore) on the labial mucosa.

See Table 12-6, Findings in the Pharynx, Palate and Oral Mucosa (pp. 317–319).

The Gums and Teeth

Note the color of the gums which are normally pink. Patchy brownness may be present, especially but not exclusively in darker-skinned people.

Redness of *gingivitis*, black line of *lead poisoning*

Inspect the gum margins and the interdental papillae for swelling or ulceration.

Inspect the teeth as they can be indicative of development, hygiene, nutritional deficits, and cultural differences. Individuals with larger teeth may have protruding jaws, although does not present a problem.

Assess for missing, discolored, misshapen, or abnormally positioned teeth. Note *malocclusion* of the teeth, facial or jaw pain. Check for loose teeth with your gloved thumb and index finger. Loose fitting dentures may contribute to ulcers in the mouth or tooth decay and ultimately cause halitosis (bad breath).[21]

Swollen interdental papillae in *gingivitis*. See Table 12-7, Findings in the Gums and Teeth (pp. 320–321).

Overall, whites have more decay and 51% have complete tooth loss compared to 39% in African Americans, although there is a more periodontal disease in African Americans.[20]

Breath odor is indicative of many issues, such as diabetic ketoacidosis, renal failure, or mouth, nose, or pharynx infection.[21]

The Roof of the Mouth

Inspect the color and architecture and continuity of the hard palate.

Cleft lip is a separation or split of the upper lip, which can extend down from the base of the nose.

Cleft palate is an opening or split of the roof of the mouth, involving the hard and/or the soft palate (see photo below).

Cleft palate

The Tongue and the Floor of the Mouth

Ask the patient to put out his or her tongue. Inspect it for symmetry—a test of the hypoglossal nerve (CN XII).

Note the color and texture of the dorsum of the tongue.

Inspect the entire oral cavity, especially the sides and undersurface of the tongue and the floor of the mouth. These are the areas where cancer most often develops. Note any white or reddened areas, nodules, or ulcerations.

Asymmetric protrusion suggests a lesion of CN XII, as shown below. The tongue points "toward" the lesion.

Torus mandibularis is a bony protrusion from the medial mandible near the surface close to the tongue.

Wearing gloves, palpate all lesions. Ask the patient to protrude the tongue. With your right hand, grasp the tip of the tongue with a square of gauze and gently pull it to the patient's left. Inspect the side of the tongue, and then palpate it with your gloved left hand, feeling for any induration. Reverse the procedure for the right side.

Men older than 50 years of age, smokers, and heavy users of chewing tobacco and alcohol are at highest risk for cancers of the tongue and oral cavity, usually *squamous cell carcinomas* on the side or base of the tongue. Any persistent nodule or ulcer, red or white, is suspect, especially if indurated. These discolored lesions represent *erythroplakia* and *leukoplakia* and should be biopsied.[21,22]

See Table 12-8, Findings in or Under the Tongue (pp. 322–323).

The Pharynx

With the patient's mouth open but the tongue not protruded, ask the patient to say "ah" or yawn. This action helps you see the pharynx well. If you are not able to visualize the pharynx, press a tongue blade firmly down on the midpoint of the arched tongue—back far enough to see the pharynx but not so far that you cause gagging. Simultaneously, ask for an "ah" or a yawn. Note the rise of the soft palate and the uvula—a test of CN X (the vagal nerve).

Inspect the soft palate, anterior and posterior pillars, uvula, tonsils, and pharynx. Note their color and symmetry and look for exudate, swelling, ulceration, or tonsillar enlargement. Tonsils have crypts, or deep folds of squamous epithelium where whitish spots of normal exfoliating epithelium may sometimes be seen.

Tonsils are graded based on size:

+1: Tonsils are visible.

+2: Tonsils are between the tonsillar pillars and the uvula.

+3: Tonsils are touching the uvula.

+4: Tonsils are touching each other.

If possible, palpate any suspicious area for induration or tenderness.

Discard your tongue blade and gloves after use and wash hands.

In CN X paralysis, the soft palate fails to rise and the uvula deviates to the opposite side (points "away" from the lesion).

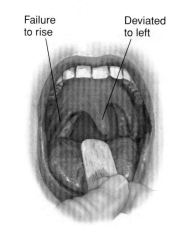

Failure to rise   Deviated to left

See Table 12-6, Findings in the Pharynx, Palate, and Oral Mucosa (pp. 317–319).

RECORDING YOUR FINDINGS

Case: Med-Surg: Simulation in Nursing Education – Medical-Surgical Scenarios (NLN, 2014): Medical Scenario 1, Core: Acute Strep Throat/Moderate Reaction to Antibiotic: Kenneth Bronson

[Show Learning Tips] [Return to Case Info]

Thursday, July 28, 2016 08:04

Bronson, Kenneth
MRN: PCS10500
Allergies **1** : No Known Allergies

Gender: Male
DOB: 10/5/1988
Age: 27 Years
Height: 72 in
Weight: 163 lb

Diagnosis: Pharyngitis
Isolation Precaution: Standard
Adv Directive: Full Code

Adm Provider:
Facility: Clinic
Adm On: 7/28/2016 07:49 [0 day(s)]

Patient Info | **Assessment** | ADLs | Notes | Nursing Dx | Orders | MAR | I/O | Vital Signs | Diagnostics | Immunizations | Flowsheet

HEENT | Neuro | Cardio | Respiratory | GI | GU | Musculoskeletal | Mental Health | Pain Scale | Integumentary | Vascular Access

[Save Assessment] [Delete] [Cancel]   [Past Assessments ▾]

Edit HEENT Assessment (Charted by Susan Fletcher, RN, Registered Nurse on 7/28/2016 08:19)

Documented By:
[Susan Fletcher, RN, Registered Nurse   ▾]

Documented At:
[0] days [0] hours [30] minutes [after admission   ▾]

Additional Notes
[Complains of severe sore throat, reports he was exposed to child with strep throat 2 days ago.]

Head

Size/Shape
- ☑ Symmetric
- ☐ Asymmetric
- ☐ Enlarged
- ☐ Decreased size

Recent Trauma
- ○ Yes
- ◉ No
- ○ Unknown

Hair
- ☑ Fine
- ☐ Coarse
- ☐ Balding
- ☐ Facial hair

Ears

- ☐ Not assessed

	Left Ear	Right Ear
Pain	☐	☐
Drainage	☐	☐
Hearing		
Intact	☑	☑
Impaired	☐	☐
Hearing device present	☐	☐
Interior		
Normal	☐	☐
Redness	☐	☐
Cerumen present	☑	☑
Swollen	☐	☐

Eyes

	Left Eye	Right Eye
Sclera		
Normal/clear	☑	☑
Jaundice	☐	☐
Redness	☐	☐
Swelling	☐	☐
Movement		
Symmetrical	☑	☑
Intact	☐	☐
Nystagmus	☐	☐
Lid lag	☐	☐
Asymmetrical corneal reflections	☐	☐
Convergence		
Average	◉	◉
Poor	○	○

Nose

Character
- ☑ Symmetrical
- ☐ Asymmetrical
- ☐ Deformity

Obstruction
- ☑ Absent
- ☐ Present left
- ☐ Present right

Septum
- ☑ Intact
- ☐ Perforated
- ☐ Deviated

Abnormalities
- ☐ Ulcers present
- ☐ Polyps present
- ☐ Blood present
- ☐ Recent trauma

Mouth/Throat

Teeth
- ☑ Present
- ☐ Absent
- ☐ Tooth decay
- ☑ Cavity(ies)
- ☐ Implant(s)
- ☐ Cap(s)
- ☐ Bridge(s)
- ☐ Dentures

Oral Mucosa
- ☑ Normal
- ☐ Ulcers
- ☑ Pink
- ☐ White
- ☐ Pale
- ☐ Dusky
- ☐ Swelling
- ☐ Moist
- ☐ Dry

Pharynx
- ☐ Normal
- ☐ Exudate
- ☑ Swelling
- ☐ Ulceration
- ☐ Tonsillar enlargement
- ☐ Pain

Lymph Nodes
- ☐ Non-tender
- ☑ Tender
- ☐ Shotty

Location:
[tonsillar lymph nodes BL]

Notes:
[ears - small amount of tan, sticky cerumen
ears - patent BL
teeth - cavity visible in upper left second molar
pharynx - red, inflamed throat with white exudate
lymph nodes - tonsillar lymph nodes BL tender, 1
cm, round, tender, non-mobile]

Ears—Acuity to whispered voice: L, "4-P-9"; R, "2-K-6." Tympanic membranes (TMs) intact, pearly grey, with cone of light at 7:00, L ear; 5:00, R ear. Weber midline. AC > BC. *Nose*—Nasal mucosa pink, septum midline; no sinus tenderness. *Throat (or Mouth)*—Oral mucosa pink, dentition 32 teeth, white, visible decay, pharynx without exudates.

OR

Ears—Acuity diminished to whispered voice; intact to spoken voice, L decreased to "4-P-9," TMs intact, pearly grey. *Nose*—Mucosa swollen with erythema and clear drainage. Septum midline. Tender over maxillary sinuses. *Throat*—Oral mucosa pink, dental caries in lower molars, pharynx erythematous, no exudates.

HEALTH PROMOTION, DISEASE PREVENTION, AND EDUCATION: EARS

Important Topics

- Hearing screening
- Ear protection

Hearing is a critical sense for experiencing the world around us, and areas of importance are health promotion and disease prevention. Nursing education is vital in maintaining hearing and a healthy outlook for clients.

Hearing Screening

Since 2008, the standard of care has become universal screening for newborns in the United States. This is the initial step in the Early Hearing Detection and Intervention (EHDI) program which includes not only screening but evaluations to diagnose infants who do not pass the initial screening and interventions for those with hearing loss.[23] This early detection will assist with early interventions in language and communication. Additional information can be obtained from the National Institute for Deafness and Communication Disorders at www.nidcd.nih.gov/directory.

Hearing Loss

Hearing loss can happen at any time and at any age. The Center for Disease Control (CDC) has determined that 15% of Americans between 20 to 69 years of age have hearing loss from noise in leisure or job-related activities and 16% of teens 12 to 19 years of age, note hearing loss related to noise.[23] Sound is measured in decibels. Sound at or above 85 dB will cause hearing loss and even sounds less than 75 dB with repeated exposure are likely to cause loss. Normal conversation is 60 dB. African

Americans have been shown to have a higher amount of melanin in the cochlea and research has thought this is why they may have less hearing loss due to loud sounds such as music or noise related to the environment.[20] Prevention is key, and patients should be reminded to use ear protection when exposed to loud noises in their daily lives (e.g., lawnmowers, leaf blowers, chainsaws, concerts, train stations, battlefields, and sirens) and to limit exposure (concerts, ear buds, and cell phones). A key to remember is to avoid noises that are too close, too loud, or too long.

Hearing loss can also trouble the later years not only from noise exposure but also from presbycusis which affects many older adults.[24] Adults older than 50 years have a 20% to 40% chance of a detectable hearing deficits and almost 80% of those 80 and older have a hearing loss, both deficits are usually greater for high-pitched sounds.[24] Hearing loss can contribute to emotional isolation and social withdrawal. Loss of hearing may go undetected if it is gradual as many do not realize their hearing is decreasing. Unlike vision prerequisites for driving, there is no mandate for widespread testing of hearing, and many seniors avoid use of hearing aids. Questionnaires and handheld audiometers work well for periodic screening. Less sensitive are the clinical "whisper test," rubbing fingers, or use of the tuning fork.

HEALTH PROMOTION, DISEASE PREVENTION, AND EDUCATION: MOUTH AND THROAT

Important Topics

- Oral and dental screening
- Cancer prevention

More than one third (36.8%) of poor children ages 2 to 19 have one or more untreated decayed primary teeth, compared to 17.3% of nonpoor children.[25] This issue persists, as the 50 to 69-year-old age group has at least one tooth with periodontal disease. The rate is highest for non-Hispanic blacks (31.2%), Mexican Americans (28.2%), and non-Hispanic whites (16.9%). As these groups age, the percentages rise to 47.1%, 32.0%, and 24.1%, respectively.[25]

Oral Health

Nurses play an active role in promoting oral health. Health disparities in regards to oral health greatly affect certain racial and ethnic groups. Overall Non-Hispanic black, Hispanics, American Indians, and Alaska Natives have poorer oral health. Untreated tooth decay and periodontal disease is three times as likely in adults, 35 to 44 years of age with less than a high school education.

Effective screening begins with careful examination of the mouth. Inspect the oral cavity for decayed or loose teeth, inflammation of the gingiva, and signs of periodontal disease (bleeding, pus, recession of the gums, and bad breath). Inspect the mucous membranes, the palate, the oral floor, and the surfaces of the tongue for ulcers and leukoplakia, warning signs for oral cancer and HIV disease. Use of dental dams during oral sex will act as a barrier to bodily fluids and help reduce transmission of sexually transmitted infections (STIs) such as herpes, genital warts, and HIV.

To improve oral health, counsel patients to adopt daily hygiene measures. Use of fluoride-containing toothpaste reduces tooth decay, and brushing and flossing daily delays periodontal disease by removing bacterial plaques. Urge patients to seek dental care at least annually to receive the benefits of more specialized preventive care such as scaling, planing of roots, and topical fluorides.[26]

Diet, tobacco and alcohol use, changes in salivary flow from medication, and proper use of dentures should also be addressed. As with children, adults should avoid excessive intake of foods high in refined sugars such as sucrose, which enhance attachment and colonization of cariogenic bacteria. Use of all tobacco products and excessive alcohol, the principal risk factors for oral cancers, should be avoided.

Saliva cleanses and lubricates the mouth. Many medications reduce salivary flow, increasing risk for tooth decay, mucositis, and gum disease from *xerostomia*, especially for the elderly. For those wearing dentures, dental examinations should be scheduled annually, and patients should be counseled about the importance of removing and cleaning the dentures each night to reduce bacterial plaque and risk of malodor. Regular massage of the gums relieves soreness and pressure from dentures on the underlying soft tissue.

TABLE

12-1

Dizziness and Vertigo[27–31]

"Dizziness" is a nonspecific term used by patients encompassing several disorders that clinicians must carefully sort out. A detailed history usually identifies the primary etiology. It is important to learn the specific meanings of the following terms or conditions:

- *Vertigo*—a spinning sensation accompanied by nystagmus and ataxia; usually from *peripheral vestibular dysfunction* (~40% of "dizzy" patients) but may be from a *central brainstem lesion* (~10%; causes include atherosclerosis, multiple sclerosis, vertebrobasilar migraine, or transient ischemic attack [TIA])
- *Presyncope*—a near faint from "feeling faint or lightheaded"; causes include orthostatic hypotension, especially from medication, arrhythmias, and vasovagal attacks (~5%)
- *Dysequilibrium*—unsteadiness or imbalance when walking, especially in older patients, causes include fear of walking, visual loss, weakness from musculoskeletal problems, and peripheral neuropathy (up to 15%)
- *Psychiatric*—causes include anxiety, panic disorder, hyperventilation, depression, somatization disorder, and alcohol and substance abuse (~10%)
- *Multifactorial or unknown*—(up to 20%)

Peripheral and Central Vertigo					
	Onset	Duration and Course	Hearing	Tinnitus	Additional Features
Peripheral Vertigo					
• *Benign Positional Vertigo*	Sudden, often when rolling onto the affected side or tilting up the head	Onset a few seconds to <1min. Lasts a few weeks, may recur	Not affected	Absent	Sometimes nausea, vomiting nystagmus
• *Vestibular Neuronitis (acute labyrinthitis)*	Sudden	Onset hours to up to 2 wks. May recur over 12–18 mo	Not affected	Absent	Nausea, vomiting, nystagmus
• *Ménière Disease*	Sudden	Onset several hours to ≥1 day. Recurrent	Sensorineural hearing loss—recurs, eventually progresses	Present, fluctuating	Pressure or fullness in affected ear; nausea, vomiting, nystagmus
• *Drug Toxicity*	Insidious or acute—linked to loop diuretics, aminoglycosides, salicylates, alcohol	May or may not be reversible. Partial adaptation occurs	May be impaired	May be present	Nausea, vomiting
• *Acoustic Neuroma*	Insidious from CN VIII compression, vestibular branch	Variable	Impaired, one side	Present	May involve CN V and VII
Central Vertigo	Often sudden (see causes above)	Variable but rarely continuous	Not affected	Absent	Usually with other brainstem deficits—dysarthria, ataxia, crossed motor and sensory deficits

Sources: Chan Y. Differential diagnosis of dizziness. *Curr Opin Otolaryngol Head Neck Surg*. 2009;17:200; Kroenke K, Lucas CA, Rosengerg ML, et al. Causes of persistent dizziness: a prospective study of 100 patients in ambulatory care. *Ann Intern Med*. 1992;117:898–904; Tusa RJ. Vertigo. *Neurol Clin*. 2001;19:23–55; Lockwood AH, Salvi RJ, Burkard RF. Tinnitus. *N Engl J Med*. 2002;347:904.

TABLE
12-2

Lumps on or Near the Ear

Keloid. A firm, nodular, hypertrophic mass of scar tissue extending beyond the area of injury. It may develop in any scarred area but is most common on the shoulders and upper chest. A keloid on a pierced earlobe may have troublesome cosmetic effects. Keloids are more common in darker-skinned people and may recur following treatment.

Chondrodermatitis Helicis. This chronic inflammatory lesion starts as a painful, tender papule on the helix or antihelix. Here the upper lesion is at a later stage of ulceration and crusting. Reddening may occur. Biopsy is needed to rule out carcinoma.

Tophi. A deposit of uric acid crystals characteristic of chronic tophaceous gout. It appears as hard nodules in the helix or antihelix and may discharge chalky white crystals through the skin. It also may appear near the joints, hands (p. 641), feet, and other areas. It usually develops after chronic sustained high blood levels of uric acid.

Basal Cell Carcinoma. This raised nodule shows the lustrous surface and telangiectatic vessels of basal cell carcinoma, a common slow-growing malignancy that rarely metastasizes. Growth and ulceration may occur. These are more frequent in fair-skinned people overexposed to sunlight.

Cutaneous Cyst. Formerly called a *sebaceous cyst,* a dome-shaped lump in the dermis forms a benign closed firm sac attached to the epidermis. A dark dot (blackhead) may be visible on its surface. Histologically, it is usually either (1) an *epidermoid* cyst, common on the face and neck, or (2) a *pilar (trichilemmal)* cyst, common in the scalp. Both may become inflamed.

Rheumatoid Nodules. In chronic rheumatoid arthritis, look for small lumps on the helix or antihelix and additional nodules elsewhere on the hands, along the surface of the ulna distal to the elbow, and on the knees and heels. Ulceration may result from repeated injuries. These nodules may antedate the arthritis.

Sources of photos: *Keloid*—Sams WM Jr, Lynch PJ, eds. *Principles and Practice of Dermatology.* Edinburgh: Churchill Livingstone; 1990; *Tophi*—du Vivier A. *Atlas of Clinical Dermatology.* 2nd ed. London: Gower Medical Publishing; 1993; *Cutaneous Cyst, Chondrodermatitis Helicis*—Young EM, Newcomer VD, Kligman AM. *Geriatric Dermatology: Color Atlas and Practitioner's Guide.* Philadelphia: Lea & Febiger; 1993; *Basal Cell Carcinoma*—*N Engl J Med.* 1992;326:169–170; *Rheumatoid Nodules*—Champion RH, Burton JL, Ebling FJG, eds. *Rook/Wilkinson/Ebling Textbook of Dermatology.* 5th ed. Oxford, UK: Blackwell Scientific; 1992.

TABLE

12-3   Abnormalities of the Eardrum

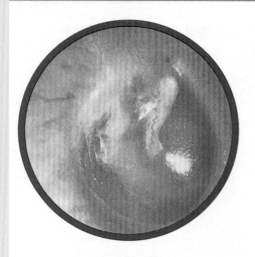

Normal Eardrum (Right)

This normal right eardrum (tympanic membrane) is pinkish gray. Note the malleus lying behind the upper part of the drum. Above the short process lies the *pars flaccida*. The remainder of the drum is the *pars tensa*. From the umbo, the bright cone of light fans anteriorly and downward. Posterior to the malleus, part of the incus is visible behind the drum. The small blood vessels along the handle of the malleus are normal.

Perforation of the Drum

Perforations are holes in the eardrum that usually result from purulent infections of the middle ear. They may be *central,* if not involving the margin of the drum, or *marginal,* when the margin is involved. The membrane covering the perforation may be notably thin and transparent.

The more common central perforation is illustrated here. A reddened ring of granulation tissue surrounds the perforation, indicating chronic infection. The eardrum itself is scarred, and no landmarks are visible. Discharge from the infected middle ear may drain out through such a perforation. A perforation often closes in the healing process, as in the next photo. There may be associated earache or even hearing loss, especially if the perforations are large.

Tympanosclerosis

Tympanosclerosis is a scarring process of the middle ear from otitis media that involves deposition of hyaline and calcium and phosphate crystals in the eardrum and middle ear. When severe it may entrap the ossicles and cause conductive hearing loss.

In the inferior portion of this left eardrum, note the large, chalky white patch with irregular margins. Other abnormalities in this eardrum include a *healed perforation* (the large oval area in the upper posterior drum) and signs of a *retracted drum*. A retracted drum is pulled medially, away from the examiner's eye, and the malleolar folds are tightened into sharp outlines. The short process often protrudes sharply, and the handle of the malleus, pulled inward at the umbo, looks foreshortened and more horizontal.

Serous Effusion

Serous effusions are usually caused by viral upper respiratory infections (*otitis media with serous effusion*) or by sudden changes in atmospheric pressure as from flying or diving (*otitic barotrauma*). The eustachian tube cannot equalize the air pressure in the middle ear with that of the outside air. Air is partly or completely absorbed from the middle ear into the bloodstream, and serous fluid accumulates there instead. Symptoms include fullness and popping sensations in the ear, mild conduction hearing loss, and perhaps some pain.

Amber fluid behind the eardrum is characteristic, as in this patient with otic barotrauma. A fluid level, a line between air above and amber fluid below, can be seen on either side of the short process. Air bubbles (not always present) can be seen here within the amber fluid.

Acute Otitis Media With Purulent Effusion

Acute otitis media with purulent effusion is caused by bacterial infection from *S. pneumoniae* or *H. influenzae*. Symptoms include earache, fever, and hearing loss. The eardrum reddens, loses its landmarks, and bulges laterally, toward the examiner's eye.

Here the eardrum is bulging, and most landmarks are obscured. Redness is most obvious near the umbo, but dilated vessels can be seen in all segments of the drum. A diffuse redness of the entire drum often develops. Spontaneous rupture (perforation) of the drum may follow, with discharge of purulent material into the ear canal.

Hearing loss is of the conductive type. Acute purulent otitis media is much more common in children than in adults.

Bullous Myringitis

Bullous myringitis is a viral infection characterized by painful hemorrhagic vesicles that appear on the tympanic membrane, the ear canal, or both. Symptoms include earache, blood-tinged discharge from the ear, and hearing loss of the conductive type.

In this right ear, at least two large vesicles (bullae) are discernible on the drum. The drum is reddened, and its landmarks are obscured.
This condition is caused by mycoplasma, viral, and bacterial otitis media.

Sources of photos: *Normal Eardrum*—Hawke M, Keene M, Alberti PW. Clinical Otoscopy: A Text and Colour Atlas. Edinburgh: Churchill Livingstone, 1984; *Perforation of the Drum, Tympanosclerosis*—Courtesy of Michael Hawke, MD, Toronto, Canada.
Sources of photos: *Serous Effusion*—Hawke M, Keene M, Alberti PW. Clinical Otoscopy: A Text and Colour Atlas. Edinburgh: Churchill Livingstone, 1984; *Acute Otitis Media, Bullous Myringitis*—The Wellcome Trust, National Medical Slide Bank, London, UK.

TABLE
12-4

Patterns of Hearing Loss

	Conductive Loss	Sensorineural Loss
Pathophysiology	External or middle ear disorder impairs sound conduction to inner ear. Causes include foreign body, *otitis media,* perforated eardrum, and otosclerosis of ossicles.	Inner ear disorder involves cochlear nerve and neuronal impulse transmission to the brain. Causes include loud noise exposure, inner ear infections, trauma, tremors, congenital and familial disorders, and aging.
Usual Age of Onset	Childhood and young adulthood, up to age 40	Middle or later years
Ear Canal and Drum Effects	Abnormality usually visible, except in otosclerosis • Little effect on sound • Hearing seems to improve in noisy environment • Voice becomes soft because inner ear and cochlear nerve are intact	Problem not visible • Higher registers are lost, so sound may be distorted. • Hearing worsens in noisy environment. • Voice may be loud because hearing is difficult.
Weber Test *(in unilateral hearing loss)*	• Tuning fork at vertex • Sound lateralizes to *impaired ear*—room noise not well heard, so detection of vibrations *improves*.	• Tuning fork at vertex • Sound lateralizes to *good ear*—inner ear or cochlear nerve damage impairs transmission to affected ear.
Rinne Test	• Tuning fork at external auditory meatus then on mastoid bone • Bone conduction longer than or equal to air conduction (BC ≥ AC). While air conduction through the external or middle ear is impaired, vibrations through bone bypass the problem to reach the cochlea.	• Tuning fork at external auditory meatus then on mastoid bone • Air conduction longer than bone conduction (AC > BC). The inner ear or cochlear nerve is less able to transmit impulses regardless of how the vibrations reach the cochlea. The normal pattern prevails.

TABLE
12-5

Abnormalities of the Lips

Angular Cheilitis

Angular cheilitis starts with softening of the skin at the angles of the mouth, followed by fissuring. It may be due to nutritional deficiency or, more commonly, to over closure of the mouth, as in people with no teeth or with ill-fitting dentures. Saliva wets and macerates the infolded skin, often leading to secondary infection with *Candida,* as seen here.

Actinic Cheilitis

Actinic cheilitis is a precancerous condition that results from excessive exposure to sunlight and affects primarily the lower lip. Fair-skinned men who work outdoors are most often affected. The lip loses its normal redness and may become scaly, somewhat thickened, and slightly everted. Because solar damage also predisposes to carcinoma of the lip, be alert to this possibility.

Herpes Simplex *(Cold Sore, Fever Blister)*

The herpes simplex virus (HSV) produces recurrent and painful vesicular eruptions of the lips and surrounding skin. A small cluster of vesicles first develops. As these break, yellow-brown crusts form, healing takes 10–14 days. Both new and erupted vesicles are visible here.

Angioedema

Angioedema is a localized subcutaneous or submucosal swelling caused by leakage of intravascular fluid into interstitial tissue. Two types are common. When vascular permeability is triggered by mast cells in allergic and NSAID reactions, look for associated urticaria and pruritus. These are uncommon in angioedema from bradykinin and complement-derived mediators, the mechanism in ACE-inhibitor reactions. Angioedema is usually benign and resolves within 24–48 h. It can be life-threatening when it involves the larynx, tongue, or upper airway or develops into anaphylaxis.

(table continues on page 316)

TABLE
12-5

Abnormalities of the Lips (continued)

Hereditary Hemorrhagic Telangiectasia (Osler–Weber–Rendu syndrome)

Multiple small red spots on the lips strongly suggest hereditary hemorrhagic telangiectasia, an autosomal dominant endothelial disorder causing vascular fragility and arteriovascular malformations (AVMs). Telangiectasias are also visible on the oral mucosa, nasal septal mucosa, and fingertips. Nosebleeds, gastrointestinal bleeding, and iron deficiency anemia are common. AVMs in the lungs and brain can cause life-threatening hemorrhage and embolic disease.

Peutz–Jeghers Syndrome

Look for prominent small brown pigmented spots in the dermal layer of the lips, buccal mucosa, and perioral area. These spots may also appear on the hands and feet. In this autosomal dominant syndrome, these characteristic skin changes accompany numerous intestinal polyps. The risk of gastrointestinal and other cancers ranges from 40–90%. Note that these spots rarely appear around the nose and mouth.

Chancre of Syphilis

This ulcerated papule with an indurated edge usually appears after 3–6 wks of incubating infection from the spirochete *Treponema pallidum*. These lesions may resemble a carcinoma or crusted cold sore. Similar primary lesions are common in the pharynx, anus, and vagina but may escape detection since they are painless, nonsuppurative, and usually heal spontaneously in 3–6 wks. Wear gloves during palpation since these chancres are infectious.

Carcinoma of the Lip

Like actinic cheilitis, *squamous cell carcinoma* usually affects the lower lip. It may appear as a scaly plaque, as an ulcer with or without a crust, or as a nodular lesion, as illustrated here. Fair skin and prolonged exposure to the sun are common risk factors.

Sources of photos: *Angular Cheilitis, Herpes Simplex, Angioedema*—Neville B, et al. *Color Atlas of Clinical Oral Pathology*. Philadelphia: Lea & Febiger; 1991, Used with permission; *Actinic Cheilitis, Hereditary Hemorrhagic Telangiectasia*—Langlais RP, Miller CS. *Color Atlas of Common Oral Diseases*. Philadelphia: Lea & Febiger; 1992, Used with permission; *Peutz–Jeghers Syndrome*—Robinson HBG, Miller AS. *Colby, Kerr, and Robinson's Color Atlas of Oral Pathology*. Philadelphia: JB Lippincott; 1990; *Chancre of Syphilis*—Wisdom A. *A Colour Atlas of Sexually Transmitted Diseases*. 2nd ed. London: Wolfe Medical Publications; 1989; *Carcinoma of the Lip*—Tyldesley WR. *A Colour Atlas of Orofacial Diseases*. 2nd ed. London: Wolfe Medical Publications; 1991.

TABLE
12-6

Findings in the Pharynx, Palate, and Oral Mucosa

Large Normal Tonsils

Normal tonsils may be large without being infected, especially in children. They may protrude medially beyond the pillars and even to the midline. Here they touch the sides of the uvula and obscure the pharynx. Their color is pink. The white marks are light reflections, not exudate.

Exudative Tonsillitis

This red throat has a white exudate on the tonsils. This, together with fever and enlarged cervical nodes, increases the probability of *group A streptococcal infection* or *infectious mononucleosis*. Anterior cervical lymph nodes are usually enlarged in the former, posterior nodes in the latter.

Pharyngitis

These two photos show reddened throats without exudate.

In **A**, redness and vascularity of the pillars and uvula are mild to moderate.

In **B**, redness is diffuse and intense. Each patient would probably complain of a sore throat, or at least a scratchy one. Possible causes include several kinds of viruses and bacteria. If the patient has no fever, exudate, or enlargement of cervical lymph nodes, the chances of infection by either of two common causes—*group A streptococci* and *Epstein–Barr virus* (infectious mononucleosis)—are reduced.

(table continues on page 318)

TABLE 12-6

Findings in the Pharynx, Palate, and Oral Mucosa (continued)

Diphtheria

Diphtheria, an acute infection caused by *Corynebacterium diphtheriae* is now rare but still important. The throat is dull red, and a gray exudate (pseudomembrane) is present on the uvula, pharynx, and tongue. The airway may become obstructed. Prompt diagnosis may lead to lifesaving treatment.

Thrush on the Palate (Candidiasis)

Thrush is a yeast infection due to *Candida*. Shown here on the palate, it may appear elsewhere in the mouth (see p. 322). Thick, white plaques are somewhat adherent to the underlying mucosa. Predisposing factors include (1) prolonged treatment with antibiotics or corticosteroids and (2) AIDS.

Kaposi Sarcoma in AIDS

The deep purple color of these lesions suggests Kaposi sarcoma, a low-grade vascular tumor associated with human herpesvirus 8. The lesions may be raised or flat. About a third of patients with Kaposi sarcoma have lesions in the oral cavity; other affected sites are the gastrointestinal tract and the lungs. Antiretroviral therapy has markedly reduced the prevalence of this disease.

Torus Palatinus

A torus palatinus is a midline bony growth in the hard palate that is fairly common in adults. Its size and lobulation vary. Although alarming at first glance, it is harmless. In this example, an upper denture has been fitted around the torus.

Sources of photos: *Large Normal Tonsils, Exudative Tonsillitis, Pharyngitis (**A** and **B**), Koplik Spots, Petechiae, Thrush on the Palate*—The Wellcome Trust, National Medical Slide Bank, London, UK; *Diphtheria*—Harnisch JP, et al. Diphtheria among alcoholic urban adults. *Ann Intern Med.* 1989;111:77; *Kaposi Sarcoma in AIDS*—Ioachim HL. *Textbook and Atlas of Disease Associated With Acquired Immune Deficiency Syndrome.* London: Gower Medical Publishing; 1989; *Fordyce Spots*—Neville B, et al. *Color Atlas of Clinical Oral Pathology.* Philadelphia: Lea & Febiger; 1991, Used with permission; *Leukoplakia*—Robinson HBG, Miller AS. *Colby, Kerr, and Robinson's Color Atlas of Oral Pathology.* Philadelphia: JB Lippincott; 1990.

Fordyce Spots *(Fordyce Granules)*

Fordyce spots are normal sebaceous glands that appear as small yellowish spots in the buccal mucosa or on the lips. A worried person who has suddenly noticed them may be reassured. Here they are seen best anterior to the tongue and lower jaw. These spots are usually not so numerous.

Koplik Spots

Koplik spots are an early sign of measles (rubeola). Search for small white specks that resemble grains of salt on a red background. They usually appear on the buccal mucosa near the first and second molars. In this photo, look also in the upper third of the mucosa. The rash of measles appears within a day.

Petechiae

Petechiae are small red spots that result when blood escapes from capillaries into the tissues. Petechiae in the buccal mucosa, as shown, are often caused by accidentally biting the cheek. Oral petechiae may be due to infection or decreased platelets, as well as to trauma.

Leukoplakia

A thickened white patch (*leukoplakia*) may occur anywhere in the oral mucosa. The extensive example shown on this buccal mucosa resulted from frequent chewing of tobacco, a local irritant. This benign reactive process of the squamous epithelium may lead to cancer and should be biopsied. Another risk factor is human papillomavirus infection.

TABLE
12-7

Findings in the Gums and Teeth

Marginal Gingivitis

Marginal gingivitis is common during adolescence, early adulthood, and pregnancy. The gingival margins are reddened and swollen, and the interdental papillae are blunted, swollen, and red. Brushing the teeth often makes the gums bleed. *Plaque*—the soft white film of salivary salts, protein, and bacteria that covers the teeth and leads to gingivitis—is not readily visible.

Acute Necrotizing Ulcerative Gingivitis

This uncommon form of gingivitis occurs suddenly in adolescents and young adults and is accompanied by fever, malaise, and enlarged lymph nodes. Ulcers develop in the interdental papillae. Then the destructive (necrotizing) process spreads along the gum margins, where a grayish pseudomembrane develops. The red, painful gums bleed easily; the breath is foul.

Gingival Hyperplasia

Gums enlarged by hyperplasia are swollen into heaped-up masses that may even cover the teeth. The redness of inflammation may coexist, as in this example. Causes include phenytoin (dilantin) therapy (as in this case), puberty, pregnancy, and leukemia.

Pregnancy Tumor (Pregnancy Epulis, Pyogenic Granuloma)

Red purple papules of granulation tissue form in the gingival interdental papillae, in the nasal cavity, and sometimes on the fingers. They are red and soft and usually bleeds easily. They occur in 1–5% of pregnancies and usually regress after delivery. Note the accompanying gingivitis in this example.

Sources of photos: *Marginal Gingivitis, Acute Necrotizing Ulcerative Gingivitis*—Tyldesley WR. *A Colour Atlas of Orofacial Diseases.* 2nd ed. London: Wolfe Medical Publications; 1991; *Gingival Hyperplasia*—Courtesy of Dr. James Cottone; *Pregnancy Tumor, Attrition of Teeth, Erosion of Teeth*—Langlais RP, Miller CS. *Color Atlas of Common Oral Diseases.* Philadelphia: Lea & Febiger; 1992, Used with permission; *Abrasion of Teeth, Hutchinson Teeth*—Robinson HBG, Miller AS. *Colby, Kerr, and Robinson's Color Atlas of Oral Pathology.* Philadelphia: JB Lippincott; 1990.

Attrition of Teeth; Recession of Gums

In many elderly people, the chewing surfaces of the teeth have been worn down by repetitive use so that the yellow-brown dentin becomes exposed—a process called *attrition*. Note the *recession of the gums*, which has exposed the roots of the teeth, giving a "long in the tooth" appearance.

Erosion of Teeth

Teeth may be eroded by chemical action. Note here the erosion of the enamel from the lingual surfaces of the upper incisors, exposing the yellow-brown dentin. This results from recurrent regurgitation of stomach contents, as in bulimia.

Abrasion of Teeth With Notching

The biting surface of the teeth may become abraded or notched by recurrent trauma, such as holding nails or opening bobby pins between the teeth. Unlike Hutchinson teeth, the sides of these teeth show normal contours; size and spacing of the teeth are unaffected.

Hutchinson Teeth

Hutchinson teeth are smaller and more widely spaced than normal and are notched on their biting surfaces. The sides of the teeth taper toward the biting edges. The upper central incisors of the permanent (not the deciduous) teeth are most often affected. These teeth are a sign of congenital syphilis.

TABLE

12-8

Findings in or Under the Tongue

Geographic Tongue. In this benign condition, the dorsum shows scattered smooth red areas denuded of papillae. Together with the normal rough and coated areas, they give a map-like pattern that changes over time.

Hairy Tongue. Note the "hairy" yellowish to brown or black hypertrophied and elongated papillae on the tongue's dorsum. This benign condition is associated with *Candida* and bacterial overgrowth, antibiotic therapy, and poor dental hygiene. It may occur spontaneously.

Fissured Tongue. Fissures appear with increasing age, sometimes termed *furrowed tongue*. Food debris may accumulate in the crevices and become irritating, but a fissured tongue is benign.

Smooth Tongue (Atrophic Glossitis). A smooth and often sore tongue that has lost its papillae, sometimes just in patches, suggests a deficiency in riboflavin, niacin, folic acid, vitamin B_{12}, pyridoxine, or iron, or treatment with chemotherapy.

Candidiasis. Note the thick white coating from *Candida* infection. The raw red surface is where the coat was scraped off. Infection may also occur without the white coating. It is seen in immunosuppression from chemotherapy or prednisone therapy.

Hairy Leukoplakia. These whitish raised asymptomatic plaques with a feathery or corrugated pattern commonly occur on the sides of the tongue. Unlike candidiasis, these areas cannot be scraped off. This condition is caused by Epstein–Barr virus infection and is seen with HIV and AIDS.

Sources of photos: *Fissured Tongue, Candidiasis, Mucous Patch, Leukoplakia, Carcinoma*—Robinson HBG, Miller AS. *Colby, Kerr, and Robinson's Color Atlas of Oral Pathology.* Philadelphia: JB Lippincott; 1990; *Smooth Tongue*—Courtesy of Dr. R. A. Cawson, from Cawson RA. *Oral Pathology.* 1st ed. London, UK: Gower Medical Publishing; 1987; *Geographic Tongue*—The Wellcome Trust, National Medical Slide Bank, London, UK; *Hairy Leukoplakia*—Ioachim HL. *Textbook and Atlas of Disease Associated With Acquired Immune Deficiency Syndrome.* London, UK: Gower Medical Publishing, 1989; *Varicose Veins*—Neville B, et al. *Color Atlas of Clinical Oral Pathology.* Philadelphia, Lea & Febiger; 1991, Used with permission.

Varicose Veins. Small purplish or blue-black round swellings appear under the tongue with age. These dilatations of the lingual veins have no clinical significance.

Aphthous Ulcer (Canker Sore). A painful, round or oval shallow whitish-gray oval ulceration surrounded by a halo of reddened mucosa. It may be single or multiple and may also occur on the gingiva and oral mucosa. It heals in 7–10 days, but may recur, for example, in Behcet disease.

Mucous Patch of Syphilis. This painless lesion in the secondary stage of syphilis is highly infectious. It is slightly raised, oval, and covered by a grayish membrane. It may be multiple and occur elsewhere in the mouth.

Leukoplakia. With this persisting painless white patch in the oral mucosa, the undersurface of the tongue appears painted white. Patches of any size raise the possibility of squamous cell carcinoma and require a biopsy.

Tori Mandibulares. Rounded bony growths on the inner surfaces of the mandible are typically bilateral, asymptomatic, and harmless.

Carcinoma, Floor of the Mouth. This ulcerated lesion is in a common location for carcinoma. Medially, note the reddened area of mucosa, called *erythroplakia,* suggesting possible malignancy.

BIBLIOGRAPHY

CITATIONS

1. Uy J, Forciea MA. In the clinic. Hearing loss. *Ann Intern Med.* 2013;158:ITC4–ITC1.

2. Willems PJ. Genetic causes of hearing loss. *N Engl J Med.* 2000;342(15):1101–1109.

3. Kozin ED, Sethi RK, Remenschneider AK, et al. Epidemiology of otologic diagnoses in United States emergency departments. *Laryngoscope.* 2015;(8):1926–1933.

4. Kim SH, Kim TH, Byun JY, et al. Clinical differences in types of otalgia. *J Audiol Otol.* 2015;(1):34–38.

5. Prokop-Prigge KA, Mansfield CJ, Parker MR, et al. Ethnic/racial and genetic influences on cerumen odorant profiles. *J Chem Ecol.* 2015;41(1):67–74.

6. Wheatley LM, Togias A. Clinical practice. Allergic rhinitis. *N Engl J Med.* 2015;372:456.

7. Piccirillo JF. Acute bacterial sinusitis. *N Engl J Med.* 2004;351(9):902–910.

8. Spector SL, Bernstein IL, Li JT, et al. Parameters for the diagnosis and management of sinusitis. *J Allergy Clin Immunol.* 1998;102(6, Part 2):S107–S144.

9. Cooper RJ, Hoffman JR, Bartlett JG, et al. Principles of appropriate antibiotic use for acute pharyngitis in adults: background. *Ann Intern Med.* 2001;134(6):509–517.

10. McGinn TG, Deluca J, Ahlawat SK, et al. Validation and modification of streptococcal pharyngitis clinical prediction rules. *Mayo Clin Proc.* 2003;78(3):289–293.

11. Schwartz SR, Cohen SM, Dailey SH, et al. Clinical practice guideline: hoarseness (dysphonia). *Otolaryngol Head Neck Surg.* 2009;141(3 Suppl 2):S1–S31.

12. Pichichero ME. Otitis media. *Pediatr Clin North Am.* 2013;60:391.

13. Bagai A, Thavendiranathan P, Detsky AS. Does this patient have hearing impairment? *JAMA.* 2006;295:416.

14. McShefferty D, Whitmer WM, Swan IR, et al. The effect of experience on the sensitivity and specificity of the whispered voice test: a diagnostic accuracy study. *BMJ Open.* 2013;18;3(4):pii: e002394.

15. Pirozzo S, Papinczak T, Glasziou P. Whispered voice test for screening for hearing impairment in adults and children: systematic review. *BMJ.* 2003;327:967.

16. Krouse H. Allergic rhinitis. *Nurse Pract.* 2014;39(4):9–10.

17. Hayden ML, Womack C. Caring for patients with allergic rhinitis. *J Am Acad Nurse Pract.* 2007;19(6):290–298.

18. Aring AM, Chan MM. Acute rhinosinusitis in adults. *Am Fam Physician.* 2011;83:1057.

19. Pearce L. Managing allergic rhinitis. *Nurs Times.* 2012;108:17, 20–22.

20. Andrews MA, Boyle JS. *Transcultural Concepts in Nursing Care.* 7th ed. Philadelphia, PA: Lippincott Williams & Wilkins; 2015.

21. Neville BW, Day TA. Oral cancer and precancerous lesions. *CA Cancer J Clin.* 2002;52:195.

22. Brocklehurst P, Kujan O, O'Malley LA, et al. Screening programmes for the early detection and prevention of oral cancer. *Cochrane Database Syst Rev.* 2013;11:CD004150. http://www.ncbi.nlm.nih.gov/pubmed/24254989 Accessed Oct 8, 2015.

23. Biernath K, Holstrum WJ, Eichwald J. Hearing screening for newborns: the midwife's role in early hearing detection and intervention. *J Midwifery Womens Health.* 2009;54(1):18–26.

24. U.S. Preventive Services Task Force. Screening for hearing impairment. Available at: http://www.uspreventiveservicestaskforce.org/Page/Document/RecommendationStatementFinal/hearing-loss-in-older-adults-screening. Accessed Oct 8, 2015.

25. Centers for Disease Control and Prevention. Untreated dental caries (cavities) in children ages 2–19, United States. Updated February 2011. Available at http://www.cdc.gov/Features/dsUntreatedCavitiesKids/. Accessed Oct 8, 2015.

26. Finnegan DA, Rainchuso L, Jenkins S, et al. Immigrant caregivers of young children: oral health beliefs, attitudes, and early childhood caries knowledge. *J Community Health.* 2016;41(2):250–257. Available at: http://www.ncbi.nlm.nih.gov/pubmed/26370378. Accessed Oct 8, 2015.

27. Kroenke K, Lucas CA, Rosengerg ML, et al. Causes of persistent dizziness: a prospective study of 100 patients in ambulatory care. *Ann Intern Med.* 1992;117(11):898–904.

28. Kroenke K, Hoffman RM, Einstadter D. How common are various causes of dizziness? A critical review. *South Med J.* 2000;93(2):160–167.

29. Tusa RJ. Vertigo. *Neurol Clin.* 2001;19(1):23–55.

30. Lockwood AH, Salvi RJ, Burkard RF. Tinnitus. *N Engl J Med.* 2002;347(12):904–910.

31. Matthies C, Samii M. Management of 1000 vestibular schwannomas (acoustic neuromas): clinical presentation. *Neurosurgery.* 1997;1:1–10.

The Respiratory System

LEARNING OBJECTIVES

The student will:

1. Describe the structure and functions of the airways, alveoli, lungs, and pleura.

2. Identify the locations of each lung lobe using landmarks on the thorax.

3. Describe the mechanics of breathing.

4. Obtain an accurate history of the respiratory system.

5. Identify the percussion and auscultation sites for assessment of the lungs.

6. Describe the normal lung sounds and their location.

7. Describe adventitious sounds and voice sounds and their origin.

8. Appropriately prepare and position the patient for the respiratory examination.

9. Describe the equipment necessary to perform a respiratory examination.

10. Correctly inspect, palpate, percuss, and auscultate the thorax.

11. Discuss risk factors for respiratory disease.

12. Discuss risk reduction and health promotion strategies to reduce respiratory disease.

ANATOMY AND PHYSIOLOGY

Review the *anatomy of the chest wall,* identifying the structures illustrated. Note the intercostal space between two ribs has the same number as the rib above it.

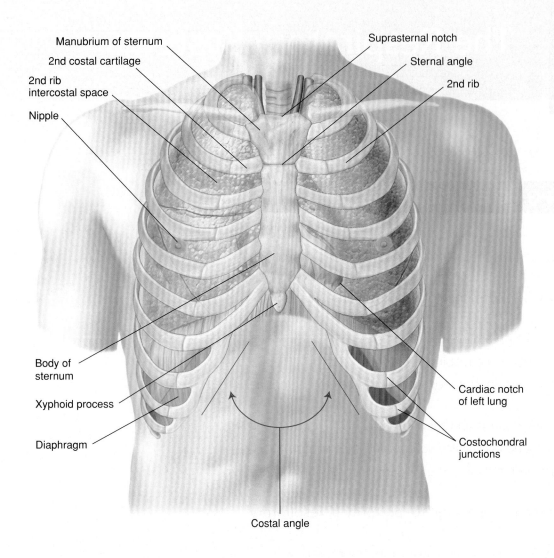

Manubrium of sternum

2nd costal cartilage

2nd rib intercostal space

Nipple

Suprasternal notch

Sternal angle

2nd rib

Body of sternum

Xyphoid process

Diaphragm

Cardiac notch of left lung

Costochondral junctions

Costal angle

Locating Findings on the Chest

Vertical Axis

Chest findings are described in two dimensions: *along the vertical axis* and *around the circumference of the chest*.

To identify *vertical* locations, count the ribs and intercostal spaces. Begin by finding the *sternal angle*, also termed the angle of Louis. Place your finger in the hollow curve of the suprasternal notch, and then move your finger down approximately 5 cm to the horizontal bony ridge joining the manubrium to the body of the sternum. Then move your finger laterally and find the adjacent 2nd rib. From here, using two fingers, "walk down" the intercostal spaces, one space at a time, on an oblique line, illustrated by the red numbers on p. 327. It is easier to identify intercostal spaces in women when they lie down, as the supine position displaces breast tissue across the chest. Avoid pressing too hard on tender breast tissue.

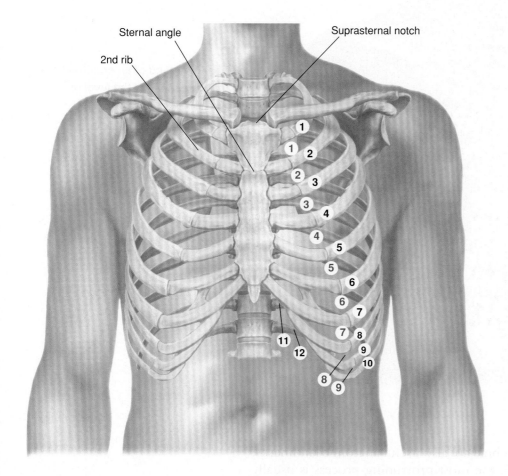

The costal cartilages of the first seven ribs articulate with the sternum; the cartilages of the 8th, 9th, and 10th ribs articulate with the costal cartilages just above them. The 11th and 12th ribs, the "floating ribs," have no anterior attachments. The cartilaginous tip of the 11th rib usually can be felt laterally, and the 12th rib may be felt posteriorly. On palpation, costal cartilages and ribs feel identical.

Posteriorly, the 12th rib is another possible starting point for counting ribs and intercostal spaces: it helps locate findings on the lower posterior chest and provides an option when the anterior approach is unsatisfactory. With the fingers of one hand, press in and up against the lower border of the 12th rib, then "walk up" the intercostal spaces numbered in red on page 328, or follow a more oblique line up and around to the front of the chest.

The inferior tip of the scapula is another useful bony landmark—it usually lies at the level of the 7th rib or intercostal space.

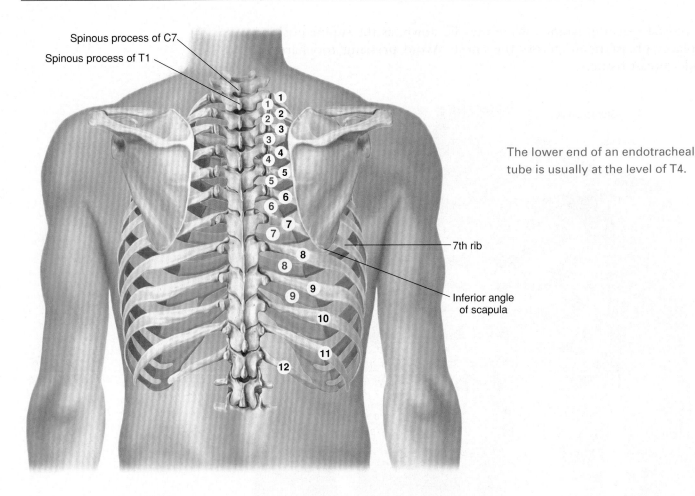

Spinous process of C7

Spinous process of T1

7th rib

Inferior angle of scapula

The lower end of an endotracheal tube is usually at the level of T4.

The spinous processes of the vertebrae are also useful anatomic landmarks. When the neck is flexed forward, the most protruding process is usually the vertebra of C7, known as the vertebral prominens. If two processes are equally prominent, they are C7 and T1. You can often palpate and count the processes below them, especially when the spine is flexed.

Circumference of the Chest

To locate findings around the *circumference of the chest*, use a series of vertical lines, shown in the adjacent illustrations. The *midsternal* and *vertebral lines* are easily seen. The others are estimated. The *midclavicular line* drops vertically from the midpoint of the clavicle. To find it, identify both ends of the clavicle accurately (See Chapter 18, The Musculoskeletal System, p. 579).

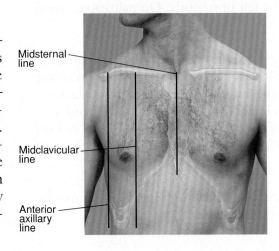

Midsternal line

Midclavicular line

Anterior axillary line

The *anterior* and *posterior axillary lines* drop vertically from the anterior and posterior axillary folds, which are the muscle masses that border the axilla. The *midaxillary line* drops from the apex of the axilla.

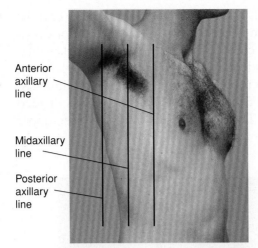

Anterior axillary line

Midaxillary line

Posterior axillary line

Posteriorly, the *vertebral line* overlies the spinous processes of the vertebrae. The scapular line drops from the inferior angle of the scapula.

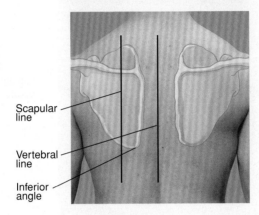

Scapular line

Vertebral line

Inferior angle

Lungs, Fissures, and Lobes

Using exterior landmarks picture the lungs and their fissures and lobes on the chest. Anteriorly, the apex of each lung rises approximately 2 to 4 cm above the inner third of the clavicle. The lower border of the lung crosses the 6th rib at the midclavicular line and the 8th rib at the midaxillary line. Posteriorly, the lower border of the lung lies at about the level of the T10 spinous process. On inspiration, it descends farther.

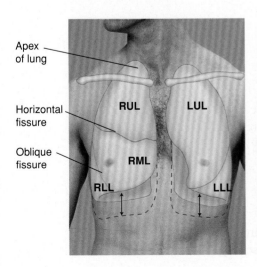

Apex of lung

Horizontal fissure

Oblique fissure

RUL

LUL

RML

RLL

LLL

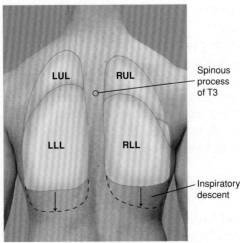

LUL

RUL

Spinous process of T3

LLL

RLL

Inspiratory descent

Each lung is divided roughly in half by an *oblique (major) fissure*. This fissure may be approximated by a string that runs from the T3 spinous process obliquely down and around the chest to the 6th rib at the midclavicular line. The right lung is further divided by the *horizontal (minor) fissure.* Anteriorly, this fissure runs close to the 4th rib and meets the oblique fissure in the midaxillary line near the 5th rib. The *right lung* is thus divided into *upper, middle,* and *lower lobes.* The *left lung* has only *two lobes,* upper and lower.

 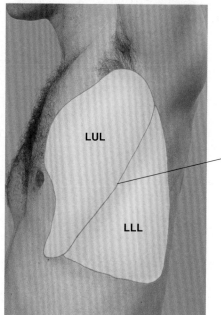

RUL - Right Upper Lobe
RML - Right Middle Lobe
RLL - Right Lower Lobe
LUL - Left Upper Lobe
LLL - Left Lower Lobe

Left oblique fissure

Locations on the Chest

Learn the general anatomic terms used to locate chest findings, such as:

Supraclavicular—above the clavicles
Infraclavicular—below the clavicles
Interscapular—between the scapulae
Infrascapular—below the scapulae
Bases of the lungs—the lowermost portions
Upper, middle, and lower lung fields

Usually physical examination findings correlate with the underlying lobe. Signs in the right upper lung field, for example, almost certainly originate in the right upper lobe. Signs in the right middle lung field laterally, however, could come from any of three different lobes.

The Trachea and Major Bronchi

Breath sounds over the trachea and bronchi have a harsher quality than breath sounds over the lung parenchyma. Know the location of these structures. The trachea bifurcates into its mainstem bronchi at the levels of the sternal angle anteriorly and the T4 spinous process posteriorly. The right main bronchus is wider, shorter, and more vertical than the left man bronchus, which extends more laterally.

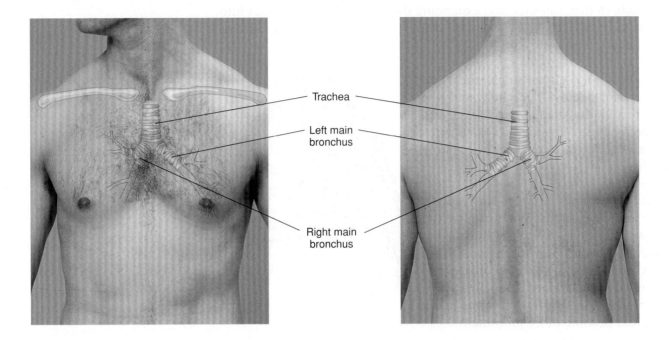

The Pleurae

The pleurae are two serous membranes that cover the outer surface of each lung. The *visceral pleura* lies next to the lung and the *parietal pleura* lines the inner rib cage and upper surface of the diaphragm. Their smooth opposing surfaces, lubricated by pleural fluid, allow the lungs to move easily within the rib cage during inspiration and expiration. The *pleural space* is the potential space between visceral and parietal pleurae

Accumulation of fluid between the pleurae is called a plural effusion.

The visceral pleura lacks sensory nerves, but the parietal pleura is richly innervated by the intercostal and phrenic nerves.

Inflammation of the parietal pleura produces pleuritic pain with deep inspiration, for example, in *pleurisy, pneumonia, and pulmonary embolism.*

Breathing

Breathing is largely an automatic act, controlled by the respiratory center in the brainstem and mediated by the muscles of respiration. The *diaphragm* is the primary muscle of inspiration. When it contracts during inhalation, it descends in the chest and enlarges the thoracic cavity. At the same time, it compresses the abdominal contents, pushing the abdominal wall outward. The muscles in the rib cage and neck also expand the thorax during inspiration, especially the intercostal muscles, and the *scalenes,* which run from the cervical vertebrae to the first two ribs.

During inspiration, as these muscles contract, the thorax expands. Intrathoracic pressure decreases, drawing air through the tracheobronchial tree into the *alveoli,* or distal air sacs, and expanding the lungs. Oxygen diffuses into the blood of adjacent pulmonary capillaries, and carbon dioxide diffuses from the blood into the alveoli.

After inspiratory effort stops, the expiratory phase begins. The chest wall and lungs recoil, the diaphragm relaxes and rises passively, air flows outward, and the chest and abdomen return to their resting positions.

Normal breathing is quiet and easy—barely audible near the open mouth as a faint whish. When a healthy person lies supine, the breathing movements of the thorax are relatively slight. In contrast, the abdominal movements are usually easy to see. In the sitting position, movements of the thorax become more prominent.

During exercise and in certain diseases, extra work is required to breathe, and accessory muscles join the inspiratory effort. The *sternocleidomastoids* are the most important of these, and the *scalenes* may become visible. Abdominal muscles assist in expiration.

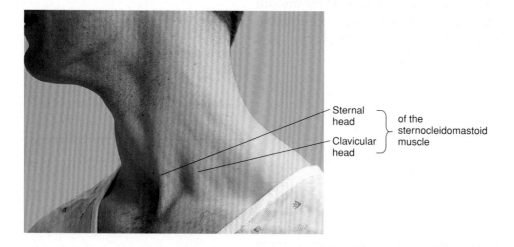

Sternal head ⎤
           ⎬ of the
Clavicular ⎦ sternocleidomastoid
head   muscle

Changes in the thorax and lungs due to age are described later in the textbook. The older adult changes are in Chapter 24, The Older Adult, pp. 932–933; infant in Chapter 23, Assessing Children: Infancy through Adolescence, infant p. 834, and child p. 875.

THE HEALTH HISTORY

Common or Concerning Symptoms

- Shortness of breath (dyspnea)
- Wheezing
- Cough
- Blood-streaked sputum (hemoptysis) or purulent sputum
- Chest pain

The thorax houses several organs and structures, and the nurse must use astute questioning to ascertain the patient's problem. Dyspnea, wheezing, cough, and hemoptysis usually point to a respiratory problem; however, they may also indicate a cardiac condition. Chest pain may be caused by cardiac, respiratory, gastrointestinal, or musculoskeletal etiologies.

The initial history questions should be as broad as possible.

Dyspnea is air hunger, a nonpainful but uncomfortable awareness of breathing that is inappropriate to the level of exertion, commonly termed shortness of breath. This is a serious symptom that warrants a full explanation and assessment. It can result from pulmonary or cardiac disease. Ask:

See Table 13-1, Chapter 13, pp. 360–361.

Have you had any difficulty breathing?

O*nset:* When did you first feel short of breath?
- Did anything bring on the shortness of breath (e.g., exposure to an allergen)?

L*ocation:* Is the difficulty in your throat or neck area or chest?

D*uration:* Does this occur at a particular time of day?
- Did it come on suddenly or gradually?

Sudden onset may indicate anaphylaxis or pulmonary embolism (both emergencies), spontaneous pneumothorax, or anxiety.

- Is it continuous or intermittent?
- Does it occur at rest or with exertion or activity?

C*haracteristic Symptoms:* Can the patient talk in full sentences or only short phrases?

Determine the severity of the dyspnea based on the patient's ability to talk and complete daily activities.

Is the shortness of breath worse when you are lying down or upright? Has shortness of breath altered your lifestyle or daily activities?
- How many steps or flights of stairs can you climb before pausing for breath?
- Can you carry groceries, vacuum the floor, or make the bed without dyspnea?

Associated *Manifestations:* Are there any associated symptoms, such as wheezing or cough? Chest pain? Nausea?
Relieving *Factors:* Does anything make it better?
Treatment: Have you seen anyone or tried any medications or treatments?

Anxious patients present a different picture. They may describe difficulty taking a deep-enough breath, or a smothering sensation with the inability to get enough air. If they are hyperventilating they may report *paresthesias,* which are sensations of tingling or "pins and needles" around the lips or in the hands and feet.

Wheezes are musical respiratory sounds that may be audible to the patient and others. Wheezes are caused by partial obstruction of the lower airways. The airway may be narrowed by bronchoconstriction, edema, secretions as in asthma or a foreign body.

Do you have any wheezing?

O*nset:* When did you first notice the wheeze?
- Did anything precipitate the wheezing (e.g., exposure to an allergen, cold, etc.)?

L*ocation:* Is it from your throat area or chest?
D*uration:* Does this occur at a particular time of day?
- Did it come on suddenly or gradually?
- Is it continuous or intermittent?
- Does it occur at rest or with exercise or activity?

C*haracteristic Symptoms:* Does the wheeze occur when you inhale, exhale or both?
A*ssociated Manifestations:* Are there any associated symptoms, such as shortness of breath or cough?
R*elieving Factors:* Does anything make it better?
T*reatment:* Have you seen anyone? Tried any medicines? Any treatments?

Cough is typically a reflex response to stimuli that irritate receptors in the larynx, trachea, or large bronchi. These stimuli include mucus, pus, blood, dust, foreign bodies, and even extremely hot or cold air. Coughing may also be caused by inflammation of the respiratory mucosa or tension in the air passages from a tumor or enlarged peribronchial lymph nodes. Patients with asthma may experience a cough without wheezing. The narrowed airways trigger a cough on expiration as the patient tries to fully exhale the trapped air. Duration of a cough is important to document. An *acute cough* lasts less than 3 weeks, *subacute cough* lasts 3 to 8 weeks, and a *chronic cough* lasts over 8 weeks.

Do you have a cough?

O*nset:* When did you first notice the cough?
- Did anything precipitate the cough (e.g., a cold or respiratory infection)?

Anxious patients may have episodic dyspnea during both rest and exercise, and hyperventilation, or rapid shallow breathing. At other times, they may sigh frequently.

See Table 13-2, chapter 13, Cough and Hemoptysis, p. 362.

Cough may also be a symptom of *left-sided heart failure.*

Viral upper respiratory infections are the most common cause of *acute cough;* other causes include acute bronchitis, pneumonia, asthma, pertussis or foreign body.

- Have you begun any new medicines recently?

Some medications such as angiotensin-converting enzyme (ACE) inhibitors produce a persistent dry cough as a side effect.

Location: Does your cough come from your throat or chest?
Duration: Does this happen at a particular time of day?
- Did it come on suddenly or gradually?
- Does it come and go or last all the time?
- Does it occur at rest or with exercise or activity?
- Does it wake you at night?

Characteristic Symptoms: Do you feel the urge to cough when you inhale or exhale?

Does the cough come in spasms that make breathing difficult?'

Paroxysms of coughing followed by a "whooping" intake of breath occur with pertussis.

Do you cough up mucus or phlegm?

Mucoid sputum is translucent, white or grey; *purulent* sputum is yellowish or greenish.

Foul-smelling sputum is seen in anaerobic lung abscess; tenacious sputum in cystic fibrosis.

Large volumes of purulent sputum may occur in bronchiectasis or lung abscess.

- If yes, ask the patient to describe the color, odor, consistency, and amount.
- To quantify mucus volume, ask: How much mucus do you think you cough up in 24 hours: a teaspoon, tablespoon, quarter cup, half cup, cupful?
- Have you noticed blood in the mucus?

Hemoptysis is coughing up of blood from the lungs; it may vary from blood-streaked phlegm to frank blood. Blood or blood-streaked material may originate in the mouth, pharynx, or gastrointestinal tract and is easily misidentified. Blood originating in the stomach is usually darker than blood from the respiratory tract and food particles may be mixed in. Hemoptysis is rare in infants, children, and adolescents, although common in cystic fibrosis.

- Describe the color and amount of blood.
- Have you had any mouth injuries or nosebleeds recently? Any ulcers?

- If the patient is actively coughing ask him or her to cough into a tissue in order to examine its characteristics.

Associated *Manifestations:* Do you have any other symptoms like shortness of breath or wheezing?

Relieving *Factors:* Does anything make it better?

Treatment: Have you seen anyone or tried any medicines? Or treatments?

Chest pain may be caused by cardiac, respiratory, gastrointestinal, or musculoskeletal etiologies. See Table 13-3, Chest Pain, pp. 363–364. The nurse should carefully ask follow-up questions using the "OLD CART" mnemonic to identify the source of the pain. Lung tissue itself has no pain fibers. Pain in lung conditions, such as pneumonia or pulmonary infarction, usually arises from inflammation of the adjacent parietal pleura. Sources of chest pain are listed below.

Sources of Chest Pain and Related Causes	
• Trachea and large bronchi	Bronchitis
• Parietal pleura	Pericarditis, pneumonia
Chest wall, including the musculoskeletal system and skin	Costochondritis, herpes zoster
• Myocardium	Angina pectoris, myocardial infarction
• Pericardium	Pericarditis
• Aorta	Dissecting aortic aneurysm
• Esophagus	Gastric esophageal reflux disease, esophageal spasm
Extrathoracic structures: neck, gallbladder, and stomach	Cervical arthritis, biliary colic, gastritis
Anxiety	The mechanism of pain remains obscure

- Extrathoracic structures: neck, gallbladder, and stomach

This chapter will focus on pulmonary complaints. See Chapter 14, The Cardiovascular System, and Chapter 16, The Gastrointestinal and Renal Systems for history questions related to nonpulmonary chest pain.

Do you have chest pain?

Onset: When did the pain begin?
- Have you had chest pain previously? When?
- Is this the same pain?
- Did you fall or have any chest injuries prior to the pain?

Location: Where in your chest do you feel the pain?

Duration: Does it occur with breathing? Does the pain come and go or last all the time?

Characteristic Symptoms: Describe your pain. Is your chest tender to touch? Rate the pain on a scale of 1 to 10.

Associated Manifestations: When you have the chest pain, does anything else happen, for example, loss of consciousness, nausea, numbness, or tingling?

Relieving Factors: Does anything make it better?

Treatment: Have you seen anyone or tried any medicines or treatments?

Past History

- Have you had any prior lung problems, such as infections, asthma, bronchitis, emphysema, pneumonia, tuberculosis, collapsed lung (pneumothorax), or cystic fibrosis?

  - If yes, ask about onset, duration, treatment, and sequelae.

- Have you had chest surgery, biopsy, or trauma to your chest?

  - If yes, ask the purpose, date, and outcome of the event.

- Do you have any allergies that affect your breathing or respiratory system?

  - If yes, ask the patient to describe his or her symptoms and treatment.

- Have you had tuberculosis skin testing (purified protein derivative [PPD]) or a chest x-ray? When? What were the results?

  Ask clients born outside the United States if they received the bacillus Calmette–Guerin (BCG) vaccine. This vaccine is given in some countries to reduce the risk of contracting tuberculosis.

- Have you had any other lung function testing? When? What were the results?

- Have you had the flu vaccine? When?

- Have you had the Tdap version of the tetanus immunization?

  Immunity to pertussis from the childhood (DPT) vaccine has been shown to be weakening. Vaccination with the Tdap vaccine is recommended.

- If the patient is over 65 years, inquire: did you have the pneumonia (pneumococcal) vaccines?

- Have you traveled outside the United States within the last 6 months? If yes, where?

Family History

- Does anyone in your family currently have a lung infection or disease?

- Has anyone had lung cancer, asthma, or cystic fibrosis?

- Did anyone smoke in your home when you were growing up? Who?

Lifestyle and Personal Habits

- Do you smoke or have you ever smoked tobacco or marijuana?

  - How many cigarettes or packs per day do you smoke?

  - When did you start? How long have you smoked/did you ever smoke?

- Do you use or have you ever used snuff?

- Do you chew or have you ever chewed tobacco?

- Are you exposed to second-hand smoke? Where?

  - How many hours per day? For how many years?

- Are you exposed to any environmental conditions at home or work that affect your breathing (e.g., mold, sawdust, asbestos, coal dust, insecticides, radon, paint, or pollution)?

- Are you taking any prescription, herbal, or over-the-counter (OTC) medications for breathing or respiratory problems?

- Do you use oxygen or other treatments for breathing problems (e.g., nebulizer treatments)?

PHYSICAL EXAMINATION

For best results examine the posterior and lateral thorax and lungs while the patient is sitting, and the anterior thorax and lungs with the patient supine. Proceed in an orderly fashion: inspect, palpate, percuss, and auscultate the entire chest. Try to visualize the underlying lobes, and compare one side with the other, noting any asymmetrical findings. For men, arrange the patient's gown so that you can see the chest fully. For women, cover the anterior chest when you examine the back and sides. For the anterior examination, drape the gown over each half of the chest as you examine the other half.

- *With the patient sitting,* examine the posterior and lateral thorax and lungs. The patient's arms should be folded across the chest with hands resting, if possible, on the opposite shoulders. This position moves the scapulae laterally and increases your access to the lung fields. Following the complete posterior and lateral thorax examination, ask the patient to lie down.

- *With the patient supine,* examine the anterior thorax and lungs. The supine position makes it easier to examine women because the breasts can be gently displaced. Furthermore, wheezes, if present, are more likely to be heard. (Some clinicians examine both the back and the front of the chest with the patient sitting. This technique is also satisfactory.)

- *For patients who cannot sit up without aid,* obtain assistance so that you can examine the posterior chest in the sitting position. If this is impossible, roll the patient to one side and then to the other. Percuss the upper lung, and auscultate both lungs in each position. Because ventilation is relatively greater in the dependent (i.e., lower) lung, your chances of hearing abnormal wheezes or crackles are greater on the dependent side (see Chapter 13, Characteristics of Breath Sounds, p. 346).

Hospitalized or long-term care patients who cannot sit up for routine lung assessment every shift may be examined using this technique.

Initial Survey of Respiration and the Thorax

Observe and document the rate, rhythm, depth, and effort of breathing. This may have been done already with the vital signs. A healthy adult breathes quietly and regularly about 12 to 20 times a minute. An occasional sigh is to be expected. Note whether expiration lasts longer than usual. See Chapter 7, Beginning the Physical Examination: General Survey, Vital Signs, and Pain, p. 135 for information on assessing respiratory rate and rhythm.

See Table 13-4, Abnormalities in Rate and Rhythm of Breathing, p. 365.

Inspect the patient for signs of respiratory difficulty.

- *Observe the patient's facial expression*—it should be relaxed and calm.

Low oxygenation produces anxiety and restlessness.

- *Observe level of consciousness.*

Decreased level of consciousness indicates poor oxygenation to the brain and other disease processes.

- *Assess the patient's color* for cyanosis, especially the face, mucous membranes, and nail beds (shown in the toes in the photo; note the contrast with the normal fingers).

Cyanosis signals hypoxia. Clubbing of the nails (see Table 9-14, Findings In or Near the Nails, p. 208) in *cystic fibrosis,* or *congenital heart disease.*

- *Listen to the patient's breathing.* Are there any audible sounds (e.g., *wheezing* or *stridor*)? If so, do they occur during inhalation exhalation or both?

Audible stridor, a high-pitched inspiratory sound, is an ominous sign of airway obstruction in the larynx or trachea. Audible wheezing indicates severe asthma.

- *Inspect the neck.* During inspiration, is there contraction of the accessory muscles, namely, the sternocleidomastoid and scalene muscles, or supraclavicular retraction? Is the trachea midline?

Inspiratory contraction of the sternocleidomastoids and scalenes at rest signals severe difficulty in breathing. Lateral displacement of the trachea may be seen in *pneumothorax, pleural effusion,* or *atelectasis.*

Observe the shape of the chest, which is normally wider than it is deep. The ratio of the anteroposterior (AP) diameter to the lateral chest diameter is usually 0.70–0.75 up to 0.90, and increases with aging.[1]

The AP diameter also may increase in *chronic obstructive pulmonary disease* (COPD).

Examination of the Posterior Chest

Refer to Chapter 6, Physical Examination: Getting Started, pp. 116–117, for a description of how to perform the four assessment techniques.

Inspection

From a midline position behind the patient, note the *shape of the chest* and *how the chest moves,* including:

- Deformities or asymmetry.

See Table 13-5, Chapter 13, Deformities of the Thorax, p. 366.

- Intercostal retractions during inspiration. Retractions are most apparent in the lower intercostal spaces.

Retraction is seen in severe *asthma, COPD,* or upper airway obstruction.

- Impaired respiratory movement on one or both sides or a unilateral lag (or delay) in movement.

Unilateral impairment or lagging of respiratory movement suggests disease of the underlying lung or pleura.

Palpation

As you palpate the chest, focus on areas of tenderness and abnormalities in the overlying skin, muscles and ribs, respiratory expansion, and fremitus.

Intercostal tenderness over inflamed pleura.

- *Identify tender areas.* Gently palpate any area where pain has been reported or where lesions or bruises are evident.

Bruises or tenderness over a fractured rib.

- *Assess any observed abnormalities* such as masses.

- *Test chest expansion.* Place your thumbs at about the level of the 10th ribs, with your fingers loosely grasping and parallel to the lateral rib cage. As you position your hands, slide them medially just enough to raise a loose fold of skin on each side between your thumb and the spine.

Ask the patient to inhale deeply. Watch the distance between your thumbs as they move apart during inspiration, and feel for the range and symmetry of the rib cage as it expands and contracts. Your thumbs should move equally apart.

Causes of unilateral decrease or delay in chest expansion include *pleural effusion, lobar pneumonia,* pleural pain with associated splinting, unilateral bronchial obstruction, and *chronic fibrosis* of the underlying lung or pleura.

- *Feel for tactile fremitus.* Fremitus refers to the palpable vibrations transmitted through the bronchopulmonary tree to the chest wall as the patient is speaking. To detect fremitus, use either the ball (the bony part of the palm at the base of the fingers) or the ulnar surface of your hand to optimize the vibratory sensitivity of the bones in your hand. Ask the patient to repeat the words "ninety-nine" or "one-one-one." If fremitus is faint, ask the patient to speak more loudly or in a deeper voice. The simultaneous use of both hands to compare sides, increases your speed and may facilitate detection of asymmetry.

Fremitus is decreased or absent when the voice is soft or when the transmission of vibrations from the larynx to the surface of the chest is impeded. Causes include a very thick chest wall; an obstructed bronchus; *COPD;* and pleural effusion, fibrosis (*pleural thickening*), air (*pneumothorax*), or an infiltrating tumor.

- *Palpate and compare symmetric areas* of the lungs in the pattern shown in the photograph. Identify and locate any areas of increased, decreased, or absent fremitus. Fremitus is typically more prominent in the interscapular area than in the lower lung fields and sides. For the #4 location in the photo, place your hands on the lateral chest below the axillae. Fremitus is often more prominent on the right side than on the left. It disappears below the diaphragm. Tactile fremitus is a somewhat imprecise assessment tool, but as

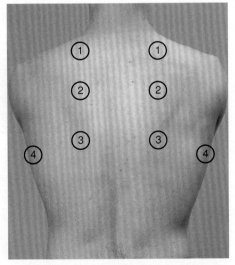

LOCATIONS FOR FEELING FREMITUS

Look for *asymmetric* fremitus: asymmetric *decreased* fremitus is seen in unilateral pleural effusion, pneumothorax, neoplasm from decreased transmission of low-frequency sounds; asymmetric *increased* fremitus is seen in unilateral pneumonia from increased transmission.[1]

a scouting technique, it directs your attention to possible abnormalities. Later in the examination you will check any suggested findings by listening for breath sounds, voice sounds, and whispered voice sounds. All these attributes tend to increase or decrease together.

Percussion

Percussion sets the chest wall and underlying tissues in motion, producing audible sound. Percussion helps to establish whether the underlying tissues are air filled, fluid filled, or solid. It penetrates only 5 to 7 cm into the chest, however, and will not help detect deep-seated lesions.

The technique of percussion can be practiced on any surface. As you practice, listen for changes in percussion notes over different types of materials or different parts of the body. The key points for good technique, described for a right-handed person, are as follows:

- Hyperextend the middle finger of your left hand, known as the *pleximeter finger.* Press its distal interphalangeal joint firmly on the surface to be percussed. *Avoid surface contact by any other part of the hand, because this dampens out vibrations.* Note that the thumb and 2nd, 4th, and 5th fingers are not touching the chest.

- Position your right forearm quite close to the surface, with the hand cocked upward. The middle finger should be partially flexed, relaxed, and poised to strike.

- With a *quick, sharp but relaxed wrist motion,* strike the pleximeter finger with the right middle finger, or plexor finger. Aim at your distal interphalangeal joint. You are trying to transmit vibrations through the bones of this joint to the underlying chest wall.

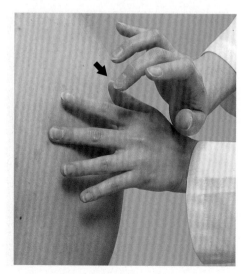

- Strike using the *tip of the plexor finger*, not the finger pad. Your finger should be almost at right angles to the pleximeter. A short fingernail is recommended to avoid self-injury.

- Withdraw your striking finger quickly to avoid damping the vibrations you have created.

In summary, the movement is at the wrist. It is directed, brisk yet relaxed, and slightly bouncy.

Percussion Notes

With your plexor or tapping finger, use the lightest percussion that produces a clear note. A thick chest wall requires stronger percussion than a thin one. However, if a *louder* note is needed, apply more pressure with the *pleximeter* finger (this is more effective for increasing percussion note volume than tapping harder with the plexor finger).

- *When percussing the lower posterior chest*, stand somewhat to the side rather than directly behind the patient. This allows you to place your pleximeter finger more firmly on the chest and your plexor strike is more effective, making a better percussion note.

- *When comparing two areas*, use the same percussion technique in both areas. Percuss or strike twice in each location comparing percussion notes.

- *Learn to identify five percussion notes.* You can practice four of them on yourself. These notes differ in their basic qualities of sound: intensity, pitch, and duration. Train your ear to distinguish these differences by concentrating on one quality at a time as you percuss first in one location, then in another. Review the table below. Healthy lungs are *resonant*.

Percussion Notes and Their Characteristics				
	Relative Intensity	Relative Pitch	Relative Duration	Example of Location	Pathologic Examples
Flatness	Soft	High	Short	Thigh	Large pleural effusion
Dullness	Medium	Medium	Medium	Liver	Lobar pneumonia
Resonance	Loud	Low	Long	Healthy lung	Simple chronic bronchitis
Hyperresonance	Very loud	Lower	Longer	Usually none	COPD, pneumothorax
Tympany	Loud	High[a]	Longer	Gastric air bubble or puffed-out cheek	Large pneumothorax

[a]Distinguished mainly by its musical timbre.

While the patient keeps both arms crossed in front of the chest, percuss the thorax in symmetric locations from the apex to the base.

- *Alternate percussing one side of the chest and then the other at each level* in a ladder-like pattern, as shown in the photograph below. Begin above the scapula. Omit the areas over the scapulae—the thickness of muscle and bone alters the percussion notes of the lungs. The lateral numbers 6 and 7 should be percussed on the midaxillary line. Identify and locate the area and quality of any abnormal percussion note.

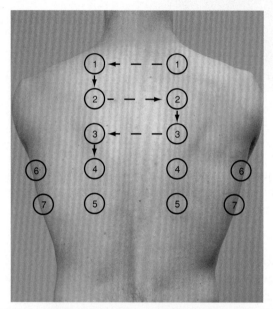

"LADDER" PATTERN FOR PERCUSSION AND AUSCULTATION

Dullness replaces resonance when fluid or solid tissue replaces air-containing lung or occupies the pleural space beneath your percussing fingers. Examples include *lobar pneumonia,* in which the alveoli are filled with fluid and blood cells; and pleural accumulations of serous fluid (*pleural effusion*), blood (*hemothorax*), pus (*empyema*), fibrous tissue, or tumor.

Generalized hyperresonance may be heard over the hyperinflated lungs of COPD or *asthma,* but is not a reliable sign. *Unilateral hyperresonance* suggests a large pneumothorax or possibly a large air-filled bulla in the lung.

- *Identify the descent of the diaphragm,* or **diaphragmatic excursion.** First, *determine the level of diaphragmatic dullness* during quiet respiration. Holding the pleximeter finger *above and parallel* to the expected level of dullness, percuss downward in progressive steps until dullness clearly replaces resonance. Confirm this level of change by percussion near the scapular line and more laterally.

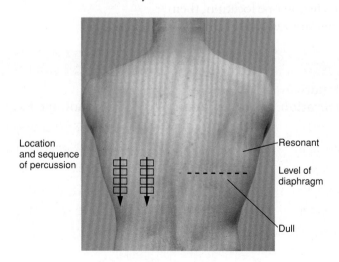

Location and sequence of percussion

Resonant

Level of diaphragm

Dull

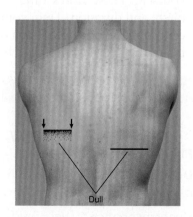

Dull

An abnormally high level suggests *pleural effusion,* or a high diaphragm as in *atelectasis* or *diaphragmatic paralysis.*

Note that with this technique, you are identifying the boundary between the resonant lung tissue and the duller structures below the diaphragm. You are not percussing the diaphragm itself. You can infer the probable location of the diaphragm from the level of dullness.

Now, *estimate the extent of diaphragmatic excursion* by determining the distance between the level of dullness on full expiration and the level of dullness on full inspiration, normally about 3 to 5 cm.

- Ask the patient to breathe in, then out fully and hold his or her breath.

- Percuss down to dullness and mark this point on the patient's back with a pen.

- Next ask the patient to breathe in fully and hold his or her breath, and continue percussing down until dullness is heard; mark this point.

- Repeat on the opposite side.

- Measure the distances; they should be equal through the right side, may be 1 cm higher due to the liver.

The diaphragmatic excursion should be 3 to 5 cm in adults, although in athletes it may be up to 7 to 8 cm.

Auscultation

Auscultation is the most important examination technique for assessing air flow through the tracheobronchial tree. Together with percussion, it also helps the nurse assess the condition of the surrounding lungs and pleural space. Auscultation involves (1) listening to the sounds generated by breathing, (2) listening for any adventitious (extra) sounds, and (3) if abnormalities are suspected, listening to the sounds of the patient's spoken or whispered voice as they are transmitted through the chest wall.

Sounds from bedclothes, paper gowns, and the chest itself can generate confusion in auscultation. Hair on the chest may cause crackling sounds. Either press harder or wet the hair. If the patient is cold or tense, you may hear muscle contraction sounds—muffled, low-pitched rumbling or roaring noises. A change in the patient's position may eliminate this noise. You can reproduce this sound on yourself by doing a Valsalva maneuver (straining down) as you listen to your own chest.

Breath Sounds (Lung Sounds)

Learn to identify patterns of breath sounds by their intensity, their pitch, and the relative duration of their inspiratory and expiratory phases. Normal breath sounds are:

- *Vesicular,* or soft and low pitched. They are heard throughout inspiration, continue without pause through expiration, and then fade away about one third of the way through expiration.

- *Bronchovesicular,* with inspiratory and expiratory sounds about equal in length, at times separated by a silent interval. Detecting differences in pitch and intensity is often easier during expiration.

- *Bronchial,* or louder and higher in pitch, with a short silence between inspiratory and expiratory sounds. Expiratory sounds last longer than inspiratory sounds.

- *Tracheal,* very loud, harsh sounds with inspiratory and expiratory sounds equal in length, over the trachea in the neck.

The characteristics of breath sounds are summarized in the table below.

Characteristics of Breath Sounds[2,3]

	Duration of Sounds	Intensity of Expiratory Sound	Pitch of Expiratory Sound	Locations Where Heard Normally
Vesicular[a]	Inspiratory sounds last longer than expiratory ones.	Soft	Relatively low	Over most of both lungs
Bronchove-sicular	Inspiratory and expiratory sounds are about equal.	Intermediate	Intermediate	Often in the 1st and 2nd intercostal spaces anteriorly and between the scapulae
Bronchial	Expiratory sounds last longer than inspiratory ones.	Loud	Relatively high	Over the manubrium, if heard at all
Tracheal	Inspiratory and expiratory sounds are about equal.	Very loud	Relatively high	Over the trachea in the neck

[a]The thickness of the bars indicates intensity; the steeper their incline, the higher the pitch.

If bronchovesicular or bronchial breath sounds are heard in locations distant from those listed, suspect that air-filled lung has been replaced by fluid-filled or solid lung tissue. See Table 13-6, Chapter 13, Normal and Altered Breath and Voice Sounds, p. 367.

Listen to the breath sounds with the diaphragm of a stethoscope. Tell the patient to breathe deeply through an open mouth. Always place the stethoscope directly on the skin. Clothing may alter the quality of the breath sounds and introduce extra friction sounds. Use the pattern suggested for percussion, moving from one side to the other and comparing symmetric areas of the lungs. If you hear or suspect abnormal sounds, auscultate adjacent areas so that you can fully describe the extent of any abnormality. Listen to at least one full breath in each location. Be alert for patient discomfort resulting from hyperventilation (e.g., lightheadedness, faintness), and allow the patient to rest as needed.

Note the *intensity* of the breath sounds. Breath sounds are usually louder in the lower posterior lung fields and may also vary from area to area. If the breath sounds seem faint, ask the patient to breathe more deeply. You may then hear them easily. When patients do not breathe deeply enough or have a thick chest wall, as in obesity, breath sounds may remain diminished.

> Breath sounds may be decreased when air flow is decreased (as in obstructive lung disease or muscular weakness) or when the transmission of sound is poor (as in *pleural effusion, pneumothorax,* or *COPD*).

Is there a *silent gap* between the inspiratory and expiratory sounds?

> A gap suggests bronchial breath sounds.

Listen for the *pitch, intensity, and duration of the expiratory and inspiratory sounds.* Are vesicular breath sounds distributed throughout the chest wall? Or are there bronchovesicular or bronchial breath sounds in unexpected places? If so, where are they?

Adventitious (Extra) Sounds

Listen for any extra, or adventitious, sounds that are superimposed on the usual breath sounds. Detection of adventitious sounds—*crackles* (sometimes called *rales*), *wheezes,* and *rhonchi*—is an important part of your examination, often leading to diagnosis of cardiac and pulmonary conditions. The most common kinds of these sounds are described below.

> For further discussion and other added sounds, see Table 13-7, pp. 368–369.

Adventitious or Added Breath Sounds[2,3]	
Crackles (or Rales)	**Wheezes and Rhonchi**
Discontinuous	Continuous
• Intermittent, nonmusical, and brief • Like dots in time • *Fine crackles:* soft, high-pitched, very brief (5–10 msec) • *Coarse crackles:* somewhat louder, lower in pitch, brief (20–30 msec)	• ≥250 msec, sinusoidal prolonged (but not necessarily persisting throughout the respiratory cycle) • Like dashes in time • *Wheezes:* musical, relatively high pitched (≥400 Hz) with hissing or shrill quality • *Rhonchi:* relatively low pitched (≤200 Hz) with snoring quality

> Crackles may be from abnormalities of the lungs (*pneumonia, fibrosis, early congestive heart failure*) or of the airways (bronchitis, bronchiectasis).
>
> Wheezes suggest narrowed airways, as in *asthma, COPD,* or *bronchitis.*
>
> Rhonchi suggest secretions in large airways.

If you hear *crackles,* especially those that do not clear after coughing, listen carefully for the following characteristics.[2,4–6] These are clues to the underlying condition:

- Loudness, pitch, and duration (summarized as fine or coarse crackles)

- Number (few to many)

- Timing in the respiratory cycle

- Location on the chest wall

- Persistence of their pattern from breath to breath

- Any change after a cough or a change in the patient's position

Fine late inspiratory crackles that persist from breath to breath suggest abnormal lung tissue.

Clearing of crackles, wheezes, or rhonchi after coughing or position change suggests thickened secretions, as in *bronchitis* or *atelectasis.*

In some normal people, crackles may be heard at the lung bases anteriorly after maximal expiration. Crackles in dependent portions of the lungs may also occur after prolonged time lying flat.

If you hear *wheezes* or *rhonchi,* note their timing (inspiratory, expiratory, or both) and location. Do they change with deep breathing or coughing?

During a severe asthma exacerbation wheezing may decrease or cease due to lack of air flow in the bronchial tree. This is a clinical emergency.

Transmitted Voice Sounds

Sound waves travel better through consolidated tissue as when airways are blocked by inflammation and secretions. If you hear abnormally located bronchovesicular or bronchial breath sounds or adventitious sounds, assess transmitted voice sounds. With the diaphragm of the stethoscope, listen in symmetric areas over the chest wall as you:

See Table 13-6, Chapter 13, Normal and Altered Breath and Voice Sounds, p. 367.

- Ask the patient to say "ninety-nine." Normally the sounds transmitted through the chest wall are muffled and indistinct.

Louder, clearer voice sounds are called **bronchophony.**

- Ask the patient to say "ee." You will normally hear a muffled long E sound.

When "ee" is heard as "ay," an *E-to-A change* (**egophony**) is present, as in lobar consolidation from *pneumonia.* The quality sounds nasal.

- Ask the patient to whisper "ninety-nine" or "one-two-three." The whispered voice is normally heard faintly and indistinctly, if at all.

Louder, clearer whispered sounds are called ***whispered pectoriloquy.***

Examination of the Anterior Chest

When examined in the supine position, the patient should lie comfortably with arms somewhat abducted. A patient who is having difficulty breathing should be examined in the sitting position or with the head of the bed elevated to a comfortable level.

Persons with severe asthma or *COPD* may prefer to sit leaning forward, with lips pursed during exhalation and arms supported on their knees or a table. This is called *tripod* position.

Inspection

Observe *the shape of the patient's chest* and the *movement of the chest wall.* Note:

- Deformities or asymmetry of the thorax

  See Table 13-4, Deformities of the Chest, p. 365.

- Work of breathing: intercostal, supraclavicular and/or substernal retractions during inspiration

  Severe *asthma, COPD,* or upper airway obstruction.

- Local lag or impairment in respiratory movement

  Underlying disease of lung or pleura.

- Bruising or other skin lesions

Palpation

Palpation has four potential uses:

- *Identification of tender areas*

  Tender pectoral muscles or costal cartilages corroborate, but do not prove, that chest pain has a musculoskeletal origin.

- *Assessment of observed abnormalities*

- *Assessment of chest expansion.* Place your thumbs along each costal margin, your hands along the lateral rib cage. As you position your hands, slide them medially a bit to raise loose skin folds between your thumbs. Ask the patient to inhale deeply (as the thorax expands; see photograph on p. 350). Observe how far your thumbs diverge and feel for the extent and symmetry of respiratory movement.

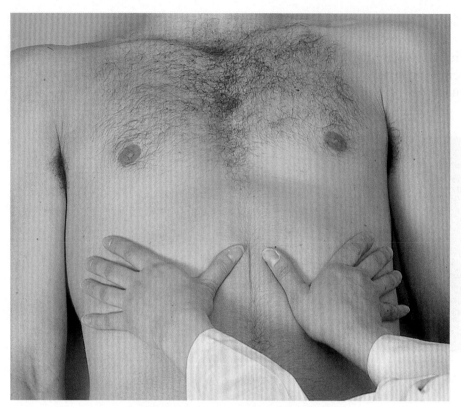

CHEST EXPANSION HAND POSITION

- *Assessment of tactile fremitus.* Compare both sides of the chest, using the ball or ulnar surface of your hand. Fremitus is usually decreased or absent over the precordium. When examining a woman, gently displace the breasts as necessary.

LOCATIONS FOR FEELING FREMITUS

Percussion

- Percuss the anterior and lateral chest, again comparing both sides. The heart normally produces an area of dullness to the left of the sternum from the 3rd to the 5th intercostal spaces. Percuss the left lung lateral to it. Identify and locate any area with an abnormal percussion note.

Dullness replaces resonance when fluid or solid tissue replaces air-containing lung or occupies the pleural space. Because pleural fluid usually sinks to the lowest part of the pleural space (posteriorly in a supine patient), only a very large effusion can be detected anteriorly.

The hyperresonance of *COPD* may totally replace cardiac dullness.

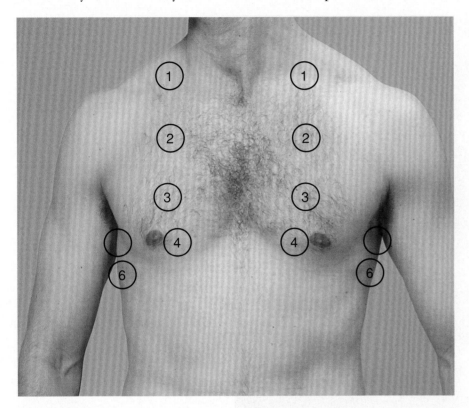

In a woman, to enhance percussion, gently displace the breast with your left hand while percussing with the right. Alternatively, you may ask the patient to move her breast for you.

The dullness of right middle lobe pneumonia typically occurs behind the right breast. Unless you displace the breast, you may miss the abnormal percussion note.

- With your pleximeter finger above and parallel to the expected upper border of liver dullness, percuss in progressive steps downward in the right midclavicular line. Identify the upper border of liver dullness. Later, during the abdominal examination, you will use this method to estimate the size of the liver. As you percuss down the chest on the left, the resonance of normal lung usually changes to the tympany of the gastric air bubble.

A lung affected by *COPD* often displaces the upper border of the liver downward. It also lowers the level of diaphragmatic dullness posteriorly.

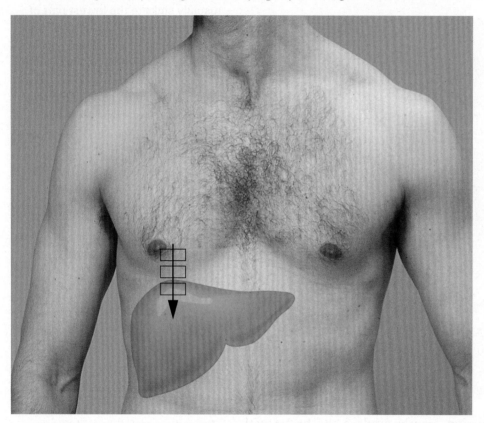

Auscultation

Listen to the chest anteriorly and laterally as the patient breathes with mouth open, more deeply than normal. Compare symmetric areas of the lungs, using the pattern suggested for percussion and extending it to adjacent areas as indicated.

- *Listen to the breath sounds,* noting their intensity and identifying any variations from normal vesicular breathing. Breath sounds are usually louder in the upper anterior lung fields. Bronchovesicular breath sounds may be heard over the large airways, especially on the right.

- *Identify any adventitious sounds,* time them in the respiratory cycle, and locate them on the chest wall. Do they clear with deep breathing?

See Table 13-7, Adventitious Sounds: Causes and Qualities, pp. 368–369 and Table 13-8, Physical Findings om Selected Chest Disorders, pp. 370–371.

- If indicated, *listen for transmitted voice sounds.*

SPECIAL TECHNIQUES

Pulse Oximetry

Pulse oximetry measures the arterial oxygenation saturation, or SpO_2. A probe is placed on the patient's finger or earlobe. The toe is used for infants and young children. A diode emits light and a detector on the opposite side of the probe measures the amount of light absorbed by oxyhemoglobin. The oximeter compares the amount of light emitted to the amount absorbed and calculates the percentage of oxygen saturation. A healthy person has an SpO_2 of 95% to 100%. Poor perfusion, hypotension, dyshemoglobinemias, dyes in some nail polishes, and excessive ambient light may cause inaccurate readings.

Peak Flow Assessment

A peak flow meter assesses the maximum volume of air expelled from the lungs during a vigorous exhalation. A decrease in peak flow volume occurs in diseases that reduce outflow of air, for example, asthma. As peak flow decreases the severity of an exacerbation increases. Regular monitoring of a patient's peak flow can evaluate the effectiveness of treatment for chronic asthma.

Peak flow rate can be accurately performed by most people over 5 years of age.

To measure peak flow move the marker on the meter to the bottom of the numbered scale and instruct the patient to:

- Stand up straight. Remove gum or candy from the mouth.

- Take a deep breath. Fill your lungs all the way.

- Hold your breath and place the mouthpiece in your mouth, between your teeth. Close your lips around it. Do not put your tongue against or inside the hole.

- Blow out as hard and fast as you can in a single blow.

The patient's first burst of air is the most important. So blowing for a longer time will not improve the result.

Note the number. Move the marker back to the bottom and repeat these steps 2 more times. The highest of the 3 numbers is recorded as the patient's peak flow.

NIH, MedLine Plus. How to Use your Peak Flow Meter. Available at: https://www.nlm.nih.gov/medlineplus/ency/patientinstructions/000043.htm. Accessed May 25, 2016.

If the patient coughs, disregard that attempt and have the patient repeat the steps again.

Identification of a Fractured Rib

Local pain and tenderness of one or more ribs raise the question of fracture. By anteroposterior compression of the chest, you can help to distinguish a fracture from soft tissue injury. With one hand on the sternum and the other on the thoracic spine, squeeze the chest. Is this painful, and where?

An increase in the local pain (distant from your hands) suggests rib fracture rather than just soft tissue injury.

RECORDING YOUR FINDINGS

Recording the Physical Examination—The Thorax and Lungs

"Thorax is symmetric with equal expansion. Lungs resonant. Anterior and posterior breath sounds clear bilaterally. Diaphragm descends 4 cm bilaterally."

OR

"Thorax symmetric with moderate kyphosis and increased AP diameter, decreased expansion. Lungs are hyperresonant. Breath sounds distant with delayed expiratory phase and scattered expiratory wheezes. Fremitus decreased; no bronchophony, egophony, or whispered pectoriloquy. Diaphragm descends 2 cm bilaterally."

Suggests *COPD*.

HEALTH PROMOTION AND COUNSELING

Important Topics for Health Promotion and Counseling

- Tobacco cessation
- Immunizations

Tobacco Cessation

According to the CDC tobacco use is the leading cause of preventable disease and death in the United States. Cigarette smoking causes more than 480,000 deaths each year. This is about one in five deaths. Although the proportion of adult smokers declined from 20.9% in 2005 to 17.8% in 2013, millions of adults still smoke. Cigarette smoking remains high among adults who are male, younger, multiracial or American Indian/Alaska Native, lesbian, gay and bisexual (LGB), have less education, live below the poverty level, live in the South or Midwest, or have a disability/limitation.[7] Tobacco use and addiction most often begin during middle school and high school years. Nicotine use during adolescence, a critical window for brain development, might have lasting adverse consequences for brain development, cause addiction, and lead to continued tobacco use. In 2014, a total of 24.6% of high school students and 7.7% of middle school students reported using a tobacco product. This translates into an estimated 4.6 million youths who are exposed to tobacco. In this population, e-cigarettes were the most common tobacco product used, followed by hookahs.[8]

Adverse Effects of Smoking on Health and Disease

Condition	Increased Risk Compared With Nonsmokers
• Coronary artery disease	2–4 times higher
• Stroke	2–4 times higher
• COPD mortality	12–13 times higher
• Lung cancer mortality	23 times higher in men 25.7 times higher in women

Source: Centers for Disease Control and Prevention, DHHS. Smoking and tobacco use. Fact sheet. Health effects of cigarette smoking. Available at: http://www.cdc.gov/tobacco/data_statistics/fact_sheets/health_effects/effects_cig_smoking/index.htm. Accessed May 27, 2016.

In addition to respiratory tract cancers, smoking contributes to cancers of the bladder, cervix, colon and rectum, kidney, oropharynx, larynx, esophagus, stomach, liver, and pancreas, as well as acute myeloid leukemia.[9] Smoking increases risk of infertility, preterm birth, low birth weight, and sudden infant death syndrome. Smoking is associated with developing diabetes, cataracts, and rheumatoid arthritis. Nonsmokers exposed to smoke also have increased risk of lung cancer, ear and respiratory infections, asthma and residential fires.

Nearly 7 out of every 10 (68.8%) U.S. adult cigarette smokers, reported in 2010 that they wanted to quit smoking completely.[10] Nurses should focus on smoking prevention and cessation, especially in adolescents and pregnant women.[11] Health care providers should advise smokers to quit during every visit. This advice has been shown to raise quit rates by 30%.[12] Use the "5 As" framework or the Stages of Change model (precontemplation, contemplation, preparation, action, maintenance)[13] to assess readiness to quit.

Nicotine is highly addicting, comparable to heroin and cocaine, and quitting tobacco use is difficult. Cognitive therapy techniques will help patients recognize signs of withdrawal such as irritability, difficulty concentrating, anxiety, and depressed mood.[14] Guide patients to better understand craving, triggers for smoking, and strategies for managing withdrawal, coping with stress, and preventing relapse. Combining counseling with pharmacotherapy is more effective than either therapy alone.[15] Three drugs have been shown to improve and sustain quit rates: nicotine replacement therapies; bupropion, a norepinephrine and dopamine reuptake inhibitor and nicotinic receptor antagonist; and varenicline, a nicotinic receptor partial agonist that stimulates dopamine release, thought to relieve craving.[16]

Assessing Readiness to Quit Smoking[13,17]

The 5 A's
1. **Ask** about tobacco use.
2. **Advise** to quit through clear, personalized messages.
3. **Assess** willingness to quit.
4. **Assist** to quit.
5. **Arrange** follow-up and support.

Stages of Change Model
- **Precontemplation**—"I don't want to quit."
- **Contemplation**—"I am concerned but not ready to quit now."
- **Preparation**—"I am ready to quit."
- **Action**—"I just quit."
- **Maintenance**—"I quit 6 months ago."

Immunizations (Adults)

Influenza Vaccine

Influenza can cause substantial morbidity and mortality, especially during the late fall and winter, peaking in February. The numbers of annual deaths related to influenza varies depending on the virus type and subtype, ranging from a few thousand to nearly 50,000 deaths. The CDC Advisory Committee on Immunization Practices (ACIP) updates its recommendations for vaccination annually. Two types of vaccine are available: the "flu shot," an inactivated vaccine containing killed virus, and a nasal-spray vaccine containing attenuated live viruses, approved only for healthy people between 2 and 49 years of age.[18] Because influenza viruses mutate from year to year, each vaccine contains three to four vaccine strains and is modified yearly.

Annual vaccination is recommended for all people ages 6 months and older, especially the groups listed below.

- Adults with chronic pulmonary conditions and chronic medical conditions; adults who are immunosuppressed or morbidly obese

- Adults 50 years of age or older

- Women who are or will be pregnant during influenza season

- Residents of nursing homes and chronic care facilities

- American Indians and Alaska natives

- Health care personnel

- Household contacts and caregivers of children 5 years of age or younger (especially infants age 6 months or younger) and of adults 50 years of age or older with medical conditions placing them at higher risk for complications of influenza

Pneumococcal Vaccine

Approximately 400,000 hospitalizations from pneumococcal pneumonia (*streptococcal pneumonia*) are estimated to occur annually in the United States. Pneumococci account for up to 36% of adult community-acquired pneumonia. About 25% to 30% of patients with pneumococcal pneumonia also experience pneumococcal bacteremia. Pneumococcal pneumonia may complicate influenza infection. Pneumococci cause over 50% of all cases of bacterial meningitis in the United States.[19]

Since 2010, infants younger than 2 have routinely been vaccinated with the 13-valent pneumococcal conjugate vaccine (PCV13). In 2014, the ACIP recommended vaccinating adults aged 65 years or older using the PCV13 along with the 23-valent inactivated pneumococcal polysaccharide vaccine (PPSV23). The vaccines should not be coadministered. Adults in this age range who never received the PPSV23 should first receive the PCV13 followed 6 to 12 months later by the PPSV23. Adults aged 65 years or older previously vaccinated with PPSV23 should receive a dose of PCV13 no earlier than 1 year following the most recent PPSV23. The ACIP recommends using PCV13 and PPSV23 for high-risk groups listed.

The CDC recommends the pneumococcal vaccine for these groups:

- Adults 65 years of age or older

- Children and adults from 2 years to 64 years old with chronic illnesses specifically associated with increased risk of pneumococcal infection (sickle cell disease, cardiovascular and pulmonary disease, diabetes, alcoholism, cirrhosis, cochlear implants, and leaks of cerebrospinal fluid)

- Any adult 19 to 64 years old who is a smoker or has asthma

- Adults and children older than 2 years who are immunocompromised (including from HIV infection, AIDS, long-term steroids, Hodgkin disease; lymphoma or leukemia; kidney failure; multiple myeloma; nephrotic syndrome; organ transplant; damaged spleen or no spleen; radiation, or chemotherapy)

- Residents of nursing homes or long-term care facilities

Pertussis Vaccine

Pertussis (*Bordetella pertussis*) is an acute respiratory infectious illness that remains endemic in the United States despite routine childhood vaccination. Immunity to pertussis wanes approximately 5 to 10 years after completion of the childhood vaccination series, leaving adolescents and adults susceptible to pertussis. Since the 1980s, the number of reported pertussis cases has steadily increased, especially among adolescents and adults. Pertussis poses the most risk to infants and young children. Therefore, to protect them, the CDC recommends:

- Adults 19 years and older who have not received a dose of Tdap (*Tetanus, diphtheria, & acellular pertussis*) should get one as soon as possible, to protect themselves and infants. The Tdap booster can replace one of the 10-year Td booster vaccines.

- For adolescents 11 through 18 years of age, Tdap is routinely recommended as a single dose with preferred administration at 11 through 12 years of age.

- Infants should receive the five-dose series of DTaP (pediatric Diphtheria, Tetanus, and acellular Pertussis) vaccine.

TABLE 13-1 Dyspnea[20]

Problem	Process	Timing
Asthma[21]	Bronchial hyperresponsiveness involving release of inflammatory mediators, increased airway secretions, and bronchoconstriction	Acute episodes, separated by symptom-free periods. Nocturnal episodes common.
Pneumonia[22]	Infection of lung parenchyma from the respiratory bronchioles to the alveoli	An acute illness, timing varies with the causative agent
Spontaneous Pneumothorax	Leakage of air into pleural space through blebs on visceral pleura, with resulting partial or complete collapse of the lung	Sudden onset of dyspnea
Acute Pulmonary Embolism[23]	Sudden occlusion of part of pulmonary arterial tree by a blood clot that usually originates in deep veins of legs or pelvis	Sudden onset of tachypnea, dyspnea
Chronic Bronchitis[a,24]	Excessive mucus production in bronchi, followed by chronic obstruction of airways	Chronic productive cough followed by slowly progressive dyspnea
Chronic Obstructive Pulmonary Disease (COPD)[a,25–29]	Overdistention of air spaces distal to terminal bronchioles, with destruction of alveolar septa and chronic obstruction of the airways	Slowly progressive dyspnea; relatively mild cough later
Diffuse Interstitial Lung Diseases *(such as sarcoidosis, widespread neoplasms, asbestosis, and idiopathic pulmonary fibrosis)*	Abnormal and widespread infiltration of cells, fluid, and collagen into interstitial spaces between alveoli. Many causes	Progressive dyspnea, which varies in its rate of development with the cause
Left-Sided Heart Failure *(left ventricular failure or mitral stenosis)*	Elevated pressure in pulmonary capillary bed with movement of fluid into interstitial spaces and alveoli, decreased compliance (increased stiffness) of the lungs, increased work of breathing	Dyspnea may progress slowly, or suddenly as in acute pulmonary edema.
Anxiety With Hyperventilation	Overbreathing, with resultant respiratory alkalosis and fall in the partial pressure of carbon dioxide in the blood	Episodic, often recurrent

[a]Chronic bronchitis and chronic obstructive pulmonary disease (COPD) may coexist.

Factors That Aggravate	Factors That Relieve	Associated Symptoms	Setting
Variable, including allergens, irritants, respiratory infections, cold and exercise, and emotion.	Separation from aggravating factors	Wheezing, cough, tightness in chest	Environmental conditions
Exertion, smoking	Rest, though dyspnea may become persistent	Pleuritic pain, cough, sputum, fever, though not necessarily present	Varied
		Pleuritic pain, cough	Often a previously healthy young adult or adult with emphysema
Exertion	Rest, though dyspnea may become persistent	Often none. Retrosternal oppressive pain if the occlusion is massive. Pleuritic pain, cough, syncope and hemoptysis, and/ or unilateral leg swelling and pain from an instigating deep vein thrombosis. Anxiety (see below). Symptoms of anxiety (see below)	Postpartum or postoperative periods; prolonged bed rest; congestive heart failure, chronic lung disease, and fractures of hip or leg; deep venous thrombosis (often not clinically apparent)
Exertion, inhaled irritants, respiratory infections	Expectoration; rest, though dyspnea may become persistent	Chronic productive cough, recurrent respiratory infections; wheezing may develop	History of smoking, air pollutants, recurrent respiratory infections
Exertion	Rest, though dyspnea may become persistent	Cough, with scant mucoid sputum	History of smoking, air pollutants, sometimes a familial deficiency in α1-antitrypsin
Exertion	Rest, though dyspnea may become persistent	Often weakness, fatigue. Cough less common than in other lung diseases	Varied. Exposure to one of many substances may be causative.
Exertion, lying down	Rest, sitting up, though dyspnea may become persistent	Often cough, orthopnea, paroxysmal nocturnal dyspnea; sometimes wheezing	History of heart disease or its predisposing factors
More often occurs at rest than after exercise. An upsetting event may not be evident.	Breathing in and out of a paper or plastic bag sometimes helps the associated symptoms.	Sighing, lightheadedness, numbness or tingling of the hands and feet, palpitations, chest pain	Other manifestations of anxiety may be present.

TABLE
13-2

Cough[30] and Hemoptysis[a]

Problem	Cough and Sputum	Associated Symptoms and Setting
Acute Inflammation		
Laryngitis	Dry cough (without sputum), may become productive of variable amounts of sputum	An acute, fairly minor illness with hoarseness. Often associated with viral nasopharyngitis
Acute Bronchitis[24]	Cough may be dry or productive	An acute, often viral illness generally without fever or dyspnea; at times with burning retrosternal discomfort
Mycoplasma and Viral Pneumonias[31]	Dry hacking cough, may become productive of mucoid sputum	An acute febrile illness, often with malaise, headache, and possibly dyspnea
Bacterial Pneumonias[31]	Sputum is mucoid or purulent; may be blood streaked, diffusely pinkish, or rusty	An acute illness with chills, often high fever, dyspnea, and chest pain. Commonly from *Streptococcus pneumoniae, Haemophilus influenzae, Moraxella catarrhalis; Klebsiella* in alcoholism, especially if there is underlying smoking, chronic bronchitis and COPD, cardiovascular disease, diabetes.
Pertussis (*Bordetella Pertussis*)	Cough comes in paroxysms; followed by a sudden forceful inhalation *(in children a whooping sound is produced.)*	Begins with coryza (runny nose), sneezing, low-grade fever.
Chronic Inflammation		
Postnasal Drip	Chronic cough; sputum mucoid or mucopurulent	Repeated attempts to clear the throat. Postnasal discharge may be sensed by patient or seen in posterior pharynx. Associated with chronic rhinitis, with or without sinusitis
Chronic Bronchitis[24]	Chronic cough; sputum mucoid to purulent, may be blood streaked or even bloody	Often with recurrent wheezing and dyspnea and prolonged history of tobacco abuse.
Bronchiectasis[32]	Chronic cough; sputum purulent, often copious and foul smelling; may be blood streaked or bloody	Recurrent bronchopulmonary infections common; sinusitis may coexist.
Pulmonary Tuberculosis[33]	Cough dry or with mucoid or purulent sputum that is mucoid or purulent; may be blood streaked or bloody	Early, no symptoms. Later, anorexia, weight loss, fatigue, fever, and night sweats
Lung Abscess	Sputum purulent and foul smelling; may be bloody	Usually from aspiration pneumonia with fever and infection from oral anaerobes and poor dental hygiene; often with dysphagia or episode of impaired consciousness
Asthma[21]	Cough, at times with thick mucoid sputum, especially near end of an attack	Episodic wheezing and dyspnea, but cough may occur alone. Often with a history of allergies.
Gastroesophageal Reflux	Chronic cough, especially at night or early in the morning	Wheezing, especially at night (often mistaken for asthma), early morning hoarseness, and repeated attempts to clear the throat. Often with heartburn and regurgitation
Neoplasm *Cancer of the Lung*	Cough dry to productive; sputum may be blood streaked or bloody	Commonly with dyspnea, weight loss, and tobacco use.
Cardiovascular Disorders		
Left Ventricular Failure or Mitral Stenosis	Often dry, especially on exertion or at night; may progress to the pink frothy sputum of pulmonary edema or to frank hemoptysis	Dyspnea, orthopnea, paroxysmal nocturnal dyspnea
Pulmonary Embolism[23,34]	Dry to productive; may be dark, bright red, or mixed with blood	Dyspnea, anxiety, chest pain, fever; factors that predispose to deep venous thrombosis
Irritating Particles, Chemicals, or Gases	Variable. There may be a latent period between exposure and symptoms.	Exposure to irritants. Eyes, nose, and throat may be affected.

[a]Characteristics of hemoptysis are printed in red.

TABLE
13-3

Chest Pain

Problem	Process	Location	Quality	Severity	Timing	Factors That Aggravate	Factors That Relieve	Associated Symptoms
Pulmonary								
Pleuritic Pain	Inflammation of the parietal pleura, as in pleurisy, pneumonia, pulmonary infarction, or neoplasm	Chest wall overlying the process	Sharp, knife-like	Often severe	Persistent	Inspiration, coughing, movements of the trunk		Of the underlying illness
Cardiovascular								
Angina Pectoris	Temporary myocardial ischemia, usually secondary to coronary atherosclerosis	Retrosternal or across the anterior chest, often radiates the shoulders, arms, neck, lower jaw, or upper abdomen	Pressing, squeezing, tight, heavy, occasionally burning	Mild to moderate, sometimes perceived as discomfort rather than pain	Usually 1–3 min but up to 10 min. Prolonged episodes up to 20 min	Often exertion, especially in the cold; meals; emotional stress. May occur at rest	Often but not always rest, nitroglycerin	Sometimes dyspnea, nausea, sweating
Myocardial Infarction	Prolonged myocardial ischemia, resulting in irreversible muscle damage or necrosis	Same as in angina	Same as in angina	Often but not always a severe pain	20 min to several hours	Not always triggered by exertion	Not relieved by rest	Nausea, vomiting, sweating, weakness
Pericarditis	Irritation of parietal pleura adjacent to the pericardium	Precordial, may radiate to the tip of the shoulder and to the neck	Sharp, knife-like Crushing	Often severe	Persistent	Breathing, changing position, coughing, lying down, sometimes swallowing	Sitting forward may relieve it.	Of the underlying illness
Dissecting Aortic Aneurysm	A splitting within the layers of the aortic wall, allowing passage of blood to dissect a channel	Anterior or posterior chest, radiating to the neck, back, or abdomen	Ripping, tearing	Very severe	Abrupt onset, early peak, persistent for hours or more	Hypertension		If thoracic, hoarseness, dysphagia, also syncope, hemiplegia, paraplegia

(table continues on page 364)

TABLE
13-3

Chest Pain (continued)

Problem	Process	Location	Quality	Severity	Timing	Factors That Aggravate	Factors That Relieve	Associated Symptoms
Gastrointestinal and Other								
Gastrointestinal Reflux Disease	Irritation or inflammation of the esophageal mucosa due to reflux of gastric acid from lowered esophageal sphincter tone	Retrosternal, may radiate to the back	Burning, may be squeezing	Mild to severe	Variable	Large meal; bending over, lying down	Antacids, sometimes belching	Sometimes regurgitation, dysphagia
Diffuse Esophageal Spasm	Motor dysfunction of the esophageal muscle	Retrosternal, may radiate to the back, arms, and jaw	Usually squeezing	Mild to severe	Variable	Swallowing of food or cold liquid; emotional stress	Sometimes nitroglycerin	Dysphagia
Chest Wall Pain, Costochondritis	Variable, including trauma, inflammation of costal cartilage	Often below the left breast or along the costal cartilages; also elsewhere	Stabbing, sticking, or dull, aching	Variable	Fleeting to hours or days	Coughing; movement of chest, trunk, arms		Often local tenderness
Anxiety (Panic Disorder)	Unclear	Precordial, below the left breast, or across the anterior chest	Stabbing, sticking, or dull, aching	Variable	Fleeting to hours or days	May follow effort, emotional stress		Breathlessness, palpitations, weakness, anxiety

Note: Chest pain may be referred from extrathoracic structures such as the neck (*arthritis*) and abdomen (*biliary colic, acute cholecystitis*). Pleural pain may be from abdominal conditions such as *subdiaphragmatic abscess*.

TABLE
13-4

Abnormalities in Rate and Rhythm of Breathing

When observing respiratory patterns, note the rate, depth, and regularity of the patient's breathing. Traditional terms, such as tachypnea, are given below so that you will understand them, but simple descriptions are recommended.

Normal
The respiratory rate is about 14–20 per min in normal adults and up to 44 per min in infants.

Slow Breathing (Bradypnea)
Slow breathing with or without an increase in tidal volume that maintains alveolar ventilation. Abnormal alveolar hypoventilation without increased tidal volume can arise from uremia, drug-induced respiratory depression, and increased intracranial pressure.

Sighing Respiration
Breathing punctuated by frequent sighs suggests *hyperventilation syndrome*—a common cause of dyspnea and dizziness. Occasional sighs are normal.

Rapid Shallow Breathing (Tachypnea)
Rapid shallow breathing has numerous causes, including salicylate intoxication, restrictive lung disease, pleuritic chest pain, and an elevated diaphragm.

Cheyne–Stokes Breathing
Periods of deep breathing alternate with periods of *apnea* (no breathing). This pattern is normal in children and older adults during sleep. Causes include heart failure, uremia, drug-induced respiratory depression, and brain injury (typically bihemispheric).

Obstructive Breathing
In obstructive lung disease, expiration is prolonged due to narrowed airways increase the resistance to air flow. Causes include asthma, chronic bronchitis, and COPD.

Rapid Deep Breathing (Hyperpnea, Hyperventilation)
In *hyperpnea*, rapid deep breathing occurs in response to metabolic demand from causes such as exercise, high altitude, sepsis, and anemia. In *hyperventilation*, this pattern is independent of metabolic demand, except in respiratory acidosis. Light-headedness and tingling may arise from decreased CO_2 concentration. In the comatose patient, consider hypoxia, or hypoglycemia affecting the midbrain or pons. *Kussmaul breathing* is compensatory overbreathing due to systemic acidosis. The breathing rate may be fast, normal, or slow.

Ataxic Breathing (Biot Breathing)
Breathing is irregular—periods of apnea alternate with regular deep breaths which stop suddenly for short intervals. Causes include meningitis, respiratory depression, and brain injury, typically at the medullary level.

TABLE
13-5

Deformities of the Thorax

Normal Adult
The thorax in the normal adult is wider than it is deep. Its lateral diameter is larger than its anteroposterior diameter.

Funnel Chest (*Pectus Excavatum*)
Note depression in the lower portion of the sternum. Compression of the heart and great vessels may cause murmurs.

Barrel Chest
There is an increased anteroposterior diameter. This shape is normal during infancy, and often accompanies aging and chronic obstructive pulmonary disease.

Anteriorly displaced sternum

Depressed costal cartilages

Pigeon Chest (*Pectus Carinatum*)
The sternum is displaced anteriorly, increasing the anteroposterior diameter. The costal cartilages adjacent to the protruding sternum are depressed.

Expiration

Inspiration

Traumatic Flail Chest
Multiple rib fractures may result in paradoxical movements of the thorax. As descent of the diaphragm decreases intrathoracic pressure, on inspiration the injured area caves inward; on expiration, it moves outward.

Spinal convexity to the right (patient bending forward)

Ribs widely separated

Ribs close together

Thoracic Kyphoscoliosis
Abnormal spinal curvatures and vertebral rotation deform the chest. Distortion of the underlying lungs may make interpretation of lung findings very difficult.

TABLE
13-6

Normal and Altered Breath and Voice Sounds

The origins of breath sounds are still unclear. Turbulent air flow in the pharynx, glottis, and subglottic region produce tracheal breath sounds, which are similar to bronchial sounds. The inspiratory component of vesicular breath sounds seems to arise in the lobar and segmental airways; the expiratory component arises in the more central larger airways. Normally, tracheal and bronchial sounds may be heard over the trachea and mainstem bronchi; vesicular breath sounds predominate throughout most of the lungs.

Fluids and solids transmit sound and vibration waves better than air. When lung tissue loses its air, it transmits high-pitched sounds much better. If the tracheobronchial tree is open, bronchial breath sounds may replace the normal vesicular sounds over airless areas of the lung. This change is seen in lobar pneumonia when the alveoli fill with fluid, red cells, and white cells—a process called consolidation. Other causes include pulmonary edema or hemorrhage. Bronchial breath sounds usually correlate with an increase in tactile fremitus and transmitted voice sounds. These findings are summarized below.

	Normal Air-Filled Lung	Airless Lung, as in Lobar Pneumonia

	Normal Air-Filled Lung	Airless Lung, as in Lobar Pneumonia
Breath Sounds	Predominantly vesicular	Bronchial or bronchovesicular over the involved area
Transmitted Voice Sounds	Spoken words muffled and indistinct	Spoken words louder, clearer (*bronchophony*)
	Spoken "ee" heard as "ee"	Spoken "ee" heard as "ay" (*egophony*)
	Whispered words faint and indistinct, if heard at all	Whispered words louder, clearer (*whispered pectoriloquy*)
Tactile Fremitus	Normal	Increased

TABLE
13-7

Adventitious (Added) Lung Sounds: Causes and Qualities[2,3]

Crackles

Inspiration Expiration

Crackles are discontinuous nonmusical sounds that can be early inspiratory (as in *COPD*), late inspiratory (as in *pulmonary fibrosis*), or biphasic (as in *pneumonia*). They are currently considered to result from a series of tiny explosions when small distal airways, deflated during expiration, pop open during inspiration. With few exceptions, recent acoustic studies indicate that the role of secretions as a cause of crackles to secretions is less likely.[1,3]

- *Fine crackles* are soft, higher pitched, and more frequent per breath than coarse crackles. They are heard from mid to late inspiration, especially in the dependent areas of the lung, and change according to body position. They have a shorter duration and higher frequency than coarse crackles. Fine crackles appear to be generated by the "sudden inspiratory opening of small airways held close by surface forces during the previous expiration".[3]

  Examples include *pulmonary fibrosis* (known for "Velcro rales") and interstitial lung disease such as *interstitial fibrosis and interstitial pneumonitis heart failure.*

- *Coarse crackles* appear in early inspiration and last throughout expiration (*biphasic*), have a popping sound, are heard over any lung region, and do not vary with body position. They have a longer duration and lower frequency than fine crackles, change or disappear with coughing, and are transmitted to the mouth. Coarse crackles appear to result from "boluses of gas passing through airways as the open and close intermittently.[3]

  Examples include *COPD, asthma,* and *bronchiectasis; pneumonia* (crackles may become finer and change from mid to late inspiratory during recovery); and *heart failure.*

Wheezes and Rhonchi

Wheezes are continuous musical sounds that occur during rapid airflow when bronchial airways are narrowed almost to the point of closure. Wheezes can be inspiratory, expiratory, or biphasic. They may be localized, due to a foreign body, mucous plug, or tumor, or heard throughout the lung. Although wheezes are typical of asthma, they can occur in a number of pulmonary diseases. Recent studies suggest that as the airways become more narrowed, wheezes become less audible, culminating finally in "the silent chest" of severe asthma that requires immediate intervention.

Rhonchi are now considered to be a variant of wheezes, arising from the same mechanism but lower in pitch. Unlike wheezes, rhonchi may disappear with coughing, so secretions may be involved.[3]

Stridor

Stridor is a continuous high-frequency high-pitched musical sound produced during airflow through a narrowing in the upper respiratory tract. Stridor is best heard over the neck during inspiration, but can be biphasic. Causes of the underlying airway obstruction include tracheal stenosis from intubation, airway edema after device removal, croup, epiglottitis, foreign body, and anaphylaxis. Immediate intervention is warranted.

Pleural Friction Rub

A *pleural friction rub* is a discontinuous low-frequency grating sound that arises from inflammation and roughening of the visceral pleura as it slides against the parietal pleura. This nonmusical sound is biphasic, heard during inspiration and expiration, and is often described as creaking or like two pieces of leather rubbing together. It is often best heard in the axilla and base of the lungs.

Mediastinal Crunch (*Hamman Sign*)

A **mediastinal crunch** is a series of precordial crackles synchronous with the heartbeat, not with respiration. Best heard in the left lateral position, it arises from air entry into the mediastinum causing mediastinal emphysema (*pneumomediastinum*). It usually produces severe central chest pain and may be spontaneous. It has been reported in cases of tracheobronchial injury, blunt trauma, pulmonary disease, use of recreational drugs, childbirth, and rapid ascent of scuba-divers.[35]

TABLE
13-8

Physical Findings in Selected Chest Disorders

This table lists the typical changes seen in respiratory disorders. The changes described vary with the extent and severity of the disorder. Use the table for the direction of typical changes, not for absolute distinctions.

Condition	Percussion Note	Trachea
Normal The tracheobronchial tree and alveoli are open; pleurae are thin and close together; mobility of the chest wall is unimpaired.	Resonant	Midline
Chronic Bronchitis The bronchi are chronically inflamed and a productive cough is present. Airway obstruction may develop.	Resonant	Midline
Left-Sided Heart Failure (*Early*) Increased pressure in the pulmonary veins causes congestion and interstitial edema (around the alveoli); bronchial mucosa may become edematous.	Resonant	Midline
Lobar Pneumonia Alveoli fill with fluid or blood cells, as in pneumonia, pulmonary edema, or pulmonary hemorrhage.	Dull over the airless area	Midline
Partial Lobar Obstruction Atelectasis When a plug in a mainstem bronchus (as from mucus or a foreign object) obstructs bronchial air flow, affected alveoli collapse and become airless.	Dull over the airless area	May be *shifted toward involved side*
Pleural Effusion Fluid accumulates in the pleural space and separates air-filled lung from the chest wall, blocking the transmission breath sounds.	Dull to flat over the fluid	*Shifted toward the unaffected side* in a large effusion
Pneumothorax When air leaks into the pleural space, usually unilaterally, the lung recoils away from the chest wall. Pleural air blocks transmission of sound.	Hyperresonant or tympanitic over the pleural air	*Shifted toward the unaffected side if* tension pneumothorax
Chronic Obstructive Pulmonary Disease (COPD) Slowly progressive disorder in which the distal air spaces enlarge and lungs become hyperinflated. Chronic may precede or follow the development of COPD.	Diffusely hyperresonant	Midline
Asthma Widespread usually reversible airflow obstruction with bronchial hyperresponsiveness and underlying inflammation. During attacks, as air flow decreases lungs hyperinflate.	Resonant to diffusely hyperresonant	Midline

Breath Sounds	Adventitious Sounds	Tactile Fremitus and Transmitted Voice Sounds
Vesicular, except perhaps bronchovesicular and bronchial sounds over the large bronchi and trachea, respectively	None, except perhaps a few transient inspiratory crackles at the bases of the lungs	Normal
Vesicular (normal)	None; or scattered coarse crackles in early inspiration and perhaps expiration; or *wheezes* or *rhonchi*	Normal
Vesicular	*Late inspiratory crackles* in the dependent portions of the lungs; possibly *wheezes*	Normal
Bronchial over the involved area	*Late inspiratory crackles* over the involved area	*Increased over* the involved area, with *bronchophony, egophony,* and *whispered pectoriloquy*
Usually absent when bronchial plug persists. Exceptions include right upper lobe atelectasis, where adjacent tracheal sounds may be transmitted.	None	Usually absent when the bronchial plug persists. In exceptions (e.g., right upper lobe atelectasis) may be increased
Decreased to absent, but bronchial breath sounds may be heard near top of large effusion.	None, except a *possible pleural rub*	*Decreased to absent, but may be increased* toward the top of a large effusion
Decreased to absent over the pleural air	None, except a *possible pleural rub*	*Decreased to absent* over the pleural air
Decreased to absent with delayed expiration	None, or the crackles, wheezes, and rhonchi of associated chronic bronchitis	Decreased
Often obscured by wheezes	*Wheezes, possibly crackles*	Decreased

BIBLIOGRAPHY

CITATIONS

1. McGee S. *Evidence-based Physical Diagnosis*. 3rd ed. Philadelphia, PA: Saunders; 2012.

2. Loudon R, Murphy LH. Lungs sounds. *Am Rev Respir Dis*. 1994;130(4):663–673.

3. Bohadana A, Izbicki G, Kraman SS. Fundamentals of lung auscultation. *N Engl J Med*. 2014;370:744.

4. Epler GR, Carrrington CB, Gaensler EA. Crackles (rales) in the interstitial pulmonary diseases. *Chest*. 1978;73(3):333–339.

5. Nath AR, Capel LH. Inspiratory crackles and mechanical events of breathing. *Thorax*. 1974;29(6):695–698.

6. Nath AR, Capel LH. Lung crackles in bronchiectasis. *Thorax*. 1980;35(9):694–699.

7. CDC, MMWR: Current Cigarette Smoking Among Adults — United States, 2005–2013 Weekly. 2014;63(47):1108–1112. Available at: http://www.cdc.gov/mmwr/preview/mmwrhtml/mm6347a4.htm?s_cid=mm6347a4_w. Accessed July 19, 2015.

8. CDC, MMWR: Tobacco Use Among Middle and High School Students—United States, 2011–2014. 2015;64(14);381–385. Available at: http://www.cdc.gov/mmwr/preview/mmwrhtml/mm6414a3.htm?s_cid=mm6414a3_e. Accessed July 19, 2015.

9. CDC Fact Sheet: Smoking and Tobacco Use: Health Effects of Cigarette Smoking. Available at: http://www.cdc.gov/tobacco/data_statistics/fact_sheets/health_effects/effects_cig_smoking/index.htm. Accessed May 27, 2016.

10. Centers for Disease Control and Prevention. Quitting Smoking Among Adults –United States, 2001-2010. Morbidity and Mortality Weekly Report 2011;60(44):1513–1519.

11. Moyer VA. Primary care interventions to prevent tobacco use in children and adolescents: U.S. Preventative Services Task Force recommenation statement. *Ann Intern Med*. 2013; 159:552.

12. Ranney L, Melvin C, Lux L, et al. Systematic review: smoking cessation intervention strategies for adults and adults in special populations. *Ann Intern Med*. 2006;145(11):845–856.

13. Norcross JC, Prochaska JO. Using the stages of change. *Harv Ment Health Lett*. 2002;18(11):5–7.

14. CDC Fact Sheet: Smoking and Tobacco Use: Quitting Smoking. Available at: http://www.cdc.gov/tobacco/data_statistics/fact_sheets/cessation/quitting/index.htm. Accessed May 27, 2016.

15. Fiore MC, Jaén CR, Baker TB, et al. Treating Tobacco Use and Dependence: 2008 Update—Clinical Practice Guidelines. Rockville, MD: U.S. Department of Health and Human Services, Public Health Service, Agency for Healthcare Research and Quality, 2008.

16. Stead LF, Lancaster T. Combined pharmacotherapy and behavioural interventions for smoking cessation. *Cochrane Database Syst Rev*. 2012;10:CD008286.

17. U.S. Preventive Services Task Force. Tobacco Smoking Cessation in Adults, Including Pregnant Women: Behavioral and Pharmacotherapy Interventions recommendation statement. Rockville, MD: Agency for Healthcare Research and Quality; 2015. Available at: http://www.uspreventiveservicestaskforce.org/Page/Document/UpdateSummaryFinal/tobacco-use-in-adults-and-pregnant-women-counseling-and-interventions1. Accessed May 27, 2016.

18. Advisory Committee on Immunization Practices (ACIP), Centers for Disease Control and Prevention. Seasonal influenza: recommendations of the ACIP,2015–2016 Flu Season. Available at: http://www.cdc.gov/flu/about/season/flu-season-2015-2016.htm. Accessed November 12, 2015.

19. Pneumococcal Disease. Centers for Disease Control and Prevention Epidemiology and Prevention of Vaccine-Preventable Diseases, 13th Edition (2015).

20. Parshall MB, Schwartzstein RM, Adams L et al; American Thoracic Society Committee on Dyspnea. An official American Thoracic Society statement: update on the mechanisms, assessment, and management of dyspnea. American journal of respiratory and critical care medicine." Am J Respir Crit Care Med 2012;185:435.

21. Panettieri RA. In the clinic. Asthma. *Ann Intern Med*. 2007; 146(11):ITC6–1–ITC6–14.

22. Neiderman M. In the clinic: community-acquired pneumonia. *Ann Intern Med*. 2009;151:ITC4–1–ITC4–16.

23. Agnelli G, Becattini C. Acute pulmonary embolism. *N Engl J Med*. 2010;363:266.

24. Wenzel RP, Fowler AA. Acute bronchitis. *N Engl J Med*. 2006; 355(20):2125–2130.

25. Badgett RG, Tanaka DJ, Hunt DK, et al. Can moderate chronic obstructive pulmonary disease be diagnosed by historical and physical findings alone? *Am J Med*. 1993;94(2):188–196.

26. Straus SE, McAlister FA, Sackett DL, et al. The accuracy of patient history, wheezing, and laryngeal measurements in diagnosing obstructive airway disease. *JAMA*. 2000;283(14):1853–1857.

27. Global Initiative for Chronic Obstructive Lung Disease. Global strategy for the diagnosis, management, and prevention of chronic obstructive pulmonary disease. Updated 2015. Available at http://www.goldcopd.org/uploads/users/files/GOLD_Report_2015_Feb18.pdf. Accessed April 6, 2015.

28. Littner M. In the clinic: chronic obstructive pulmonary disease. *Ann Intern Med*. 2011;154(7):ITC4–1–ITC4–15.

29. Neiwoehner DR. Outpatient management of severe COPD. *N Engl J Med*. 2010;362:1407.

30. Irwin RS, Madison JM. The diagnosis and treatment of cough. *N Engl J Med*. 2000;3432(3):1715–1721.

31. Metlay JP, Kapoor WN, Fine MJ. Does this patient have community-acquired pneumonia? Diagnosing pneumonia by history and physical examination. *JAMA*. 1997;378:1440.

32. Barker A. Bronchiectasis. *N Engl J Med*. 2002;346(18):1383–1393.

33. Escalante P. In the clinic: tuberculosis. *Ann Intern Med*. 2009;150:ITC6–1.

34. Kerlin MP. In the Clinic: acute pulmonary embolism. *N Engl J Med*. 2010;363:26.

35. Kouritas VK, Papagiannoupoulos K, Lazaridis G, et al. Pneumomediastinum. *J Thorac Dis*. 2015;7(Suppl 1):S44.

ADDITIONAL REFERENCES

American Thoracic Society. Dyspnea–mechanisms, assessment, and management: a consensus statement. *Am J Respir Crit Care Med*. 1999;159(1):321–340.

Cahill K, Stead LF, Lancaster T. Nicotine receptor partial agonists for smoking cessation. *Cochrane Database Syst Rev*. 2011; (2):CD006103.

Centers for Disease Control and Prevention, DHHS. Fact sheet: smoking and tobacco use. Cessation. Available at: http://www.cdc.gov/tobacco/data_statistics/Factsheets/cessation2.htm. Accessed April 10, 2011.

Centers for Disease Control and Prevention. Vaccines and preventable diseases: pneumococcal vaccination. Available at: http://www.cdc.gov/vaccines/vpd-vac/pneumo/default.htm Accessed July 21, 2015.

Holleman DR, Simel DL. Does the clinical examination predict airflow limitation? *JAMA*. 1995;273(4):63–68.

Varenicline (Chantix) for tobacco dependence. *Med Lett Drugs Ther*. 2006;48(1241–1242):66–68.

CHAPTER 14

The Cardiovascular System

The student will:

1. Describe the structure and functions of the heart and great vessels.
2. Identify the landmarks and key auscultation sites of the precordium.
3. Describe the electrical conduction system of the heart.
4. Explain the normal electrocardiogram waveform pattern.
5. Describe the two phases of the cardiac cycle.
6. Describe the normal heart sounds and their origin.
7. Describe extra heart sounds and their origin.
8. Obtain an accurate history of the cardiovascular system.
9. Appropriately prepare and position the patient for the cardiovascular examination.
10. Describe the equipment necessary to perform a cardiovascular examination.
11. Examine the jugular veins and carotid arteries of the neck.
12. Inspect, palpate, and auscultate the precordium to evaluate the cardiovascular system.
13. Discuss risk factors for coronary heart disease.
14. Discuss risk reduction and health promotion strategies to reduce coronary heart disease.

The cardiovascular system is made up of the heart and blood vessels. The main functions of this system are delivering oxygen and nutrients to the cells of the body, removing waste products, and maintaining perfusion to the organs and tissues. The heart is the pump that drives circulation of the blood and the blood vessels are the pathways to and from the tissues. To assess a patient's cardiovascular health the nurse gathers a thorough focused health history and uses this information to perform an appropriate physical examination of the patient's heart and blood vessels. This chapter will discuss the assessment of the heart and great vessels, aorta, pulmonary artery, venae cavae, and pulmonary veins. Chapter 15, The Peripheral Vascular

System and Lymphatic System, covers the assessment of the peripheral blood vessels and lymph system.

ANATOMY AND PHYSIOLOGY

In order to perform an accurate assessment of the cardiovascular system the nurse must have a thorough understanding of the anatomy and physiology of the system including the heart muscle, chambers, valves, great vessels, conduction system of the heart, peripheral arteries and veins, capillaries, and lymph system.

Location of the Heart and Great Vessels

The heart is a hollow muscular organ a little larger than the patient's fist. It lies in the pericardial cavity in the mediastinum under the sternum and between the 2nd and 5th intercostal spaces. About two thirds of the heart lies to the left of the midline of the sternum.

The area of the exterior chest that overlays the heart and great vessels is called the *precordium*. It is helpful to visualize the underlying structures of the heart as you examine the precordium. Note that the heart is rotated so that the *right ventricle* occupies most of the anterior cardiac surface. This chamber and the pulmonary artery form a wedge-shaped structure behind and to the left of the sternum, outlined in black.

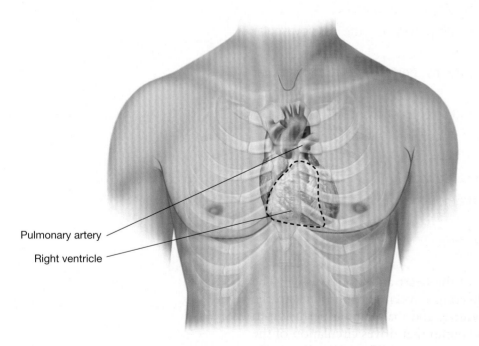

Pulmonary artery

Right ventricle

The inferior border of the right ventricle lies at the junction of the sternum and the xiphoid process. The right ventricle narrows as it rises to meet the pulmonary artery just below the sternal angle. This is called the *"base of the heart"* and is located at the right and left 2nd intercostal spaces next to the sternum.

The *left ventricle,* behind the right ventricle and to the left, outlined below in black, forms the left margin of the heart. Its tapered inferior tip is often termed the *cardiac "apex."* It is clinically important because it produces the apical impulse, identified during palpation of the precordium as the *point of maximal impulse,* or *PMI.* This impulse locates the left border of the heart and is normally found in the 5th intercostal space 7 cm to 9 cm lateral to the midsternal line, at or just medial to the left midclavicular line. The PMI may not be readily felt in a healthy patient with a normal heart, however.

- In supine patients the *diameter of the PMI* may be as large as a quarter, approximately 1 to 2.5 cm. A PMI greater than 2.5 cm is evidence of left ventricular hypertrophy (LVH), or enlargement.

- Similarly, *displacement of the PMI* lateral to the midclavicular line or greater than 10 cm lateral to the midsternal line also suggests LVH, or enlargement.

The apical impulse is easily palpated in children and slender adults, but as the anteroposterior chest diameter increases it becomes more difficult to feel. Obesity or a thick chest wall also makes palpation of the apical impulse difficult.[1]

Note that in some patients the most prominent precordial impulse may not be at the apex of the left ventricle. For example, in patients with chronic obstructive pulmonary disease, the most prominent palpable impulse or PMI may be in the xiphoid or epigastric area as a result of *right ventricular hypertrophy.*

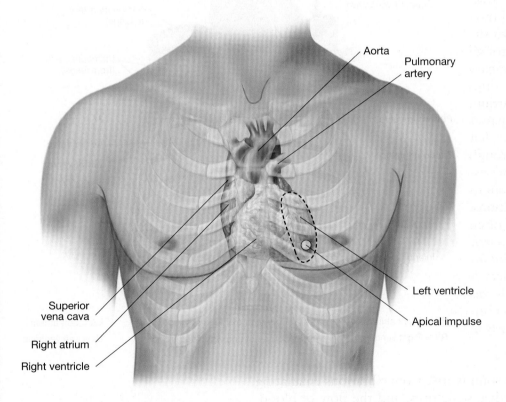

Aorta

Pulmonary artery

Left ventricle

Apical impulse

Superior vena cava

Right atrium

Right ventricle

Above the heart lie the *great vessels.* The *pulmonary artery,* which carries unoxygenated blood to the lungs, bifurcates quickly into its left and right branches. The *aorta* curves upward from the left ventricle to the level of the sternal angle, where it arches backward to the left and then downward. On the medial border, the *superior* and *inferior venae cavae* channel venous blood from the upper and lower portions of the body, respectively, into the right atrium.

The Heart Wall

The wall of the heart is composed of three layers. The *pericardium,* the outermost layer, is composed of two tough fibrous membranes that enclose and protect the heart. A few milliliters of serous fluid between the membranes provide lubrication for smooth movement of the heart. The *myocardium* is the heart muscle that does the pumping. The *endocardium* is a thin, smooth layer of endothelial tissue that lines the inner surface of the chambers and valves of the heart.

Cardiac Chambers, Valves, and Circulation

Circulation through the heart is shown in the diagram which identifies the cardiac chambers, valves, and direction of blood flow. Blood from the body's organs and tissues returns to the heart via the superior and inferior venae cavae; empties into the right atrium; and travels through the tricuspid valve into the right ventricle, which pumps it through the pulmonary valve into the pulmonary artery. After passage through the lungs the blood returns to the left atrium through the pulmonary veins and passes through the mitral valve into the left ventricle, where it is pumped through the aortic valve into the aorta for distribution of oxygenated blood throughout the body. Because of their positions, the *tricuspid* and *mitral valves* are often called *atrioventricular valves.* The *aortic* and *pulmonic valves* are called *semilunar valves* because each of their leaflets is shaped like a half moon. Although this diagram shows all valves in an open position, they do not open simultaneously in the living heart.

RA = Right atrium
RV = Right ventricle

⟹ Course of oxygenated blood
➡ Course of unoxygenated blood

LA = Left atrium
LV = Left ventricle

As the heart valves close, the heart sounds arise from vibrations emanating from the leaflets, the adjacent cardiac structures, and the flow of blood. Study carefully the positions and movements of the valves in relation to events in the cardiac cycle in order to understand the heart sounds.

The Cardiac Cycle

Ventricular Pressures

The heart serves as a pump that generates varying pressures within its chambers as they contract and relax. *Systole is the period of ventricular contraction.*

In the diagram below, pressure in the left ventricle rises from less than 5 mm Hg in its resting state to a normal peak of 120 mm Hg. After the ventricle ejects much of its blood into the aorta, the pressure levels off and starts to fall. *Diastole is the period of ventricular relaxation.* Ventricular pressure falls to below 5 mm Hg, and blood flows from atrium to ventricle. Late in diastole, ventricular pressure rises slightly during inflow of blood from atrial contraction.

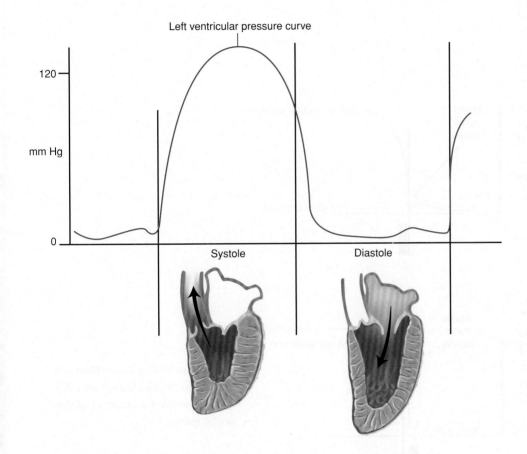

Left ventricular pressure curve

Valve Openings and Closings

Note during *systole* the aortic valve is open, allowing ejection of blood from the left ventricle into the aorta. The mitral valve is closed, preventing blood from regurgitating (leaking) back into the left atrium. In contrast, during *diastole* the aortic valve is closed, preventing regurgitation of blood from the aorta back into the left ventricle. The mitral valve is open, allowing blood to flow from the left atrium into the relaxed left ventricle.

Understanding the interrelationships of the *pressures* in the left atrium, left ventricle, and aorta together with the position and movement of the valves is fundamental to understanding heart sounds. Trace these changing pressures and sounds through one cardiac cycle. During auscultation the first and second heart sounds define the duration of *systole* and *diastole*.

During *diastole,* pressure in the blood-filled left atrium slightly exceeds that in the relaxed left ventricle, and blood flows from left atrium to left ventricle across the open mitral valve. Just before the onset of ventricular systole, atrial contraction (*the "atrial kick"*) empties the atrium and produces a slight pressure rise in both chambers.

During *systole,* the left ventricle starts to contract and ventricular pressure rapidly exceeds left atrial pressure, shutting the mitral valve. *Closure of the mitral valve produces the first heart sound, S_1.*

As left ventricular pressure continues to rise, it quickly exceeds the pressure in the aorta and forces the aortic valve open. *Normally, maximal left ventricular pressure corresponds to systolic blood pressure.*

In some pathologic conditions, an early systolic ejection sound (Ej) accompanies the opening of the aortic valve.

After the left ventricle ejects most of its blood, ventricular pressure begins to fall. When left ventricular pressure drops below aortic pressure, the aortic valve shuts. *Aortic valve closure produces the second heart sound, S_2, and another diastole begins.*

In *diastole,* left ventricular pressure continues to drop and falls below left atrial pressure. The mitral valve silently opens.

An opening snap (OS) may be heard if valve leaflet motion is restricted, as in mitral stenosis.

After the mitral valve opens, there is a period of early rapid ventricular filling as blood flows early in diastole from left atrium to left ventricle.

In children and young adults, a third heart sound, S₃, may be caused by the rapid deceleration of the column of blood against the ventricular wall. In older adults, an S₃, sometimes termed "an S₃ gallop," usually indicates a pathologic change in ventricular compliance.

Finally, although not often heard in healthy adults, a fourth heart sound, S₄, marks atrial contraction. It immediately precedes S₁ of the next beat and also reflects a pathologic change in ventricular compliance.

Compliance is the ease with which the heart muscle relaxes as it fills with blood. Poor compliance produces a stiff ventricle with reduced ability to expand as it receives blood.

The Splitting of Heart Sounds

Split S₂

While these events are occurring on the left side of the heart, similar changes are occurring on the right, involving the right atrium, right ventricle, tricuspid valve, pulmonic valve, and pulmonary artery. However, right ventricular and pulmonary arterial pressures are significantly lower than corresponding pressures on the left side.

Furthermore, right-sided events usually occur slightly later than those on the left. Instead of a single heart sound, two discernible sounds may be heard, the first from left-sided aortic valve closure, or A_2, and the second from right-sided closure of the pulmonic valve, or P_2.

S_2, and its two components, A_2 and P_2, are caused by the closure of the aortic and pulmonary valves, respectively. During inspiration the filling time of the right heart increases, thereby increasing the *stroke volume* and lengthening the duration of right ventricle emptying compared to the left ventricle. This delays closure of the pulmonic valve, P_2, *splitting* S_2 into its two audible components.[2]

During expiration, these two components fuse into a single sound, S_2.

The split S may be difficult to hear in obese individuals or people with increased anteroposterior diameter chest walls.

Stroke volume is the amount of blood ejected by the ventricle with each heartbeat.

Vein walls contain less muscle so they are more distensible than arteries and can store more blood. During inspiration the pulmonary vascular bed has more capacity, which contributes to the increased filling time and delays closure of P_2.

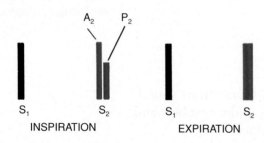

Of the two components of the S_2, A_2 is normally louder, reflecting the high pressure in the aorta. It is heard throughout the precordium. P_2, in contrast, is relatively soft, reflecting the lower pressure in the pulmonary artery. It is heard best in its own area—the 2nd and 3rd left intercostal spaces close to the sternum. It is here that you should search for splitting of the S_2. See the diagram on p. 382.

Split S₁

S_1 also has two components, an earlier mitral and a later tricuspid sound. The mitral sound, its principal component, is much louder, again reflecting the high pressures on the left side of the heart. It can be heard throughout the precordium and is loudest at the cardiac apex. The softer tricuspid component is heard best at the lower left sternal border, and it is here that you may hear a split S_1. The earlier, louder mitral component may mask the tricuspid sound, however, and splitting is not always detectable. Splitting of S_1 does not vary with respiration.

Heart Murmurs

Heart murmurs are distinguishable from heart sounds by their longer duration. They are attributed to turbulent blood flow and may be "innocent," as with flow murmurs of young adults, or diagnostic of valvular or congenital heart disease. A *stenotic valve* has an abnormally narrowed valvular orifice that obstructs blood flow, as in *aortic stenosis,* and causes a characteristic murmur. A valve that fails to fully close, as in *aortic regurgitation* or *insufficiency,* allows blood to leak backward in a retrograde direction and produces a *regurgitant* murmur.

Stenosis means narrowing, in this case the aortic valve outlet is narrowed, producing turbulent blood flow.

Normal flow

High flow rate

Incompetent valve

Valve stenosis

Abnormal opening

In the section on Physical Examination, the characteristics of murmurs, including intensity, pitch, duration, and direction of radiation, will be discussed (see pp. 409–412).

Relation of Auscultatory Findings to the Chest Wall

The locations on the chest wall where heart sounds and murmurs are heard help to identify the valve or chamber where they originate. The sounds produced by the heart valves travel with the flow of blood. As you review the locations on the diagram on p. 382, picture the direction of blood flow between the upper and lower chambers and through the pulmonary artery and aorta. Sounds and murmurs arising from the mitral valve are usually heard best at and around the cardiac apex. Those originating in the tricuspid valve are heard best at or near the lower left sternal border. Murmurs arising from the pulmonic valve are usually heard best in the 2nd and 3rd left intercostal spaces close to the sternum but at times may also be heard at higher or lower levels. Murmurs originating in the aortic valve may be heard anywhere from the right 2nd intercostal space to the apex. *These areas overlap,* as illustrated, and you will need to correlate auscultatory findings with other cardiac examination findings to identify sounds and murmurs accurately.

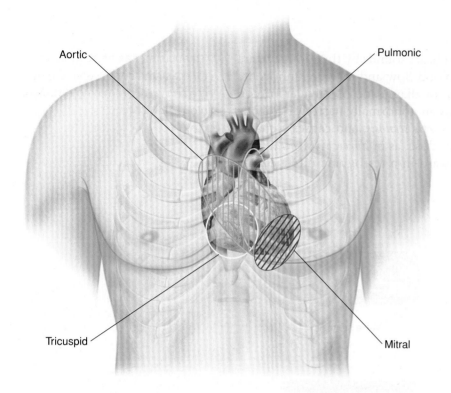

The Conduction System

An electrical conduction system stimulates and coordinates the contraction of cardiac muscle.

Each electrical impulse is initiated in the *sinus node,* a group of specialized cardiac cells located in the right atrium near the junction of the vena cava. The sinus node acts as the cardiac pacemaker and automatically discharges an impulse about 60 to 100 times a minute. This impulse travels through both atria to the *atrioventricular node,* a specialized group of cells located low in the atrial septum. Here the impulse is delayed before passing down the bundle of His and its branches to the ventricular myocardium. Muscular contraction follows: first the atria, then the ventricles. The normal conduction pathway is diagrammed above in simplified form. The electrocardiogram, or ECG, records these events. Contraction of cardiac smooth muscle produces electrical activity, resulting in a series of waves on the ECG. The ECG consists of *six limb leads* in the *frontal plane* and *six chest or precordial leads* in the *transverse plane*.

- Electrical vectors (signals) approaching a lead cause a *positive, or upward, deflection*.

- Electrical vectors moving away from the lead cause a *negative, or downward, deflection*.

- When positive and negative vectors balance, they are *isoelectric*, appearing as a straight line.

The components of the *normal ECG* and their duration are briefly summarized here, but you will need further instruction and practice to interpret recordings from patients. The term "normal sinus rhythm" (NSR) is used to describe normal ECG transmission. Note:

- The small *P wave* of atrial depolarization (duration up to 80 milliseconds; *PR interval* 120 to 200 milliseconds)

- The larger *QRS complex* of ventricular depolarization (up to 100 milliseconds), consisting of one or more of the following:

  – The *Q wave*, a downward deflection from septal depolarization
  – The *R wave*, an upward deflection from ventricular depolarization
  – The *S wave*, a downward deflection following an R wave

- A *T wave* of ventricular repolarization, or recovery (duration relates to QRS)

The electrical impulse slightly precedes the myocardial contraction that it stimulates. The relation of electrocardiographic waves to the cardiac cycle is shown below.

LIMB LEADS: FRONTAL PLANE

CHEST LEADS: TRANSVERSE PLANE

The Heart as a Pump

The left and right ventricles pump blood into the systemic and pulmonary arterial trees, respectively. *Cardiac output,* the volume of blood ejected from each ventricle during 1 minute, is the product of *heart rate* and *stroke volume.* Stroke volume (the volume of blood ejected with each heartbeat) depends in turn on preload, myocardial contractility, and afterload.

- *Preload* refers to the load that stretches the cardiac muscle before contraction. The volume of blood in the right ventricle at the end of diastole, then, constitutes its preload for the next beat. Right ventricular preload is increased by increasing venous return to the right heart. Physiologic causes include inspiration and the increased volume of blood flow from exercising muscles. The increased blood volume in a dilated right ventricle of heart failure also increases preload. Causes of decreased right ventricular preload include exhalation, decreased left ventricular output, and pooling of blood in the capillary bed or the venous system.

- *Myocardial contractility* refers to the ability of the cardiac muscle, when given a load, to contract or shorten. Contractility increases when stimulated by the sympathetic nervous system and decreases when blood flow or oxygen delivery to the myocardium is impaired.

- *Afterload* refers to the degree of vascular resistance to ventricular contraction. Sources of resistance to left ventricular contraction include the tone in the walls of the aorta, the large arteries, and the peripheral vascular tree (primarily the small arteries and arterioles), as well as the volume of blood already in the aorta. Increased arterial blood pressure causes increased afterload.

Pathologic increases in preload and afterload, called *volume overload* and *pressure overload,* respectively, produce changes in ventricular function that may be clinically detectable. These changes include alterations in ventricular impulses, detectable by palpation, and in normal heart sounds. Pathologic heart sounds and murmurs may also develop.

The term *heart failure* is now preferred over "congestive heart failure" because not all patients have volume overload on initial presentation.[3]

Arterial Pulses and Blood Pressure

With each contraction, the left ventricle ejects a volume of blood into the aorta and on to the arterial tree. The ensuing pressure wave moves rapidly through the arterial system, where it is felt as the *arterial pulse.* Although the pressure wave travels quickly—many times faster than the blood itself—a palpable delay between ventricular contraction and peripheral pulses makes the pulses in the arms and legs unsuitable for timing events in the cardiac cycle.

Blood pressure in the arterial system varies during the cardiac cycle, peaking in systole and falling to its lowest trough in diastole. These are the levels that are measured with the blood pressure cuff, or sphygmomanometer. The difference between systolic and diastolic pressures is known as the *pulse pressure.*

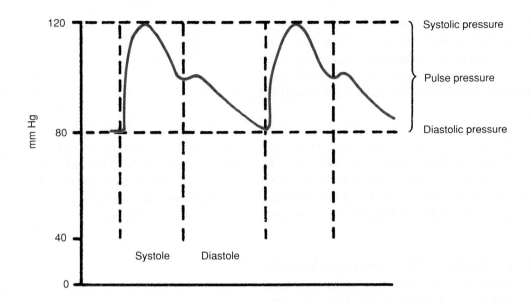

Factors Influencing Arterial Pressure

- Left ventricular stroke volume
- Distensibility of the aorta and the large arteries
- Peripheral vascular resistance, particularly at the arteriolar level
- Volume of blood in the arterial system

Changes in any of these four factors alter systolic pressure, diastolic pressure, or both. Blood pressure levels fluctuate strikingly throughout any 24-hour period, varying with physical activity; emotional state; pain; noise; environmental temperature; use of coffee, tobacco, and other drugs; and even time of day.

Jugular Venous Undulations

The oscillations visible in the internal jugular veins, and often in the externals, reflect changing pressures within the right atrium. Careful observation reveals that the undulating pulsations of the internal jugular veins, and sometimes the externals, are composed of two quick peaks (a and v) and two troughs (x and y).

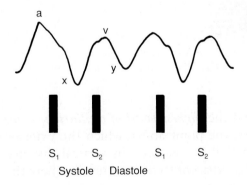

Jugular Venous Pressure

The jugular veins provide an important clinical index of right heart pressures and cardiac function. *Jugular venous pressure (JVP)* reflects right atrial pressure, which in turn equals *central venous pressure (CVP)* and right ventricular end-diastolic pressure. The JVP is best estimated from the *right internal jugular vein,* which has a more direct anatomic channel into the right atrium. Contrary to widely held views, a recent study has reaffirmed inspection of the *right external jugular vein* as a useful and accurate method for estimating CVP.[4,5]

Pressure changes from right atrial filling, contraction, and emptying cause fluctuations in the JVP and its waveforms that are visible to the examiner. Careful observation of changes in these fluctuations yields clues about volume status, right and left ventricular function, patency of the tricuspid and pulmonary valves, pressures in the pericardium, and arrhythmias.

JVP falls with loss of blood and increases with right or left heart failure, pulmonary hypertension, tricuspid stenosis, and pericardial compression or tamponade.

The internal jugular veins lie under the sternocleidomastoid muscles in the neck and are not directly visible, so the nurse must learn to identify the *undulations* of the *internal jugular vein* or *external jugular vein* that are transmitted to the surface of the neck, making sure to carefully distinguish these venous undulations from the crisp pulsations of the carotid artery.

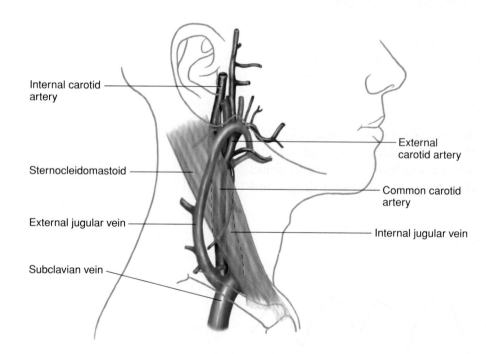

Internal carotid artery

Sternocleidomastoid

External jugular vein

Subclavian vein

External carotid artery

Common carotid artery

Internal jugular vein

To estimate the level of the JVP, find the *highest point of oscillation in the internal jugular vein* or, if necessary, the point above which the external jugular vein appears collapsed. The JVP is measured in vertical distance above the *sternal angle,* the bony ridge adjacent to the second rib where the manubrium joins the body of the sternum.

The visibility of the jugular veins varies by patient position due to gravity. Review the illustrations on p. 387. In this patient, the pressure in the internal jugular vein is elevated.

- In *Position A,* the head of the bed is raised to 30 degrees, but the JVP cannot be measured because venous undulation is above the jaw and therefore not visible.

- In *Position B,* the head of the bed is raised to 60 degrees. The "top" of the internal jugular vein is now visible, so the vertical distance from the sternal angle or right atrium can be measured.

- In *Position C,* the patient is upright and the veins are barely discernible above the clavicle, making measurement impossible.

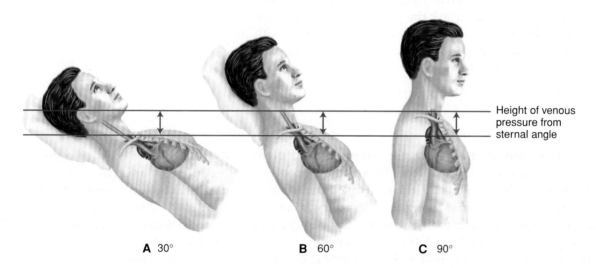

Height of venous
pressure from
sternal angle

A 30°　　　　**B** 60°　　　　**C** 90°

Note that the height of the venous pressure as measured from the sternal angle is the *same* in all three positions, but your ability to *measure* the height of the column of venous blood, or JVP, differs according to how you position the patient. The JVP measured at more than 4 cm above the sternal angle, or more than 9 cm above the right atrium, is considered abnormal. The techniques for measuring the JVP are fully described in the Physical Examination section on pp. 395–397.

THE HEALTH HISTORY

Common or Concerning Symptoms

- Chest pain or discomfort, pain or discomfort radiating to the neck, left shoulder or arm, and back
- Arrhythmias: skipped beats, palpitations
- Dyspnea
- Cough
- Edema
- Nocturia
- Fatigue
- Cyanosis or pallor

Assessing Cardiac Symptoms—Overview and Comparison With Baseline Activity Levels

Chest symptoms may be caused by cardiac, respiratory, gastrointestinal, or musculoskeletal etiologies. The nurse differentiates the cause of the symptoms through astute history questioning. This section focuses on chest symptoms from a cardiac standpoint. Cardiac symptoms reflect the heart's ability to function (i.e., to pump blood through the body and remove waste products).

Start the inquiry about the heart with broad open-ended questions. For each symptom it is important to habitually ask the patient to quantify how it affects lifestyle or baseline level of activity. For example, in patients with chest pain, does the pain occur with walking? If yes, how far can you walk before the pain begins—50 ft, one block, more?

Chest Pain

Chest pain is one of the most serious and important symptoms and often signals *coronary heart disease,* which currently affects 16.5 million people in the United States.[6] Approximately 9 million of these people have *angina pectoris,* and 8 million have had a *myocardial infarction.* Coronary heart disease (CHD) is the leading cause of death for both men and women, and accounted for one in every three U.S. deaths in 2011. Death rates are highest in African-American men and women, compared with other ethnic groups.

Classic pain on exertion, pressure, or discomfort in the chest, shoulder, back, neck, or arm in angina pectoris, seen in 50% of patients with acute myocardial infarction; atypical descriptors also are common, such as cramping, grinding, pricking; rarely, tooth or jaw pain.[7]

Women experiencing myocardial infarctions frequently complain of different symptoms than men. Rather than chest pain, they may experience upper body pain, for example, one or both arms, back, neck, jaw, or stomach. Dyspnea, cold sweats, nausea, indigestion, or lightheadedness may be the presenting symptom.[8]

Your initial questions should be broad: **Do you have any pain or discomfort in your chest?**

Acute coronary syndrome is increasingly used to refer to any of the clinical syndromes caused by acute myocardial ischemia, including unstable angina, non-ST elevation myocardial infarction, and ST elevation infarction.[9]

- Ask the patient to point to the pain and to describe its attributes.

Anterior chest pain, often tearing or ripping, often radiating into the back or neck, in *acute aortic dissection.*[10]

- Move on to more specific questions, such as:

  - Is the pain related to exertion?

  - What kinds of activities bring on the pain?

  - How intense is the pain, on a scale of 1 to 10?

  - Does it radiate into the neck, shoulder, or back or down your arm?

  - Are there any associated symptoms such as shortness of breath, sweating, palpitations, or nausea?

  - Does it ever wake you up at night?

  - What do you do to make it better?

Palpitations

Palpitations involve an unpleasant awareness of the heartbeat. When describing palpitations, patients use terms such as skipping, racing, fluttering, pounding, or stopping of the heart.

Palpitations may result from an irregular heartbeat, from rapid acceleration or slowing of the heart, or from increased forcefulness of cardiac contraction. Such perceptions also depend on how patients respond to their own body sensations. Palpitations do not necessarily mean heart disease. In contrast, the most serious dysrhythmias, such as ventricular tachycardia, often do not produce palpitations.

Do you ever have palpitations?

If the patient does not understand your question, reword it. Are you ever aware of your heartbeat? What is it like? How long did the palpitations last? Did they start and stop suddenly or come on gradually?

Shortness of Breath

Shortness of breath is a common patient concern and may represent *dyspnea, orthopnea,* or *paroxysmal nocturnal dyspnea.*

Dyspnea is an uncomfortable awareness of breathing that is inappropriate to a given level of exertion.

Do you ever have difficulty breathing or shortness of breath?

- When does it occur?

- What were you doing when you became short of breath?

- How many pillows do you use to sleep?

Orthopnea is dyspnea that occurs when the patient is lying down and improves when the patient sits up. Make sure, however, that the reason the patient uses extra pillows or sleeps upright is shortness of breath and not other causes.

- Have you ever awoken suddenly due to shortness of breath?

Paroxysmal nocturnal dyspnea, or PND, describes episodes of sudden dyspnea and orthopnea that awaken the patient from sleep, usually 1 or 2 hours after going to bed, prompting the patient to sit up, stand up, or go to a window for air. There may be associated wheezing and coughing. The episode usually subsides but may recur at about the same time on subsequent nights.

Cough

Cough can result from fluid leaking into the lungs.

Left-sided heart failure can cause fluid to leak into the lungs. Fine crackles or rales may be heard on auscultation.

- Do you ever have a cough?

- Describe your cough.

- Do you cough up mucus? If yes, describe the mucus.

- When does it occur? Any particular time of day?

Edema

Edema refers to the accumulation of excessive fluid in the extravascular interstitial space. Focus your questions on the location, timing, and setting of the swelling, and on associated symptoms.

Dependent edema appears in the lowest body parts: the feet and lower legs when sitting, or the sacrum when bedridden. Causes may be cardiac (*heart failure*), peripheral vascular disease, nutritional (*hypoalbuminemia*), or positional.

- Have you had any swelling anywhere?

- Where? Anywhere else?

- When does it occur?

- Is it worse in the morning or at night?

- Do your shoes get tight?

- Are the rings tight on your fingers?

- Are your eyelids puffy or swollen in the morning?

- Have you had to let out your belt?

Nocturia

Nocturia is urination at night. It is dependent edema that is mobilized at night and returned to the kidneys for excretion during the night when the patient is reclining.

- Do you get up more than once during the night to urinate?

- How many times?

Fatigue

Fatigue is an overwhelming sustained sense of exhaustion.

Fatigue signals that the heart is not adequately supplying the body with oxygen and nutrients.

- Do you feel more tired than previously?

- Are you able to perform your usual activities without resting?

Cyanosis or Pallor

Cyanosis or pallor indicates poor oxygenation of the body.

- Have you ever noticed your facial skin, lips, or fingers become blue or pale?

Cyanosis and pallor also indicate that the heart is not adequately circulating blood.

- How long did it last?

Past History

Do you have a history of heart problems or heart disease?
Do you have a history of:
    Heart murmur?
    Congenital heart disease?
    Rheumatic fever?
    High blood pressure? Do you know what the reading was?
    Elevated cholesterol or triglycerides?
    Peripheral arterial disease?
    Cerebral arterial disease?
    Diabetes?
When was your last ECG? Cholesterol measurement? Results?
Have you had any other heart tests? When? Results?

Family History

Is there any family history of coronary artery disease, hypertension, sudden death at younger than 60 years of age? Stroke? Diabetes? Obesity? (Family refers primarily to first-degree blood relatives [i.e., parent, sibling, or child]. However, information on grandparents, aunts, uncles, and first cousins can be useful as well.)

Lifestyle Habits

Nutrition—typical diet
Smoking
Alcohol
Exercise: Describe your daily or weekly exercise: type and amount
Medications prescribed and over-the-counter

PHYSICAL EXAMINATION

Preparation of the Patient

Appropriate preparation of the patient is essential to obtain accurate findings during the cardiovascular examination. The patient should be comfortable and calm as anxiety may elevate the blood pressure or change the heart rate or rhythm. Review the examination procedure with the patient before putting on the examination gown. Explain why visualization of the anterior chest is important for data gathering. Have the patient put on the examination gown with the opening in the front, which enables the nurse to open the gown only as necessary during the examination. Assist the patient onto the examination table, if necessary, and immediately drape with a sheet. Perform the examination from the patient's right side.

Equipment Needed for Examination

- Stethoscope with a bell and diaphragm
- Sphygmomanometer
- Two 15-cm rulers
- Watch with second hand
- Gooseneck lamp for tangential lighting

Blood Pressure and Heart Rate

As you begin the cardiovascular examination, review the blood pressure and heart rate recorded during the General Survey and Vital Signs at the start of the physical examination. If you need to repeat these measurements, or if they have not already been done, take the time to measure the blood pressure and heart rate using optimal technique (see Chapter 7, Beginning the Physical Examination: General Survey, Vital Signs, and Pain, pp. 128–135).

The components of the cardiovascular examination include:

- Examination of the face

- Examination of the great vessels of the neck

- Inspection and palpation of the precordium

- Auscultation of heart sounds

- Inspection for peripheral edema

Face

As you are taking the patient's history inspect the face, noting its color and the presence of any orbital edema. Look for signs of anxiety. Pallor or cyanosis may indicate poor perfusion of oxygen and orbital edema may indicate heart failure. Anxiety occurs during heart attacks.

Infants with cardiac disease may exhibit circumoral (around the mouth) cyanosis with feeding.

Great Vessels of the Neck

The Carotid Artery Pulse

The carotid pulse provides valuable information about cardiac function and is especially useful for detecting stenosis or insufficiency of the aortic valve.

For irregular rhythms, see Table 14-1, Selected Heart Rates and Rhythms, p. 424 and Table 14-2, Selected Irregular Rhythms, p. 425.

Amplitude and Contour

To assess *amplitude and contour* of the carotid pulse, the patient should be lying down with the head of the bed elevated to about 30 degrees. First inspect the neck for carotid pulsations. These may be visible just medial to the sternocleidomastoid muscles. Then place your index and middle fingers on the right carotid artery in the lower third of the neck, press posteriorly, and feel for pulsations.

A tortuous and kinked carotid artery may produce a unilateral pulsatile bulge.

Press just inside the medial border of a well-relaxed sternomastoid muscle, roughly at the level of the cricoid cartilage. Avoid pressing on the *carotid sinus,* which lies at the level of the top of the thyroid cartilage. For the left carotid artery, use your right fingers. Never press both carotids at the same time. This may decrease blood flow to the brain and induce syncope.

Causes of decreased pulsations include decreased stroke volume and local factors in the artery such as atherosclerotic narrowing or occlusion.

Pressure on the carotid sinus may cause a reflex drop in pulse rate or blood pressure.

Slowly increase pressure until the maximal pulsation is felt, and then slowly decrease pressure until you best sense the arterial pressure and contour. Try to assess:

- The *amplitude of the pulse*. This correlates reasonably well with the pulse pressure.

- The *contour of the pulse wave*, namely, the speed of the upstroke, the duration of its summit, and the speed of the downstroke. The normal upstroke is *brisk*. It is smooth and rapid and follows S_1 almost immediately. The summit is smooth, rounded, and roughly midsystolic. The downstroke is less abrupt than the upstroke.

- Any *variations in amplitude,* either from beat to beat or with respiration.

- *The timing of the carotid upstroke in relation to S_1 and S_2.* Note that the normal carotid upstroke follows S_1 and precedes S_2. This relationship is very helpful in correctly identifying S_1 and S_2, especially when the heart rate is increased and the duration of diastole, normally longer than systole, is shortened and approaches the duration of systole.

Thrills and Bruits

During palpation of the carotid artery, humming vibrations, or *thrills,* that feel like the throat of a purring cat may be detected. Routinely, but especially in the presence of a thrill, listen over both carotid arteries with the bell of the stethoscope for a *bruit,* a murmur-like sound of vascular rather than cardiac origin.

Listen for carotid bruits if the patient is middle-aged or elderly or if cerebrovascular disease is suspected. Ask the patient to hold breathing for a moment so that breath sounds do not obscure the vascular sound, and then listen with the bell. Heart sounds alone do not constitute a bruit.

Further examination of arterial pulses is described in Chapter 15, The Peripheral Vascular System.

The Brachial Artery

The carotid arteries reflect aortic pulsations more accurately, but in patients with carotid obstruction, kinking, or thrills, they are unsuitable. If so, assess

---

See Table 15-5, Abnormalities of the Arterial Pulse and Pressure Waves, p. 471.

Small, thready, or weak pulse in *cardiogenic shock; bounding* pulse in *aortic insufficiency* (see Table 15-5, Abnormalities of the Arterial Pulse and Pressure Waves, p. 471).

Delayed carotid upstroke is seen in *aortic stenosis.*

Pulsus alternans (see Table 15-5, Abnormalities of the Arterial Pulse and Pressure Waves, p. 471), bigeminal pulse [beat-to-beat variation]; paradoxical pulse [respiratory variation].

Note that an aortic valve murmur may radiate to the neck and sound like a carotid bruit.

The prevalence of asymptomatic carotid bruits increases with age, reaching 8% in people 75 years or older, with a threefold increased risk of ischemic heart disease and stroke. Presence of a carotid bruit does not predict the degree of underlying stenosis, so pursue further investigation.[11]

the pulse in the *brachial artery,* applying the techniques described above for determining amplitude and contour.

Use the index and middle fingers to feel for the pulse just medial to the biceps tendon. The patient's arm should rest with the elbow extended, palm up. With your free hand, you may need to flex the elbow to a varying degree to get optimal muscular relaxation.

Jugular Venous Pressure

The JVP provides valuable information about the patient's volume status and cardiac function. As you have read, the JVP reflects pressure in the right atrium, or central venous pressure, and is best assessed from undulations in the right internal jugular vein.[12]

Note, however, that the jugular veins are difficult to see in children younger than 12 years, so they are not useful for evaluating the cardiovascular system in this age group.

At the beginning of the assessment, consider the patient's volume status and how high the head of the bed or examining table needs to be elevated.

- The usual starting point for assessing the JVP is to elevate the head of the bed to 30 degrees. Identify the external jugular vein on each side, and then find the internal jugular venous undulations transmitted from deep in the neck to the overlying soft tissues. The JVP is the highest point of the jugular venous undulation that is usually evident in euvolemic patients.

- In patients who are *hypovolemic, the JVP may be low,* necessitating lowering *the head of the bed,* sometimes even to 0 degrees, to see the point of undulation best.

- Likewise, in volume-overloaded or *hypervolemic* patients, *the JVP may be high,* requiring raising *the head of the bed.*

- When documenting the JVP, record the height of the head of the bed, for example, JVP 2 cm from sternal angle with HOB elevated 45 degrees.

A hypovolemic patient may have to lie flat before you see the neck veins. In contrast, when JVP is increased, an elevation up to 45 degrees, 60 degrees, or even 90 degrees may be required. See diagram on p. 387.

Steps for Assessing the JVP

- Make the patient comfortable. *Raise the head slightly on a pillow* to relax the sternocleidomastoid muscles.
- *Raise the head of the bed or examining table to about 30 degrees. Turn the patient's head slightly away from the side you are inspecting.*
- Use *tangential lighting* and examine both sides of the neck. Identify the external jugular vein on each side, and then find the internal jugular venous pulsations.

- *If necessary, raise or lower the head of the bed* until you can see the undulations of the internal jugular vein in the lower half of the neck.
- Focus on the *right internal jugular vein.* Look for undulations in the suprasternal notch, between the attachments of the sternocleidomastoid muscle on the sternum and clavicle, or just posterior to the sternocleidomastoid. The table below helps you distinguish internal jugular undulations from those of the carotid artery.
- *Identify the highest point of undulation in the right internal jugular vein.* Extend a ruler or card horizontally from this point and a second centimeter ruler vertically from the sternal angle, making an exact right angle. Measure the vertical distance in centimeters above the sternal angle where the horizontal object crosses the ruler. *This distance, measured in centimeters above the sternal angle or the right atrium, is the JVP* (see photograph on p. 397).

The following features help to distinguish jugular undulations from carotid artery pulsations:[12]

Distinguishing Internal Jugular Undulations and Carotid Pulsations	
Internal Jugular Undulations	**Carotid Pulsations**
Rarely palpable	Palpable
Soft, biphasic, undulating quality, usually with two elevations and two troughs per heartbeat	A more vigorous thrust with a *single outward component*
Undulations can be eliminated by light pressure on the vein(s) just above the sternal end of the clavicle	Pulsations not eliminated by this pressure
Height of undulations changes with position, dropping as the patient becomes more upright	Height of pulsations unchanged by position
Height of undulations usually falls with inspiration	Height of pulsations not affected by inspiration

Establishing the true vertical and horizontal lines to measure the JVP is difficult, much like the problem of hanging a picture straight when you are close to it. Place your ruler on the sternal angle and line it up with something in the room that you know to be vertical. Then place a card or rectangular object at an exact right angle to the ruler. This constitutes your horizontal line. Move it up or down—still horizontal—so that the lower

Increased pressure suggests right-sided heart failure or, less commonly, constrictive pericarditis, tricuspid stenosis, or superior vena cava obstruction.[13,14]

edge rests at the top of the jugular pulsations, and read the vertical distance on the ruler. Round your measurement off to the nearest centimeter.

Venous pressure measured at greater than 3 cm is considered *abnormal*.

An elevated JVP is 98% specific for an increased left ventricular end-diastolic pressure and low-left ventricular ejection fraction, although its role as a predictor of hospitalization and death from heart failure is less clear.[1,15]

If undulations in the internal jugular vein cannot be seen, look for them in the external jugular vein. If there is no undulation, use *the point above which the external jugular veins appear to collapse*. Make this observation on each side of the neck. Measure the vertical distance of this point from the sternal angle.

Local kinking or obstruction is the usual cause of unilateral distention of the external jugular vein.

The highest point of venous undulations may lie below the level of the sternal angle. Under these circumstances, venous pressure is not elevated and seldom needs to be measured.

Abdominojugular Test

If heart failure is suspected from the patient history or physical examination or if the JVP is elevated, perform the abdominojugular test. Position the patient supine with the head of the bed at the same angle used for the JVP examination. With your right hand apply firm pressure on the patient's right upper quadrant (as seen on the next page) or middle abdomen for at least 10 seconds. This maneuver forces the hepatic venous blood into the vena cava, elevating the venous blood volume and pressure. While you are applying pressure, watch the patient's jugular

The abdominojugular test was formerly known as hepatojugular reflux. If heart failure is present the JVP will remain elevated as long as the pressure is maintained.

vein level. The healthy person is able to pump the extra blood through the heart within a few seconds. The jugular vein pressure will rise for a few seconds and then rapidly diminish to previous levels.

The Heart

For much of the cardiac examination, the patient should be *supine,* with the upper body raised by elevating the head of the bed or table to about 30 degrees. Two other positions are also needed: (1) the left lateral decubitus position (the patient *lays on the left side*) and (2) *sitting and leaning forward.* These positions bring the ventricular apex and left ventricular outflow tract closer to the chest wall, enhancing detection of the PMI and aortic insufficiency. *The examiner should stand at the patient's right side.*

During the cardiac examination, remember to correlate the findings with the patient's JVP and carotid pulse. It is also important to document both the anatomic location of findings with their timing in the cardiac cycle.

- Note the *anatomic location* of sounds in terms of intercostal spaces and their distance from the midsternal or midclavicular lines. The midsternal line offers the most reliable zero point for measurement, but some feel that the midclavicular line accommodates the different sizes and shapes of patients.

- Identify the *timing of impulses or sounds* in relation to the cardiac cycle. Timing of sounds is often possible through auscultation alone. In most people with normal or slow heart rates, it is easy to identify the paired heart sounds by listening through a stethoscope. S_1 is the first of these sounds, S_2 is the second, and the relatively long diastolic interval separates one pair from the next.

S_1 is sometimes called "lub" and S_2 "dub." Listen for the lub–dub sequence to distinguish the two sounds.

Lub	Dub	Lub	Dub
S_1	S_2	S_1	S_2
Systole	Diastole	Systole	

The relative intensity of these sounds is also helpful. S_1 is usually louder than S_2 at the apex; S_2 is usually louder than S_1 at the base.

Even experienced nurses are sometimes uncertain about the timing of heart sounds, especially extra sounds and murmurs. "Inching" can then be helpful. Return to a place on the chest—most often the base—where it is easy to identify S_1 and S_2. Get their rhythm clearly in mind. Then inch your stethoscope down the chest in steps until you hear the new sound.

Auscultation alone, however, can be misleading. The intensities of S_1 and S_2, for example, may be abnormal. At rapid heart rates, diastole shortens, and at about a rate of 120, the durations of systole and diastole become indistinguishable. *Use palpation of the carotid pulse or of the apical impulse to help determine whether the sound or murmur is systolic or diastolic.* Because both the carotid upstroke and the apical impulse occur in systole, right after S_1, sounds or murmurs coinciding with them are systolic; sounds or murmurs occurring after the carotid upstroke or apical impulse are diastolic.

For example, S_1 is decreased in first-degree heart block, and S_2 is decreased in aortic stenosis.

Sequence of Cardiac Examination

The table below summarizes patient positions and a suggested sequence for the examination.

Sequence of Cardiac Examination	
Patient Position	**Examination**
Supine, with the head elevated 30 degrees	Inspect and palpate the precordium: the 2nd right and left intercostal spaces; the right ventricle; and the left ventricle, including the apical impulse (diameter, location, amplitude, duration).
	Auscultate the 2nd right and left intercostal spaces, along the left sternal border, down the left sternal border to the 4th and 5th interspaces, and across to the apex with the *diaphragm*.
Left lateral decubitus	Palpate the apical impulse if not previously detected. Auscultate the apex with the *bell* of the stethoscope.
Sitting, leaning forward, after full exhalation	Auscultate the right sternal border for tricuspid murmurs and sounds with the *bell*.

Low-pitched extra sounds such as an S_3, OS, diastolic rumble of *mitral stenosis*

Soft decrescendo diastolic murmur of *aortic insufficiency*

Inspection

Carefully *inspect* the anterior chest for the location of the *apical impulse* or *point of maximal impulse* and heaves over the precordium, which indicate increased ventricular movement. Tangential light is useful for making this observation. Use *palpation* to confirm the characteristics of the apical impulse.

Palpation

- Begin with general palpation of the chest wall. First palpate for *heaves, (lifts),* using your *fingerpads.* Hold them flat or obliquely on the body surface. Ventricular impulses may heave or lift your fingers.

- Check for *thrills,* formed by the turbulence of underlying murmurs, by pressing the *ball of your hand* firmly on the chest. If subsequent auscultation reveals a loud murmur, go back to that area and check for thrills again.

Thrills may accompany loud, harsh, or rumbling murmurs as in *aortic stenosis, patent ductus arteriosus, ventricular septal defect,* and, less commonly, *mitral stenosis.* They are palpated more easily in patient positions that accentuate the murmur.

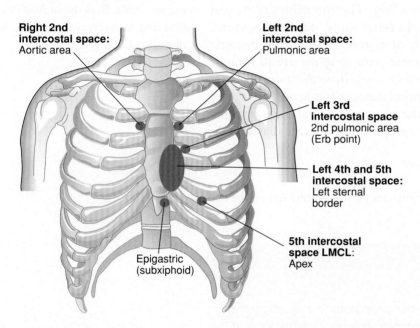

Right 2nd intercostal space: Aortic area

Left 2nd intercostal space: Pulmonic area

Left 3rd intercostal space 2nd pulmonic area (Erb point)

Left 4th and 5th intercostal space: Left sternal border

5th intercostal space LMCL: Apex

Epigastric (subxiphoid)

On rare occasions, a patient has *dextrocardia*—a heart situated on the right side. The apical impulse will then be found on the right. If you cannot find an apical impulse, percuss for the dullness of the heart and liver and for the tympany of the stomach. In *situs inversus,* all three of these structures are on opposite sides from normal. A right-sided heart with a normally placed liver and stomach is usually associated with congenital heart disease.

- Be sure to assess the *right ventricle* by palpating the right ventricular area at the lower left sternal border and in the subxiphoid area, the pulmonary artery in the left 2nd intercostal space, and the aortic area in the right 2nd intercostal space (see the diagram with palpation areas indicated).

Palpable pulsations of the right ventricle may indicate an enlarged right ventricle.

The Apical Impulse or Point of Maximal Impulse

The apical impulse represents the brief early pulsation of the left ventricle as it moves anteriorly during contraction and touches the chest wall.

Note that in most examinations the apical impulse is the point of maximal impulse, or PMI; however, some pathologic conditions may produce a pulsation that is more prominent than the apex beat, such as an enlarged right ventricle, a dilated pulmonary artery, or an aneurysm of the aorta.

If you cannot identify the apical impulse with the patient supine, ask the patient to roll partly onto the left side—this is the *left lateral decubitus* position. Palpate again, using the palmar surfaces of several fingers. If you cannot find the apical impulse, ask the patient to exhale fully and stop breathing for a few seconds. When examining a woman, it may be helpful to displace the left breast upward or laterally as necessary; alternatively, ask her to do this for you.

The apex beat is palpable in only 25% to 40% of healthy adults in the supine position and in 50% of healthy adults in the left lateral decubitus position, especially those who are thin.[1]

Once the apical impulse is found, make finer assessments with the fingertips, and then with one finger.

Obesity, a very muscular chest wall, or an increased anteroposterior diameter of the chest, however, may make it undetectable. Some apical impulses hide behind the rib cage, despite positioning.

Now assess the location, diameter, amplitude, and duration of the apical impulse. You may wish to have the patient breathe out and briefly stop breathing to check your findings.

See Table 14-3, Variations and Abnormalities of the Apical Impulse, p. 426.

- **Location.** Try to assess location with the patient *supine,* because the left lateral decubitus position displaces the apical impulse to the left. Locate two points: the intercostal spaces, usually the 5th or possibly the 4th, which give the vertical location; and the distance in centimeters from the *midsternal line,* which gives the horizontal location.

Midsternal   Midclavicular
line   line

Pregnancy or a high left diaphragm may displace the apical impulse upward and to the left.

Lateral displacement may occur with cardiac enlargement in *heart failure, cardiomyopathy, ischemic heart disease.* Displacement in deformities of the thorax and mediastinal shift, secondary to respiratory disease, may also occur.

Lateral displacement outside the midclavicular line increases the likelihood of cardiac enlargement and a low-left ventricular ejection fraction.

- **Diameter.** Palpate the diameter of the apical impulse. In the supine patient, it usually measures less than 2.5 cm and occupies only one intercostal space. It may feel larger in the left lateral decubitus position.

In the left lateral decubitus position, a *diffuse* PMI with a diameter greater than 3 cm indicates left ventricular enlargement.[16]

- **Amplitude.** Estimate the amplitude of the impulse. It is usually small and feels *brisk* and *tapping.* Some young people have an increased amplitude, or hyperkinetic impulse, especially when excited or after exercise; its duration, however, is normal.

Increased amplitude may also reflect *hyperthyroidism, severe anemia,* pressure overload of the left ventricle (as in *aortic stenosis*), or volume overload of the left ventricle (as in *mitral regurgitation*).

- **Duration.** Duration is the most useful characteristic of the apical impulse for identifying hypertrophy of the left ventricle. To assess duration, listen to the heart sounds as you feel the apical impulse, or watch the movement of your stethoscope as you listen at the apex. Estimate the proportion of systole occupied by the apical impulse. Normally it lasts through the first two thirds of systole, and often less, but does not continue to the second heart sound.

A *sustained,* high-amplitude impulse that is normally located suggests LVH from pressure overload (as in *hypertension*). If the impulse is also displaced laterally, it may indicate fluid volume overload.

A sustained low-amplitude (hypokinetic) impulse may result from *dilated cardiomyopathy.*

Right Ventricular Area—The Left Sternal Border in the 3rd, 4th, and 5th Intercostal Spaces

The patient should rest supine at 30 degrees. Place the tips of your curved fingers in the 3rd, 4th, and 5th intercostal spaces and try to feel the systolic impulse of the right ventricle. Again, asking the patient to breathe out and then briefly stop breathing improves your observation.

If an impulse or heave is palpable, assess its location, amplitude, and duration.

A marked increase in amplitude with little or no change in duration indicates chronic fluid volume overload of the right ventricle, as from an *atrial septal defect*. An impulse with increased amplitude and duration occurs with pressure overload of the right ventricle, as in *pulmonic stenosis* or *pulmonary hypertension*.

In patients with an increased anteroposterior (AP) diameter, palpation of the *right ventricle* in the *epigastric* or *subxiphoid area* is also useful. With your hand flattened, press your index finger just under the rib cage and up toward the left shoulder and try to feel right ventricular pulsations.

In obstructive pulmonary disease, hyperinflated lung may prevent palpation of an enlarged right ventricle in the left parasternal area. The impulse is felt easily, however, high in the epigastrium where heart sounds are also often heard best.

Asking the patient to inhale and briefly stop breathing is helpful. The inspiratory position moves your hand well away from the pulsations of the abdominal aorta, which might otherwise be confusing.

Pulmonic Area—The Left 2nd Intercostal Space

This intercostal space overlies the *pulmonary artery*. As the patient holds expiration, look and feel for an impulse and feel for possible heart sounds. In thin or shallow-chested patients, the pulsation of a pulmonary artery may sometimes be felt here, especially after exercise or with excitement.

Aortic Area—The Right 2nd Intercostal Space

This intercostal space overlies the aortic outflow tract. Search for pulsations and palpable heart sounds.

A prominent pulsation here often accompanies dilatation or increased flow in the pulmonary artery. A palpable S_2 suggests increased pressure in the pulmonary artery (pulmonary hypertension).

A palpable S_2 suggests systemic hypertension. A visible pulsation here suggests a dilated or aneurysmal aorta.

Percussion

Percussion is rarely used today to estimate cardiac size. X-rays, ECG, and echocardiography provide accurate measurement. Palpation of the apical impulse can provide a rough size estimate. When you cannot feel the apical impulse, however, percussion may be your only tool, but may not be reliable. Starting well to the left on the chest, percuss from resonance toward cardiac dullness in the 3rd, 4th, 5th, and possibly 6th intercostal spaces. It is especially difficult to obtain accurate findings in women. Ask the woman to lift her breast up and back before attempting percussion.

Auscultation

Auscultation of heart sounds and murmurs is an important skill of physical examination. In this section, you will learn the techniques for identifying S_1 and S_2, extra heart sounds in systole and diastole, and systolic and diastolic murmurs. Review the auscultatory areas on the Chapter 14, p. 406 with the following caveats: (1) many authorities discourage use of names such as "aortic area," because murmurs may be loudest in other areas; and (2) these areas may not apply to patients with cardiac enlargement, anomalies of the great vessels, or dextrocardia. It is best to use locations such as "base of the heart," apex, or parasternal border to describe your findings.

Know Your Stethoscope

The stethoscope has two sides, the diaphragm and the bell, which are acoustically different.

- *The diaphragm.* The diaphragm is better for picking up the relatively high-pitched sounds of S_1 and S_2, the murmurs of aortic and mitral regurgitation, and pericardial friction rubs. *Listen throughout the precordium* with the diaphragm, pressing it firmly against the chest.

- *The bell.* The bell is more sensitive to the low-pitched sounds of S_3 and S_4 and the murmur of mitral stenosis. Apply the bell lightly, with just enough pressure to produce an air seal with its full rim. *Use the bell at the apex, and then move medially along the lower sternal border.* Resting the heel of your hand on the chest like a fulcrum may help you to maintain light pressure.

Pressing the bell firmly on the chest makes it function more like the diaphragm by stretching the underlying skin. Low-pitched sounds such as S_3 and S_4 may disappear with this technique—an observation that may help to identify them. In contrast, high-pitched sounds such as a midsystolic click, an ejection sound, or an OS will persist or get louder.

There are three types of stethoscope heads. The simplest has only a diaphragm. This type is unsuitable for a full cardiac examination. The second type has a diaphragm on one side and a bell on the opposite side. The head of the stethoscope is rotated to open either the bell or the diaphragm. Lightly tapping on each side with the stethoscope in one's ears will reveal which side is open. The third type of head combines the diaphragm and bell on one side. The bell is activated by very light pressure (no ring should be seen on the skin when the stethoscope is removed) and with increased pressure it becomes a diaphragm. (A ring of blanched skin will remain for a few seconds.) This version comes as either a single-sided stethoscope or a double-sided stethoscope with a pediatric and adult side.

"Inching" Your Stethoscope

In a quiet room, listen to the heart with your stethoscope, starting at either the base or apex. Either pattern is satisfactory.

- Some experts recommend *starting at the apex and inching to the base:* move the stethoscope from the PMI medially to the left sternal border, superiorly to the 2nd intercostal space, then across the sternum to the 2nd intercostal space at the right sternal border.

- Alternatively, you can *start at the base and inch your stethoscope to the apex:* with your stethoscope in the right 2nd intercostal space close to the sternum, move along the left sternal border in each intercostal space from the 2nd through the 5th, and then to the apex.

Heart sounds and murmurs that originate in the four valves range widely, as illustrated. Use anatomic location rather than valve area to describe where murmurs and sounds are best heard.

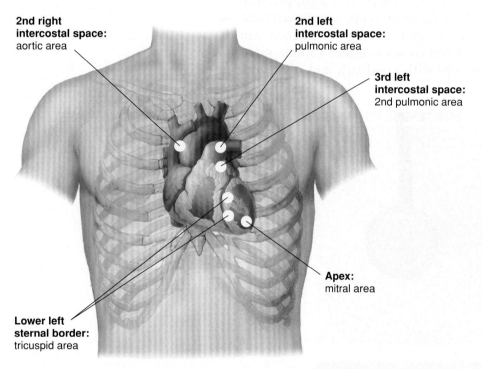

2nd right intercostal space: aortic area

2nd left intercostal space: pulmonic area

3rd left intercostal space: 2nd pulmonic area

Apex: mitral area

Lower left sternal border: tricuspid area

Aortic

Pulmonic

Tricuspid

Mitral

The Importance of Timing S₁ and S₂

Regardless of the direction you move your stethoscope, keep your left index and middle fingers on the right carotid artery in the lower third of the neck to facilitate correct identification of S_1, just before the carotid upstroke, and S_2, which follows the carotid upstroke. Be sure to compare the relative intensities of S_1 and S_2 as you move your stethoscope through the listening areas above.

- At the base S_2 is louder than S_1 and may split with respiration. At the apex, S_1 is usually louder than S_2 unless the PR interval is prolonged.

- By carefully noting the intensities of S_1 and S_2, you will confirm each of these sounds and thereby correctly identify *systole*, the interval between S_1 and S_2, and *diastole*, the interval between S_2 and S_1.

When listening to the extra sounds of S_3 and S_4 and to murmurs, timing systole and diastole is an absolute prerequisite to the correct identification of these events in the cardiac cycle.

Listen to the entire precordium with the patient supine. For new patients and patients needing a complete cardiac examination, use two other positions to listen for S_3, S_4, and the murmurs of mitral stenosis and aortic regurgitation.

Use Important Maneuvers

Ask the patient to *roll partly onto the left side into the left lateral decubitus position*, bringing the left ventricle close to the chest wall. Place the bell of your stethoscope lightly on the apical impulse.

This position accentuates or brings out a left-sided S_3 and S_4 and mitral murmurs, especially *mitral stenosis*. Otherwise, you may miss these important findings.

Next ask the patient to *sit up, lean forward, exhale completely, and stop breathing in expiration*. Pressing the diaphragm of your stethoscope on the chest, listen along the left sternal border and at the apex, pausing periodically so the patient may breathe.

This position accentuates or brings out aortic murmurs. You may easily miss the soft diastolic murmur of *aortic regurgitation* unless you listen at this position.

> **Concept Mastery Alert**
>
> Auscultating heart sounds can be challenging. To determine if an extra heart sound is heard after S_2, the nurse should observe the patient's respirations while listening to the heart. If the sound is a normal extra sound (split), then it will be heard on inspiration but not during expiration. To hear a possible diastolic murmur, the nurse would have the patient lean forward to bring the left ventricle closer to the chest wall.

Listening for Heart Sounds

Throughout your examination, take your time at each auscultatory area. Concentrate on each of the events in the cardiac cycle listed below and sounds heard in systole and diastole.

Auscultatory Sounds	
Heart Sounds	**Guides to Auscultation**
S_1	Note its intensity and any splitting. Normal splitting is detectable along the lower left sternal border.
S_2	Note its intensity.
Split S_2	Listen for splitting of this sound in the 2nd and 3rd left intercostal spaces. Ask the patient to breathe quietly, and then slightly more deeply than normal. Does S_2 split into its two components, as it normally does? If not, ask the patient to (1) breathe a little more deeply or (2) sit up. Listen again. A thick chest wall may make the pulmonic component of S_1 inaudible. ***Width of split.*** How wide is the split? It is normally quite narrow. ***Timing of split.*** When in the respiratory cycle do you hear the split? It is normally heard late in inspiration.

See Table 14-4, Variations in the First Heart Sound, S_1, p. 427. Note that S_1 is louder at more rapid heart rates (and PR intervals are shorter).

See Table 14-5, Variations in the Second Heart Sound—S_2, p. 428.

Expiratory splitting suggests an abnormality.

Persistent splitting results from delayed closure of the pulmonic valve or early closure of the aortic valve.

	Does the split disappear as it should, during exhalation? If not, listen again with the patient sitting up. Intensity of A_2 and P_2. Compare the intensity of the two components, A_2 and P_2. A_2 is usually louder.	A loud P_2 suggests pulmonary hypertension.
Extra Sounds in Systole	Such as ejection sounds or systolic clicks Note their location, timing, intensity, and pitch, and the effects of respiration on the sounds.	The systolic click of mitral valve prolapse is the most common of these sounds. See Table 14-6, Extra Heart Sounds in Systole, p. 429.
Extra Sounds in Diastole	Such as S_3, S_4, or an opening snap Note the location, timing, intensity, and pitch, and the effects of respiration on the sounds. (An S_3 or S_4 in athletes is a normal finding.)	See Table 14-7, Extra Heart Sounds in Diastole, p. 430.
Systolic and Diastolic Murmurs	Murmurs are differentiated from heart sounds by their longer duration.	See Table 14-8, Pansystolic Murmurs, p. 431; Table 14-9, Midsystolic Murmurs, pp. 432–433; Table 14-10, Diastolic Murmurs, p. 434.

Correctly Identifying Heart Murmurs

Correctly identifying heart murmurs requires a logical and systematic approach, a thorough understanding of cardiac anatomy and physiology.

- *Timing.* First decide if you are hearing a *systolic murmur,* falling between S_1 and S_2, or a *diastolic murmur,* falling between S_2 and S_1. The S_1 or S_2 sounds may be hidden by a loud murmur. Palpating the carotid pulse as you listen can help you with timing. *Murmurs that coincide with the carotid upstroke are systolic.* Murmurs can be described as occurring *early, mid, late or throughout (pan) systole or diastole.*

Diastolic murmurs usually indicate valvular heart disease. Systolic murmurs may indicate valvular disease but often occur when the heart valves are normal.

Systolic murmurs are usually *midsystolic* or *pansystolic.* Late systolic murmurs may also be heard.

Tips for Identifying Heart Murmurs

- Time the murmur—does it occur in systole or diastole?
- Locate where the murmur is loudest on the precordium—at the base, along the sternal border, at the apex?
- Conduct any necessary maneuvers, such as having the patient lean forward and exhale or turn to the left lateral decubitus position.
- Determine the shape of the murmur—for example, is it crescendo (becomes louder) or decrescendo (becomes softer), is it pansystolic?
- Grade the intensity of the murmur from 1 to 6.
- Identify associated features such as the quality of S_1 and S_2; the presence of extra sounds such as S_3, S_4, or an OS; or the presence of additional murmurs.
- Be sure to listen in a quiet room!

A *midsystolic murmur* begins after S_1 and stops before S_2. Brief gaps are audible between the murmur and the heart sounds. Listen carefully for the gap just before S_2. It is heard more easily and, if present, usually confirms the murmur as midsystolic, not pansystolic.

Midsystolic murmurs typically arise from blood flow across the semilunar (aortic and pulmonic) valves. See Table 14-9, Midsystolic Murmurs, pp. 432–433.

A *pansystolic (holosystolic) murmur* starts with S_1 and stops at S_2, without a gap between murmur and heart sounds.

Pansystolic murmurs often occur with regurgitant (backward) flow across the atrioventricular valves. See Table 14-8, Pansystolic Murmurs, p. 431.

A *late systolic murmur* usually starts in mid- or late systole and persists up to S_2.

This is the murmur of mitral valve prolapse and is often, but not always, preceded by a systolic click.

Diastolic murmurs may be early *diastolic*, *middiastolic*, or *late diastolic*.

An *early diastolic murmur* starts immediately after S_2, without a discernible gap, and then usually fades into silence before the next S_1.

Early diastolic murmurs typically accompany regurgitant flow across incompetent semilunar valves.

A *middiastolic murmur* starts a short time after S_2. It may fade away, as illustrated, or merge into a late diastolic murmur.

Middiastolic and presystolic murmurs reflect turbulent flow across the atrioventricular valves. See Table 14-10, Diastolic Murmurs, p. 434.

A *late diastolic (presystolic) murmur* starts late in diastole and typically continues up to S_1.

The murmur of a patent ductus arteriosus starts in systole and continues into diastole without a pause, but not necessarily throughout diastole. It is called a *continuous murmur*. Other cardiovascular sounds, such as pericardial friction rubs or venous hums, have *both systolic and diastolic components*. Observe and describe these sounds according to the characteristics used for systolic and diastolic murmurs.

See Table 14-11, Cardiovascular Sounds with both Systolic and Diastolic Components, p. 435.

- *Shape.* The shape or configuration of a murmur's shape is the most difficult for a novice to determine. Concentrate on learning the other characteristics of murmurs first. As your ears become attuned to listening, shape will become identifiable.

A *crescendo murmur* grows louder.

The late diastolic murmur of *mitral stenosis* in normal sinus rhythym

A *decrescendo murmur* grows softer.

The early diastolic murmur of *aortic regurgitation*

A *crescendo–decrescendo murmur* first rises in intensity, then falls.

The midsystolic murmur of aortic stenosis and innocent flow murmurs

A *plateau murmur* has the same intensity throughout.

The pansystolic murmur of *mitral regurgitation*

- *Location of Maximal Intensity.* Find the location where the murmur is heard in terms of the intercostal space and its relation to the sternum, the apex, or the midsternal, the midclavicular, or one of the axillary lines.

  For example, a murmur best heard in the 2nd right intercostal space often originates at or near the aortic valve.

- *Radiation or Transmission From the Point of Maximal Intensity.* This reflects not only the site of origin but also the intensity of the murmur and the direction of blood flow. Explore the area around a murmur and determine where else you can hear it.

  A loud murmur of *aortic stenosis* often radiates into the neck (in the direction of arterial flow), especially on the right side.

- *Intensity.* This is usually graded on a 6-point scale and expressed as a fraction. The numerator describes the intensity of the murmur wherever it is loudest; the denominator indicates the scale you are using. Intensity is influenced by the thickness of the chest wall and the presence of intervening tissue.

  An identical degree of turbulence would cause a louder murmur in a thin person than in a very muscular or obese person. Emphysematous lungs may diminish the intensity of murmurs.

Grade murmurs using the 6-point scale below. Note that Grades 4 through 6 require the added presence of a palpable thrill.

Grades of Murmurs	
Grade	**Description**
Grade 1	Very faint, heard only after listener has "tuned in"; may not be heard in all positions
Grade 2	Quiet, but heard immediately after placing the stethoscope on the chest
Grade 3	Moderately loud
Grade 4	Loud, with palpable thrill
Grade 5	Very loud, with thrill. May be heard when the stethoscope is partly off the chest
Grade 6	Very loud, with thrill. May be heard with stethoscope entirely off the chest

- *Pitch.* This is categorized as high, medium, or low.

- *Quality.* This is described in terms such as blowing, harsh, rumbling, and musical.

A fully described murmur might be: a "medium-pitched, grade 2/6, blowing decrescendo diastolic murmur, heard best in the 4th left intercostal space, with radiation to the apex" (aortic regurgitation).

Other characteristics of murmurs include variation with respiration or with the position of the patient. Document the position(s) of the patient or respiratory variation with the other characteristics.

Murmurs originating in the right side of the heart tend to vary with respiration more than left-sided murmurs.

Functional (innocent) murmurs are short, early, midsystolic murmurs that decrease in intensity with maneuvers that reduce left ventricular volume, such as standing, sitting up, and straining during the Valsalva maneuver.

Peripheral Edema

Inspect the patient's feet, ankles and legs for edema. See Chapter 15, The Peripheral Vascular System and Lymphatic System, for the examination techniques.

Peripheral edema may indicate heart failure.

Integrating Cardiovascular Assessment

Cardiovascular assessment requires more than careful examination. You need to correctly identify and interpret individual findings, fit them together in a logical pattern, and correlate your cardiac findings with the patient's blood pressure and heart rate, carotid upstroke and jugular venous pressure, the arterial pulses, the remainder of your physical examination, and the patient's history.

In a 60-year-old person with angina, you might hear a harsh 3/6 midsystolic crescendo–decrescendo murmur in the right 2nd intercostal space radiating to the neck. These findings suggest aortic stenosis but could arise from aortic sclerosis (leaflets sclerotic but not stenotic), a dilated aorta, or increased flow across a normal valve. Assess any delay in the carotid upstroke and the intensity of A_2 for evidence of aortic stenosis. Check the apical impulse for LVH. Listen for aortic regurgitation as the patient leans forward and exhales.

Evaluating the common systolic murmur illustrates this point. An asymptomatic teenager might have a grade 2/6 midsystolic murmur in the 2nd and 3rd left interspaces. Because this suggests a pulmonic murmur you should assess the right ventricle for hypertrophy by carefully palpating the left parasternal area. Because pulmonic stenosis and atrial septal defects can cause this murmur, auscultate carefully for a split S_2, any ejection sounds, and variation with inspiration. Listen to the murmur after the patient sits up. Look for evidence of anemia, hyperthyroidism, or pregnancy that could cause such a murmur by increasing the flow across the aortic or the pulmonic valve. If all your findings are normal, your patient probably has a *functional murmur*—one with no pathologic significance.

Integrating this information allows you to generate a differential diagnosis about the origin of the murmur.

RECORDING YOUR FINDINGS

Case: LPN/LVN: Med-Surg: NLN II, Case 4, Complex: Congestive Heart Failure/Fluid Overload: Charles Jones

[Show Learning Tips] [Return to Case Info]

Thursday, July 28, 2016 17:25

Jones, Charles J	**Gender:** Male	**Diagnosis:** Congestive heart failure	**Adm Provider:**
MRN: PCS42000	DOB: 6/24/1948	**Isolation Precaution:** Standard	**Facility:** Holy Cross Hospital
Allergies ❶ : No Known Allergies	Age: 68 Years	**Adv Directive:** Full Code	Room: 224 Bed: A
	Height: 72.5 in		Adm On: 7/26/2016 17:25 [2 day(s)]
	Weight: 182 lb		

Patient Info | **Assessment** | ADLs | Notes | Nursing Dx | Orders | MAR | I/O | Vital Signs | Diagnostics | Immunizations | Flowsheet

HEENT | Neuro | Cardio | Respiratory | GI | GU | Musculoskeletal | Mental Health | Pain Scale | Integumentary | Vascular Access

[Save Assessment] [Delete] [Cancel]   [Past Assessments ▼]

Edit Cardiac Assessment (Charted by Karri Babcock, Registered Nurse on 7/26/2016 17:45)

Documented By:

| Karri Babcock, Registered Nurse ▼ |

Documented At:

| 0 | days | 0 | hours | 20 | minutes | after admission ▼ |

Additional Notes

Complains of shortness of breath, cough with pink tinged sputum, fatigue and nocturia (3-4 times a night).

Heart Tones

☑ S1, S2   ☑ Regular
☐ Irregular ☐ Murmur
☐ S3   ☑ S4
☐ Gallop   ☐ Muffled
☐ Distant   ☐ Radiating

Pulses

	All	LUE	RUE	LLE	RLE
Absent	○	○	○	○	○
Intermittent	○	○	○	○	○
+1	○	○	○	●	●
+2	○	●	●	○	○
+3	○	○	○	○	○
Bounding	○	○	○	○	○
Doppler	○	○	○	○	○

Edema

	All	LUE	RUE	LLE	RLE
Absent	○	●	●	○	○
Trace	○	○	○	○	○
1+	○	○	○	○	○
2+	○	○	○	○	○
3+	○	○	○	●	●
4+	○	○	○	○	○
Non-Pitting	○	○	○	○	○
Pitting	○	○	○	○	○
Anasarca	○	○	○	○	○

Capillary Refill

	All	LUE	RUE	LLE	RLE
<3 sec	○	●	●	○	○
>3 sec	○	○	○	●	●
Absent	○	○	○	○	○

Skin Color and Description

☑ Appropriate for ethnicity   ☑ Warm
☐ Dry   ☑ Intact
☐ Cool   ☐ Clammy
☐ Cyanotic   ☐ Diaphoretic
☐ Blotchy   ☐ Dusky
☐ Flushed   ☐ Fragile
☐ Jaundiced   ☐ Moist
☐ Mottled   ☐ Pale
☐ Ashen

Skin Color Details:

Vasoactive Drips

| |

Rate Of Drip:

| |

Devices

☐ Pacer
☐ IABP
☐ CVP
☐ Pulmonary Artery Monitoring
☑ Cardiac Monitor

Cardiac Rhythm:

| Sinus tachycardia ▼ |

Notes:

Heart rate 96 - 116.
3+ edema lower extremities to mid-calf.

☐ Arterial Line

Recording the Physical Examination—The Cardiovascular Examination

"Carotid upstrokes are brisk, without bruits. JVP is 3 cm above the sternal angle with the head of bed elevated to 30 degrees. Jugular venous distension diminishes rapidly with hepatojugular reflex. The apical impulse is 2 cm in diameter, 7 cm lateral to the midsternal line in the 5th intercostal space. S_1 and S_2 crisp with regular rhythm. At the base S_2 is $>S_1$ and at the apex S_1 is $>S_2$. No murmurs or extra sounds."

OR

"Carotid upstrokes are brisk; a bruit is heard over the left carotid artery. The JVP is 5 cm above the sternal angle with the head of bed elevated to 50 degrees. Venous distension diminishes over 10 seconds with hepatojugular reflux. The apical impulse is diffuse, 3 cm in diameter, palpated at the anterior axillary line in the 5th and 6th intercostal spaces. S_1 and S_2 are soft. S_3 present at the apex. High-pitched harsh 2/6 holosystolic murmur best heard at the apex, radiating to the axilla."

Suggests *heart failure with volume overload* with partial *left carotid occlusion* and *mitral regurgitation*.[3,17–19]

HEALTH PROMOTION

Health Promotion Topics

- CHD and stroke prevention
- Hypertension prevention and management
- Hyperlipidemia prevention and management

Key roles for the nurse in health promotion are:

- Screening patients for disease and risk factors

- Teaching patients the relationship of risk factors to diseases

- Educating patients on lifestyle changes to reduce risk factors

- Encouraging patients to adhere to healthy lifestyles and medical regimens to reduce the incidence of disease morbidity

Profile of Cardiovascular Disease

Cardiovascular disease (CVD) affects 85.6 million U.S. adults and includes hypertension, CHD, heart failure, stroke, peripheral vascular disease, and congenital cardiovascular defects. CVD remains the leading cause of death for both men and women, accounting for approximately one third of all U.S. deaths.[6]

According to the U.S. Preventative Services Task Force, hypertension is a prevalent condition, affecting 29.1% of U.S. adults in 2011 to 2012. Uncontrolled hypertension is a risk factor for heart attack, stroke, and heart failure and a major contributing factor to cardiovascular and all-cause mortality in the United States. Primary hypertension has no known cause and few symptoms, but is responsible for approximately 95% of adult hypertension.[20]

Blood Pressure Classification for Adults

Category	Systolic (mm Hg)	Diastolic (mm Hg)	
Normal	<120	<80	No treatment required
Prehypertension	120–139	80–89	Lifestyle modifications advised

Stage 1 Hypertension
    Age ≥18 to <60
    Age ≥60
	
	140–159
	150–159
		
		90–99
		90–99
			Lifestyle modifications plus drug therapy

Stage 2 Hypertension	≥160	≥100	Lifestyle modifications plus drug therapy, frequently two-drug combination required
If Diabetes or Renal Disease (Including Age ≥60 years)	<140	<90	Begin drug therapy when BP is 140/90

Sources: James PA, Oparil S, Carter BL, et al. 2014 evidence-based guideline for the management of high blood pressure in adults: report from the panel members appointed to the Eighth Joint National Committee (JNC 8). *JAMA* 2014;311:507. Chobanian AV, Bakris GL, Black HR, et al. The Seventh Report of the Joint National Committee on Prevention, Detection, Evaluation, and Treatment of High Blood Pressure—The JNC 7 Report. *JAMA* 2003;289:2560–2572. Available at http://www.nhlbi.nih.gov/health-pro/guidelines/current/hypertension-jnc-7/complete-report. Accessed May 30, 2016.

Hypertension Facts

- "Individuals who are normotensive at 55 years have a 90% lifetime risk for developing hypertension."[21]
- "Prevalence rates increase with age, from 7.3% in persons aged 18 to 39 years to 32.4% in those aged 40 to 59 years and to 65.0% in those aged 60 years or older. Non-Hispanic black adults have the highest prevalence (42.1%) compared with white (28.0%), Hispanic (26.0%), and Asian (24.7%) Americans" and only 34% of those with hypertension have achieved blood pressure goals.[20]
- "For individuals aged 40 to 70 years, each increment of 20 mm Hg in systolic BP or 10 mm Hg in diastolic BP doubles the risk of CVD."[21]

- Identifying and treating people with risk factors are not enough. The American Heart Association's is expanding its focus beyond CVD prevention in adults to encouraging the development of healthy cardiovascular behaviors in childhood to lower the risk of developing cardiovascular disease in adulthood.[6]

High serum cholesterol and related lipid disorders are correlated with an elevated risk for CVD in many of the world's populations.[6]

Diabetes and metabolic syndrome increase a person's risk for CVD. Metabolic syndrome is a group of lipid and nonlipid risk factors of metabolic origin that increases the risk of heart disease, stroke, and diabetes. It is closely linked to the metabolic insulin resistance disorder.[6]

A client with three or more of these findings may have metabolic syndrome:[22]

- Large waist circumference (abdominal obesity)

   Men: waist circumference of 40 in or more
   Women: waist circumference of 35 in or more

- High blood pressure—≥130 mm Hg systolic or ≥85 mm Hg diastolic or undergoing drug treatment

- High fasting blood sugar—fasting glucose of ≥100 mg/dL or being treated for high glucose.

- High triglycerides—150 mg/dL or higher or undergoing drug treatment for elevated triglycerides

- Low high-density lipoprotein (HDL; good) cholesterol or being treated with drugs.

   Men: <40 mg/dL
   Women: <50 mg/dL

Risk Reduction

Identification of the patient's risk factors for CVD is a primary nursing function and a part of the history. The risks for cardiac disorders and hypertension overlap, as seen on the next page. The more risk factors an individual has, the greater is the chance of developing heart disease. Also, the greater the level of each risk factor, the greater is the risk (e.g., a low-density lipoprotein [LDL] cholesterol of 160 is a greater risk than 1 of 135). Decreasing the number and severity of risk factors reduces the risk of developing heart disease.

Coronary Heart Disease Risk Factors

Modifiable Risk Factors
Diabetes
Systolic and/or diastolic hypertension
Elevated cholesterol and/or triglycerides
Smoking
Obesity
Physical inactivity

Nonmodifiable Factors
Increasing age
History of cardiovascular disease
Family history of early heart disease (younger than 55 years for men and 65 years for women)

Hypertension Risk Factors[23]

Modifiable Risk Factors
Obesity
Physical inactivity
Smoking
Microalbuminuria or a glomerular filtration rate of <60 mL/min
Excess dietary sodium
Insufficient intake of potassium
Excess alcohol consumption

Nonmodifiable Factors
Age
Family history of hypertension or early CVD

The National Cholesterol Education Program (NCEP) wrote a report titled *Detection, Evaluation, and Treatment of High Cholesterol in Adults (Adult Treatment Panel III)* or ATP III that provides guidelines on how to prevent, detect, evaluate, and treat high blood cholesterol.

The 8th Report of the Joint National Committee on Prevention, Detection, Evaluation, and Treatment of High Blood Pressure (JNC-8) describes how to prevent, detect, evaluate, and treat high blood pressure.[24]

Risk assessment is a key element of the report. Screening for adults should begin at 20 years, and the American Academy of Pediatrics recommends screening all children for cholesterol levels and hypertension. Adults 40 years and older should have their *10-year global risk* for heart disease estimated to help them keep their risk as low as possible.

Risk Factors Used to Assess the 10-Year Coronary Heart Disease Risk Score

Age
Gender
Height, weight, waist circumference (or body mass index [BMI])
Smoking
History of CVD or diabetes
Systolic and diastolic blood pressure
Total cholesterol, LDL and HDL cholesterol
Triglycerides
Family history of early heart disease*

*Family is a blood-related parent, sibling, or child.

Risk assessment tools for Coronary Heart Disease (CHD) and metabolic syndrome were developed from the ATP III national guidelines based on research from the Framingham Heart Study.

The CHD tool predicts a patient's risk of suffering a heart attack or dying of heart disease over the next 10 years. For example, if the patient scores a 10% risk, it means in a group of 100 people with similar risk factors about 10 will have a heart attack or die from heart disease (CHD) in the next 10 years.

The CHD risk tool can be found on the following Websites. http://cvdrisk.nhlbi.nih.gov/http://www.heart.org/HEARTORG/Conditions/HeartAttack/HeartAttackToolsResources/Heart-Attack-Risk-Assessment_UCM_303944_Article.jsp

A more sensitive assessment tool called the Reynolds Risk Score was developed for women. This tool is based on data from both the Framingham Heart Study and the Women's Health Study from Harvard. The researchers added C-reactive protein to the risk analysis.[25,26]

This tool can be found at www.reynoldsriskscore.org.

Screening for hypertension, cardiovascular disease, hyperlipidemia, metabolic syndrome, and other risk factors should be carried out routinely. A suggested schedule is on the next page; however, if a condition is present, more frequent screening is recommended. The nurse should encourage patients to obtain regular screening.[27]

Risk Factors and Screening Frequency for Adults Beginning at 20 Years	
Risk Factor	**Frequency**
Family history of coronary heart disease (CHD)	Update regularly
Smoking status Diet Alcohol intake Physical activity	At each routine visit
Blood pressure Body mass index Waist circumference Pulse (to detect atrial fibrillation)	At each routine visit (at least every 2 years)
Fasting lipoprotein profile	Every 5 years if low risk; every 2 years if strong risk
Fasting glucose, HgA1C	If risk factors for hyperlipidemia or diabetes present

Source: Pearson TA, Blair SN, Daniels SR, et al. AHA guidelines for primary prevention of cardiovascular disease and stroke: 2002 update. *Circulation.* 2002;106(3):388–391.

Healthy Lifestyles

Educating patients about healthy lifestyle choices and encouraging them to make changes is an important nursing role. It is helpful to obtain a picture of the client's lifestyle before "preaching" changes. Many patients will already include healthy choices in their lives. A nutrition history (see Chapter 8, Nutrition and Hydration, pp. 152–153) and a "typical day" record can help the nurse identify good diet choices and where improvements can be made. Healthy choices should be affirmed. The nurse can then work with the patient to identify where further change is needed and create a mutually agreed upon change plan. The nurse can also supply resources that may help the patient achieve goals. For example, if the patient's goal is to stop smoking, the nurse can explain aids available to decrease the desire for nicotine. Prochaska and DiClemente's Stages of Change Model can be used during a patient assessment to help the nurse determine interventions appropriate to the patient's level.[28]

Lifestyle Modifications to Prevent or Manage Hypertension

- Maintenance of an optimal weight or BMI of 18.5 to 24.9
- Salt intake of <6 g of sodium chloride or 2,300 mg of sodium per day. However individuals with hypertension, diabetes or kidney disease, ≥51 years or are African American should consume no more than 1,500 mg of sodium per day.[29]
- Regular aerobic exercise, such as brisk walking for at least 30 minutes per day, most days of the week
- Moderate alcohol consumption per day of two drinks or fewer for men and one drink or fewer for women (two drinks = 1 oz ethanol, 24 oz beer, 10 oz wine, or 2 to 3 oz whiskey)
- Dietary intake of more than 3,500 mg of potassium
- Diet rich in fruits, vegetables, and low-fat dairy products with reduced content of saturated and total fat

Source: CDC. Preventing High Blood Pressure: Healthy Living Habits. Available at http://www.cdc.gov/bloodpressure/healthy_living.htm. Accessed October 30, 2015; Whelton PK, He J, Appel LJ, et al. Primary prevention of hypertension. Clinical and Public Health Advisory from the National High Blood Pressure Education Program. *JAMA.* 2002;28815:1882–1888.

Lifestyle Modifications to Prevent Cardiovascular Disease and Stroke

- Complete cessation of smoking
- Optimal blood pressure control
- Healthy eating—see diet recommendations
- Lipid management
- Regular aerobic exercise
- Optimal weight
- Diabetes management so that fasting glucose level is below 110 mg/dL and HgA1C is <7%
- Conversion of atrial fibrillation to NSR or, if chronic, anticoagulation

Source: Pearson TA, Blair SN, Daniels SR, et al. AHA guidelines for primary prevention of cardiovascular disease and stroke: 2002 update. *Circulation.*2002;106(3):388–391 and CDC. Preventing High Blood Pressure: Healthy Living Habits. Available at: http://www.cdc.gov/bloodpressure/healthy_living.htm. Accessed October 30, 2015.

Healthy Eating

Begin with a nutrition history (see Chapter 8, Nutrition and Hydration, pp. 152–153), and then target low intake of cholesterol and total fat, especially less saturated and *trans* fat. Foods with monounsaturated fats, polyunsaturated fats, and omega-3 fatty acids in fish oils help to lower blood cholesterol. Review the food sources of these healthy and unhealthy fats on the next page.

Food Sources of Healthy and Unhealthy Fats

Healthy Fats
* *Foods high in monounsaturated fat:* nuts, such as almonds, pecans, and peanuts; sesame seeds; avocados; canola oil; olive and peanut oil; peanut butter
* *Foods high in polyunsaturated fat:* corn, safflower, cottonseed, and soybean oil; walnuts; pumpkin or sunflower seeds; soft (tub) margarine; mayonnaise; salad dressings
* *Foods high in omega-3 fatty acids:* albacore tuna, herring, mackerel, rainbow trout, salmon, sardines, anchovies, shrimp, flaxseed, walnuts

Unhealthy Fats
* *Foods high in trans fat:* snacks and baked goods with hydrogenated or partially hydrogenated oil, stick margarines, shortening, fried foods
* *Foods high in cholesterol:* dairy products, liver and organ meats, high-fat meat and poultry
* *Foods high in saturated fat:* high-fat dairy products—cream, cheese, ice cream, whole and 2% milk, butter, and sour cream; bacon; chocolate; lard and gravy from meat drippings; high-fat meats like ground beef, bologna, hot dogs, and sausage

Source: U.S. Department of Agriculture and U.S. Department of Health and Human Services. Dietary Guidelines for Americans, 2010. Washington, D.C., U.S. Government Printing Office. 7th ed. Available at http://www.health.gov/dietaryguidelines/dga2010/DietaryGuidelines2010.pdf. Accessed May 31, 2016.

Counseling About Weight and Exercise

The Healthy People 2020 Nutrition and Weight Status reports that dietary factors are associated with 4 of the 10 leading causes of death—coronary heart disease, some types of cancer, stroke, and type 2 diabetes—as well as with high blood pressure and osteoporosis.[30] More than 60% of all Americans are now obese or overweight, with a BMI of 25 or greater.

Counseling about weight has become imperative for nurses. Assess BMI as described in Chapter 8, Nutrition and Hydration, pp. 157–158. Discuss the principles of healthy eating—patients with high fat intake are more likely to accumulate body fat than patients with high intake of protein and carbohydrate. Review the patient's eating habits and weight patterns in the family. Set realistic goals that will help the patient maintain healthy eating habits *for life*.

Exercise is a critical adjunct to weight control for maintaining health. *Healthy People 2020's* overview on Physical Activity notes that "Regular physical activity can improve the health and quality of life of Americans of all ages, regardless of the presence of a chronic disease or disability. Among adults and older adults, physical activity can lower the risk of early death, coronary heart disease, stroke, high blood pressure, type 2 diabetes, breast and colon cancer, falls, and depression."[31] To reduce the risk for CHD, counsel patients to pursue aerobic exercise, or exercise that increases muscle oxygen uptake, for at least 30 minutes on most days of the week. Spur motivation by emphasizing the immediate benefits to health and well-being. Deep breathing, sweating in cool temperatures, and pulse rates exceeding 60% of the maximum normal age-adjusted heart rate, or 220 minus the person's age, are markers that help patients recognize onset of aerobic metabolism. Be sure to evaluate any cardiovascular, pulmonary, or musculoskeletal conditions that present risks before selecting an exercise regimen.

TABLE

14-1

Selected Heart Rates and Rhythms

Cardiac rhythms may be classified as *regular or irregular.* When rhythms are irregular or rates are fast or slow, an ECG should be obtained to identify the origin of the beats (sinus node, AV node, atrium, or ventricle) and the pattern of conduction. The normal range for normal sinus rhythm is reported at 50 to 90 beats/minute.[32] Note that with AV (atrioventricular) block, arrhythmias may have a fast, normal, or slow ventricular rate.

	ECG Pattern	Usual Resting Rate

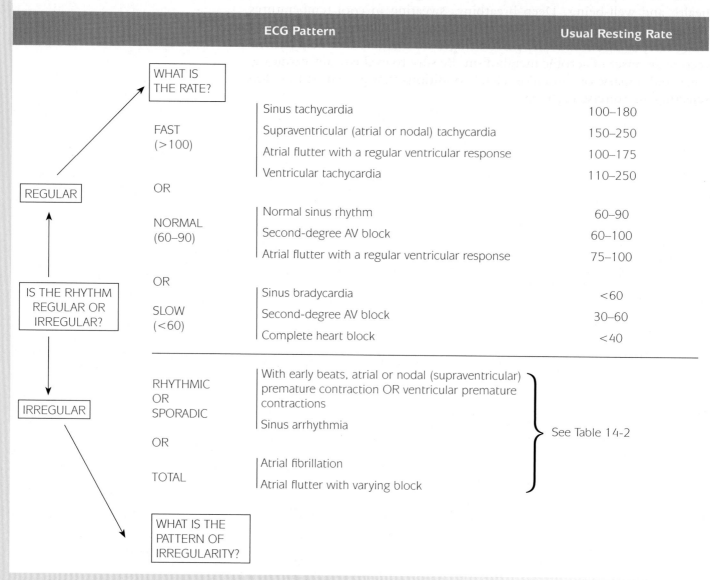

WHAT IS THE RATE?		
FAST (>100)	Sinus tachycardia	100–180
	Supraventricular (atrial or nodal) tachycardia	150–250
	Atrial flutter with a regular ventricular response	100–175
	Ventricular tachycardia	110–250
OR		
NORMAL (60–90)	Normal sinus rhythm	60–90
	Second-degree AV block	60–100
	Atrial flutter with a regular ventricular response	75–100
OR		
SLOW (<60)	Sinus bradycardia	<60
	Second-degree AV block	30–60
	Complete heart block	<40
RHYTHMIC OR SPORADIC	With early beats, atrial or nodal (supraventricular) premature contraction OR ventricular premature contractions	See Table 14-2
	Sinus arrhythmia	
OR		
TOTAL	Atrial fibrillation	
	Atrial flutter with varying block	

REGULAR

IS THE RHYTHM REGULAR OR IRREGULAR?

IRREGULAR

WHAT IS THE PATTERN OF IRREGULARITY?

TABLE
14-2

Selected Irregular Rhythms

Type of Rhythm	ECG Waves and Heart Sounds	

Atrial or Nodal Premature Contractions (Supraventricular)

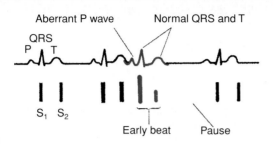

Rhythm. A beat of atrial or nodal origin comes earlier than the next expected normal beat. A pause follows, and then the rhythm resumes.

Heart Sounds. S_1 may differ in intensity from the S_1 of normal beats, and S_2 may be decreased.

Ventricular Premature Contractions

Rhythm. A beat of ventricular origin comes earlier than the next expected normal beat. A pause follows, and the rhythm resumes.

Heart Sounds. S_1 may differ in intensity from the S_1 of the normal beats, and S_2 may be decreased. Both sounds are likely to be split.

Sinus Arrhythmia

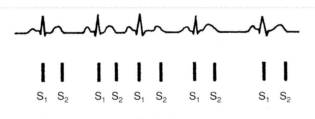

Rhythm. The heart varies cyclically, usually speeding up with inspiration and slowing down with expiration.

Heart Sounds. Normal, although S_1 may vary with the heart rate.

Atrial Fibrillation and Atrial Flutter With Varying AV Block

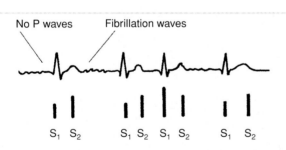

Rhythm. The ventricular rhythm is totally irregular, although short runs of the irregular ventricular rhythm may seem regular.

Heart Sounds. S_1 varies in intensity.

TABLE
14-3

Variations and Abnormalities of the Apical Impulse

In the healthy heart, the apical impulse or *left ventricular impulse* is usually the *point of maximal impulse*, or *PMI*. This brief impulse is generated by the movement of the ventricular apex against the chest wall during contraction. The classical descriptors of the apical impulse are:

- *Location:* in the 4th or 5th intercostal space, ~7–10 cm lateral to the midsternal line, depending on the diameter of the chest
- *Diameter: discrete,* or ≤2 cm
- *Amplitude:* brisk and *tapping*
- *Duration:* ≤2/3 of systole

Careful examination of the apical impulse gives you important clues about underlying cardiovascular hemodynamics. The quality of the impulse changes as the left ventricle adapts to high-output states (anxiety, hyperthyroidism, and severe anemia) and to the more pathologic conditions of chronic pressure or volume overload. Note below the distinguishing features of three types of apical impulses: the *hyperkinetic impulse* from transiently increased stroke volume—this change does not necessarily indicate heart disease; the *sustained* impulse of ventricular hypertrophy from chronic pressure load, known as *increased afterload* (see p. 384); and the *diffuse* impulse of ventricular dilation from chronic volume overload, or *increased preload*.

	Left Ventricular Impulse		
	Hyperkinetic	**Pressure Overload (Increased Afterload)**	**Volume Overload (Increased Preload)**
Examples of Causes	Anxiety, hyperthyroidism, severe anemia	Aortic stenosis, hypertension	Aortic or mitral regurgitation
Location	Normal	Normal	Displaced to the left and possibly downward
Diameter	~2 cm, though increased amplitude may make it seem larger	>2 cm	>2 cm
Amplitude	More forceful tapping	More forceful tapping	*Diffuse*
Duration	<2/3 systole	*Sustained* (up to S_2)	Often slightly sustained

TABLE
14-4

Variations in the First Heart Sound—S$_1$

Normal

S_1 is softer than S_2 at the *base* (right and left 2nd intercostal spaces).

S_1 is often but not always louder than S_2 at the *apex*.

Accentuated S$_1$

S_1 is accentuated in (1) tachycardia, rhythms with a short PR interval, and high cardiac output states (e.g., exercise, anemia, hyperthyroidism) and (2) mitral stenosis. In these conditions, the mitral valve is still open wide at the onset of ventricular systole and then closes quickly.

Diminished S$_1$

S_1 is diminished in first-degree heart block (delayed conduction from atria to ventricles). Here the mitral valve has had time after atrial contraction to float back into an almost closed position before ventricular contraction shuts it. It closes more quietly. S_1 is also diminished (1) when the mitral valve is calcified and relatively immobile, as in mitral regurgitation, and (2) when left ventricular contractility is markedly reduced, as in heart failure or coronary heart disease.

Varying S$_1$

S_1 varies in intensity (1) in complete heart block, when atria and ventricles are beating independently of each other, and (2) in any totally irregular rhythm (e.g., atrial fibrillation). In these situations, the mitral valve is in varying positions before being shut by ventricular contraction. Its closure sound, therefore, varies in loudness.

Split S$_1$

S_1 may be split normally along the lower left sternal border where the tricuspid component, often too faint to be heard, becomes audible. This split may sometimes be heard at the apex, but if heard it should be differentiated from an S_4, an aortic ejection sound, or an early systolic click. Abnormal splitting of both heart sounds may be heard in right bundle branch block and in premature ventricular contractions.

TABLE

14-5

Variations in the Second Heart Sound—S_2

Inspiration	Expiration	

Physiologic Splitting

Listen for *physiologic splitting* of S_2 in the *2nd or 3rd left intercostal space*. The pulmonic component of S_2 is usually too faint to be heard at the apex or aortic area, where S_2 is a single sound derived from aortic valve closure alone. Normal splitting is *accentuated by inspiration* and usually *disappears on expiration*. In some patients, especially younger ones, S_2 may not become single on expiration, but may merge when the patient sits up.

Pathologic Splitting *(involves splitting during expiration and suggests heart disease)*

Wide splitting of S_2 refers to an increase in the usual splitting that persists throughout the respiratory cycle. Wide splitting can be caused by delayed closure of the pulmonic valve (as in pulmonic stenosis or right bundle branch block). As illustrated here, right bundle branch block also causes splitting of S_1 into its mitral and tricuspid components. Wide splitting can also be caused by early closure of the aortic valve, as in mitral regurgitation.

Fixed splitting refers to wide splitting that does not vary with respiration. It occurs in atrial septal defect and right ventricular failure.

Paradoxical or reversed splitting refers to splitting that appears on expiration and disappears on inspiration. Closure of the aortic valve is abnormally delayed so that A_2 follows P_2 in expiration. Normal inspiratory delay of P_2 makes the split disappear. The most common cause of paradoxical splitting is left bundle branch block.

TABLE

14-6

Extra Heart Sounds in Systole

There are two kinds of extra heart sounds in systole: (1) early ejection sounds and (2) clicks, commonly heard in mid- and late systole.

**Early Systolic
Ejection Sounds**

S_1 E_j S_2

Early systolic ejection sounds occur shortly after S_1, coincident with opening of the aortic and pulmonic valves.[1] They are relatively high in pitch; have a sharp, clicking quality; and are heard better with the diaphragm of the stethoscope. An ejection sound indicates cardiovascular disease.

Listen for an *aortic ejection sound* at both the base and apex. It may be louder at the apex and usually does not vary with respiration. An aortic ejection sound may accompany a dilated aorta, or aortic valve disease from congenital stenosis or a bicuspid valve.[33,34]

A *pulmonic ejection sound* is heard best in the 2nd and 3rd left intercostal spaces. When S_1, usually relatively soft in this area, appears to be loud, you may be hearing a pulmonic ejection sound. Its intensity often *decreases with inspiration*. Causes include dilatation of the pulmonary artery, pulmonary hypertension, and pulmonic stenosis.

Systolic Clicks

S_1 C_1 S_2

Systolic clicks are usually caused by *mitral valve prolapse*—an abnormal systolic ballooning of part of the mitral valve into the left atrium. The clicks are usually mid- or late systolic. Prolapse of the mitral valve is a common cardiac condition, affecting about 2–3% of the general population. There is equal prevalence in men and women.[35–37]

The click is usually single, but you may hear more than one, usually *at or medial to the apex,* but also *at the lower left sternal border.* It is high-pitched, so listen with the diaphragm. The click is often followed by a late systolic murmur from mitral regurgitation—a flow of blood from left ventricle to left atrium. The murmur usually crescendos up to S_2. Auscultatory findings are notably variable. Most patients have only a click, some have only a murmur, and some have both. Systolic clicks may also be of extracardial or mediastinal origin.

TABLE
14-7

Extra Heart Sounds in Diastole

Opening Snap

S_1	S_2 OS	S_1

The *opening snap* is a very early diastolic sound usually produced by the opening of a *stenotic mitral valve*. It is heard best just medial to the apex and along the lower left sternal border. When it is loud, an opening snap radiates to the apex and to the pulmonic area, where it may be mistaken for the pulmonic component of a split S_2. Its high pitch and snapping quality help to distinguish it from an S_2. It is heard better with the *diaphragm*.

S_3

S_1	S_2 S_3	S_1

You will detect *physiologic* S_3 frequently in children and in young adults to the age of 35 or 40. It is common during the last trimester of pregnancy. Occurring early in diastole during rapid ventricular filling, it is later than an opening snap, dull and low in pitch, and heard best at the apex in the left lateral decubitus position. The *bell* of the stethoscope should be used with very light pressure.

A *pathologic S_3* or *ventricular gallop* sounds just like a physiologic S_3. An S_3 in a person over age 40 (possibly a little older in women) is almost certainly pathologic, arising from altered left ventricular compliance at the end of the rapid filling phase of diastole.[38,39] Causes include decreased myocardial contractility, heart failure, and volume overloading of a ventricle, as in mitral or tricuspid regurgitation. A *left-sided S_3* is heard typically at the apex in the left lateral decubitus position. A *right-sided S_3* is usually heard along the lower left sternal border or below the xiphoid with the patient supine, and is louder on inspiration. The term *gallop* comes from the cadence of three heart sounds, especially at rapid heart rates, and sounds like "Kentucky."

S_4

S_1	S_2	S_4 S_1

An S_4 (*atrial sound* or *atrial gallop*) occurs just before S_1. It is dull, low in pitch, and heard better with the bell. Listen at the lower left sternal border for a right ventricular S_4. An S_4 is heard occasionally in an apparently normal person, especially in trained athletes and older age groups. More commonly, it is due to increased resistance to ventricular filling following atrial contraction. This increased resistance is related to decreased compliance (increased stiffness) of the ventricular myocardium.[1,40]

Causes of a left-sided S_4 include hypertensive heart disease, coronary artery disease, aortic stenosis, and cardiomyopathy. A *left-sided S_4* is heard best at the apex in the left lateral position; it may sound like "Tennessee." The less common *right-sided S_4* is heard along the lower left sternal border or below the xiphoid. It often gets louder with inspiration. Causes of a right-sided S_4 include pulmonary hypertension and pulmonic stenosis.

An S_4 may also be associated with delayed conduction between the atria and ventricles. This delay separates the normally faint atrial sound from the louder S_1 and makes it audible. An S_4 is never heard in the absence of atrial contraction, which occurs with atrial fibrillation.

Occasionally, a patient has both an S_3 and an S_4, producing a *quadruple rhythm* of four heart sounds. At rapid heart rates, the S_3 and S_4 may merge into one loud extra heart sound, called a *summation gallop*.

TABLE
14-8

Pansystolic (Holosystolic) Murmurs

Pansystolic (holosystolic) murmurs are pathologic, arising from blood flow from a chamber with high pressure to one of lower pressure, through a valve or other structure that should be closed. The murmur begins immediately with S_1 and continues up to S_2.

	Mitral Regurgitation[41-44]	Tricuspid Regurgitation[1,45,46]	Ventricular Septal Defect
Murmur	*Location*. Apex	*Location*. Lower left sternal border	*Location*. 3rd, 4th, and 5th left intercostal spaces
	Radiation. To the left axilla, less often to the left sternal border	*Radiation*. To the right of the sternum, to the xiphoid area, and perhaps to the left midclavicular line, but not into the axilla	*Radiation*. Often wide
	Intensity. Soft to loud; if loud, associated with an apical thrill	*Intensity*. Variable	*Intensity*. Often very loud, with a thrill
	Pitch. Medium to high	*Pitch*. Medium	*Pitch*. High, holosystolic
	Quality. Harsh, holosystolic	Quality. Blowing, holosystolic	*Quality*. Often harsh
	Aids. Unlike tricuspid regurgitation, it does not become louder in inspiration.	*Aids*. Unlike mitral regurgitation, the intensity may increase slightly with inspiration.	
Associated Findings	S_1 normal (75%), loud (12%), soft (12%)	The right ventricular impulse is increased in amplitude and may be sustained.	S_2 may be obscured by the loud murmur.
	An apical S_3 reflects volume overload of the left ventricle.	An S_3 may be audible along the lower left sternal border. The jugular venous pressure is often elevated, with large *v* waves in the jugular veins.	Findings vary with the severity of the defect and with associated lesions.
	The apical impulse is increased in amplitude (diffuse), is laterally displaced, and may be sustained.		
Mechanism	When the *mitral valve fails to close fully in systole,* blood regurgitates from left ventricle to left atrium, causing a murmur. This leakage creates volume overload on the left ventricle, with subsequent dilatation.	When the *tricuspid valve fails to close fully in systole,* blood regurgitates from right ventricle to right atrium, producing a murmur. The most common cause is right ventricular failure and dilatation, with resulting enlargement of the tricuspid orifice. Either pulmonary hypertension or left ventricular failure is the usual initiating cause.	A ventricular septal defect is a congenital abnormality in which *blood flows from the relatively high-pressure left ventricle into the low-pressure right ventricle through a hole.*

TABLE
14-9

Midsystolic Murmurs

Midsystolic ejection murmurs are the most common kind of heart murmur. They may be (1) *innocent*—without any detectable physiologic or structural abnormality; (2) *physiologic*—from physiologic changes in body metabolism; or (3) *pathologic*—arising from a structural abnormality in the heart or great vessels.[1,47,48] Midsystolic murmurs tend to peak near midsystole and usually stop before S_2. The crescendo–decrescendo or "diamond" shape is not always audible, but the gap between the murmur and S_2 helps to distinguish midsystolic from pansystolic murmurs.

	Innocent Murmurs	Physiologic Murmurs
	S_1 S_2	S_1 S_2
Murmur	*Location*. 2nd to 4th left intercostal spaces between the left sternal border and the apex	Similar to innocent murmurs
	Radiation. Little	
	Intensity. Grades 1–2, possibly 3	
	Pitch. Soft to medium	
	Quality. Variable	
	Aids. Usually decreases or disappears on sitting	
Associated Findings	None: normal splitting, no ejection sounds, no diastolic murmurs, and no palpable evidence of ventricular enlargement. Occasionally, both an innocent murmur and another kind of murmur are present.	Possible signs of a likely cause
Mechanism	Innocent murmurs result from turbulent blood flow, probably generated by ventricular ejection of blood into the aorta from the left and occasionally the right ventricle. Very common in children and young adults—may also be heard in older people. There is no underlying cardiovascular disease.	Turbulence due to a temporary increase in blood flow in predisposing conditions such as anemia, pregnancy, fever, and hyperthyroidism.

Pathologic Murmurs		
Aortic Stenosis[49]	**Hypertrophic Cardiomyopathy**[50]	**Pulmonic Stenosis**[51]
Location. Right 2nd intercostal space	*Location.* 3rd and 4th left intercostal spaces	*Location.* 2nd and 3rd left intercostal spaces
Radiation. Often to the carotids, down the left sternal border, even to the apex	*Radiation.* Down the left sternal border to the apex, possibly to the base, but not to the neck	*Radiation.* If loud, toward the left shoulder and neck
Intensity. Sometimes soft but often loud, with a thrill	*Intensity.* Variable	*Intensity.* Soft to loud; if loud, associated with a thrill
Pitch. Medium, harsh; crescendo–decrescendo may be higher at the apex	*Pitch.* Medium	*Pitch.* Medium; crescendo–decrescendo
Quality. Often harsh; may be more musical at the apex	*Quality.* Harsh	*Quality.* Often harsh
Aids. Heard best with the patient sitting and leaning forward	*Aids.* Decreases with squatting, increases with straining down from Valsalva and standing	
A_2 decreases as aortic stenosis worsens. A_2 may be delayed and merge with $P_2 \rightarrow$ single S_2 on expiration or paradoxical S_2 split. Carotid upstroke may be *delayed*, with slow rise and small amplitude. Hypertrophied left ventricle may $\rightarrow$ *sustained* apical impulse and an S_4 from decreased compliance.	S_3 may be present. An S_4 is often present at the apex (unlike mitral regurgitation). The apical impulse may be *sustained* and have two palpable components. The carotid pulse rises *quickly,* unlike the pulse in aortic stenosis.	In severe stenosis, S_2 is widely split, and P_2 is diminished or inaudible. An early pulmonic ejection sound is common. May hear a right-sided S_4. Right ventricular impulse often increased in amplitude and *sustained.*
Significant aortic valve stenosis impairs blood flow across the valve, causing turbulence, and increases left ventricular afterload. Causes are congenital, rheumatic, and degenerative; findings may differ with each cause. Other conditions mimic aortic stenosis without obstructing flow: *aortic sclerosis,* a stiffening of aortic valve leaflets associated with aging; a *bicuspid aortic valve,* a congenital condition that may not be recognized until adulthood; a *dilated aorta,* as in arteriosclerosis, syphilis, or Marfan syndrome; *pathologically increased flow across the aortic valve* during systole can accompany aortic regurgitation.	Massive ventricular hypertrophy is associated with unusually rapid ejection of blood from the left ventricle during systole. Outflow tract obstruction of flow may coexist. Accompanying distortion of the mitral valve may cause mitral regurgitation.	Pulmonic valve stenosis impairs flow across the valve, increasing right ventricular afterload. Congenital and usually found in children. In an *atrial septal defect,* the systolic murmur from pathologically increased flow across the pulmonic valve may mimic pulmonic stenosis.

TABLE

14-10

Diastolic Murmurs

Diastolic murmurs almost always indicate heart disease. There are two basic types. *Early decrescendo diastolic murmurs* signify regurgitant flow through an incompetent semilunar valve, more commonly the aortic. *Rumbling diastolic murmurs in mid- or late* diastole suggest stenosis of an atrioventricular valve, usually the mitral.

	Aortic Regurgitation[1,44,52,53]	Mitral Stenosis[1,52]
	S_2 S_1	Accentuated S_2 OS S_1
Murmur	*Location*. 2nd to 4th left intercostal spaces	*Location*. Usually limited to the apex
	Radiation. If loud, to the apex, perhaps to the right sternal border	*Radiation*. Little or none
	Intensity. Grades 1–3	*Intensity*. Grades 1–4
	Pitch. High. *Use the diaphragm.*	*Pitch*. Decrescendo low-pitched rumble. *Use the bell.*
	Quality. Blowing decrescendo; may be mistaken for breath sounds	
	Aids. The murmur is heard best with the *patient sitting, leaning forward,* with breath held after exhalation.	*Aids*. Placing the bell exactly on the apical impulse, turning the patient into a *left lateral position,* and mild exercise all help to make the murmur audible. It is heard better in exhalation.
Associated Findings	An ejection sound may be present.	S_1 is accentuated and may be palpable at the apex.
	An S_3 or S_4, if present, suggests severe regurgitation.	An opening snap (OS) often follows S_2 and initiates the murmur.
	Progressive changes in the apical impulse include increased amplitude, displacement laterally and downward, widened diameter, and increased duration.	If pulmonary hypertension develops, P_2 is accentuated, and the right ventricular impulse becomes palpable.
	The pulse pressure increases, and *arterial pulses are often large and bounding*. A midsystolic flow murmur or an Austin Flint murmur suggests large regurgitant flow.	Mitral regurgitation and aortic valve disease may be associated with mitral stenosis.
Mechanism	The leaflets of the aortic valve fail to close completely during diastole, and blood regurgitates from the aorta back into the left ventricle. Volume overload on the left ventricle results. Two other murmurs may be associated: (1) a midsystolic murmur from the resulting increased forward flow across the aortic valve and (2) a mitral diastolic (*Austin Flint*) murmur, attributed to diastolic impingement of the regurgitant flow on the anterior leaflet of the mitral valve.	When the leaflets of the mitral valve thicken, stiffen, and become distorted from the effects of rheumatic fever, the *mitral valve fails to open sufficiently in diastole*. The resulting murmur has two components: (1) middiastolic (during rapid ventricular filling) and (2) presystolic (during atrial contraction). The latter disappears if atrial fibrillation develops, leaving only a middiastolic rumble.

TABLE
14-11

Cardiovascular Sounds With Both Systolic and Diastolic Components

Some cardiovascular sounds extend beyond one phase of the cardiac cycle. Three examples, further described below, are: (1) a *venous hum*, a benign sound produced by turbulence of blood in the jugular veins—common in children; (2) a *pericardial friction rub*, produced by inflammation of the pericardial sac; and (3) *patent ductus arteriosus*, a congenital abnormality in which an open channel persists between the aorta and pulmonary artery. *Continuous murmurs* begin in systole and extend through S_2 into all or part of diastole, as in *patent ductus arteriosus*.

	Venous Hum	Pericardial Friction Rub[1,54]	Patent Ductus Arteriosus
Timing	Continuous murmur without a silent interval. Loudest in diastole	May have three short components, each associated with friction from cardiac movement in the pericardial sac: (1) atrial systole, (2) ventricular systole, and (3) ventricular diastole. Usually the first two components are present; all three make diagnosis easy; only one (usually the systolic) invites confusion with a murmur.	Continuous murmur in both systole and diastole, often with a silent interval late in diastole. Loudest in late systole, obscures S_2, and fades in diastole
Location	Above the medial third of the clavicles, especially on the right	Variable, but usually heard best in the 3rd interspace to the left of the sternum	Left 2nd intercostal space
Radiation	1st and 2nd intercostal spaces	Little	Toward the left clavicle
Intensity	Soft to moderate. Can be obliterated by pressure on the jugular veins	Variable. May increase when the patient leans forward, exhales, and holds breath (in contrast to pleural rub)	Usually loud, sometimes associated with a thrill
Quality	Humming, roaring	Scratchy, scraping	Harsh, machinery-like
Pitch	Low (heard better with the *bell*)	High (heard better with the *diaphragm*)	Medium

BIBLIOGRAPHY

CITATIONS

1. McGee S. Palpation of the heart. In: *Evidence-Based Physical Diagnosis*. 3rd ed. St. Louis, MO: Saunders, 2012.

2. O'Gara PT, Loscalzo J. Physical examination of the cardiovascular system. In: Kasper D, Fauci A, Hauser S, et al., eds. *Harrison's Principles of Internal Medicine*. 19th ed. New York, NY: McGraw-Hill; 2015. Available at http://accesspharmacy.mhmedical.com.uri.idm.oclc.org/content.aspx?bookid=1130&Sectionid=79741626. Accessed October 31, 2015.

3. Hunt SA, Abraham WT, Chin MH, et al. 2009 Focused guidelines for the diagnosis and management of heart failure in adults: A report of the American College of Cardiology Foundation/American Heart Association Task Force on Practice Guidelines: Developed in collaboration with the international society for heart and lung transplantation. *Circulation*. 2009;119:e391–e479.

4. Vinayak AG, Levitt J, Gehlbach B, et al. Usefulness of the external jugular vein examination in detecting abnormal central venous pressure in critically ill patients. *Arch Intern Med*. 2006;166(19):2132–2137.

5. Chua J, Parikh N, Fergusson D. The jugular venous pressure revisited. *Cleve Clin J Med*. 2013;80(10):638–644.

6. Mozaffarian D, Benjamin EJ, Go AS, et al. Heart disease and stroke statistics—2015 update: A report from the American Heart Association. *Circulation*. 2015;131:e29–e322.

7. Abrams J. Chronic stable angina. *N Engl J Med*. 2005;352(24):2524–2533.

8. American Heart Association. *Heart Attack Symptoms in Women*. Available at http://www.heart.org/HEARTORG/Conditions/HeartAttack/WarningSignsofaHeartAttack/Heart-Attack-Symptoms-in-Women_UCM_436448_Article.jsp#.ViqGlSse-ok8. Accessed October 23, 2015.

9. Gibbons RJ, Abrams J, Chatterjee K, et al. ACC/AHA 2002 ACC/AHA 2002 guideline update for the management of patients with chronic stable angina—summary article. *Circulation*. 2003;107(1):149–158.

10. Klompas M. Does this patient have an acute thoracic aortic dissection? *JAMA*. 2002;287(17):2262–2272.

11. Sauve JS, Laupacis A, Feagan B, et al. Does this patient have a clinically important carotid bruit? *JAMA*. 1993;270(23):2843–2845.

12. Cook DJ, Simel DL. Does this patient have abnormal central venous pressure? *JAMA*. 1996;275(8):630.

13. Lange RA, Hillis LD. Acute pericarditis. *N Engl J Med*. 2004;351(21):2195–2202.

14. Aurigemma GP, Gasach WH. Diastolic heart failure. *N Engl J Med*. 2004;351(11):1097–1104.

15. Drazner MH, Rame E, Stevenson LW, et al. Prognostic importance of elevated jugular venous pressure and a third heart sound in patients with heart failure. *N Engl J Med*. 2001;345(8):574–581.

16. Dans AL, Bossone EF, Guyatt GH, et al. Evaluation of the reproducibility and accuracy of apex beat measurement in the detection of echocardiographic left ventricular dilation. *Can J Cardiol*. 1995;11(6):493–407.

17. McMurray JJ. Systolic heart failure. *N Engl J Med*. 2010;362:228–238.

18. Goldberg LR. In the clinic. Heart failure. *Ann Intern Med*. 2010;152:ITC 6-1.

19. Meyer T, Shih J, Aurigemma G. In the clinic. Heart failure with preserved ejection fraction (diastolic dysfunction). *Ann Intern Med*. 2013;158:ITC 5-1.

20. U.S. Preventive Services Task Force. Final Recommendation Statement: *Hypertension in Adults: Screening and Home Monitoring*, 2015. Available at: http://www.uspreventiveservicestaskforce.org/Page/Document/RecommendationStatementFinal/high-blood-pressure-in-adults-screening. Accessed May 30, 2016.

21. NIH. National Heart, Lung and Blood Institute. JNC 7 Complete Report: The Science Behind the New Guidelines. 2004. Available at: http://www.nhlbi.nih.gov/health-pro/guidelines/current/hypertension-jnc-7/complete-report. Accessed May 31, 2016.

22. Alberti KG, Eckel RH, Grundy SM, et al. Harmonizing the metabolic syndrome: a joint interim statement of the International Diabetes Federation Task Force on Epidemiology and Prevention; National Heart, Lung, and Blood Institute; American Heart Association; World Heart Federation; International Atherosclerosis Society; and International Association for the Study of Obesity. *Circulation*. 2009;120:1640.

23. Chobanion AV, Bakris GL, Black HR, et al. The Seventh Report of the Joint National Committee on Prevention, Detection, Evaluation, and Treatment of High Blood Pressure: the JNC 7 report. *JAMA*. 2003;289(19):2560–2572. Available at http://www.nhlbi.nih.gov/guidelines/hypertension/jnc7full.htm. Accessed October 31, 2015. April 13, 2011.

24. James PA, Oparil S, Carter BL, et al. 2014 evidence-based guideline for the management of high blood pressure in adults: report from the panel members appointed to the Eighth Joint National Committee (JNC 8). *JAMA*. 2014;311:507.

25. Bassuk SB. The Reynolds risk score—improving cardiovascular risk prediction in women. *AAOHN J*. 2008;56(4):180.

26. Ridker PM, Buring JE, Rifai N, et al. Development and validation of improved algorithms for the assessment of global cardiovascular risk in women. *JAMA*. 2007;297(6):611–619.

27. Pearson TA, Blair SN, Daniels SR, et al. AHA guidelines for primary prevention of cardiovascular disease and stroke: 2002 update. *Circulation*. 2002;106(3):388–391.

28. Prochaska JO, DiClemente CC. Stages and processes of self-change in smoking: towards an integrative model of change. *J Consult Clin Psychol*. 1983;51:390–395.

29. Center for Disease Control and Prevention. *CDC Features: Most Americans Should Consume Less Sodium (1,500 mg./Day or Less*. Available at http://www.cdc.gov/Features/Sodium/. Accessed October 30, 2015.

30. Healthy People 2020. *2020 Topics and Objectives: Nutrition and Weight Status U.S. Department of Health and Human Services*. Available at http://www.healthypeople.gov/2020/topics-objectives/topic/nutrition-and-weight-status. Accessed October 30, 2015.

31. Healthy People 2020. *2020 Topics and Objectives: Physical Activity*. U.S. Department of Health and Human Services. Available at

http://www.healthypeople.gov/2020/topics-objectives/topic/physical-activity. Accessed October 30, 2015.

32. Spodick DH. Normal sinus heart rate: appropraite rate thresholds for sinus tachycardia and bradycardia. *S Med J.* 1996;89:666.

33. Kari FA, Beyersdorf F, Siepe M. Pathophysiological implications of different bicuspid aortic valve configurations. *Cardiol Res Pract.* 2012;2012:735829.

34. Siu SC, Silversides CK. Bicuspid aortic valve disease. *J Am Coll Cardiol.* 2010;55:2789.

35. Topilsky Y, Michelena H, Bichara V, et al. Mitral valve prolapse with mid-late systolic mitral regurgitation: pitfalls of evaluation and clinical outcome compared with holosystolic regurgitation. *Circulation.* 2012;125:1643.

36. Foster E. Mitral regurgitation due to degenerative mitral-valve disease. *N Engl J Med.* 2010;363:156.

37. Hayek E, Gring CN, Griffin BP. Mitral valve prolapse. *Lancet.* 2005;365:507.

38. Shah SJ, Michaels AD. Hemodynamic correlates of the third heart sound and systolic time intervals. *CHF.* 2006;12(4 suppl 1):8.

39. Shah SJ, Marcus GM, Gerber IL, et al. Physiology of the third heart sound: novel insights from tissue Doppler imaging. *J Am Soc Echocardiogr.* 2008;21:394.

40. Shah SJ, Nakamura K, Marcus GM, et al. Association of the fourth heart sound with increased left ventricular end-diastolic stiffness. *J Card Fail.* 2008;14:431.

41. Asgar AW, Mack MJ, Stone GW. Secondary mitral regurgitation in heart failure: pathophysiology, prognosis, and therapeutic considerations. *J Am Coll Cardiol.* 2015;65:1231.

42. Bonow RO. Chronic mitral regurgitation and aortic regurgitation: have indications for surgery changed? *J Am coll Cardiol.* 2013;61:693.

43. Foster E. Mitral regurgitation due to degenerative mitral-valve disease. *N Engl J Med.* 2010;363:156.

44. Enriquez-Sarano M, Akins CW, Vahanian A. Mitral regurgitation. *Lancet.* 2009;373(9672):1382.

45. Irwin RB, Luckie M, Khattar RS. Tricuspid regurgitation: contemporary management of a neglected valvular lesion. *Postgrad Med J.* 2010:86:648.

46. Mutlak D, Aronson D, Lessick J, Functional tricuspid regurgitation in patients with pulmonary hypertension: is pulmonary artery pressure the only determinant of regurgitation severity? *Chest.* 2009;135:115.

47. Felker GM, Cuculich PS, Gheorghiade M. The Valsalva maneuver: a bedside "biomarker" for heart failure. *Am J Med.* 2006;119:117.

48. Lembo NJ, Dell'Italia LJ, Crawford MH, et al. Bedside diagnosis of systolic murmurs. *N Engl J Med.* 1988;318:1572.

49. Otto CM, Prendergast B. Aortic-valve stenosis–from patients at risk to severe valve obstruction. *N Engl J Med.* 2014;371:744.

50. Ho CY. Hypertrophic cardiomyopathy in 2012. *Circulation.* 2012;125:1432.

51. Fitzgerald KP, Lim MJ. The pulmonary valve. *Cardiol Clin.* 2011;29:223.

52. Maganti K, Rigolin VH, Sarano ME, et al. Valvular heart disease: diagnosis and management. *Mayo Clin Proc.* 2010;85:483.

53. Babu AN, Kymes SM, Carpenter Fryer SM. Eponyms and the diagnosis of aortic regurgitation: what says the evidence? *Ann Intern Med.* 2003;138:736.

54. Chizner MA. Cardiac auscultation: rediscovering the lost art. *Curr Probl Cardiol.* 2008;33:326.

ADDITIONAL REFERENCES

Crane PB, Wallace DC. Cardiovascular risks and physical activity in middle-aged and elderly African American women. *J Cardiovasc Nurs.* 2007;22(4):297–303.

Dennis K, Anthony F, Stephen H, et al. *Harrison's Principles of Internal Medicine.* 19th ed. New York, NY; McGraw-Hill Medical; 2015.

Fischer Aggarwal BA, Liao M, Mosca L. Physical activity as a potential mechanism through which social support may reduce cardiovascular disease risk. *J Cardiovasc Nurs.* 2008;23(2):90–96.

Goldstein BI, Carnethon MR, Matthews KA, et al. Atherosclerosis and early cardiovascular disease: A scientific statement from the major depressive disorder and bipolar disorder predispose youth to accelerated atherosclerosis and early cardiovascular disease: A scientific statement from the American Heart Association. *Circulation.* published online August 10, 2015; Available at http://circ.ahajournals.org/content/early/2015/08/10/CIR.0000000000000229

McSweeney JC, Fischer MA, Moser EP, et al. Predicting coronary heart disease events in women: A longitudinal cohort study. *J Cardiovasc Nurs.* 2014;29(6):482–492.

Ritchie SK, Murphy EC, Ice C, et al. Universal versus targeted blood cholesterol screening among youth: The CARDIAC project. *Pediatrics.* 2010126(2):260–265.

Schroetter SA, Peck SD. Women's risk of heart disease: promoting awareness and prevention—a primary care approach. *Medsurg Nurs.* 2008;17(2):107–113.

Sherman C. Reducing the risk of heart disease in women. *The Clinical Advisor: For Nurse Practitioners.* 2008;111:49–50, 53.

Wenger NK. Women and coronary heart disease: a century after Herrick: understudied, underdiagnosed, and undertreated. *Circulation.* 2012;126(5):604–611.

The Peripheral Vascular System and Lymphatic System

The student will:

1. Describe the structure and functions of arteries, veins, and lymph vessels and nodes.

2. Obtain an accurate history of the peripheral vascular system.

3. Identify the locations of and palpate the peripheral pulses for rate, rhythm, and amplitude.

4. Appropriately prepare and position the patient for the peripheral vascular examination.

5. Describe the equipment necessary to perform a peripheral vascular examination.

6. Evaluate and interpret variations in pulse rhythm, rate, and amplitude.

7. Discuss risk factors for peripheral artery disease, chronic venous stasis, and thromboembolic disease.

8. Discuss risk reduction and health promotion strategies to reduce peripheral vascular disease.

Careful assessment of the peripheral vascular system is essential for detection of **peripheral arterial disease** (PAD). PAD affects roughly 8 million Americans, with estimates ranging from 5.8% to 12% of the population over age 40, but is "silent" in 20% to 50% of those affected.[1–3] Prevalence increases with age, rising from 7% of adults ages 60 to 69 to 23% of adults 80 years of age and older.[4] Detection is doubly important because PAD is both a marker for cardiovascular morbidity and mortality, and a harbinger of functional decline. Risk of death from myocardial infarction and stroke triples in adults with PAD. PAD is defined by the American Heart Association as stenotic, occlusive, and aneurysmal disease of the aorta, its visceral arterial branches, and the arteries of the lower extremities, but not the coronary arteries.

Venous thrombosis or thrombophlebitis is the presence of a thrombus or clot in a vein that is accompanied by an inflammatory response in the vein wall. Thrombi in the superficial veins are usually a response to vessel injury and rarely cause complications. Deep vein thrombosis (DVT) poses

Dislodgement of the thrombus produces an *embolus* that can travel to the lungs, causing pulmonary embolism and possible death.

a grave danger to patients. Lower extremity DVT is seen in an estimated 1% of adults above age 60.[5,6] DVT in the upper extremity now represents about 10% of cases of DVT, reflecting complications from increased placement of central venous catheters, cardiac pacemakers, and defibrillators.[7]

Chronic venous insufficiency is caused by incompetent vein valves secondary to DVT or prolonged increased venous pressure as seen in prolonged standing or pregnancy. This can lead to varicose veins and skin changes.

The term *venous thromboembolism* (VTE) is also used for DVT.

ANATOMY AND PHYSIOLOGY

Arteries

Arteries contain three concentric layers of tissue: the *intima*, the *media*, and the *adventitia* (or the externa). The *internal elastic membrane* borders the intima and the media; the *external elastic membrane* separates the media from the adventitia.

Atherosclerosis is a chronic inflammatory disease initiated by injury to vascular endothelial cells, provoking atheromatous plaque formation and the vascular lesions of hypertension.

Labels: Smooth muscle; Internal elastic membrane; External elastic membrane; Endothelium; Artery; Tunica externa; Tunica media; Tunica intima

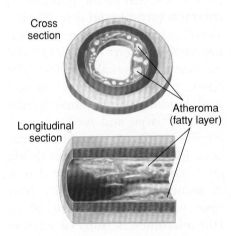

Labels: Cross section; Longitudinal section; Atheroma (fatty layer)

The innermost layer of all blood vessels is the *intima,* a single continuous lining of the endothelial cells, which synthesize regulators of clotting, modulate blood flow through synthesis of vasoconstrictors and vasodilators, and regulate immune and inflammatory reactions.

An atheroma is a fatty thickening in the walls of arteries. It begins in the intima as lipid-filled foam cells, then fatty streaks. Complex atheromas are thickened asymmetric plaques that narrow the lumen, reducing blood flow, and weaken the underlying media. They have a soft lipid core and a fibrous cap of smooth muscle cells and a collagen-rich matrix. Plaque rupture may precede thrombosis formation and lead to arterial occlusions in peripheral coronary or cerebral arteries.[8,9]

The *media* is composed of smooth muscle cells that dilate and constrict to accommodate blood pressure and flow. Its inner and outer boundaries are membranes of elastic fibers, or *elastin*, called *internal and external elastic laminae*. Small arterioles called the *vasa vasorum* perfuse the media. The outer layer of the artery is the *adventitia*, connective tissue containing nerve fibers and the vasa vasorum.

Arteries must respond to the variations that cardiac systole and diastole generate in cardiac output. Their anatomy and size vary according to their distance from the heart. The aorta and its immediate branches are large highly elastic arteries such as the pulmonary, common carotid, and iliac arteries. These arteries course into *medium-sized muscular arteries* like the coronary and renal arteries. The elastic recoil and smooth muscle contraction and relaxation in the media of large and medium-sized arteries propagate arterial pulsatile flow. Medium-sized arteries divide into *small arteries* less than 2 mm in diameter and even smaller *arterioles* with diameters from 20 to 100 micrometers (μm) or microns. Resistance to blood flow occurs primarily in the arterioles. Resistance is inversely proportional to the vessel radius. From the arterioles blood flows into the vast network of *capillaries*. The diameter of each capillary is only 7 to 8 microns, the same diameter as a single red blood cell. Capillaries have an endothelial cell lining but no media, facilitating rapid diffusion of oxygen and carbon dioxide.

Brachial artery

Radial artery

Ulnar artery

Arterial arches

Arterial pulses are palpable in arteries lying close to the body surface. In the arms, note pulsations in:

* The *brachial artery* at the bend of the elbow just medial to the biceps tendon

* The *radial artery* on the lateral flexor surface

* The *ulnar artery* on the medial flexor surface, although overlying tissues may obscure the ulnar artery

Two vascular arches within the hand interconnect the radial and ulnar arteries, doubly protecting circulation to the hand and fingers against possible arterial occlusion.

In the legs, palpate pulsations in:

- The *femoral artery* just below the inguinal ligament, midway between the anterior superior iliac spine and the symphysis pubis

- The *popliteal artery,* an extension of the femoral artery that passes medially behind the femur, palpable just behind the knee. The popliteal artery divides into the two arteries perfusing the lower leg and foot, namely:

  - The *dorsalis pedis artery* on the dorsum of the foot just lateral to the extensor tendon of the big toe

  - The *posterior tibial artery* behind the medial malleolus of the ankle. An interconnecting arch between its two chief arterial branches protects circulation to the foot.

Veins

Anterior superior iliac spine

Inguinal ligament

Femoral artery

Symphysis pubis

Popliteal artery

Posterior tibial artery

Dorsalis pedis artery

Arterial arch

Artery

Vein

Elastic tissue

Inner tunic (endothelium)

Middle tunic (smooth muscle)

Outer tunic (connective tissue)

Valve

Blood flow

Arteriole

Venule

Capillary

Unlike arteries, veins are thin-walled and highly distensible, with a capacity for up to two thirds of circulating blood flow. The *venous intima* consists of nonthrombogenic endothelium. Protruding into the lumen are valves that promote unidirectional venous return to the heart. The *media* contains circumferential rings of elastic tissue and smooth muscle that change vein diameter in response to even minor changes in venous pressure.[8,10] The smallest veins, or *venules,* drain capillary beds.

Veins from the arms, upper trunk, and head and neck drain into the *superior vena cava,* which empties into the right atrium. Veins from the legs and lower trunk drain upward into the *inferior vena cava.* Because of their weaker wall structure, the leg veins are susceptible to irregular dilatation (varicosities), compression, ulceration, and invasion by tumors and warrant special attention.

Deep and Superficial Venous System of the Legs

The *deep veins* of the legs carry approximately 90% of the venous return from the lower extremities. They are well supported by surrounding tissues.

In contrast, the *superficial veins* are subcutaneous, with relatively poor tissue support. They include:

• The *great saphenous vein,* which originates on the dorsum of the foot, passes just anterior to the medial malleolus, continues up the medial aspect of the leg, and joins the femoral vein of the deep venous system below the inguinal ligament and

• The *small saphenous vein,* which begins at the side of the foot, passes upward along the posterior calf, and joins the deep venous system in the popliteal fossa

Anastomotic veins connect the two saphenous veins that are readily visible when dilated. Bridging or *perforating* connect the superficial system with the deep system.

When competent, the one-way valves of the deep, superficial, and perforating veins propel blood toward the heart, preventing pooling, venous stasis, and backward flow. Contraction of the calf muscles during walking also serves as a venous pump, propelling blood upward against gravity.

Femoral vein

Great saphenous vein

Small saphenous vein

Femoral vein

Great saphenous vein

Perforating vein

Small saphenous vein

The Lymphatic System and Lymph Nodes

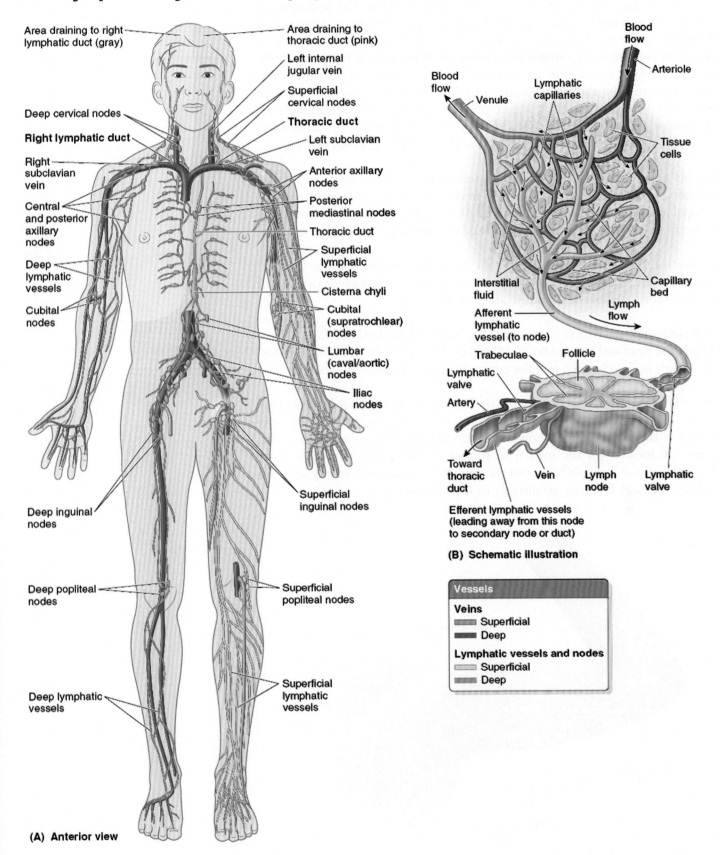

Area draining to right lymphatic duct (gray)

Area draining to thoracic duct (pink)

Left internal jugular vein

Superficial cervical nodes

Thoracic duct

Deep cervical nodes

Right lymphatic duct

Left subclavian vein

Right subclavian vein

Anterior axillary nodes

Central and posterior axillary nodes

Posterior mediastinal nodes

Thoracic duct

Deep lymphatic vessels

Superficial lymphatic vessels

Cubital nodes

Cisterna chyli

Cubital (supratrochlear) nodes

Lumbar (caval/aortic) nodes

Iliac nodes

Deep inguinal nodes

Superficial inguinal nodes

Deep popliteal nodes

Superficial popliteal nodes

Deep lymphatic vessels

Superficial lymphatic vessels

(A) Anterior view

Blood flow

Arteriole

Blood flow

Venule

Lymphatic capillaries

Tissue cells

Interstitial fluid

Capillary bed

Afferent lymphatic vessel (to node)

Lymph flow

Trabeculae

Follicle

Lymphatic valve

Artery

Toward thoracic duct

Vein

Lymph node

Lymphatic valve

Efferent lymphatic vessels (leading away from this node to secondary node or duct)

(B) Schematic illustration

Vessels		
Veins		
	Superficial	
	Deep	
Lymphatic vessels and nodes		
	Superficial	
	Deep	

The lymphatic system is an extensive vascular network that drains lymph fluid from body tissues and returns it to the venous circulation. The system starts peripherally as blind lymphatic capillaries; continues centrally as thin vascular channels, then collecting ducts; and empties into the major veins at the neck. The *right lymphatic duct* drains fluid from the right side of the head, neck, thorax, and right upper limb and empties into the junction of the right internal jugular and the right subclavian veins. The *thoracic duct* collects lymph fluid from the rest of the body and empties into the junction of the left internal jugular and the left subclavian veins. Lymph fluid transported through these channels is filtered through lymph nodes interposed along the way.

Lymph nodes are round, oval, or bean-shaped structures that vary in size according to their location. Some lymph nodes, such as the preauricular nodes, if palpable at all, are typically very small. The inguinal nodes, in contrast, are relatively larger—often 1 cm in diameter and occasionally even 2 cm in an adult.

In addition to its vascular functions, the lymphatic system plays an important role in the body's immune system. Cells within the lymph nodes engulf cellular debris and bacteria and produce antibodies.

Only the superficial lymph nodes are accessible to physical examination. These include the head and cervical nodes (Chapter 10, p. 217), the clavicular nodes, the axillary nodes (below), and the epitrochlear and inguinal nodes.

The axillary lymph nodes drain most of the arm. Lymphatics from the ulnar surface of the forearm and hand, the little and ring fingers, and the adjacent surface of the middle finger, however, drain first into the *epitrochlear nodes*. These are located on the medial surface of the arm approximately 3 cm above the elbow. Lymphatics from the rest of the arm drain mostly into the axillary nodes. A few may go directly to the infraclavicular nodes.

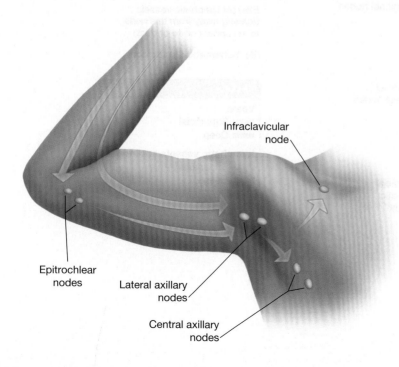

Infraclavicular node

Epitrochlear nodes

Lateral axillary nodes

Central axillary nodes

The lymphatics of the lower limb follow the veins and consist of both deep and superficial systems. Only the superficial nodes are palpable. The *superficial inguinal nodes* include two groups. The *horizontal group* lies in a chain high in the anterior thigh below the inguinal ligament. It drains the superficial portions of the lower abdomen and buttock, the external genitalia (but not the testes), the anal canal and perianal area, and the lower vagina.

The *vertical group* clusters near the upper part of the saphenous vein and drains a corresponding region of the leg.

In contrast, lymphatics from the heel and outer aspect of the foot join the deep system at the level of the popliteal space. Lesions in this area, therefore, are not usually associated with palpable inguinal lymph nodes.

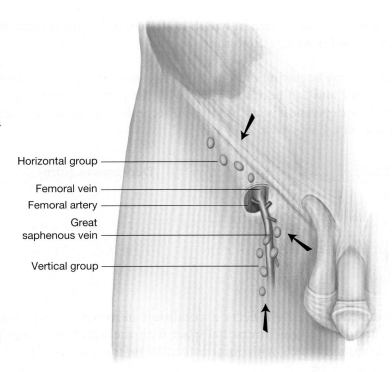

Fluid Exchange and the Capillary Bed

Blood circulates from arteries to veins through the capillary bed. Here fluids diffuse across the capillary membrane, maintaining a dynamic equilibrium between the vascular and interstitial spaces. Most filtered fluid returns to the circulation not as fluid resorbed at the venous end of the capillaries, but as lymph through the lymphatic system.[11]

Lymphatic dysfunction or disturbances in capillary bed fluid exchange commonly result in **edema**, the presence of excess fluid in the interstitial spaces. Four mechanisms produce edema: (1) increased plasma volume from sodium retention; (2) increased capillary membrane permeability may be caused by burns, snake bites, angioedema, or allergic reactions; (3) low plasma protein levels (creating low colloid osmotic pressure), caused by renal disorders; and (4) blockage or inadequate removal of

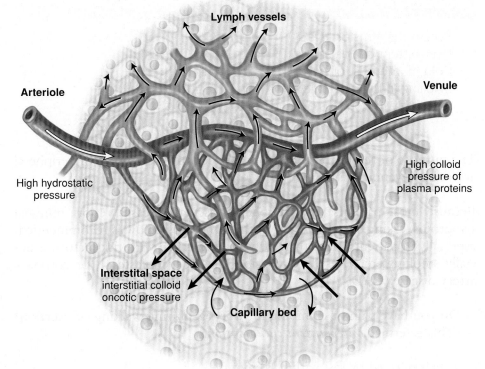

lymphatic fluid, as seen in lymph node removal. This is termed as lymph-edema and is usually nonpitting.

Edema may be pitting or nonpitting. In pitting edema, the interstitial water is mobile and can be translocated with the pressure exerted by a finger. A "pit" or depression is left for 5 to 30 seconds. The degree of pitting is measured on a 1 to 4 scale.

Scale	Depression (mm)
1+	2
2+	4
3+	6
4+	8

Nonpitting edema reflects a condition in which serum proteins have accumulated in the interstitial space with the water and coagulated. This is frequently seen with local infection or trauma and is called brawny edema.

THE HEALTH HISTORY

Common or Concerning Symptoms

- Pain in the arms or legs
- Intermittent claudication
- Cold, numbness, or pallor in the legs; hair loss
- Swelling in the calves, legs, or feet
- Swelling with redness or tenderness

The purpose of the history questions is to identify symptoms of peripheral arterial and venous disease.

Because most patients with peripheral vascular diseases report minimal symptoms, asking specifically about the symptoms below is recommended, especially in patients older than 50 years and those with risk factors, especially smoking, diabetes, hypertension, elevated cholesterol, or coronary artery disease (CAD):

- Do you have pain or cramping in your legs during walking or exertion? (This is termed *intermittent claudication*.)

  - Is it relieved by rest within 10 minutes?

  - Where is the pain felt? How far can you walk before the pain occurs?

These symptoms are caused by insufficient arterial supply to the legs, which may be caused by atherosclerosis.

- Do you have coldness or numbness in your legs or feet? Are your feet pale?

- Do you have hair on your shins?

- Do you have aching or pain at rest in the lower leg or foot?

  - Is the pain alleviated by elevating the legs?

- Do you have fatigue or aching in the lower legs with prolonged standing?

- Do you have swelling of the feet or legs? If present, identify:

  - Location

  - Time of day it is present

  - Whether it is bilateral or unilateral

Edema, varicose veins, and aching in the legs are symptoms of venous stasis.

- Do you have any varicose veins?

  - Where are they located?

  - How long have you had them?

  - Do you have any discomfort from them?

- Do you have any wounds of the legs or feet that will not heal or heal very slowly?

  - Where is the wound located?

  - How long have you had the wound?

  - Did anything cause the wound (e.g., an injury)?

Ulcers may be of venous or arterial origin.

- Do your fingertips or toes change color in cold weather?

May be caused by Raynaud disease: the small arteries spasm in response to cold.

- Have you experienced erectile dysfunction?

Poor blood supply to the penile arteries can cause erectile dysfunction.

- Do you have abdominal pain after meals?

  - Does it prevent you from eating?

Atherosclerosis of the mesenteric or celiac arteries can cause intestinal ischemia, producing abdominal pain and "food fear," where the patient is fearful of eating.

- Do you have tender or swollen lymph nodes (glands)?

Swollen nodes may indicate an infection or tumor.

Past History

- Medications, especially oral contraceptives or hormone replacement therapy

Estrogen use and pregnancy increase one's risk for blood clots.

- Pregnancy or recent childbirth

- Inflammatory diseases such as lupus, rheumatoid arthritis, or irritable bowel disease

Inflammation contributes to clot formation.

- Active cancer

- Coronary artery disease (CAD)

CAD and cerebral artery disease are also caused by atherosclerosis; an individual with either is at risk for PAD.

- Heart attack

- Congestive heart failure

- Stroke (cerebral arterial disease)

- Clotting disorders

- Hypertension

- Diabetes

- Problems in circulation, such as blood clots, leg ulcers, swelling, or poor healing of wounds

- Major surgery or fracture of a long bone in the last 4 weeks

- **Risk factors**

  - Obesity

  - Smoking

  - Hyperlipidemia

  - Constrictive clothing

  - Central venous lines

Family History

- Peripheral vascular disease

- Varicose veins

- Abdominal aortic aneurysm

- CAD

- Sudden death younger than 60 years of age

- Diabetes

Lifestyle or Health Patterns

- Prolonged standing or sitting (sedentary/stationary job, long distance travel)

- Sedentary lifestyle

- Decreased mobility such as paralysis or cast

PHYSICAL EXAMINATION

Equipment List

- Tape measure
- Doppler ultrasound device
- Tourniquet or blood pressure cuff

Important Areas of Examination

The Arms	The Legs
• Size, symmetry, skin color • Radial pulse, brachial pulse • Epitrochlear lymph nodes	• Size, symmetry, skin color, tenderness • Femoral pulse and inguinal lymph nodes • Popliteal, dorsalis pedis, and posterior tibial pulses • Peripheral edema

The American College of Cardiology and the American Heart Association have urged close examination of the peripheral vascular system, because PAD is often asymptomatic and underdiagnosed, leading to significant morbidity and mortality.[12,13]

Arms

Inspection

Inspect both arms from the fingertips to the shoulders. Note:

1. Their size, symmetry, any edema and lesions.

Lymphedema of the arm and hand may follow axillary node dissection and radiation therapy.

2. The venous pattern

Prominent veins in an edematous arm suggest venous obstruction, such as a DVT.

3. The color of the skin and nail beds and the texture of the skin

Source of photo: Effeney, DJ, Stoney, RJ. *Wylie's Atlas of Vascular Surgery: Disorders of the Extremities.* Philadelphia, PA: Lippincott Williams & Wilkins; 1993.

Palpation

1. Palpate the temperature of the arms and hands simultaneously with the backs of your fingers. Compare the temperature of the arms simultaneously.

2. *Palpate the radial pulse* with the pads of your fingers on the flexor surface of the wrist laterally. Partially flexing the patient's wrist may help you feel this pulse. Compare the pulses in both arms. Pulses may be palpated simultaneously to facilitate comparison.

In Raynaud disease, wrist pulses are typically normal, but spasm of more distal arteries causes episodes of sharply demarcated pallor of the fingers (see Table 15-1, Painful Peripheral Vascular Disorders and Their Mimics, pp. 466–467).

There are two common systems for grading the amplitude of the arterial pulses. One system uses a scale of 0 to 3, as below.[12] The other system uses a scale of 0 to 4. You should check to see what scale your institution uses.

Recommended Grading of Pulses[12]	
3+	Bounding
2+	Brisk, expected (normal)
1+	Diminished, weaker than expected
0	Absent, unable to palpate

Document pulse amplitude as a fraction with the denominator indicating, which scale is being used, for example, 2+/3 indicates a normal pulse in this scale.

If you cannot obtain the radial pulse, feel for the *brachial pulse*. Flex the patient's elbow slightly, and palpate the artery just medial to the biceps tendon at the antecubital crease. The brachial artery can also be felt higher in the arm in the groove between the biceps and triceps muscles.

Bounding carotid, radial, and femoral pulses in aortic insufficiency; asymmetric diminished pulses in arterial occlusion from atherosclerosis or embolism

Feel for the *epitrochlear nodes*. With the patient's elbow flexed to about 90 degrees and the forearm supported by your hand, reach around behind the arm and feel in the groove between the biceps and triceps muscles, about 3 cm above the medial epicondyle. If a node is present, note its size, consistency, and tenderness.

Epitrochlear nodes are nonpalpable in most normal people.

An enlarged epitrochlear node may arise from local or distal infection or may be associated with generalized lymphadenopathy.

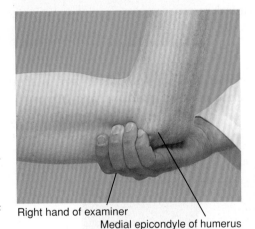

Right hand of examiner
Medial epicondyle of humerus

Concept Mastery Alert

Identifying the characteristics of a pulse is important to determine if palpation reveals a normal finding, a finding associated with aging, or a problem. A bounding pulse may indicate decreased elasticity of the arterial walls, most commonly seen with aging. However, a bisferiens pulse, for example (one in which there is an increased arterial pulse with double systolic beats), suggests aortic stenosis.

Legs

The patient should be lying down and draped so that the external genitalia are covered and the legs fully exposed. A good examination is impossible through stockings or socks.

Inspection

Inspect both legs from the groin and buttocks to the feet. Note:

1. Their size, symmetry, and edema. Measure leg circumferences in centimeters if discrepancy is suspected.

See Table 15-2, Chronic Insufficiency of Arteries and Veins, p. 468.

2. The venous pattern and any venous enlargement or varicosities

3. Pigmentation, rashes, scars, or ulcers

See Table 15-3, Common Ulcers of the Ankles and Feet, p. 470.

4. The color and texture of the skin and the color of the nail beds

5. The distribution of hair on the lower legs, feet, and toes.

Tight socks may rub off the hair. If hair is absent, look for a clean demarcation where the top of the sock ends.

6. Look for brownish areas (or increased pigmentation on dark-skinned clients) near the ankles. The brown discoloration is caused by hemosiderin released from the red blood cells that seep into the skin with edema and break down.

Brownish discoloration or ulcers just above the malleolus suggest chronic venous insufficiency.

7. Note the location, size, and depth of any ulcers in the skin. Note whether the edges of the wound are well demarcated or uneven and if there is bleeding?

Palpation

1. Palpate the temperature of both legs and feet simultaneously with the backs of your hands. Compare the temperature of the legs. Bilateral coolness is may be caused by a cold environment or anxiety.

Coldness, especially when unilateral or associated with other signs, suggests arterial insufficiency from inadequate arterial circulation.

2. Palpate for edema. Compare one foot and leg with the other, noting their relative size and the prominence of veins, tendons, and bones.

Edema causes swelling that may obscure the veins, tendons, and bony prominences.

Palpate for pitting edema. Press firmly but gently with your thumb for at least 5 seconds (1) over the dorsum of each foot, (2) behind each medial malleolus, and (3) over the shins. Look for *pitting*—a depression caused by pressure from your thumb. Normally pitting edema is not detected. If found, the severity of edema is graded on a four-point scale (see p. 446).

See Table 15-4, Some Peripheral Causes of Edema, p. 471.

Shown below is 3+ pitting edema

If you suspect edema, *measure the legs* to identify the edema and to follow its course. With a flexible tape, measure (1) the forefoot, (2) the smallest possible circumference above the ankle, (3) the largest circumference at the calf, and (4) the midthigh, a measured distance above the patella with the knee extended. Compare one side with the other. A difference of more than 1 cm just above the ankle or 2 cm at the calf is unusual and suggests edema.

If edema is present, look for possible causes in the peripheral vascular system. These include (1) recent DVT, (2) chronic venous insufficiency from previous DVT or incompetence of the venous valves, and (3) lymphedema. Note the extent of the swelling and how far up the leg it goes.

In *DVT,* the extent of edema suggests the location of the occlusion: the popliteal vein when the lower leg or the ankle is swollen; the iliofemoral veins when the entire leg is swollen.

Is the swelling unilateral or bilateral?

Unilateral calf and ankle swelling and edema suggest DVT, chronic venous insufficiency from prior DVT, or incompetent venous valves; or may be lymphedema.

Bilateral edema is present in *heart failure, cirrhosis,* and *nephrotic syndrome.*

Venous distention suggests a venous cause of edema.

If risk factors for DVT are present, try to identify any venous tenderness that may accompany DVT. Very gently palpate the groin just medial to the femoral pulse for tenderness of the femoral vein. Next, with the patient's leg flexed at the knee and relaxed, palpate the calf by very gently compressing the calf muscles against the tibia with your fingerpads. Search for any tenderness or cords. DVT may have no demonstrable signs, and diagnosis often depends on high clinical suspicion and other testing. *Firm palpation or massage over a DVT should be avoided as it may dislodge the clot, causing a pulmonary embolus or death.*

A painful, pale swollen leg, together with tenderness in the groin over the femoral vein, suggests deep *iliofemoral thrombosis.* Only half of patients with *DVT* in the calf have tenderness and cords deep in the calf. Calf tenderness is nonspecific and may be present without thrombosis.

3. Feel the thickness of the skin.

Thickened brawny skin suggests lymphedema and advanced venous insufficiency.

4. Palpate areas of local redness, noting the skin temperature, and then gently palpate for the firm cord of a thrombosed vein in the area. The calf is most often involved.

Local swelling, redness, warmth, and a subcutaneous cord suggest *superficial thrombophlebitis.*

5. *Palpate the pulses* to assess the arterial circulation.

A diminished or absent pulse indicates partial or complete occlusion proximally; for example, at the popliteal level, the dorsalis pedis and posterior tibial pulses are typically affected. Chronic arterial occlusion, usually from atherosclerosis, causes *intermittent claudication.*

- *The femoral pulse.* Press deeply, below the inguinal ligament and about midway between the anterior superior iliac spine and the symphysis pubis. As in deep abdominal palpation, the use of two hands, one on top of the other, may facilitate this examination, especially in obese patients.

An exaggerated, widened femoral pulse suggests a *femoral aneurysm,* a pathologic dilatation of the artery.

- *The popliteal pulse.* The patient's knee should be somewhat flexed, with the leg relaxed. Place the fingertips of both hands so that they meet in the midline behind the knee and press deeply into the popliteal fossa. The popliteal pulse is often more difficult to find than other pulses. It is deeper and feels more diffuse.

An exaggerated, widened popliteal pulse suggests an aneurysm of the popliteal artery. Popliteal and femoral aneurysms are not common. They are usually caused by atherosclerosis and occur primarily in men older than 50 years.

If you cannot palpate the popliteal pulse with this approach, try with the patient prone. Flex the patient's knee to about 90 degrees, let the lower leg relax against your shoulder or upper arm, and press your two thumbs deeply into the popliteal fossa.

Atherosclerosis (arteriosclerosis obliterans) most commonly obstructs arterial circulation in the thigh. The femoral pulse is then normal, the popliteal decreased or absent.

• *The dorsalis pedis pulse.* Palpate the dorsum of the foot (not the ankle) just lateral to the extensor tendon of the great toe. If you cannot feel a pulse, explore the dorsum of the foot more laterally.

The dorsalis pedis artery may be congenitally absent or may branch higher in the ankle.

Decreased or absent pedal pulses (assuming a warm environment) with normal femoral and popliteal pulses suggest occlusive disease in the lower popliteal artery or its branches, often seen in *diabetes mellitus.*

- *The posterior tibial pulse.* Curve your fingers behind and slightly below the medial malleolus of the ankle. (This pulse may be hard to feel in an ankle that is enlarged due to fat deposits or edema.)

Sudden arterial occlusion from embolism or thrombosis causes pain and numbness or tingling. The limb distal to the occlusion becomes cold, pale, and pulseless. Emergency treatment is required. If collateral circulation is good, only numbness and coolness may result.

Tips for Feeling Difficult Pulses

1. Position your body and examining hand comfortably; awkward positions decrease your tactile sensitivity.
2. Once your hand is positioned properly, linger and vary the pressure of your fingers to pick up a weak pulsation. If unsuccessful, then gently explore the area more deliberately.
3. Do not confuse the patient's pulse with your own pulsating fingertips. If you are unsure, count your own heart rate and compare it with the patient's. The rates are usually different. Your carotid pulse is convenient for this comparison.

6. Palpate the *superficial inguinal nodes,* including both the horizontal and the vertical groups. Note their size, consistency, and discreteness, and note any tenderness. Nontender, discrete inguinal nodes up to 1 cm or even 2 cm in diameter are frequently palpable in normal people. See p. 445.

Lymphadenopathy refers to enlargement of the nodes, with or without tenderness.

Varicose veins are dilated and tortuous. Their walls may feel somewhat thickened. Many varicose veins can be seen in the leg in the picture on the left.

At the end of the examination, ask the patient to stand, and *inspect the saphenous system for varicosities.* The standing posture allows any varicosities to fill with blood and makes them visible. You can easily miss them when the patient is in a supine position. Feel for any varicosities, noting any signs of thrombophlebitis.

RECORDING YOUR FINDINGS

Recall that the written description of lymph nodes appears in Chapter 10, The Head and Neck, p. 225. Likewise, assessment of the carotid pulse is recorded in Chapter 14, The Cardiovascular System, p. 415.

Recording the Physical Examination—The Peripheral Vascular System

"Extremities are warm and without edema. No varicosities or stasis changes. Calves are supple and nontender. No femoral or abdominal bruits. Brachial, radial, femoral, popliteal, dorsalis pedis (DP), and posterior tibial (PT) pulses are 2+ and symmetric."

OR

"Extremities are pale below the midcalf, with notable hair loss. Rubor noted when legs are dependent but no edema or ulceration. Bilateral femoral bruits; no abdominal bruits heard. Brachial and radial pulses 2+; femoral, popliteal, DP, and PT pulses 1+ bilaterally." (Alternatively, pulses can be recorded as below.)

Suggests atherosclerotic peripheral arterial disease.

	Radial	Brachial	Femoral	Popliteal	Dorsalis Pedis	Posterior Tibial
RT	2+	2+	1+	1+	1+	1+
LT	2+	2+	1+	1+	1+	1+

OR

"Bilateral pitting edema 2+ and brownish pigmentation present to midcalf bilaterally. 2-cm × 1-cm shallow ulcer with irregular edges and moderate exudate on right leg superior to medial malleolus. Granulation tissue visible in ulcer. Varicose veins posterior upper legs bilaterally."

Suggests venous ulcer.

SPECIAL TECHNIQUES

Evaluating the Arterial Supply to the Hand

To assess for arterial insufficiency in the arm or hand, try to palpate the *ulnar pulse* as well as the radial and brachial pulses. Press deeply on the flexor surface of the medial wrist. Partially flexing the patient's wrist may help you. The pulse of a normal ulnar artery, however, may not be palpable.

Arterial occlusive disease is much less common in the arms than in the legs. Absent or diminished pulses at the wrist occur in acute embolic occlusion and in Buerger disease, or thromboangiitis obliterans.

Allen Test

The *Allen test* compares patency of the ulnar and radial arteries. It also ensures the patency of the ulnar artery before puncturing the radial artery for blood samples or arterial lines. The patient should rest with hands in lap, palms up.

Ask the patient to make a tight fist with one hand; then compress both radial and ulnar arteries firmly between your thumbs and fingers.

Next, ask the patient to open the hand into a relaxed, slightly flexed position. The palm is pale.

Extending the hand fully may cause pallor and a falsely positive test.

Release your pressure over the ulnar artery. If the ulnar artery is patent, the palm flushes within 3 to 5 seconds.

Persisting pallor indicates occlusion of the ulnar artery or its distal branches.

Patency of the radial artery may be tested by repeating the test and releasing the radial artery while still compressing the ulnar artery.

Evaluating Arterial Supply to the Legs

If pain or diminished pulses suggest arterial insufficiency, look for postural color changes. With the patient lying down, raise both legs, as shown to about 60 degrees until maximal pallor of the feet develops—usually within a minute. Have the patient flex the ankles up and down to drain venous blood. In light-skinned persons, either maintenance of normal color, as seen in this right foot, or slight pallor is normal. In dark-skinned persons, evaluate the soles of the feet or nail beds for pallor.

Marked pallor on elevation suggests *arterial insufficiency.*

Then ask the patient to sit up and dangle the legs over the side of the examination table. Compare both feet, noting the time required for:

* Return of pinkness to the skin, normally about 10 seconds or less

* Filling of the veins of the feet and ankles, normally about 15 seconds

This right foot has normal color and the veins on the foot have filled. These normal responses suggest an adequate circulation.

The patient's left foot is still pale, and the veins are just starting to fill—signs of arterial insufficiency.

Source of foot photos: Kappert A, Winsor T. *Diagnosis of Peripheral Vascular Disease.* Philadelphia, PA: FA Davis; 1972.

Look for any unusual *rubor* (dusky redness) to replace the pallor of the dependent foot. Rubor may take a minute or more to appear.

Normal responses accompanied by diminished arterial pulses suggest that a good collateral circulation has developed around an arterial occlusion.

Persisting-dependent rubor on dependency suggests arterial insufficiency. If the patient's veins are incompetent, dependent rubor and the timing of color return and venous filling are not reliable tests of arterial insufficiency.

Ankle–Brachial Index

If the patient has risk factors for peripheral artery disease, an ankle–brachial index (ABI) screening should be performed. ABI is a noninvasive method to assess lower extremity arterial blood flow by comparing systolic blood pressure in the ankle to arm systolic pressure.

Equipment

Doppler device with 8-MHz probe (For obese individuals, a 4-MHz probe may be necessary.)

Doppler gel

Blood pressure cuffs for arm and leg; cuffs should be 40% of limb circumference (or 20% of the limb diameter).

Procedure

1. Advise patients to avoid caffeine, tobacco, and heavy activity for at least 1 hour prior to the procedure.
2. Perform the ABI in a quiet, warm environment to prevent vasoconstriction.
3. Have patient empty his bladder and remove tight or restrictive clothing, shoes, and socks.
4. Explain the procedure to the patient and position him or her in the supine position. The patient should rest supine for 10 to 20 minutes before the procedure.
5. Apply the blood pressure cuff to the patient's arm and palpate the brachial pulse.
6. Apply a small mound of gel over the pulse; turn on the Doppler.
7. Place the tip of the Doppler probe in the gel at a 45-degree angle and listen for the "whooshing" sound, indicating the pulse. (The probe may be adjusted between 30 and 60 degrees to maximize the sound.)
8. Inflate the blood pressure cuff until the sound is no longer heard, and then inflate it 20 to 30 mm Hg above that point.
9. Deflate the cuff at a rate of 2 to 3 mm Hg/sec until the sound returns. This is the systolic blood pressure. Repeat the procedure in the other arm.
10. Place the ankle blood pressure cuff just above the malleoli. Locate the posterior tibial pulse with the Doppler and inflate the cuff 20 to 30 mm Hg above the number the pulse is last heard. Slowly release the pressure until the pulse is heard. This is the systolic pressure. Repeat the procedure using the dorsalis pedis pulse.

11. Obtain the systolic pressure for both pulses on the opposite ankle.

NOTE: The ankle blood pressure cuff must be the appropriate size in order to obtain accurate readings. Artery pressure is measured at the site of the cuff; if the cuff is placed higher on the leg a false high systolic reading will be obtained.

Calculation
Divide the higher systolic pressure from each leg by the higher brachial systolic pressure to obtain the ABI for each leg.

Documentation
Describe the patient's tolerance of the procedure and any problems encountered during the test. Document all brachial and ankle pressures, the ABI value and the interpretation of perfusion status.

Interpretation

ABI	Interpretation
>1.3	Unreliable. Calcium in arterial walls prevents compression of the artery during the test. Frequently seen in diabetic patients.
1.0	Normal
≤0.9	Lower extremity arterial disease (LEAD)
0.6–0.8	Borderline perfusion
0.50–0.75	Severe ischemia
≤0.49	Critical ischemia, limb threatened
	Refer to a vascular surgeon for further vascular testing.

Wound Ostomy and Continence Nurses Society. Ankle brachial index: Quick reference guide for clinicians. *J Wound Ostomy Continence Nurs.* 2012;39(25);S21–S29.

Ann Intern Med 2013 Sep 3;159(5):342–348. doi: 10.7326/0003–4819–159–5–201309030–00008. Screening for peripheral artery disease and cardiovascular disease risk assessment with the ankle-brachial index in adults: U.S. Preventive Services Task Force recommendation statement. http://www-ncbi-nlm-nih-gov.uri.idm.oclc.org/pubmed/24026320

Ghannam M, Rodriguez Y, Ehrmann D, Grossman PM. Ankle-brachial index as a clinical tool. *Amer J Med.* 2012;125(12):1171–1172.

Evaluating the Competency of Venous Valves

By the *retrograde filling (Trendelenburg) test,* you can assess the valvular competency in both the penetrating veins and the saphenous system.

- With the patient supine. Elevate one leg to about 90 degrees to empty it of venous blood.

- Occlude the great saphenous vein in the upper thigh by manual compression or tourniquet, using enough pressure to occlude this vein but not the deeper vessels.

- Ask the patient to stand. While you keep the vein occluded, watch for venous filling in the leg. Normally the saphenous vein fills from below, taking about 35 seconds as blood flows through the capillary bed into the venous system.

Rapid filling of the superficial veins during occlusion of the saphenous vein indicates incompetent valves in the penetrating veins, which allows rapid retrograde flow from the deep to the saphenous system.

After the patient stands for 20 seconds, release the compression and look for sudden additional venous filling. Normally slow venous filling continues since competent valves in the saphenous vein block retrograde flow.

Sudden additional filling of superficial veins after release of compression indicates incompetent valves in the saphenous vein.

When both steps of this test are normal, the response is termed negative–negative. Negative–positive and positive–negative responses may also occur.

When both steps are abnormal, the test is positive–positive.

Pulsus Alternans

In *pulsus alternans,* the rhythm of the pulse remains regular, but the *force* of the arterial pulse alternates because of alternating strong and weak ventricular contractions. *Pulsus alternans* almost always indicates severe left-sided heart failure and is usually best felt by applying light pressure on the radial or femoral arteries.[14] Use a blood pressure cuff to confirm your finding. After raising the cuff pressure, lower it slowly to the systolic level—the initial Korotkoff sounds are the strong beats. As you lower the cuff, you will hear the softer sounds of the alternating weak beats.

Alternately loud and soft Korotkoff sounds or a sudden doubling of the apparent heart rate as the cuff pressure declines indicates a pulsus alternans (see Table 15-5, Abnormalities of he Arterial Pulse and Pressure Waves, p. 471.)

The alternation may be more noticeable with the patient in an upright position.

Paradoxical Pulse

Paradoxical pulse means the pulse beat amplitude is weaker during inspiration and stronger during expiration. This is due to a greater than normal drop in systolic blood pressure during inspiration. Normally, systolic blood pressure decreases slightly during inspiration, less than 10 mm Hg. In the presence of certain diseases, for example, cardiac tamponade, pericarditis, or obstructive airway disease, the fall in systolic pressure is greater than 10 mm Hg due to decreased left ventricular volume producing decreased LV output and systolic pressure. The *paradox* in *pulsus paradoxus* is that, on clinical examination, you can detect beats on cardiac auscultation during inspiration that cannot be palpated at the radial pulse.

The level identified by first hearing Korotkoff sounds is the highest systolic pressure during the respiratory cycle. The level identified by hearing sounds throughout the cycle is the lowest systolic pressure. A difference between these levels of more than 10 mm Hg indicates a paradoxical pulse.

To test for a paradoxical pulse:

- Inflate the BP cuff above the patient's usual systolic pressure.

See Table 15-5, Abnormalities of he Arterial Pulse and Pressure Waves, p. 471.

- As the patient breathes lower the cuff pressure slowly to the systolic level. Note the pressure level at which the first sounds can be heard.

- Then drop the pressure very slowly until sounds can be heard throughout the respiratory cycle. Again note the pressure level. The difference between these two levels is normally no greater than 3 or 4 mm Hg.

HEALTH PROMOTION AND COUNSELING

Important Topics for Health Promotion and Counseling

Arterial Disease
- Smoking cessation
- Weight control
- Exercise program
- Hypertension control
- Hyperlipidemia control
- Diabetes management
- Limiting alcohol intake
- Foot care

Venous Disease
- Avoidance of prolonged sitting and standing
- Avoidance of constrictive clothing, including girdles and tight hose
- Exercise program
- Weight control
- Foot care
- Dehydration prevention

Diseases of the peripheral vascular system, peripheral arterial disease, venous stasis, and thromboembolic disorders can severely affect the life-style and quality of life of patients. Identifying modifiable risk factors and providing health promotion counseling can prevent or delay long-term complications, such as decreased mobility and amputation. Helping the patient understand the effects of smoking, obesity, hypertension, hyper-lipidemia, and diabetes and the need for exercise encourages the patient to institute lifestyle changes that promote peripheral and cardiovascular health.

PAD has the same underlying pathology as CAD and is a common mani-festation of atherosclerosis. Approximately 8 million people in the United States have PAD, including 12% to 20% of individuals older than age 60. Men and woman are equally affected by PAD; however, black race/ethnic-ity is associated with an increased risk of PAD. People of Hispanic origin may have similar to slightly higher rates of PAD compared to non-His-panic whites.[15] An estimated 40% to 60% of PAD patients have coexisting CAD and/or cerebral artery disease, and the presence of PAD significantly increases the risk for cardiovascular events. Controlling risk factors will help prevent or decrease the complications of both diseases.[16]

Early identification of peripheral vascular diseases and modification of risk factors are important nursing functions. Careful and thorough history taking is essential to identify early peripheral vascular disease, especially in patients older than 50 years of age. Identification of risk factors should be performed with every patient. The nurse can use the ABI to assess peripheral arterial disease. Serial ABI testing will document any progression of the disease.

Since atherosclerotic renal arterial disease and abdominal aortic aneurysm often accompany peripheral vascular disease, patients with risk factors should be referred to their physicians for screening of these diseases.[17] Atherosclerotic renal arterial disease affects 7% of adults older than 65 years of age, and that rate rises to 22% to 55% of those with PAD and 30% of those with documented CAD.[12,18] Patients with worsening hypertension despite medication or new worsening of renal function should be evaluated. Abdominal aortic aneurysms (AAAs) are rarely symptomatic and the mortality rate for ruptured aneurysms is high. Risk factors for AAA include a history of ever smoking, family history, PAD, CAD, hypertension, elevated cholesterol, and age older than 65 years.

Prevention and early identification of DVT are critical nursing responsibilities, especially in the care of hospitalized patients and patients with reduced mobility. The Virchow triad—venous stasis, hypercoagulability, and vessel wall damage—set the stage for the development of a DVT. Most commonly immobility, compression of the vein, and increased blood viscosity (as seen in dehydration) lead to blood stasis, usually within the pockets of the vein valves. A thrombus forms and the patient is at risk for an embolism. The Homan sign, with the patient's knee flexed and the ankle forcibly dorsiflexed, was the classic assessment maneuver; however, research has found this test very unreliable, yielding many false positives and negatives.[19] It should not be used. Almost every hospitalized patient is at risk for DVT. DVT risk assessment tools for hospitalized patients have been developed. The tools identify and rank risk factors and become part of the patient chart. Prevention strategies can then be initiated.[20]

Patients should be educated about the risk of DVT outside the hospital as well. Conditions that produce dehydration, cramped positioning, or immobility, such as long plane travel, can cause a DVT to form. Patients with sedentary jobs should be advised to walk or flex their legs at their desks at least every hour. Ergonomic furniture may reduce the effects of prolonged flexion of the legs.

TABLE
15-1

Painful Peripheral Vascular Disorders and Their Mimics[12,21]

Problem	Process	Location of Pain
Arterial Disorders		
Peripheral Arterial Disease	Atherosclerotic disease leading to obstruction of peripheral arteries causing exertional claudication (muscle pain relieved by rest) and atypical leg pain. May progress to ischemic pain at rest.	Usually calf muscles, but also occurs in the buttock, hip, thigh, or foot, depending on the level of obstruction. Rest pain may be distal in the toes or forefoot.
Acute Arterial Occlusion	Embolism or thrombosis, possibly superimposed on arteriosclerosis obliterans	Distal pain, usually involving the foot and leg
Raynaud Phenomenon: Primary and Secondary[22]	*Raynaud phenomenon—primary:* Episodic reversible vasoconstriction in the fingers and toes, usually triggered by cold temperatures (capillaries are normal; no definable cause).	Distal portions of one or more fingers. Pain is usually not prominent unless fingertip ulcers develop. Numbness and tingling are common.
	Raynaud phenomenon—secondary: Symptoms/signs related to autoimmune diseases—scleroderma, lupus, mixed connective tissue disease; cryoglobulinemia; also to occupational vascular injury; drugs	
Venous Disorders		
Superficial Phlebitis	In the lower extremity: inflammation of a superficial vein.	Pain and tenderness in a local area along the course of a superficial vein, most often in the saphenous system
Superficial Vein Thrombosis	A clot is confirmed by imaging	
Deep Venous Thrombosis (DVT)	DVT and PE are disorders of venous thromboembolic disease (VTE). DVTs are distal, limited to the deep calf veins, or proximal, in the popliteal, femoral, or iliac veins.	Classically, painful calf swelling with erythema but can be painless; signs correlate poorly with site of thrombosis.
Chronic Venous Insufficiency (deep)	More severe form of chronic venous disease, with chronic venous engorgement from venous occlusion or incompetency of venous valves	Diffuse aching of the leg(s)
Compartment Syndrome	Pressure builds from trauma or bleeding into one of the four major muscle compartments between the knee and ankle. Each compartment is enclosed by fascia that limits expansion and thus cannot expand to accommodate increasing pressure.	Tight, bursting pain in calf muscles, usually in the anterior tibial compartment, sometimes with overlying dusky red skin
Acute Lymphangitis	Acute bacterial infection from *Streptococcus pyogenes* or *Staphylococcus aureus,* spreading up the lymphatic channels from a distal portal of entry such as a skin abrasion, dog bite or an ulcer	An arm or a leg
Mimics[a]		
Acute Cellulitis	Acute bacterial infection of the skin and subcutaneous tissues, most commonly from β hemolytic streptococci (erysipelas) and *Staphylococcus aureus*	Arms, legs, or elsewhere

[a]Mistaken primarily for acute superficial thrombophlebitis.

Timing	Factors That Aggravate	Factors That Relieve	Associated Manifestations
May be brief if relieved by rest. If there is *rest pain*, may be persistent and worse at night.	Exercise such as walking If *rest pain*, leg elevation and bedrest	Rest usually stops the pain in 1–3 min. *Rest pain* may be relieved by walking (increases perfusion), sitting with legs dependent	Local fatigue, numbness, progressing to cool dry hairless skin, trophic nail changes, diminished to absent pulses, pallor with elevation, ulceration, gangrene. (See p. 469)
Sudden onset; associated symptoms may occur without pain.			Coldness, numbness, weakness, absent distal pulses
Relatively brief (minutes) but recurrent	Exposure to cold, emotional upset	Warm environment	*Primary RP:* distinct digital color changes of pallor, cyanosis, and hyperemia (redness); no necrosis. *Secondary RP:* more severe, with ischemia, necrosis, and loss of digits. Capillary loops are distorted.
An acute episode lasting days or longer	Immobility, venous stasis and chronic venous disease, venous procedure, obesity	Supportive care, walking. Measures prompted by further testing.	Local induration, erythema. If palpable nodules or cords, consider superficial or deep vein thrombosis, both associated with significant risk of DVT and PE.
Often hard to determine due to lack of symptoms. One third of untreated calf DVTs extend proximally.	Immobilization or recent surgery, lower extremity trauma, pregnancy or post-partum state, hypercoagulable state (i.e., nephrotic syndrome, malignancy)	Antithrombotic and thrombolytic therapy	Asymmetric calf diameters more diagnostic than palpable cord or tenderness over femoral triangle. Homan sign unreliable. High risk of PE (50% with proximal DVT).
Chronic, increasing as the day wears on	Prolonged standing or sitting with legs dependent	Leg elevation, walking	Chronic edema, pigmentation, swelling, and possibly ulceration especially if advanced age, pregnancy, increased weight, prior history or trauma (see p. 469)
Several hours if *acute* (pressure must be relieved to overt necrosis). During exercise if *chronic*	*Acute:* anabolic steroids; surgical complication; crush injury. *Chronic:* occurs with exercise	*Acute:* surgical incision to relieve pressure *Chronic:* avoiding exercise; ice elevation	Tingling, burning sensations in calf; muscles may feel tight, full, numbness, paralysis if unrelieved
An acute episode lasting days or longer			Red streak(s) on the skin, with tenderness, enlarged, tender lymph nodes, and fever
An acute episode lasting days or longer			A local area of diffuse swelling, redness, and tenderness with enlarged, tender lymph nodes and fever; no palpable cord

TABLE
15-2

Chronic Insufficiency of Arteries and Veins

Chronic Arterial Insufficiency (advanced)	Chronic Venous Insufficiency (advanced)

Rubor

Ischemic ulcer

	Chronic Arterial Insufficiency (advanced)	**Chronic Venous Insufficiency (advanced)**
Pain	Intermittent claudication, progressing to pain at rest	Ulcer often painful[21]; generalized leg aching, especially at end of day
Mechanism	Tissue ischemia	Venous stasis and hypertension
Pulses	Decreased or absent	Normal, though may be difficult to feel through edema
Color	Pale, especially on elevation; dusky red on dependency	Normal, or cyanotic on dependency. Petechiae and then brown pigmentation appear with chronicity.
Temperature	Cool	Normal
Edema	Absent or mild; may develop as the patient tries to relieve rest pain by lowering the leg	Present, often marked
Skin Changes	Trophic changes: thin, shiny, atrophic skin; loss of hair over the foot and toes; nails thickened and ridged	Often brown pigmentation around the ankle, stasis dermatitis, and possible thickening of the skin and narrowing of the leg as scarring develops
Ulceration	If present, involves toes or points of trauma on feet	If present, develops at sides of ankle, especially medially
Gangrene	May develop	Does not develop

Sources of photos: *Arterial Insufficiency*—Kappert A, Winsor T. *Diagnosis of Peripheral Vascular Disease.* Philadelphia, PA: FA Davis; 1972; *Venous Insufficiency*—Marks R. *Skin Disease in Old Age.* Philadelphia, PA: JB Lippincott; 1987.

TABLE
15-3

Common Ulcers of the Ankles and Feet

Chronic Venous Insufficiency Ulcer

This condition usually appears over the medial and sometimes the lateral malleolus. The ulcer contains small, painful granulation tissue and fibrin; necrosis or exposed tendons are rare. Borders are irregular, flat, or slightly steep. Pain affects quality of life in 75% of patients. Associated findings include edema, reddish pigmentation and purpura, venous varicosities, the eczematous changes of stasis dermatitis (redness, scaling, and pruritus), and at times cyanosis of the foot when dependent. Gangrene is rare.[21]

Arterial Insufficiency Ulcer

This condition occurs in the toes, feet, or possibly areas of trauma (e.g., the shins). Surrounding skin shows no callus or excess pigment, although it may be atrophic. Pain often is severe unless masked by neuropathy. Gangrene may occur, along with decreased pulses, trophic changes, foot pallor on elevation, and dusky rubor on dependency.

Neuropathic Ulcer

This condition develops in pressure points of areas with diminished sensation; seen in diabetic neuropathy, neurologic disorders, and Hansen disease. The surrounding skin is calloused. There is no pain, so the ulcer may go unnoticed. In uncomplicated cases, there is no gangrene. Associated signs include decreased sensation and absent ankle jerks.

Source of photos: Marks R. *Skin Disease in Old Age*. Philadelphia, PA: JB Lippincott; 1987.

TABLE
15-4

Some Peripheral Causes of Edema

Approximately one third of total body water is extracellular. Approximately 25% of extracellular fluid is plasma; the remainder is interstitial fluid. Normally fluid diffuses out of the capillaries, where most of it is returned to the vascular system by lymphatic drainage. Several clinical conditions disrupt this balance, resulting in *edema,* or a clinically evident accumulation of interstitial fluid. Pitting characteristics reflect the viscosity of the edema fluid, based primarily on its protein concentration.[23] When protein concentration is low, as in heart failure, pitting and recovery occur within a few seconds. In lymphedema protein levels are higher and nonpitting is more typical. Not depicted below is *capillary leak syndrome,* in which protein leaks into the interstitial space, seen in burns, angioedema, snake bites, and allergic reactions.[23,24]

Pitting

Swollen foot

Pitting Edema

Edema is a soft bilateral palpable swelling from increased interstitial fluid volume and retention of salt and water, demonstrated by pitting on pressure, on the anterior tibiae and feet. There is no skin thickening, ulceration, or pigmentation. Pitting edema occurs in several conditions: when legs are dependent from prolonged standing or sitting, which leads to increased hydrostatic pressure in the veins and capillaries; congestive heart failure leading to decreased cardiac output; nephrotic syndrome, cirrhosis, or malnutrition leading to low albumin and decreased intravascular colloid oncotic pressure; and drug use.

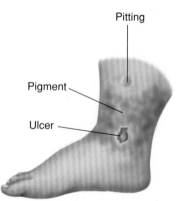

Pitting

Pigment

Ulcer

Chronic Venous Insufficiency

Edema is soft, with pitting on pressure, and occasionally bilateral. Look for brawny changes and skin thickening, especially near the ankle. Ulceration, brownish pigmentation, and edema in the feet are common. Arises from chronic obstruction and from incompetent valves in the deep venous system.

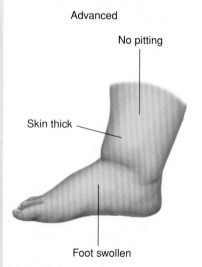

Advanced

No pitting

Skin thick

Foot swollen

Lymphedema

Edema is initially soft and pitting, then becomes indurated, hard, and nonpitting. Skin is markedly thickened; ulceration is rare. There is no pigmentation. Edema often occurs bilaterally in the feet and toes. Lymphedema arises from interstitial accumulation of protein-rich fluid when lymph channels are infiltrated or obstructed by tumor, fibrosis, or inflammation, or disrupted by axillary node dissection and/or radiation.

TABLE
15-5

Abnormalities of the Arterial Pulse and Pressure Waves

Normal

mm Hg

The pulse pressure is approximately 30–40 mm Hg. The pulse contour is smooth and rounded. (The notch on the descending slope of the pulse wave is not palpable.)

Weak

The pulse pressure is diminished, and the pulse feels weak and small. The upstroke may feel slowed, the peak prolonged. Causes include (1) decreased stroke volume, as in heart failure, hypovolemia, and severe aortic stenosis, and (2) increased peripheral resistance, as in exposure to cold and severe congestive heart failure.

Bounding

The pulse pressure is increased, and the pulse feels strong and bounding. The rise and fall may feel rapid, the peak brief. Causes include (1) increased stroke volume, decreased peripheral resistance, or both, as in fever, anemia, hyperthyroidism, aortic regurgitation, arteriovenous fistulas, and patent ductus arteriosus; (2) increased stroke volume because of slow heart rates, as in bradycardia and complete heart block; and (3) decreased compliance (increased stiffness) of the aortic walls, as in aging or atherosclerosis.

Bisferiens

A bisferiens pulse is an increased arterial pulse with a double systolic peak. Causes include pure aortic regurgitation and aortic stenosis with regurgitation.

Pulsus Alternans

The pulse alternates in amplitude from beat to beat even though the rhythm is regular. When the difference between stronger and weaker beats is slight, it can be detected only by sphygmomanometry. Pulsus alternans indicates left ventricular failure and is usually accompanied by a left-sided S3.

Bigeminal Pulse

Premature contractions

This disorder of rhythm may mimic pulsus alternans. A bigeminal pulse is caused by a normal beat alternating with a premature contraction. The stroke volume of the premature beat is diminished in relation to that of the normal beats, and the pulse varies in amplitude accordingly.

Paradoxical Pulse

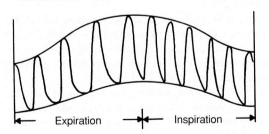

Expiration   Inspiration

A palpable decrease in the pulse's amplitude with quiet inspiration. A blood pressure cuff may be needed to detect the difference in amplitude. Systolic pressure decreases by more than 10 mm Hg during inspiration. A paradoxical pulse is found in pericardial tamponade, constrictive pericarditis (though less commonly), and obstructive lung disease.

BIBLIOGRAPHY

CITATIONS

1. Lin JS, Olson CM, Johnson ES, et al. The ankle-brachial index for peripheral artery disease screening and cardiovascular disease prediction among asymptomatic adults: a systematic evidence review for the U.S. Preventive Services Task Force. *Ann Intern Med.* 2013;159;333–341.

2. Olin JW, Allie DE, Belkin M, et al. ACCF/AHA/ACR/SCAI/SIR/SVM/SVN/SVS 2010 performance measures for adults with peripheral artery disease: a report of the American College of Cardiology Foundation/American Heart Association Task Force on performance measures, the American College of Radiology, the Society for Cardiac Angiography and Interventions, the Society for Interventional Radiology, the Society for Vascular Medicine, the Society for Vascular Nursing, and the Society for Vascular Surgery (Writing Committee to Develop Clinical Performance Measures for Peripheral Artery Disease). *Circulation.* 2010;122:2583–2618.

3. Allison MA, Ho E, Denenberg JO, et al. Ethnic-specific prevalence of peripheral arterial disease in the United States. *Am J Prev Med.* 2007;32:328–333.

4. Ostchega Y, Paulose-Ram R, Dillon CF, et al. Prevalence of peripheral arterial disease and risk factors in persons aged 60 or older: data from the National Health and Nutrition Examination Survey 1999–2004. *J am Geriatir Soc.* 2007;55:583.

5. Heit JA. The epidemiology of venous thromboembolism in the community. *Arterioscler Thromb Vasc Biol.* 2008;28:370–372.

6. Bates SM, Ginsberg JS. Treatment of deep-vein thrombosis. *N Engl J Med.* 2004;351:268–277.

7. Kucher N. Clinical practice. Deep-vein thrombosis of the upper extremities. *N Engl J Med.* 2011;364:861–869.

9. Hansson GK. Inflammation, atherosclerosis, and coronary artery disease. *N Engl J Med.* 2005;352(16):1685–1689.

8. Schoen FJ. Blood vessels. In: Kumar VK, Fausto N, Abbas AK, eds. *Robbins and Cotran Pathologic Basis of Disease.* 7th ed. Philadelphia, PA: Elsevier; 2005.

10. Lam EY, Giswold ME, Moneta GL. Venous and lymphatic disease. In: Brunicardi C, Anderson DA, Billiar TR, et al., eds. *Schwartz's Principles of Surgery.* 8th ed. New York, NY: McGraw Hill; 2005.

11. Levick JR, Michel CC. Microvascular fluid exchange and the revised Starling principle. *Cardiovasc Res.* 2010;87:198–210.

12. Hirsch AT, Haskal ZJ, Hertzer NR, et al. ACC/AHA 2005 guidelines for the management of patients with peripheral arterial disease (lower extremity, renal, mesenteric, and abdominal aortic): a collaborative report from the American Association for Vascular Surgery/Society for Vascular Surgery, Society for Cardiovascular Angiography and Interventions, Society for Vascular Medicine and Biology, Society of Interventional Radiology, and the ACC/AHA Task Force on Practice Guidelines (Writing Committee to Develop Guidelines for the Management of Patients With Peripheral Arterial Disease). Available at: http://circ.ahajournals.org/cgi/reprint/113/11/e463. Accessed June 14, 2016.

13. Rooke TW, Hirsch AT, Misra S, et al. 2011 ACCF/AHA Focused Update of the Guideline for the Management of Patients With Peripheral Artery Disease (Updating the 2005 Guideline). *Circulation.* 2011;124:2020–2045. Available at http://circ.ahajournals.org.uri.idm.oclc.org/content/124/18/2020.full?sid=ba523fd1–9738–4839-b67a-5e82ee46da4f#content-block. Accessed June 14, 2016.

14. Cha K, Falk RH. Images in clinical medicine: pulsus alternans. *N Engl J Med.* 1996;334(13):834.

15. CDC, Division of Heart Disease and Stroke Prevention. Peripheral Arterial Disease (PAD) Fact Sheet. Available at http://www.cdc.gov/dhdsp/data_statistics/fact_sheets/fs_pad.htm. Accessed June 14, 2016.

16. Norgren L, Hiatt WR, Dormandy JA, et al. Inter-Society Consensus for the Management of Peripheral Arterial Disease (TASC II). *J Vasc Surg.* 2007;45(Suppl S):S5.

17. de Mast Q, Beutler JJ. The prevalence of atherosclerotic renal artery stenosis in risk groups: a systematic literature review. *J Hypertens.* 2009;27:1333.

18. Balk E, Raman G, Chung M, et al. Effectiveness of management strategies for renal artery stenosis: a systematic review. *Ann Intern Med.* 2007;146(10):699–706.

19. Urbano FL. Homan's sign in the diagnosis of deep vein thrombosis. *Hospital Physician.* 2001.

21. De Araujo T, Valencia I, Federman D, et al. Managing the patient with venous ulcers. *Ann Intern Med.* 2003;138(4):326–334.

20. McCaffrey R, Bishop M, Adonis-Rizzo M, et al. Development and testing of a DVT risk assessment tool: providing evidence of validity and reliability. *Worldviews Evid Based Nurs.* 2007;4(1):14–20.

22. Varga J. Chapter 382: Systemic sclerosis (scleroderma) and related disorders. In: Kasper DL, Fauci AS, Hauser SL, et al., eds. *Harrison's Principles of Internal Medicine.* 19th ed. New York: McGraw-Hill Education; 2015.

23. McGee S. Chapter 52: Peripheral vascular disease; Chapter 54: Edema and deep vein thrombosis. *Evidence-Based Physical Diagnosis.* 3rd ed. Philadelphia, PA: Elsevier; 2012.

24. Lawenda BD, Mondry TE, Johnstone PA. Lymphedema: a primer on the identification and management of a chronic condition in oncologic treatment. *CA Cancer J Clin.* 2009;59:8.

ADDITIONAL REFERENCES

Aboyans V, Criqui MH, Abraham P, et al. Measurement and Interpretation of the Ankle-Brachial Index A Scientific Statement From the American Heart Association. *Circulation.* 2012;126:2890–2909.

Bonham P, Cappuccio M, Hulsey T, et al. Determining the validity of using a pocket Doppler to measure ankle brachial index (ABI) and toe brachial index (TBI) for noninvasive assessment of lower extremity arterial disease (LEAD). *J Wound Ostomy Continence Nurs.* 2006;33(3):S5–S5.

Bonham PA. Get the LEAD out: noninvasive assessment for lower extremity arterial disease using ankle brachial index and tow brachial index measurements. *J Wound Ostomy Continence Nurs.* 2006;33(1):30–41.

Bonham PA, Kelechi T. Evaluation of lower extremity arterial circulation and implications for nursing practice. *J Cardiovasc Nurs.* 2008;23(2):144–152.

Wound Ostomy and Continence Nurses Society. Ankle brachial index: Quick reference guide for clinicians. *J Wound Ostomy Continence Nurs.* 2012;39(25):S21–S29.

The Gastrointestinal and Renal Systems

LEARNING OBJECTIVES

The student will:

1. Identify the structures and function of the gastrointestinal and renal systems.

2. Identify the four quadrants and the organs in each quadrant.

3. Collect an accurate health history of the gastrointestinal and renal systems.

4. Describe the physical examination techniques and the order performed to evaluate the gastrointestinal and renal system.

5. Determine the health promotion and counseling measures related to alcohol abuse, hepatitis, colorectal cancer, and urinary incontinence.

6. Perform a complete gastrointestinal and renal system examination.

7. Document a complete gastrointestinal and renal system assessment utilizing information from the health history and the physical examination.

ANATOMY AND PHYSIOLOGY

The gastrointestinal and renal systems encompass many organs of the body. It is important to be familiar with the site and function of each organ and in which quadrant of the abdomen each is located for the assessment. The landmarks of the abdominal wall and pelvis are illustrated. The rectus abdominis muscles become more prominent when the patient raises the head and shoulders from the supine position.

Rectus abdominis
muscle

Umbilicus

Inguinal ligament

Pubic tubercle

Xiphoid process

Costal margin

Midline, overlying
linea alba

Iliac crest

Anterior superior
iliac spine

Symphysis pubis

For descriptive purposes, the abdomen is often divided by imaginary lines crossing at the umbilicus, forming the right upper quadrant (RUQ), right lower quadrant (RLQ), left upper quadrant (LUQ), and left lower quadrant (LLQ).

Examine the abdomen, moving in a clockwise rotation. Several organs are often palpable, with the exception of the stomach and much of the liver and spleen. These lie high in the abdominal cavity close to the diaphragm, where they are protected by the thoracic ribs, beyond the reach of the palpating hand. The dome of the diaphragm lies at approximately the 5th anterior intercostal space.

In the *RUQ*, the soft consistency of the *liver* makes it difficult to palpate through the abdominal wall. The lower margin of the liver, the liver edge, is often palpable at the right costal margin. The *gallbladder*, which rests against the inferior surface of the liver, and the more deeply lying *duodenum* are generally not palpable. Moving medially, the examiner encounters the rib cage with its xiphoid process, which protects the stomach. The *abdominal aorta* often has visible pulsations and is usually palpable in the upper abdomen. At a deeper level, the *lower pole of the right kidney* may be felt, especially in children or a thin person with relaxed abdominal muscles.

In the *LUQ*, the *spleen* is lateral to and behind the stomach, just above the left kidney in the left midaxillary line. Its upper margin rests against the dome of the diaphragm. The 9th, 10th, and 11th ribs protect most of the spleen. The tip of the spleen may be palpable below the left costal margin in a small percentage of adults. In healthy people, the *pancreas* cannot be detected. In the *LLQ* the firm, narrow, tubular sigmoid *colon* is often felt and portions of the transverse and descending colon may also be palpable, especially if stool is present.

In the lower midline the *bladder* may be palpated and in women, the *uterus* and *ovaries*. In the *RLQ* are bowel loops and the *appendix* at the base of the cecum near the junction of the small and large intestines. In healthy people, these are not palpable.

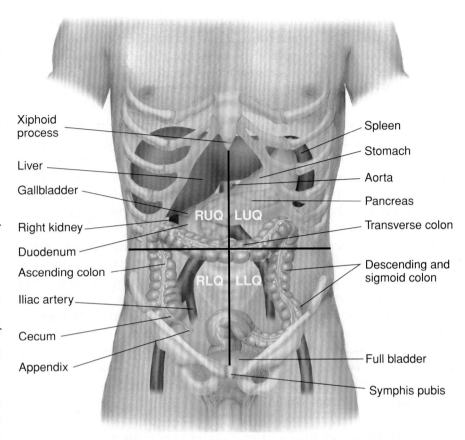

Right Upper Quadrant (RUQ)	Left Upper Quadrant (LUQ)
Ascending colon	Descending colon
Duodenum	Left kidney
Gallbladder	Pancreas (body and tail)
Right kidney	Spleen
Liver	Stomach
Pancreas (head)	Transverse colon
Transverse colon	Ureter (left)
Ureter (right)	
Right Lower Quadrant (RLQ)	**Left Lower Quadrant (LLQ)**
Appendix	Bladder
Ascending colon	Descending colon
Bladder	Ovary, uterus, fallopian tube (female)
Cecum	Prostate and spermatic cord (male)
Rectum	Small intestine
Overy, uterus and fallopian tube (female)	Sigmoid colon
Prostate and spermatic cord (male)	Ureter (left)
Small intestine	
Ureter (right)	

The *kidneys* are retroperitoneal (posterior) organs. The ribs protect their upper portions. The *costovertebral angle* is formed by the lower border of the 12th rib and the transverse processes of the upper lumbar vertebrae. This defines the region to assess for kidney tenderness, called costovertebral angle tenderness, or CVAT.

The *bladder* is a hollow reservoir with strong smooth muscle walls composed chiefly of *detrusor muscle*. The bladder distends as it fills with urine, at which time, it may be palpable above the symphysis pubis. The bladder accommodates roughly 400 to 500 mL (~1.5 to 2 cups) of urine filtered by the kidneys into the renal pelvis and the ureters. Bladder expansion stimulates parasympathetic innervation at relatively low pressures, resulting in detrusor contraction and inhibition (relaxation) of the *internal urethral sphincter*, also under autonomic control. Voiding further requires relaxation of the *external urethral sphincter*, composed of striated muscle under voluntary control. Rising pressure triggers the conscious urge to void. Increased *intraurethral* pressure can overcome rising pressures in the bladder and prevent incontinence. Intraurethral pressure is related to factors such as smooth muscle tone in the internal urethral sphincter, the thickness of the urethral mucosa, and in women, sufficient support to the bladder and proximal urethra from pelvic muscles and ligaments to maintain proper anatomic relationships. Striated muscle around the urethra can also contract voluntarily to interrupt voiding.[1]

Neuroregulatory control of the bladder functions at several levels. In infants, the bladder empties by reflex mechanisms in the sacral spinal cord. Voluntary control of the bladder depends on higher centers in the brain and on motor and sensory pathways connecting the brain and the reflex arcs of the sacral spinal cord. When voiding is inconvenient, higher centers in the brain can inhibit detrusor contractions until the capacity of the bladder, approximately 400 to 500 mL, is exceeded. The integrity of the sacral nerves that innervate the bladder can be tested by assessing perirectal and perineal sensation in the S2, S3, and S4 dermatomes (see dermatome maps, Chapter 20, The Nervous System, pp. 702–703).

POSTERIOR VIEW

THE HEALTH HISTORY

Common or Concerning Symptoms	
Gastrointestinal	**Urinary and Renal**
• Abdominal pain, acute and chronic • Indigestion, nausea, vomiting including blood (*hematemesis*), loss of appetite, early satiety • Difficulty swallowing (*dysphagia*) • Painful swallowing (*odynophagia*) • Change in bowel function • Diarrhea, constipation • Jaundice	• Suprapubic pain • Difficulty urinating (*dysuria*), urgency, or frequency • Hesitancy, decreased stream in males • Excessive urination (*polyuria*) or excess urination at night (*nocturia*) • Urinary incontinence • Blood in the urine (*hematuria*) • Flank pain and ureteral colic

Gastrointestinal complaints rank high among reasons for office and emergency room visits. Patients complain of a wide variety of upper gastrointestinal symptoms, including abdominal pain, heartburn, nausea and vomiting, difficulty or pain with swallowing, vomiting of stomach contents or blood, loss of appetite, and jaundice. Lower gastrointestinal complaints are also common: diarrhea, constipation, change in bowel habits, and blood in the stool, often described as either bright red or dark and tarry.

Numerous symptoms also originate in the *genitourinary tract*: difficulty urinating, urgency and frequency, hesitancy and decreased stream in men, high urine volume, urinating at night, incontinence, blood in the urine, and flank pain and colic from renal stones or infection. These are often accompanied by gastrointestinal symptoms such as abdominal pain, nausea, and vomiting.

Often you will need to cluster several findings from both the patient's story and your examination as you sort through various explanations for the patient's symptoms. Your skills in history taking and examination are needed for sound clinical reasoning.

Patterns and Mechanisms of Abdominal Pain

Before exploring gastrointestinal and genitourinary symptoms, review the mechanisms and clinical patterns of abdominal pain. Be familiar with the three broad categories of abdominal pain:

See Table 16-1, Chapter 16, Abdominal Pain, pp. 518–519.

• *Visceral pain* occurs when hollow abdominal organs such as the intestine or biliary tree contract unusually forcefully or are distended or stretched. Solid organs such as the liver can also become painful when their capsules are stretched. Visceral pain may be difficult to localize. It is typically palpable near the midline at levels that vary according to the structure involved, as illustrated on the next page.

Visceral pain in the RUQ suggests liver distention against its capsule from various causes of hepatitis, such as, *alcoholic hepatitis*.

Visceral pain varies in quality and may be gnawing, burning, cramping, or aching. When it becomes severe, it may be associated with sweating, pallor, nausea, vomiting, and restlessness.

Visceral periumbilical pain suggests early *acute appendicitis* from distention of an inflamed appendix. It gradually changes to parietal pain in the *RLQ* from inflammation of the adjacent parietal peritoneum.

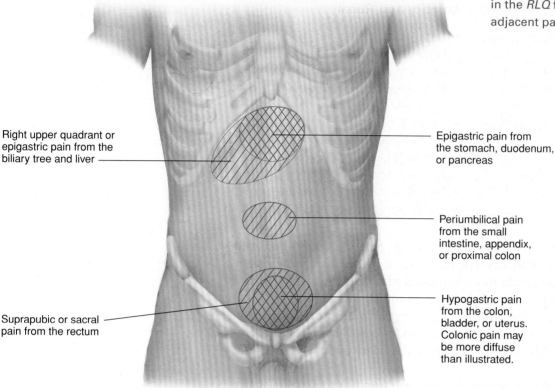

Right upper quadrant or epigastric pain from the biliary tree and liver

Epigastric pain from the stomach, duodenum, or pancreas

Periumbilical pain from the small intestine, appendix, or proximal colon

Suprapubic or sacral pain from the rectum

Hypogastric pain from the colon, bladder, or uterus. Colonic pain may be more diffuse than illustrated.

- *Parietal pain* originates from inflammation in the parietal peritoneum, also known as *peritonitis*. It is a steady, aching pain that is usually more severe than visceral pain and more precisely localized over the involved structure. It is typically aggravated by movement or coughing. Patients with parietal pain usually prefer to lie still.

- *Referred pain* is felt in more distant sites, which are innervated at approximately the same spinal levels as the inflamed structures. Referred pain often develops as the initial pain becomes more intense and thus seems to radiate or travel from the initial site. It may be palpated superficially or deeply but is usually well localized.

Pain of duodenal or pancreatic origin may be referred to the back; pain from the biliary tree, to the right scapular region or the right posterior thorax.

Pain may also be referred to the abdomen from the chest, spine, or pelvis, and complicate the assessment of abdominal pain.

Pain from *pleurisy* or inferior wall myocardial infarction may be referred to the epigastric area.

The Gastrointestinal Tract

Upper Abdominal Pain, Discomfort, and Heartburn

The prevalence of recurrent upper abdominal discomfort or pain in the United States and other Western countries is approximately 25%.[2]

Acute Upper Abdominal Pain or Discomfort

For patients with abdominal pain, causes range from benign to life threatening, so take the time to conduct a careful history. Ask the patient to describe the pain in their own words and use "OLD CART" to fill in areas the patient did not mention or to clarify the details for accuracy.

Onset: Determine the *timing of the pain*. Is it *acute or chronic*? Acute abdominal pain has many patterns. Did the pain start suddenly or gradually? When did it begin?

In emergency rooms 40% to 45% of patients have nonspecific pain, but 15% to 30% need surgery, usually for appendicitis, intestinal obstruction, or cholecystitis.[3]

Location: Ask the patient to *point to the pain*. Patients are not always able to clearly articulate their pain, especially when it is intense or radiates. The quadrant where the pain is located helps to identify which of the underlying organs are involved. If clothing interferes with the person's ability to point to the pain, repeat the question during the physical examination.

Epigastric pain occurs with gastritis, gastroesophageal reflux disease (GERD), pancreatitis and perforated ulcers. RUQ pain occurs with cholecystitis, duodenal ulcer, or hepatitis.[4]

Duration: How long does it last?
What is the pattern over a 24-hour period? Over weeks or months? Is the pain constant? or Does the pain come and go? Are you dealing with an acute illness or a chronic and recurring one?

Characteristic Symptoms:
- Ask the patient to *describe the pain in his/her own words*. Pursue important details: "Where does the pain start?"

  "Does it radiate or travel anywhere?"

  "What is the pain like?"

  If the patient has trouble describing the pain, try offering several choices:

  "Is it aching, burning, gnawing… ?"

- Ask the patient to rank the *severity of the pain* on a scale of 1 to 10. Note that severity does not always help to identify the cause. Sensitivity to abdominal pain varies widely and tends to diminish in older adults, masking acute abdominal conditions. Pain threshold varies for each individual and how patients accommodate to pain during daily activities also affect ratings of severity.

Doubling over with cramping colicky pain may signal a *renal stone*. Sudden knife-like epigastric pain can occur in *pancreatitis*.[5–7]

Associated Manifestations: Ask the patient if he or she is experiencing any other symptoms (e.g., nausea, vomiting, indigestion, constipation, diarrhea, gastrointestinal bleeding, or fever).

Relieving Factors: As you explore factors that aggravate or relieve the pain, pay special attention to nonverbals, including body position and movement, changes in eating patterns, alcohol, medications (including antacids, aspirin and aspirin-like drugs or over-the-counter medications), stress, and change in defecation or urinary patterns. Ask if indigestion or discomfort is related to exertion and relieved by rest.

Treatment: Determine what remedies the patient has tried and the results of each.

Note that angina from inferior wall coronary artery disease may present as "indigestion," but is typically precipitated by exertion and relieved by rest. See Table 13-3, Chapter 13, Chest Pain, pp. 363–364.

Chronic Upper Abdominal Discomfort or Pain

Dyspepsia is a chronic or recurrent discomfort or pain centered in the upper abdomen which is characterized by postprandial fullness, early satiety, and epigastric pain or burning.[2,8] *Discomfort* is defined as a subjective negative feeling that is nonpainful. It can include various symptoms such as bloating, nausea, upper abdominal fullness, and heartburn.

- Note that bloating, nausea, or belching can occur alone or be associated with other disorders. When they occur alone they do not meet the criteria for dyspepsia.

Bloating may occur with inflammatory bowel disease, lactose intolerance, or ovarian cancer. Belching results from aerophagia or swallowing air.

- Many patients with upper abdominal discomfort or pain will have *functional, or nonulcer dyspepsia,* defined as a 3-month history of nonspecific upper abdominal discomfort or nausea not attributable to structural abnormalities or peptic ulcer disease. Symptoms are usually recurring and typically present for more than 6 months.[8]

Multifactorial causes include delayed gastric emptying (20% to 40%), gastritis from *Helicobacter (H.) pylori* (20% to 60%), peptic ulcer disease (up to 15% if *H. pylori* is present), *irritable bowel disease,* and psychosocial factors.[2]

- Many patients with chronic upper abdominal discomfort or pain complain of *heartburn, dysphagia,* or *regurgitation.* If patients report heartburn and regurgitation together more than once a week, the accuracy of diagnosing *GERD* is over 90%.[2,9,10]

These symptoms or mucosal damage on endoscopy are the diagnostic criteria for GERD. Risk factors include reduced salivary flow, which prolongs acid clearance by damping action of the bicarbonate buffer; delayed gastric emptying; selected medications; obesity; and hiatal hernia.

- *Heartburn* is a rising retrosternal burning pain or discomfort occurring weekly or more often. It is typically aggravated by food such as alcohol, chocolate, citrus fruits, coffee, onions, and peppermint; or positions like bending over, exercising, lifting, or lying supine.

Note that angina from inferior wall coronary ischemia along the diaphragm may present as heartburn. See Table 13-3, Chapter 13, Chest Pain, pp. 363–364.

- Some patients with GERD have *atypical respiratory symptoms* such as chest pain, cough, wheezing, or aspiration pneumonia. Others complain of *pharyngeal symptoms,* such as hoarseness and chronic sore throat.[7]

- Some patients may have "*alarm symptoms*," such as difficulty swallowing (*dysphagia*), pain with swallowing (*odynophagia*), recurrent vomiting, evidence of gastrointestinal bleeding, weight loss, anemia, or risk factors for gastric cancer or painless jaundice.

Patients with uncomplicated GERD who do not respond to empiric therapy, patients older than 55 years, and those with "alarm symptoms" warrant endoscopy to detect *esophagitis*, peptic strictures, *Barrett esophagus* or esophageal cancer.[6,8,9] Approximately, 50% to 85% of those with suspected GERD have no disease on endoscopy.[11,12] Approximately, 10% of patients with chronic heartburn have Barrett esophagus, a metaplastic change in the esophageal lining from normal squamous to columnar epithelium. In those affected, dysplasia on endoscopy increases the risk of esophageal cancer from 0.1% to 0.5% (no dysplasia) to 6% to 19% per patient year (high-grade dysplasia).[11]

Lower Abdominal Pain and Discomfort—Acute and Chronic

Lower abdominal pain and discomfort may be acute or chronic. Asking the patient to point to the pain and characterize all its features, combined with findings on physical examination, will help identify possible causes. Some acute pain, especially in the suprapubic area or radiating from the flank, originates in the genitourinary tract (see pp. 489–490).

Acute Lower Abdominal Pain

Patients may complain of *acute pain* localized to the *RLQ*. Find out if it is sharp and continuous or intermittent and cramping, causing them to double over.

RLQ pain or pain that migrates from the periumbilical region, combined with abdominal wall rigidity on palpation, is suspicious for appendicitis. In women, consider causes such as *pelvic inflammatory disease, ruptured ovarian follicle, and ectopic pregnancy*.[13–15]

Cramping pain radiating to the RLQ or LLQ or groin could signify a renal stone.

When patients report acute pain in the *LLQ* or *diffuse abdominal pain,* investigate associated symptoms such as fever and loss of appetite.

LLQ pain, especially with a palpable mass, signals *diverticulitis.* Diffuse abdominal pain with abdominal distention, hyperactive high-pitched bowel sounds, and tenderness on palpation marks *small or large bowel obstruction.* Pain with absent bowel sounds, rigidity, percussion tenderness, and guarding points to *peritonitis.* See Table 16-1, Abdominal Pain, p. 518–519.

Chronic Lower Abdominal Pain

If there is *chronic pain* in the quadrants of the lower abdomen, ask about change in bowel habits and alternating diarrhea and constipation.

Change in bowel habits with a mass lesion indicates the possibility of *colon cancer.* Intermittent pain for 12 weeks of the preceding 12 months with relief from defecation, change in frequency of bowel movements, or change in form of stool (loose, watery, pellet-like), without structural or biochemical abnormalities are symptoms of *irritable bowel syndrome.*[16]

Abdominal Pain Associated With Gastrointestinal Symptoms

Patients often experience abdominal pain in conjunction with other symptoms. Ask questions that relate, beginning with; "How is your appetite?" as this may lead to other symptoms such as *indigestion, nausea, vomiting,* or *anorexia. Indigestion* is a general term for distress associated with eating that can have many meanings. Urge your patient to be more specific.

Anorexia, nausea, and vomiting accompany many gastrointestinal disorders; including pregnancy, diabetic ketoacidosis, adrenal insufficiency, hypercalcemia, uremia, liver disease, emotional states, and adverse drug reactions. Induced vomiting without nausea is more indicative of anorexia/bulimia.

- *Nausea,* often described as "feeling sick to my stomach," may progress to retching and vomiting. *Retching* describes involuntary spasm of the stomach, diaphragm, and esophagus that precedes and culminates in *vomiting,* the forceful expulsion of gastric contents out of the mouth.

Some patients may not actually vomit but raise esophageal or gastric contents without nausea or retching, called *regurgitation.*

Regurgitation occurs in GERD, esophageal stricture, and esophageal cancer.

Ask about any vomitus or regurgitated material and inspect it, if possible. Note the color, odor and quantity. Assist the patient with the amount: a teaspoon? Two teaspoons? A cupful?

Vomiting and pain indicate small bowel obstruction. Fecal odor occurs with small bowel obstruction and gastrocolic fistula.

Ask specifically if the vomitus contains any blood, and quantify the amount. Gastric juice is clear and mucoid. Small amounts of yellowish or greenish bile are common and have no special significance. Brownish or blackish vomitus with a "coffee grounds" appearance suggests blood altered by gastric acid. Coffee-grounds emesis or red blood is termed *hematemesis*.

Is there any dehydration or electrolyte imbalance from prolonged vomiting, or significant blood loss? Do the patient's symptoms suggest any complications of vomiting, such as aspiration into the lungs, seen in debilitated, obtunded, or elderly patients?

- *Anorexia* is loss or lack of appetite. Find out if it arises from intolerance to certain foods, distortion of self-image, abdominal discomfort (real or perceived) or a fear of food (*cibophobia*). Check for associated symptoms of nausea, vomiting, or excessive exercise.

- "Food fear" with abdominal pain and a slightly distended soft nontender abdomen are hallmarks of *mesenteric ischemia*. Patients may complain of unpleasant *abdominal fullness* after light or moderate meals, or *early satiety*, the inability to eat a full meal. A dietary assessment or recall may be warranted (see Chapter 8, Nutrition and Hydration).

Other Gastrointestinal Symptoms

Difficulty Swallowing (*Dysphagia*) and/or Painful Swallowing (*Odynophagia*)

Less commonly, patients may report difficulty swallowing from impaired passage of solid foods or liquids from the mouth to the stomach, or *dysphagia*. Food seems to stick, or "not go down right," suggesting motility disorders or structural anomalies. The sensation of a lump or foreign body in the throat unrelated to swallowing, called a *globus* sensation, is not true dysphagia.

Do you have any difficulty/pain swallowing? Ask the patient to point to where the dysphagia occurs.

Hematemesis may accompany esophageal or gastric varices, gastritis, or peptic ulcer disease.

Symptoms of blood loss such as lightheadedness or syncope depend on the rate and volume of bleeding and are rare until blood loss exceeds 500 mL.

If a person has fullness or early satiety, consider *diabetic gastroparesis,* anticholinergic medications, *gastric outlet obstruction, or gastric cancer;* if early satiety also consider, *hepatitis.*

For types of dysphagia, see Table 16-2, Chapter 16, Dysphagia, p. 520.

Indicators of *oropharyngeal dysphagia* include drooling, nasopharyngeal regurgitation, and cough from aspiration. Gurgling or regurgitation of undigested food occurs in GERD, motility disorders, and structural disorders like *esophageal stricture* and *Zenker diverticulum.* Causes are generally mechanical/obstructive in younger adults and neurologic/muscular in older adults (stroke, Parkinson disease).[17]

Pointing to below the sternoclavicular notch indicates *esophageal dysphagia.*

Pursue which types of foods provoke symptoms: solid foods, or solids and liquids? Establish the timing. When does the dysphagia start? Is it intermittent or persistent? Is it progressing? If so, over what time period? Are there associated symptoms and medical conditions?

If solid foods, consider structural esophageal causes such as *esophageal stricture,* webbing or *Schatzki ring,* neoplasm; if solids and liquids, a motility disorder, such as *achalasia,* is more likely.

Is there *odynophagia,* or pain on swallowing?

Consider esophageal ulceration from ingestion of aspirin or nonsteroidal anti-inflammatory agents, caustic ingestion, radiation, or infection from *Candida, cytomegalovirus, herpes simplex,* or *HIV.*

Change in Bowel Function

To assess *bowel function* start with open-ended questions: "Have you noticed any change in your bowel movements?" "How often do they occur?" "Have you noticed any change in stool appearance?" The range of normal bowel movements varies from a few a day to only a few per week depending on the individual. Some patients may complain of passing excessive gas, or *flatus,* normally about 600 mL per day.

Causes may include *aerophagia,* eating gas-producing foods (e.g., legumes, *intestinal lactase deficiency,* or *irritable bowel syndrome.)*

Diarrhea and Constipation

Patients vary widely in their views of diarrhea and constipation. Increased water content of the stool results in *diarrhea,* or stool volume >200 g in 24 hours. Patients, however, usually focus on the change to loose watery stools or increased frequency during ≥75% of defecations.[18,19]

See Table 16-3, Chapter 16, Constipation, p. 521 and Table 16-4, Chapter 16, Diarrhea, pp. 522–523.

Ask about the duration. *Acute diarrhea* lasts 2 weeks or less. *Chronic diarrhea* is defined as lasting 4 weeks or more.

Acute diarrhea is usually caused by infection[16]; chronic diarrhea is typically noninfectious in origin, as in *Crohn disease* and *ulcerative colitis.*

Ask about the characteristics of the diarrhea, including volume, frequency, and consistency.

Is there mucus, pus, or blood? Is there associated *tenesmus,* a constant urge to defecate, accompanied by pain, cramping, and involuntary straining?

High-volume, frequent watery stools usually are from the small intestine; small-volume stools with *tenesmus,* or diarrhea with mucus, pus, or blood occurs in rectal inflammatory conditions.

Does diarrhea occur at night?

Nocturnal diarrhea usually has pathologic significance.

Are the stools greasy or oily? Frothy? Foul-smelling? Floating on the surface because of excessive gas?

Oily residue, sometimes frothy or floating, occurs with *steatorrhea*, or fatty diarrheal stools, from malabsorption in *celiac sprue*, *pancreatic insufficiency, cystic fibrosis*, or *small bowel bacterial overgrowth*.

Associated features should be considered when identifying possible causes. These include current and or alternative medications, especially antibiotics, recent travel, diet patterns, baseline bowel habits, and risk factors for immunocompromise.

Diarrhea is common with use of penicillins and macrolides, magnesium-based antacids, metformin, and herbal and alternative medicines. Also, consider *Clostridium difficile* infection if recently in the hospital.[20]

Another common symptom is *constipation*. Recent definitions stipulate that constipation should be present for at least 12 weeks of the prior 6 months with at least two of the following conditions: fewer than three bowel movements per week; 25% or more defecations with either straining or sensation of incomplete evacuation; lumpy or hard stools; or manual facilitation.[18,19]

Ask about frequency of bowel movements, passage of hard or painful stools, straining, and a sense of incomplete rectal emptying or pressure. Types of primary or functional constipation are normal transit, slow transit, impaired expulsion (from pelvic floor disorders), and constipation-predominant irritable bowel syndrome. Secondary causes include medications and conditions like amyloidosis, diabetes, and CNS disorders.[21,22]

Check if the patient actually looks at the stool and can describe its color and bulk.

Thin, pencil-like stool occurs in an obstructing "apple core" lesion of the sigmoid colon.

What remedies has the patient tried? Do medications or stress play a role? Are there associated systemic disorders?

Causes of constipation may include medications such as anticholinergic agents, calcium channel blockers, iron supplements, and opiates. Constipation also occurs with *diabetes, hypothyroidism, hypercalcemia, multiple sclerosis, Parkinson disease*, and *systemic sclerosis*.

Occasionally there is no passage of either feces or gas, or *obstipation*.

Obstipation signifies intestinal obstruction.

Inquire about the color of stools. Is there *melena,* or black tarry stools, or *hematochezia* (stools that are red or maroon-colored)? Pursue such important details as quantity and frequency of any blood.

See Table 16-5, Chapter 16, Black and Bloody Stools, p. 524.

Melena may appear with as little as 100 mL of *upper gastrointestinal bleeding,* and *hematochezia,* is usually from *lower gastrointestinal bleeding,* but may occur with brisk upper gastrointestinal bleeding.

Is it mixed in with stool or on the surface? Is it streaks on the toilet paper or more copious?

Blood on the surface or toilet paper may occur with *hemorrhoids.*

Jaundice

In some patients, you will find jaundice or icterus, the yellowish discoloration of the skin and sclerae from increased levels of bilirubin, a bile pigment derived chiefly from the breakdown of hemoglobin. Normally the hepatocytes conjugate, or combine, unconjugated bilirubin with other substances, making the bile water soluble, and then excrete the conjugated bilirubin into the bile. The bile passes through the cystic duct into the common bile duct, which also drains the extrahepatic ducts from the liver. More distally the common bile duct and the pancreatic ducts empty into the duodenum at the ampulla of Vater (hepatopancreatic duct).

Mechanisms of Jaundice

- Increased production of bilirubin
- Decreased uptake of bilirubin by the hepatocytes
- Decreased ability of the liver to conjugate bilirubin
- Decreased excretion of bilirubin into the bile, resulting in absorption of *conjugated* bilirubin back into the blood

Predominantly unconjugated bilirubin occurs from the first three mechanisms, as in *hemolytic anemia* (increased destruction) and *Gilbert syndrome.*

Impaired excretion of conjugated bilirubin occurs with *viral hepatitis, cirrhosis, primary biliary cirrhosis,* and drug-induced cholestasis, from medications such as oral contraceptives, methyl testosterone, and chlorpromazine.

Intrahepatic jaundice can be *hepatocellular,* from damage to the hepatocytes, or *cholestatic,* from impaired excretion as a result of damaged hepatocytes or intrahepatic bile ducts. *Extrahepatic* jaundice arises from obstruction of the extrahepatic bile ducts, most commonly the cystic and common bile ducts.

Gallstones or pancreatic, cholangio, or duodenal carcinoma may obstruct the common bile duct.

As the patient with jaundice is assessed, pay special attention to the associated symptoms and the setting in which the illness occurred. What was the *color of the urine* as the patient became ill? When the level of conjugated bilirubin increases in the blood, it may be excreted into the urine, turning the urine a dark yellowish brown or tea color. Unconjugated bilirubin is not water soluble, so it is not excreted into urine. Is there any associated pain?

Dark urine from bilirubin indicates impaired excretion of bilirubin into the gastrointestinal tract. Painless jaundice points to malignant obstruction of the bile ducts, seen in *duodenal* or *pancreatic carcinoma;* painful jaundice is commonly infectious in origin, as in *hepatitis A* and *cholangitis.*

Ask also about the *color of the stools*. When excretion of bile into the intestine is completely obstructed, the stools become gray or light colored, or *acholic*, without bile.

Does the skin itch without other obvious explanation? Is there associated pain? What is its pattern? Has it been recurrent in the past?

Acholic stools may occur briefly in *viral hepatitis;* they are common in obstructive jaundice.

Itching indicates cholestatic or obstructive jaundice; pain may signify a distended liver capsule, biliary cholic, or pancreatic cancer.

Ask About Risk Factors for Liver Diseases, Such As

- *Hepatitis:* Travel or meals in areas of poor sanitation, ingestion of contaminated water or food (hepatitis A); parenteral or mucous membrane exposure to infectious body fluids such as blood, serum, semen, and vaginal fluid, especially through sexual contact with an infected partner or use of shared needles for injection drug use (hepatitis B); sharing needles of infected persons or tainted blood transfusion (hepatitis C)
- *Alcoholic hepatitis* or *alcoholic cirrhosis* (screen the patient carefully about alcohol use, e.g., CAGE questionnaire; see Chapter 4, The Health History, pp. 74–75.)
- *Toxic liver damage* from medications, industrial solvents, or environmental toxins
- *Gallbladder disease* or *surgery* that may result in extrahepatic biliary obstruction
- *Hereditary disorders* in the Family History

The Renal System

General questions for a urinary history include:

> Do you have any difficulty passing your urine?
> How often do you go?
> Do you have to get up at night? How often?
> How much urine do you pass at a time?
> Is there any pain or burning?
> Do you ever feel rushed getting to the toilet in time?
> Do you ever leak any urine? Or wet yourself unintentionally?
> Can you sense when your bladder is full and when voiding occurs?

See Table 16-6, Chapter 16, Frequency, Nocturia, and Polyuria, p. 525.

Involuntary voiding or lack of awareness suggests cognitive or neurosensory deficits.

Ask women:

Does sudden coughing, sneezing, or laughing cause loss of urine?

Almost half of young women report this experience even before bearing children. Occasional leakage is not necessarily significant.

Stress incontinence arises from decreased intraurethral pressure (see Table 16-7, Chapter 16, Urinary Incontinence, pp. 526–527).

Ask older men:

Do you have trouble starting your stream?
Do you have to stand close to the toilet to void?
Is there a change in the force or size of your stream, or straining to void?
Do you hesitate or stop in the middle of voiding?
Is there dribbling when you are through?

These problems are common in men with partial bladder outlet obstruction from *benign prostatic hyperplasia* or *urethral stricture*.

Suprapubic Pain

Disorders in the urinary tract may cause pain in either the abdomen or the back. Bladder disorders may cause *suprapubic pain*. In *bladder infection*, pain in the lower abdomen is typically dull and pressure-like. In sudden overdistention of the bladder, pain is often agonizing; in contrast, chronic bladder distention is usually painless.

Pain from sudden overdistention accompanies acute urinary retention.

Dysuria, Urgency, or Frequency

Infection or irritation of either the bladder or urethra often leads to *pain on urination*, usually felt as a burning sensation. Some clinicians refer to this as *dysuria*, whereas others reserve the term *dysuria* for difficulty voiding. Women may report internal urethral discomfort, sometimes described as a pressure or an external burning from the flow of urine across irritated or inflamed labia. Men typically feel a burning sensation proximal to the glans penis. In contrast, *prostatic pain* is felt in the perineum and occasionally in the rectum.

Painful urination accompanies cystitis (bladder infection), *urethritis* and *urinary tract infections*, bladder stones, tumors and in men, acute *prostatitis*. Women report, internal burning occurs in *urethritis*, and external burning in *vulvovaginitis*.

Other commonly associated urinary symptoms are *urgency* and *frequency*. Urgency is an unusually intense and immediate desire to void, sometimes leading to involuntary voiding or urge incontinence. Frequency is abnormally frequent voiding. Ask about any related fever or chills, blood in the urine, or any pain in the abdomen, flank, or back (see illustration on p. 490). Men with partial obstruction to urinary outflow often report *hesitancy* in starting the urine stream, straining to void, reduced caliber and force of the urinary stream, or dribbling as voiding is completed.[23,24]

Urgency suggests urinary tract infection or irritation from possible urinary calculi. Frequency is common in *urinary tract infection* and *bladder neck obstruction*. In men, painful urination without frequency or urgency suggests *urethritis*. Associated flank or back pain suggests *pyelonephritis*.[26,26]

Polyuria or Nocturia

Additional terms are used to describe important alterations in the pattern of urination. *Polyuria* refers to a significant increase in 24-hour urine volume, roughly defined as exceeding 3 L. It should be distinguished from urinary frequency, which can involve voiding in high amounts, seen in polyuria, or in small amounts, as in infection. *Nocturia* refers to urinary frequency at night, sometimes defined as awakening the patient more than once; urine volumes may be large or small. Clarify the patient's daily total fluid intake. Note any change in nocturnal voiding patterns and the number of trips to the bathroom to void.

Causes of polyuria include the high fluid intake of *psychogenic polydipsia* and poorly controlled *diabetes,* the decreased secretion of antidiuretic hormone (ADH) of *central diabetes insipidus,* and the decreased renal sensitivity to ADH of *nephrogenic diabetes insipidus.*

Urinary Incontinence

Up to 30% of older adults are concerned about *urinary incontinence,* an involuntary loss of urine that can be socially limiting or cause problems with hygiene. If the patient reports incontinence, ask questions to ascertain when this occurs and how often.

See Table 16-7, Chapter 16, Incontinence, pp. 526–527.

Bladder control involves complex neuroregulatory and motor mechanism**s.** Several central or peripheral nerve lesions affecting S2–4 can affect normal voiding. Does the patient sense when the bladder is full? And when voiding occurs? There are five broad categories of incontinence, including *stress, urge, overflow, functional,* and *mixed incontinence.*

> Do you leak small amounts of urine with increased intra-abdominal pressure from coughing, sneezing, laughing, or lifting?
> Is it difficult to hold the urine once there is an urge to void?
> Is a large amount of urine lost?
> Is there a sensation of bladder fullness? Frequent leakage?
> Do you void small amounts of urine but have difficulty emptying the bladder?

Stress incontinence with increased intra-abdominal pressure suggests decreased contractility of urethral sphincter or poor support of bladder neck; *urge incontinence,* if unable to hold the urine, suggests detrusor over activity; *overflow incontinence,* neurologic disorders, or anatomic obstruction from pelvic organs or the prostate limit bladder emptying until the bladder becomes over distended.[27–29]

In addition, the patient's functional status may significantly affect voiding behaviors even when the urinary tract is intact. Is the patient mobile? Alert? Able to respond to voiding cues and reach the bathroom? Is alertness or voiding affected by medications?

Functional incontinence may arise from impaired cognition, musculoskeletal problems, or immobility.

Mixed incontinence may arise from a combination of the types of incontinence.

Hematuria

Blood in the urine, or *hematuria,* is an important cause for concern. When visible to the naked eye, it is called *gross hematuria.* The urine may appear frankly bloody. Blood may be detected only during microscopic urinalysis, known as *microscopic hematuria.* Smaller amounts of blood may tinge the urine with a pinkish or brownish cast. In women, be sure to distinguish menstrual blood from hematuria. If the urine is reddish, ask about ingestion of beets or medications that might discolor the urine. Test the urine with a dipstick and microscopic examination before you settle on the term *hematuria.*

Kidney or Flank Pain; Ureteral Colic

Disorders of the urinary tract may also cause *kidney pain,* often reported as *flank pain,* at or below the posterior costal margin near the costovertebral angle. It may radiate anteriorly toward the umbilicus. Kidney pain is a visceral pain usually produced by distention of the renal capsule and typically dull, aching, and steady. *Ureteral colic* is dramatically different, severe, colicky pain originating at the costovertebral angle and radiating around the trunk into the lower quadrant of the abdomen and groin, or possibly into

Flank pain, fever, and chills suggest *acute pyelonephritis.*

Renal or ureteral colic is caused by sudden obstruction of a ureter, for example, from urinary stones or blood clots.

the upper thigh, testicle, or labium. Ureteral pain results from sudden distention of the ureter and associated distention of the renal pelvis. Ask about any associated fever, chills, or hematuria.

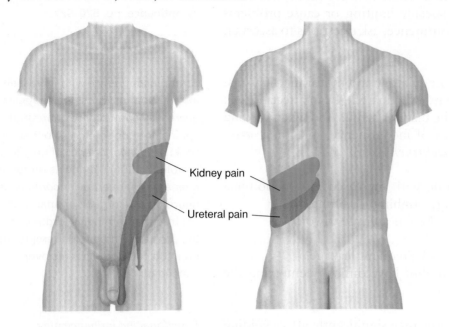

Kidney pain

Ureteral pain

PHYSICAL EXAMINATION

Equipment

- Good lighting
- Stethoscope
- Tape measure with centimeter markings

For the abdominal examination, the patient should be relaxed and have an empty bladder. Explain the steps of the examination and optimize lighting for the examination. The patient should be draped, with exposure of the abdomen.

Tips for Examining the Abdomen

- Make the patient comfortable in the supine position, with a pillow under the head and perhaps another under the knees. Slide your hand under the low back to see if the patient is relaxed and lying flat on the table.
- Ask the patient to keep the arms at the sides or folded across the chest. When the arms are above the head, the abdominal wall stretches and tightens, which hinders palpation.
- *Draping the patient.* To expose the abdomen, place the drape or sheet at the level of the symphysis pubis, then raise the gown to below the

An arched back thrusts the abdomen forward and tightens the abdominal muscles.

nipple line just above the xiphoid process. The groin should be visible but the genitalia should remain covered. The abdominal muscles should be relaxed to enhance all aspects of the examination, especially palpation.

- Before you begin palpation, ask the patient to point to any areas of pain so you can examine these areas last.
- Warm your hands and stethoscope. To warm your hands, rub them together or place them under warm water. Approach the patient calmly and avoid quick, unexpected movements. Avoid having long fingernails which could inadvertently scratch the patient.
- Stand at the patient's *right side* and proceed in a systematic fashion with inspection, auscultation, percussion, and palpation. Visualize each organ in the region you are examining. *Watch the patient's face for any signs of pain or discomfort.*
- If necessary, distract the patient with conversation or questions. If the patient is frightened or ticklish, begin palpation with the patient's hand under yours. After a few moments, slip your hand underneath to palpate directly.

The Abdomen

Inspection

First observe the general appearance of the patient. Are they lying quietly or walking guarding the abdomen, are they gripping the handrail, clenching their fists or their side, or do you notice other nonverbals that suggest abdominal pain or discomfort.

Starting from the usual standing position at the right side of the bed, inspect the surface, contours and movements of the abdomen. Watch for peristalsis or bulges. It may be helpful to sit or bend down to view the abdomen tangentially.

- During the *skin* assessment note:

  Scars. Describe or diagram their location.

  Striae. Old silver striae or stretch marks are normal.

  Pink–purple striae are found in *Cushing syndrome.*

  Dilated veins. A few small veins may be visible normally.

  Dilated veins suggest portal hypertension from *hepatic cirrhosis* or *inferior vena cava obstruction.*

  Rashes and lesions. Describe and/or diagram.

  Ecchymosis. Describe the color discoloration and location.

  Ecchymosis of the abdominal wall is seen in intraperitoneal or retroperitoneal hemorrhage.

- *The umbilicus.* Observe its contour and location and any inflammation or bulges suggesting a hernia.

  See Table 16-8, Chapter 16, Localized Bulges in the Abdominal Wall, p. 528.

- The contour of the abdomen

  Is the abdomen flat, rounded, protuberant, or scaphoid (markedly concave or hollowed)?

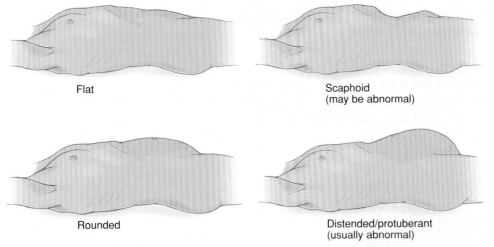

Flat

Scaphoid (may be abnormal)

Rounded

Distended/protuberant (usually abnormal)

See Table 16-9, Chapter 16, Protuberant Abdomens, p. 529.

  Observe for the bulging flanks of *ascites,* the suprapubic bulge of a distended bladder or pregnant uterus, or femoral, umbilical, or inguinal hernias.
  Inspect for abdominal symmetry. Asymmetry suggests a hernia, enlarged organ, or mass.
  Inspect for the lower abdominal mass of an ovarian or uterine tumor.

- Inspect for increased peristaltic waves which suggest an *intestinal obstruction.*

- Inspect for the increased pulsations of an *abdominal aortic aneurysm (AAA)* or of *increased pulse pressure.*

- Note: *Peristalsis* may be visible normally in very thin people and the normal aortic pulsation is frequently visible in the epigastrium.

Auscultation

Auscultation provides important information about bowel motility. Auscultate the abdomen before performing percussion or palpation because these maneuvers may alter the frequency of bowel sounds. Learn to identify variations in normal bowel sounds and to detect changes suggestive of peritoneal inflammation or obstruction. Auscultation may also reveal bruits, or vascular sounds resembling heart murmurs, over the aorta or other arteries in the abdomen.

Place the diaphragm of your stethoscope gently on the abdomen. Listen for bowel sounds and note their frequency and character. Normal sounds consist of clicks and gurgles, occurring at an estimated frequency of 5 to 34 per minute. Occasionally you may hear the prolonged gurgles of hyperperistalsis from "stomach growling, called *borborygmi.*" Bowel sounds are transmitted throughout the abdomen and listening in the RLQ should be sufficient to hear bowel sounds. If unable to hear bowel sounds, then proceed to listen in all four quadrants and question why this alteration exists.

Abdominal Bruits and Friction Rubs

If the patient has high blood pressure, listen in the epigastrium and in each upper quadrant for *bruits.* Later in the examination, when the patient sits up, listen also in the costovertebral angles. Epigastric bruits confined to systole may be heard normally.

See Table 16-10, Chapter 16, Sounds in the Abdomen, p. 530.

Bruits suggest vascular occlusive disease.

Altered bowel sounds are common in diarrhea, intestinal obstruction, *paralytic ileus,* and *peritonitis.*

A bruit in the midclavicular line that has both systolic and diastolic components strongly suggests *renal artery stenosis* as the cause of hypertension.

Concept Mastery Alert

When evaluating a patient for a possible intestinal obstruction, the nurse needs to assess the patient's bowel sounds, auscultating in each abdominal quadrant for five minutes. This time frame is necessary before determining whether or not a patient has bowel sounds. Typically, in a patient with an intestinal obstruction, the nurse would auscultate a change in pitch or rushes of high-pitched sounds.

Aorta

Renal artery

Iliac artery

Femoral artery

Listen for bruits over the aorta, the iliac arteries, and the femoral arteries. Bruits confined to systole are relatively common, however, and do not necessarily signify occlusive disease.

Listen over the liver and spleen for *friction rubs*.

Bruits with both systolic and diastolic components suggest the turbulent blood flow of partial arterial occlusion or arterial insufficiency.

Friction rubs are present in hepatoma, gonococcal infection around the liver, splenic infarction, and pancreatic carcinoma.

Percussion

Percussion helps you assess the amount and distribution of gas in the abdomen, viscera, and masses that are solid or fluid-filled, and the size of the liver and spleen.

Percuss the abdomen lightly in all four quadrants to assess the distribution of *tympany* and *dullness*. Tympany usually predominates because of gas in the gastrointestinal tract, but scattered areas of dullness from fluid and feces are also common.

Note any large dull areas that might indicate an underlying mass or enlarged organ. This observation will guide palpation.

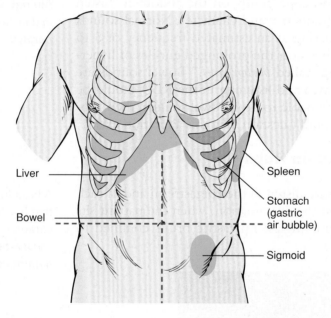

A protuberant abdomen that is tympanic throughout suggests *intestinal obstruction* or *paralytic ileus*. See Table 16-9, Chapter 16, Protuberant Abdomens, p. 529.

Dull areas are heard over a pregnant uterus, ovarian tumor, distended bladder, or large liver or spleen.

On each side of a protuberant abdomen, note where abdominal tympanic changes to the dullness of solid posterior structures.

Dullness in both flanks prompts further assessment for ascites (see pp. 506–507).

Briefly percuss the lower anterior chest, between the lungs above and costal margins. On the right, you will usually find the dullness of the liver; on the left, the tympany that overlies the gastric air bubble and the splenic flexure of the colon.

In the rare condition of situs inversus, organs are reversed: the air bubble on the right, liver dullness on the left.

Palpation

Light Palpation

Gentle palpation aids detection of abdominal tenderness, muscular resistance, and some superficial organs and masses. It also serves to reassure and relax the patient.

Keeping your hand and forearm on a horizontal plane, with fingers together and flat on the abdominal surface, palpate the abdomen with a light, gentle, dipping motion, approximately 1 cm. As you move your hand, raise it just off the skin and glide smoothly, palpating in all four quadrants.

Identify any superficial organs or masses and any area of tenderness or increased resistance to palpation. If resistance is present, try to distinguish voluntary guarding from involuntary muscular spasm. Voluntary guarding usually decreases with the techniques listed below.

Involuntary rigidity (muscular spasm) typically persists despite these maneuvers, suggesting peritoneal inflammation.

Use methods described earlier to assist the patient relax (see Chapter 16, p. 490–491).

Ask the patient to exhale and then palpate to aid in the relaxation of abdominal muscles.

Ask the patient to mouth-breathe with the jaw wide open.

Deep Palpation

Deep palpation is usually required to delineate the liver edge, the kidneys, and abdominal masses. Again using the palmar surfaces of your fingers, press down about 5 to 8 cm (2 to 3 inches) in all four quadrants. Identify any masses and note their location, size, shape, consistency, tenderness, pulsations, and any mobility with respiration or with the examining hand. Correlate your findings from palpation with the percussion notes.

Abdominal masses may be categorized in several ways: physiologic (pregnant uterus), inflammatory (diverticulitis of the colon), vascular (an AAA), neoplastic (carcinoma of the colon), or obstructive (a distended bladder or dilated loop of bowel).

TWO-HANDED DEEP PALPATION

Assessment for Peritoneal Inflammation

Abdominal pain and tenderness, especially when associated with muscular spasm, suggest inflammation of the parietal peritoneum, or *peritonitis*. Signs of peritonitis include a positive cough test, guarding, rigidity, rebound tenderness, and percussion tenderness. Even before palpation, ask the patient to cough and determine where the cough produces pain. Then, palpate gently with one finger to localize the area of pain. Pain produced by light percussion has similar localizing value. These maneuvers may establish the area of peritoneal inflammation.

Sign of Peritonitis

Guarding. Guarding is a voluntary contraction of the abdominal wall, often accompanied by a grimace that may diminish when the patient is distracted.

Rigidity. Rigidity is an involuntary reflex contraction of the abdominal wall from peritoneal inflammation that persists over several examinations.

Rebound tenderness. Rebound tenderness refers to pain expressed by the patient after the examiner presses down on an area of tenderness and suddenly removes the hand. To assess rebound tenderness, ask the patient "Which hurts more, when I press or let go?" Press down with your fingers firmly and slowly, then withdraw your hand quickly. The maneuver is positive if withdrawal produces pain. Percuss gently to check for percussion tenderness.

When positive, these signs roughly double the likelihood of *peritonitis;* rigidity makes peritonitis almost four times more likely.[30] Causes include *appendicitis, cholecystitis,* and a perforation of the bowel wall.

See Table 16-12, Tender Abdomen, pp. 532–533.

The Liver

The rib cage shelters most of the liver and can make assessment difficult. Liver size and shape can be estimated by percussion and palpation. Liver consistency, and tenderness is examined by palpation.

Percussion

Measure the vertical span of liver dullness in the right midclavicular line. First, locate the midclavicular line carefully to improve accurate measurement. Use a light to moderate percussion stroke, because a heavier stroke can underestimate liver size.[37] Starting at a level below the umbilicus (in an area of tympany, not dullness), percuss upward toward the liver. Identify the *lower border of dullness* in the midclavicular line.

Next, identify the *upper border of liver dullness* in the midclavicular line. Starting at the nipple line, percuss downward in the midclavicular line until lung resonance shifts to liver dullness. Gently displace a woman's breast as necessary to be sure to start in a resonant area. The course of percussion is shown in the picture below.

The span of liver dullness is *increased* when the liver is enlarged.

The span of liver dullness is *decreased* when the liver is small, or when free air is present below the diaphragm, as from a *perforated bowel or hollow viscus*. Liver span may decrease with resolution of *hepatitis* or *congestive heart failure* or, less commonly, with progression of *fulminant hepatitis*.

Liver dullness may be displaced downward by the low diaphragm of *chronic obstructive pulmonary disease*. Span, however, remains normal.

PERCUSSING LIVER SPAN

Now measure in centimeters the distance between the two points—the vertical span of liver dullness. Normal the liver span, shown on next page, is generally greater in men than in women and greater in taller compared to shorter people. If the liver seems to be enlarged, outline the lower edge by percussing medially and laterally.

Dullness of a right pleural effusion or consolidated lung, if adjacent to liver dullness, may falsely *increase* estimated liver size.

Gas in the colon may produce tympany in the RUQ, obscure liver dullness, and falsely *decrease* estimated liver size.

4–8 cm in
midsternal line

6–12 cm
in right
midclavicular
line

NORMAL LIVER SPANS

Measurements of liver span by percussion are more accurate when the liver is enlarged with a palpable edge.[31–33]

In *chronic liver disease* finding an enlarged palpable liver edge roughly doubles the likelihood of *cirrhosis*.[30]

Palpation

Place your left hand behind the patient, parallel to and supporting the right 11th and 12th ribs and adjacent soft tissues below. Remind the patient to relax on your hand if necessary. By pressing the left hand forward, the patient's liver may be felt more easily by the examining hand.

Place your right hand on the patient's right abdomen lateral to the rectus muscle, with the fingertips well below the lower border of liver dullness. Some examiners point their fingers up toward the patient's head, whereas others prefer a somewhat more oblique position. In either case, press gently in and up.

Ask the patient to take a deep breath. Try to feel the liver edge as it slides down to meet the fingertips. When palpable, the normal liver edge is soft, sharp, and regular with a smooth surface. If you feel the edge, slightly lighten the pressure of the palpating hand slightly so that the liver can slip under the finger pads and you can feel its anterior surface. Note any tenderness. The normal liver may be slightly tender.

Firmness or hardness of the liver, bluntness or rounding of its edge, and surface irregularity are suspicious for liver disease.

On inspiration, the liver is palpable about 3 cm below the right costal margin in the midclavicular line. Some people breathe more with the chest than with the diaphragm. It may be helpful to train such a patient to "breathe with the abdomen," which brings the liver, as well as the spleen and kidneys, into a palpable position during inspiration.

An obstructed, distended gallbladder may merge with the liver, forming a firm oval mass below the liver's edge and is dull to percussion.

Palpate the liver edge, altering the examining pressure according to the thickness and resistance of the abdominal wall. If you cannot feel the edge, move your palpating hand closer to the costal margin and try again.

Starting palpation too close to the right costal margin risks missing the lower edge of an enlarged liver that extends into the RLQ, as shown.

Try to trace the liver edge both laterally and medially. Palpation through the rectus muscles, can be difficult. A palpable liver edge does not reliably indicate hepatomegaly.

See Table 16-11, Liver Enlargment: Apparent and Real, p. 531.

The "*hooking technique*" may be helpful, especially when the patient is obese. Stand to the right of the patient's chest. Place both hands, side by side, on the right abdomen below the border of liver dullness. Press in with your fingers and up toward the costal margin. Ask the patient to take a deep breath. The liver edge shown on the next page is palpable with the finger pads of both hands.

Tenderness over the liver suggests inflammation, found in *hepatitis,* or congestion, from *heart failure.*

(AP) The Spleen

When a spleen enlarges, it expands anteriorly, downward, and medially, often replacing the tympany of the stomach and colon with the dullness of a solid organ. It then becomes palpable below the costal margin. Dullness to percussion suggests splenic enlargement, but may be absent when an enlarged spleen lies above the costal margin.

Percussion

Two techniques may help to detect *splenomegaly,* an enlarged spleen:

- *Percus the left lower anterior chest wall* from the border of cardiac dullness at the 6th rib to the anterior axillary line and down the costal margin, an area termed the *Traube space.* As you percuss along the routes shown by the arrows in the following figures, note the lateral extent of tympany. Percussion is moderately accurate in detecting splenomegaly (sensitivity, 60% to 80%; specificity, 72% to 94%).[34]

If percussion dullness is present, palpation correctly detects splenomegaly more than 80% of the time.[34]

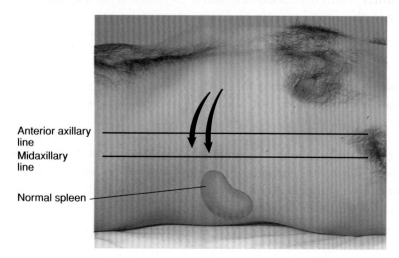

Anterior axillary line
Midaxillary line
Normal spleen

If tympany is prominent, especially laterally, splenomegaly is not likely. The dullness of a normal spleen is usually hidden within the dullness of other posterior tissues.

- *Check for a splenic percussion sign.* Percuss the lowest interspace in the left anterior axillary line, as shown next. This area is usually tympanic. Then ask the patient to take a deep breath, and percuss again. When spleen size is normal, the percussion note usually remains tympanic.

Fluid or solids in the stomach or colon may also cause dullness in the Traube space.

A change in percussion note from tympany to dullness on inspiration is a *positive splenic enlargement;* however, this is only moderately useful in detecting splenomegaly.

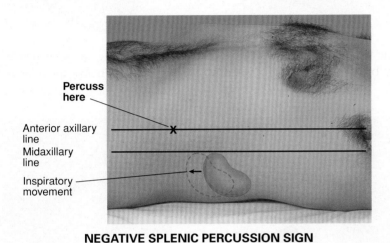

Percuss here

Anterior axillary line

Midaxillary line

Inspiratory movement

NEGATIVE SPLENIC PERCUSSION SIGN

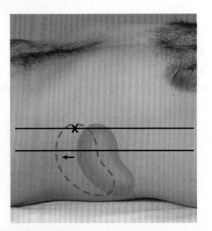

POSITIVE SPLENIC PERCUSSION SIGN

If either or both of these tests are positive, pay extra attention to palpation of the spleen.

Palpation

To enhance relaxation of the abdominal wall, the patient should keep the arms at the sides and flex the neck and legs for comfort, as necessary. With your left hand, reach over and around the patient to support and press forward the lower left rib cage and adjacent soft tissue. With your right hand below the left costal margin, press in toward the spleen. Begin palpation low enough so that you can detect an enlarged spleen. If your hand is too close to the costal margin, you will not be able to reach under the rib cage.

Ask the patient to take a deep breath. Try to feel the tip or edge of the spleen as it comes down to meet your fingertips. Note any tenderness, assess the splenic contour, and measure the distance between the spleen's lowest point and the left costal margin. Approximately 5% of normal adults have a palpable spleen tip.

An enlarged spleen may be missed if the examiner starts palpation too high in the abdomen to feel the lower edge.

Splenomegaly is eight times more likely when the spleen is palpable.[30] Causes include portal hypertension, hematologic malignancies, HIV infection, and splenic infarct or hematoma.

The spleen tip below is just palpable deep to the left costal margin.

Repeat with the patient lying on the right side with legs somewhat flexed at hips and knees. In this position, gravity may bring the spleen forward and to the right into a palpable location.

The enlarged spleen is palpable about 2 cm below the left costal margin on deep inspiration.

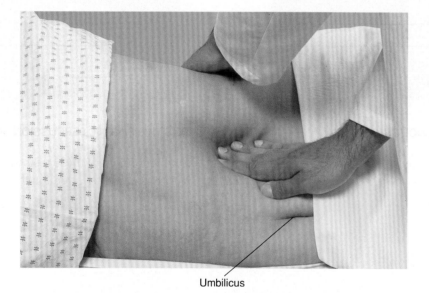

Umbilicus

PALPATING THE SPLEEN—PATIENT LYING ON RIGHT SIDE

The Kidneys

Palpation

The kidneys are retroperitoneal and usually not palpable, but learning the techniques for examination helps you distinguish enlarged kidneys from other organs and abdominal masses.

A left flank mass may represent either *splenomegaly* or an enlarged left kidney. Suspect *splenomegaly* if there is a palpable notch on the medial border, the edge extends beyond the midline, percussion is dull, and the fingers can probe deep to the medial and lateral borders but *not* between the mass and the costal margin. Confirm the findings with further evaluation.

Palpation of the Left Kidney

Move to the patient's *left side*. Place your right hand behind the patient, just below and parallel to the 12th rib, with your fingertips just reaching the costovertebral angle. Lift, trying to displace the kidney anteriorly. Place the left hand gently in the LUQ, lateral and parallel to the rectus muscle. Ask the patient to take a deep breath. At the peak of inspiration, press your left hand firmly and deeply into the LUQ, just below the costal margin, and try to "capture" the kidney between your two hands. Ask the patient to breathe out and then to stop breathing briefly. Slowly release the pressure of your left hand, feeling at the same time for the kidney to slide back into its expiratory position. If the kidney is palpable, describe its size, contour, and any tenderness.

Alternatively, try to palpate for the left kidney using the deep palpation technique similar to feeling for the spleen. Standing to the patient's right side, with your left hand, reach over and around the patient to lift up beneath the left kidney, and with your right hand, feel deep in the LUQ. Ask the patient to take a deep breath, and feel for a mass. A normal left kidney is rarely palpable.

Suspect an enlarged kidney if there is normal tympany in the LUQ and you can probe with your fingers between the mass and the costal margin, but not deep to its medial and lower borders.

Palpation of the Right Kidney

A normal right kidney may be palpable especially when the patient is thin and the abdominal muscles are relaxed. To capture the right kidney, return to the patient's right side. Use your left hand to lift up from in back, and your right hand to feel deep in the LUQ. Proceed as before. The kidney may be slightly tender. The patient is usually aware of a capture and release. Occasionally, a right kidney is more anterior and must be distinguished from the liver. The lower pole of the kidney is rounded and the liver edge, if palpable, tends to be sharper and extend farther medially and laterally. It cannot be captured.

Causes of kidney enlargement include hydronephrosis, cysts, and tumors. Bilateral enlargement suggests *polycystic kidney disease*.

Assessing Percussion Tenderness of the Kidneys

Assess percussion tenderness over the costovertebral angles. Pressure from your fingertips may be enough to elicit tenderness, if not, use fist percussion. Place the ball of one hand in the costovertebral angle and strike it with the ulnar surface of your fist. Use enough force to cause a perceptible but painless jar or thud.

To save the patient needless exertion and repositioning, integrate this assessment into your examination of the posterior lungs or back.

Pain with pressure or fist percussion suggests *pyelonephritis* associated with fever and dysuria, but may also be musculoskeletal.

**ASSESSING COSTOVERTEBRAL
ANGLE TENDERNESS**

The Bladder

The bladder cannot normally be palpated unless it is distended above the symphysis pubis. Percuss to check for dullness and to determine the height of the bladder above the symphysis pubis. Bladder volume must be 400 to 600 mL before dullness appears.[30] On palpation, the dome of the distended bladder feels smooth and round. Check for tenderness.

Bladder distention from outlet obstruction caused by *urethral stricture*, or *prostatic hyperplasia*, medication side effects, and neurologic disorders such as *stroke*, *multiple sclerosis*.

Suprapubic tenderness may be assessed in *bladder infection*.

The Aorta

Press firmly deep in the upper abdomen, slightly to the left of the midline, and identify the aortic pulsations. In people older than age 50, assess the width of the aorta by pressing deeply in the upper abdomen with one hand on each side of the aorta, as illustrated on the next page. In this age group,

Risk factors for Abdominal Aortic Aneurysm (AAA) are age of 65 years or older, history of smoking, male gender, and having a first-degree relative with a history of AAA repair.[35]

a normal aorta is not more than 3.0 cm wide (average, 2.5 cm). This measurement does not include the thickness of the abdominal wall. The ease of feeling aortic pulsations varies greatly with the thickness of the abdominal wall and with the anteroposterior diameter of the abdomen.

A periumbilical or upper abdominal mass with expansile pulsations that is 3 cm or larger suggests an AAA. Sensitivity of palpation increases as AAAs enlarge: for widths of 3.0 to 3.9 cm, 29%; 4.0 to 4.9 cm, 50%; 5.0 cm or greater, 76%.[35,36]

Screening by palpation followed by ultrasound decreases mortality, especially in male smokers older than 65 years of age. Pain may signal rupture. Rupture is 15 times more likely in AAAs that are larger than 4 cm than it is in smaller aneurysms, and it carries an 85% to 90% mortality rate.[35,36]

Note that the U.S. Preventive Services Task Force (USPSTF) recommends ultrasound screening for men over 65 years who have "ever smoked."[37]

SPECIAL TECHNIQUES

Assessment Techniques for

Ascites
Appendicitis
Acute cholecystitis
Ventral hernia
Mass in abdominal wall

Assessing Possible Ascites

A protuberant abdomen with bulging flanks is suspicious for ascites, the most common complication of cirrhosis.[38] Because ascitic fluid characteristically sinks with gravity, whereas gas-filled loops of bowel rise, dullness appears in the dependent areas of the abdomen. Percuss for dullness outward in several directions from the central area of tympany. Map the border between tympany and dullness.

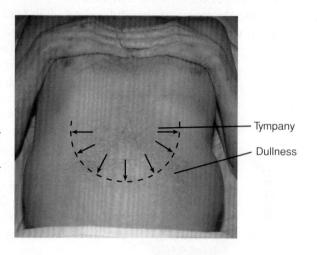

Ascites can be a clue to *increased hydrostatic pressure* in cirrhosis (most common), heart failure, constrictive pericarditis, or inferior vena cava or hepatic vein obstruction. This may be from decreased osmotic pressure in nephrotic syndrome, malnutrition, or ovarian cancer.

Two additional techniques help to confirm ascites, although both signs may be misleading.

Test for shifting dullness. Percuss the border of tympany and dullness with the patient supine, then ask the patient to roll onto one side. Percuss and mark the borders again. In a person without ascites, the borders between tympany and dullness usually stay relatively constant.

Dullness at the left abdominal border toward the right (patient turned on right sider).

PATIENT LYING ON RIGHT SIDE

Test for a fluid wave. Ask the patient or an assistant to press the edges of both hands firmly down the midline of the abdomen. This pressure helps to stop the transmission of a wave through fat. While you tap one flank sharply with your fingertips, feel on the opposite flank for an impulse transmitted through the fluid, as shown on the next page. Unfortunately, this sign is often negative until ascites is obvious, and it is sometimes positive in people without ascites.

In ascites, dullness shifts to the more dependent side, whereas tympany shifts to the top.

An easily palpable impulse suggests ascites. A positive fluid wave, shifting dullness, and peripheral edema make the diagnosis of ascites 3 to 6 times more likely.[39]

Assessing Possible Appendicitis

Appendicitis is a common cause of acute abdominal pain. Assess carefully for the peritoneal signs of acute abdomen and the additional signs of McBurney point tenderness, Rovsing sign, the psoas sign, and the obturator sign described on pp. 506–507.

Appendicitis is twice as likely in the presence of RLQ tenderness, Rovsing sign, and the psoas sign; it is three times more likely if there is McBurney point tenderness.[30]

The pain of *appendicitis* classically begins near the umbilicus, then migrates to the RLQ. Older adults are less likely to report this pattern.[10]

Ask the patient to point to where the pain began and where it is now. Ask the patient to cough and determine where pain occurs.

Palpate carefully for an area of local tenderness. *McBurney point* lies 2 inches from the anterior superior spinous process of ilium on a line drawn from that process to the umbilicus.

Localized tenderness anywhere in the RLQ, even in the right flank, suggests *appendicitis.*

Palpate the tender area for guarding, muscular rigidity, and rebound tenderness.

Early voluntary guarding may be replaced by involuntary muscular rigidity and signs of peritoneal inflammation. There may also be RLQ pain on quick withdrawal or deferred rebound tenderness.

Palpate for the *Rovsing sign* and for referred rebound tenderness. Press deeply and evenly in the *left* lower quadrant. Then quickly withdraw your fingers.

Pain in the RLQ during *left*-sided pressure is a positive Rovsing sign.

Assess for a *psoas sign*. Place your hand just above the patient's right knee and ask the patient to raise that thigh against your hand. Alternatively, ask the patient to turn onto the left side. Then extend the patient's right leg at the hip. Flexion of the leg at the hip makes the psoas muscle contract; extension stretches it.

Increased abdominal pain on either maneuver is a positive psoas sign, suggesting irritation of the psoas muscle by an inflamed appendix.

Assess for the *obturator sign*. (This sign has very low sensitivity.) Flex the patient's right thigh at the hip, with the knee bent, and rotate the leg internally at the hip. This maneuver stretches the internal obturator muscle. (Internal rotation of the hip is described on p. 613.)

Right hypogastric pain is a positive obturator sign, suggesting irritation of the obturator muscle by an inflamed appendix.

Localized pain with this maneuver, in all or part of the RLQ, may accompany appendicitis.

Perform a rectal examination and, in women, a pelvic examination. These maneuvers have low sensitivity and specificity, but they may help identify an inflamed appendix atypically located within the pelvic cavity. They may also suggest other causes of the abdominal pain.

Right-sided rectal tenderness may also be caused by an inflamed adnexa or an inflamed seminal vesicle.

Assessing Possible Acute Cholecystitis

When RUQ pain and tenderness suggest *acute cholecystitis*, assess *Murphy sign*. Hook your left thumb or the fingers of your right hand under the costal margin at the point where the lateral border of the rectus muscle intersects with the costal margin. Alternatively, palpate the RUQ with the fingers of your right hand near the costal margin. If the liver is enlarged, hook your thumb or fingers under the liver edge at a comparable point below. Ask the patient to take a deep breath, which forces the liver and gall bladder down toward the examining fingers. Watch the patient's breathing and note the degree of tenderness.

A sharp increase in tenderness with inspiratory effort is a positive Murphy sign. When positive, Murphy sign triples the likelihood of *acute cholecystitis*.[30]

Assessing Ventral Hernias

Ventral hernias are hernias in the abdominal wall exclusive of groin hernias. If you suspect but do not see an umbilical or incisional hernia, ask the patient to raise both head and shoulders off the table.

The bulge of a hernia will usually appear with this action, but should not be confused with *diastasis recti*, which is a benign 2- to 3-cm gap in the rectus muscles often seen in obese and post-partum patients.

Inguinal and femoral hernias are discussed in Chapter 21, Reproductive Systems, Hernias, pp. 773–774. They can give rise to important abdominal problems and should not be overlooked.

The cause of intestinal obstruction or peritonitis may be missed by overlooking a strangulated femoral or inguinal hernia.

Mass in the Abdominal Wall

Occasionally there is a mass in the abdominal wall rather than inside the abdominal cavity. To distinguish an abdominal mass from a mass in the abdominal wall, ask the patient either to raise the head and shoulders or to strain down, thus tightening the abdominal muscles. Feel for the mass again.

A mass in the abdominal wall remains palpable; an intra-abdominal mass is obscured by muscular contraction.

RECORDING YOUR FINDINGS

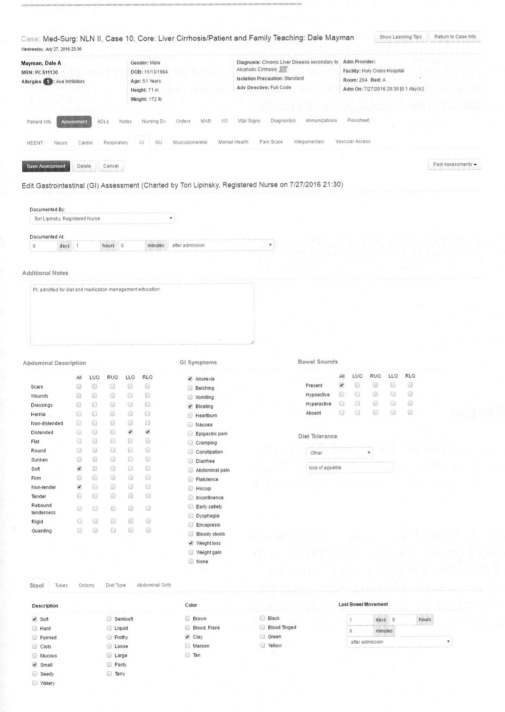

Recording the Physical Examination—The Abdomen

On the electronic health record (EHR) you will add specific findings in the free text area. Note that initially you may use sentences to describe your findings; later you will use phrases and abbreviations. For descriptive purposes the notes have included some information that would be included in the checked boxes of the EHR.

"Abdomen protuberant with active bowel sounds. Soft, nontender; no palpable masses or hepatosplenomegaly. Liver span 7 cm in right midclavicular line; edge smooth and palpable 1 cm below the right costal margin. Spleen and kidneys not palpable. No costovertebral angle tenderness."

OR

"Abdomen flat. No bowel sounds. Firm, board-like, increased tenderness, guarding, and rebound tenderness in the right midquadrant. Liver percusses 7 cm in the right MCL; edge not felt. Spleen and kidneys not palpable. No palpable masses. No CVA tenderness."

Suggests peritonitis from possible *appendicitis*.

HEALTH PROMOTION

Health Promotion Topics

- Screening for alcohol abuse
- Risk factors for hepatitis A, B, and C
- Screening for colon cancer
- Prevention of urinary incontinence

Screening for Alcohol Abuse

According to the National Institute on Alcohol Abuse and Alcoholism, 86.8% of people over 18 years, report drinking in their lifetime.[41] Binge drinking was reported by 24.6% in the past year and 6.8% report heavy drinking in the past month.[42]

Approximately 17 million adults in the United States have an *alcohol use disorder* (AUD) which is the latest diagnosis used in the DSM-5 combining alcohol abuse and alcohol dependence into a single disorder.[43] Addictions are increasingly viewed as chronic relapsing behavioral disorders with substance-induced alterations of brain neurotransmitters resulting in tolerance, physical dependence, sensitization, craving, and relapse.

Alert clinicians often notice clues of unhealthy alcohol use from social patterns and behavioral problems that emerge during the history. The patient may report past episodes of substance abuse, unstable relationships, difficulty holding jobs, or legal problems related to violent behaviors or driving under the influence.[10,45] Excessive alcohol use has numerous short-term health risks, including injuries, violence (homicide, suicide, sexual assault, intimate partner violence), alcohol poisoning, and adverse effects on reproductive health (risky sexual behaviors, miscarriage, and fetal alcohol disorders). Medical issues are often associated with chronic alcohol abuse such as cirrhosis, pancreatitis or cancer, other gastrointestinal or cardiovascular diseases, neurologic disorders, nutritional deficiencies, or additional mental health problems. Examination of the abdomen may reveal such classic findings of liver disease such as hepatosplenomegaly, ascites, or even *caput medusa* (dilated abdominal vein).

Other classic findings include jaundice, spider angiomas, palmar erythema, asterixis, and gynecomastia.

See Chapter 19, Mental Status, pp. 665–666.

Because early detection of at-risk behaviors may be difficult to identify, knowledge of basic alcohol screening criteria is critical. The USPSTF recommends screening and behavioral counseling interventions for adolescents and adults in primary care settings, including pregnant women.[44] Learn the best approach to identify problem drinking. If your patient reports drinking alcoholic beverages, ask the initial screening question about heavy drinking (see below) and follow-up with one of the well-validated screening tools: the CAGE questionnaire, the Alcohol Use Disorders Identification Test (AUDIT), or the shorter AUDIT-C questionnaire.[45] Keep in mind cutoffs for problem drinking.

See Chapter 4, The Health History, pp. 74–75.

Screening for Problem Drinking

Standard Drink Equivalents: 1 standard drink is equivalent to 12 oz of regular beer or wine cooler, 8 oz of malt liquor, 5 oz of wine, or 1.5 oz of 80-proof spirits

Initial Screening Question: "How many times in the past year have you had 4 or more drinks a day (women), or 5 or more drinks a day (men)?"

National Institute of Alcohol Abuse and Alcoholism: Definitions of Drinking-Levels for Adults[46]

	Women	Men
Moderate drinking	≤1 drink/day	≤2 drinks/day
Unsafe drinking levels (increased risk for developing an alcohol use disorder)	>3 drinks /day and >7 drinks/week[a]	>4 drinks/day and >14 drinks/week
Binge drinking[b]	≥4 drinks on one occasion	≥5 drinks on one occasion

[a]Pregnant women and those with health problems that could be worsened by drinking should not drink any alcohol.
[b]Brings blood alcohol level to 0.08%, usually within 2 hours.

Tailor your recommendations to the severity of the drinking problem, ranging from brief behavioral counseling interventions to inpatient detoxification and/or long-term rehabilitation.

Health Prevention: Hepatitis A, B, and C

The best strategy for protection and prevention of transmission and infection of hepatitis A and B is adherence to the vaccination guidelines. Education about how the hepatitis viruses spread, behavioral strategies to reduce the risk of infection, and the benefits of vaccination for groups at risk is important.

Hepatitis A

Transmission of the hepatitis A virus (HAV) is the fecal–oral route. Fecal shedding followed by inadequate hand washing can contaminate water and food. Those at highest risk include travel to or live in countries where hepatitis A is common, sex with infected person, use of recreational drugs, eating raw or undercooked shellfish from contaminated waters, have clotting disorder or live with or care for a person with hepatitis A. Infected children are often asymptomatic and play a key role in spreading infection. For immediate protection and prophylaxis for household contacts and travel and to reduce transmission, advise handwashing with soap and water after bathroom use or changing diapers, and before preparing or eating food.[47] HAV infection is rarely fatal—fewer than 100 deaths occur each year—and usually only in people with other liver diseases; it does not cause chronic hepatitis.[48]

CDC Recommendations for Hepatitis A Vaccination

- All children at age 1 year
- Individuals with chronic liver disease
- Groups at increased risk of acquiring HAV: travel or live in areas with high endemic rates of infection, men who have sex with men, injection and illicit drug users, individuals working with HAV-infected animals or work with HAV in research setting, and persons who have clotting-factor disorders and receive blood products.[49]

The vaccine alone may be administered at any time before traveling to endemic areas.

Postexposure Prophylaxis

Healthy unvaccinated individuals should receive either a hepatitis A vaccine or a single dose of *immune globulin* (preferred for those ≥age 40) within 2 weeks of being exposed to HAV. These recommendations apply to close personal contacts of persons with confirmed HAV, co-workers of infected food handlers, and staff and attendees (and their household members) of child care centers where HAV has been diagnosed in children, staff, or households of attendees.

Hepatitis B

Hepatitis B virus (HBV) poses more serious threats to patient health than infection with hepatitis A. Approximately 95% of infections in healthy adults are self-limited, with elimination of the virus from blood and development of immunity.[50] Chronic infection occurs in 5% of those older than 5 years, and approximately 15% of those infected after childhood die prematurely from cirrhosis or liver cancer. Most people (approximately 70%) with chronic infections are asymptomatic until they develop advanced liver disease.

Screening and Vaccination

The USPSTF recommends screening for HBV in persons at high risk for infection, including those born in countries with a high endemic prevalence of HBV infection, persons with HIV, injection drug users, men who have sex with men, and household contacts or sexual partners of HBV infected persons.[51] The CDC recommends screening all pregnant women, ideally in the first trimester, and universal vaccination for all infants beginning at birth.[50] For adults, vaccine recommendations also target high-risk groups, including those in high-risk settings (see below).

CDC Recommendations for Hepatitis B Vaccination: High-Risk Groups and Settings[50]

- *Sexual contacts,* including sex partners of hepatitis B surface antigen positive persons, people with more than one sex partner in the prior 6 months, people seeking evaluation and treatment for sexually transmitted infections, and men who have sex with men.
- *People with percutaneous (through the skin) or mucosal exposure to blood,* including injection drug users, household contacts of antigen-positive persons, residents and staff of facilities for the developmentally disabled, health care workers, and people on dialysis.
- *Others,* including travelers to endemic areas, people with chronic liver disease or HIV infection, and people seeking protection from hepatitis B infection.
- *All adults in high-risk settings,* such as sexually transmitted infection (STI) clinics, HIV testing and treatment programs, drug-abuse treatment programs and programs for injection drug users, correctional

facilities, programs for men having sex with men, chronic hemodialysis facilities and end-stage renal disease programs, and facilities for people with developmental disabilities.

- In primary care and specialty settings, adults in at-risk groups or requesting the hepatitis B vaccine even without acknowledging a specific risk factor.
- Adults in occupations involving exposure to blood or other potentially infectious body fluids.

Hepatitis C

There is no vaccination for hepatitis C, so prevention targets counseling to avoid risk factors. Screening should be recommended for high-risk groups.

Hepatitis C virus (HCV) is primarily transmitted by percutaneous exposure to blood, primarily via exposure to contaminated needles or syringes or receiving blood or blood products that have not been checked for HCV. Anti-HVC antibody is present in approximately 2% of U.S. adults. However, prevalence increases significantly in groups at high risk, particularly injection drug users who share needles.[52] Additional risk factors for HCV infection include health care workers with needle stick injury or mucosal exposure to HCV-positive blood, HIV infection, and birth from an HCV positive mother. *Sexual transmission is rare.* Hepatitis C becomes a chronic disease in over 75% of those infected and is a major risk factor for cirrhosis, hepatocellular carcinoma, and the need for liver transplant for end-stage liver disease.[53–55]

The majority of persons with chronic HCV are unaware of being infected. Response to antiviral therapy ranges from 40% to over 90% depending on the viral genotype and the combination of drugs used for treatment. Consequently, the USPSTF has concluded that screening for hepatitis C infection is of moderate benefit for persons at high risk for infection as well as those born between 1945 and 1965.[56]

Screening for Colorectal Cancer

Colorectal cancer is the third most common cancer in both men and women. Most cases occur between 65 and 74 years and the median age of colorectal cancer death is 73 years.[57]

Mortality rates have been declining, reflecting improvements in early detection and treatment. Evidence supports screening guidelines by multisociety task forces, including the American Cancer Society and the USPSTF placing emphasis on risk stratification, and endorsement of colorectal cancer screening.[58,59]

Risk Factors

The strongest risk factors for colorectal cancer are increasing age; personal history of colorectal cancer, adenomatous polyps, or long-standing inflammatory bowel disease; and family history of colorectal neoplasia—particularly those with affected multiple first-degree relatives, a single first-degree relative diagnosed before age 60, or a hereditary colorectal cancer syndrome. Weaker risk factors include male sex, African-American race, tobacco use, excessive alcohol use, red meat consumption, and obesity. Aside from age, persons without any strong risk factors are considered average risk—even if they have some of the weak risk factors.

Prevention

The most effective prevention strategy is to screen for and remove precancerous adenomatous polyps. Screening programs using fecal blood testing or flexible sigmoidoscopy have been shown in randomized trials to reduce the risk of developing colorectal cancer by about 15% to 20%.[60,61] Physical activity, aspirin and nonsteroidal anti-inflammatory drugs (NSAIDs), and postmenopausal combined hormone replacement therapy (estrogen and progestin) are also associated with decreased risk of colorectal cancer.[62-65] However, the USPSTF recommends against routinely using aspirin and NSAIDs for prevention in average-risk persons because the potential harms, including gastrointestinal bleeding, hemorrhagic stroke, and renal impairment, outweigh the benefits.[66]

Screening Tests

Evidence

Screening tests include stool tests that detect occult fecal blood, such as fecal immunochemical tests, high-sensitivity guaiac-based tests, and tests that detect abnormal DNA. Endoscopic tests are also used for screening, including colonoscopy, which visualizes the entire colon and can remove polyps, and flexible sigmoidoscopy, which visualizes the distal 60 cm of the bowel. Imaging tests include the double-contrast barium enema and CT colonography. Any abnormal finding on a stool test, imaging study, or flexible sigmoidoscopy warrants further evaluation with colonoscopy. Screening programs using fecal blood testing or flexible sigmoidoscopy have been shown in randomized trials to reduce the risk colorectal cancer death by about 15% to 30%.[60,61] Although colonoscopy is the gold standard diagnostic test for screening, there is no direct evidence from randomized trials that screening with colonoscopy reduces colorectal cancer incidence or mortality. Complications of colonoscopy include perforation and bleeding.[67] Patients are usually sedated during the procedure but extensive bowel preparation is required beginning the day before the procedure.

Screening Recommendations for Colorectal Cancer: U.S. Preventive Services Task Force (current proposal and under revision) Health Prevention: Hepatitis A, B, and C

- **Adults ages 50 to 75**—options
  - High-sensitivity fecal occult blood testing (FOBT) annually, either a guaiac-based or fecal immunochemical test
  - Sigmoidoscopy every 5 years with high-sensitivity FOBT every 3 years
  - Screening colonoscopy every 10 years
- **Adults ages 76 to 85**—individual decision based on overall health and prior screening
  - If patient is healthy and can withstand treatment if cancer detected
  - Do not have comorbid conditions that would limit life expectancy
  - If never screened, more likely to benefit

Urinary Incontinence

Urinary incontinence is the involuntary loss of bladder control. Incontinence is inconvenient and a disruption to daily activities, it can be physically uncomfortable and emotionally can cause embarrassment and be socially isolating.[68]

Women experience urinary incontinence more often than men. Those at higher risk for urinary incontinence, include women who are postpartum and women between the ages of 60 and 80 years. Men experience urinary incontinence more frequently after prostate surgery. Many patients believe incontinence is "normal." Information should be disseminated and patients need to be aware urinary incontinence is reversible. Nurses play an integral part during the health history in screening for patients who are experiencing urinary incontinence. The Sandvik Scale, also known as the Bladder Incontinence Severity Index (ISI), is based on two questions: How often do you experience urine leakage? How much urine do you lose each time you are incontinent?

Bladder Incontinence Severity Index (ISI)[69]

1. How often do you experience urine leakage (incontinence)?
   0—never
   1—less than once a month?
   2—one or several times a month
   3—one or several times a week
   4—every day/night

2. How much urine do you lose each time?
  1—drops/little
  2—more
3. Total score (multiply question 1 by question 2).
  0—dry
  1–2—slight incontinence
  3–5—moderate incontinence
  6–8—severe incontinence

Identification and education of patients with urinary incontinence is key. Teaching pelvic muscle exercises, behavioral changes, use of a pessary or biofeedback, are used in reducing and eliminating urinary incontinence.[70] This will promote healthy lifestyles and quality of life for these individuals.

TABLE
16-1

Abdominal Pain

Problem	Process	Location	Quality
Gastroesophageal reflux disease (GERD)[10,11]	Prolonged exposure of esophagus to gastric acid due to impaired esophageal motility or excess relaxations of the lower esophageal sphincter. *Helicobacter pylori* may be present.	Chest or epigastric	Heartburn, regurgitation
Peptic ulcer and dyspepsia[2,8]	Mucosal ulcer in stomach or duodenum >5 mm	Epigastric, may radiate straight to the back	Variable: epigastric gnawing or burning (dyspepsia); may also be boring, aching, or hunger-like. No symptoms up to 20%
Acute appendicitis[14,15]	Acute inflammation of the appendix with distention or obstruction	Poorly localized *periumbilical pain*, usually migrates to the right lower quadrant	Mild but increasing, possibly cramping Steady and more severe
Acute cholecystitis[73]	Inflammation of the gallbladder, usually from obstruction of the cystic duct by a gallstone in 90%	Right upper quadrant or epigastrium; may radiate to the right shoulder of interscapular area	Steady, aching
Biliary colic	Sudden obstruction of the cystic duct or common bile duct by a gallstone	Epigastric or right upper quadrant; may radiate to the right scapula and shoulder	Steady, aching; *not* colicky. Usually lasts longer than 3 hours
Acute bowel obstruction	Obstruction of the bowel lumen, commonly caused by (1) adhesions or hernias (small bowel) or (2) cancer or diverticulitis (colon)	*Small bowel:* periumbilical or upper abdominal *Colon:* lower abdominal or generalized	*Small bowel:* Cramping *Colon:* Cramping
Acute pancreatitis[5,7]	Intrapancreatic trypsinogen activation to trypsin and other enzymes, resulting in autodigestion and inflammation of the pancreas	Epigastric, may radiate straight to the back or other areas of the abdomen; 20% with severe sequelae of organ failure	Usually steady
Chronic pancreatitis	Irreversible destruction of the pancreatic parenchyma from recurrent inflammation of either large ducts or small ducts	Epigastric, radiating through to the back	Severe, persistent, deep
Pancreatic cancer[71,72]	Predominantly adenocarcinoma (95%). 5% 5-year survival	Epigastric in either upper quadrant; often radiates to the back	Steady, deep
Gastric cancer	Adenocarcinoma in 90–95%, either intestinal (older adults) or diffuse (younger adults, worse prognosis)	Increasingly in "cardia" and GE junction; also in distal stomach	Variable
Acute diverticulitis[74]	Acute inflammation of a colonic diverticula, outpouching a 5–10 mm in diameter, usually in sigmoid or descending colon	Left lower quadrant	May be cramping at first, then becomes steady
Mesenteric ischemia[75,76]	Occlusion of blood flow to small bowel, from arterial or venous thrombosis (especially superior mesenteric artery), cardiac embolus, or hypoperfusion. Can be colonic	May be periumbilical at first, then diffuse. May be postprandial, classically inducing "food fear"	Cramping at first, then steady. Pain disproportionate to examination findings

Timing	Factors That May Aggravate	Factors That May Relieve	Associated Symptoms and Setting
After meals, especially spicy foods	Lying down, bending over. Physical activity. Diseases such as scleroderma, gastroparesis. Drugs like nicotine that relax the lower esophageal sphincter.	Antacids; proton pump inhibitors; avoiding alcohol, smoking, fatty meals, chocolate, selected drugs such as theophylline, calcium channel blockers	Wheezing, chronic cough, shortness of breath, hoarseness, choking sensation, dysphagia, regurgitation, halitosis, sore throat. Increases risk of Barrett esophagus and esophageal cancer.
Intermittent. Duodenal ulcer is more likely than gastric ulcer or dyspepsia to cause pain that (1) wakes the patient at night and (2) occurs intermittently over a few weeks, then disappears for months, and then recurs.	Variable	Food and antacids may bring relief	Nausea, vomiting, belching, bloating; heartburn (more common in duodenal ulcer); weight loss (more common in gastric ulcer). Dyspepsia is more common in the young (20–29 years), gastric ulcer in those over 50 years, and duodenal ulcer in those 30–60 years.
Lasts roughly 4–6 hours depending on intervention	Movement or cough		Anorexia, nausea, possibly vomiting, which typically follow the onset of pain; low fever
Gradual onset; course longer than in biliary colic	Jarring, deep breathing		Anorexia, nausea, vomiting, fever. No jaundice.
Rapid onset over a few minutes, lasts 1 to several hours and subsides gradually. Often recurrent	Fatty meals but also fasting. Often precedes cholecystitis, cholangitis, pancreatitis		Anorexia, nausea, vomiting, restlessness
Small bowel: Paroxysmal; may decrease as bowel mobility is impaired *Colon:* Paroxysmal, though typically milder	Ingestion of food or liquids		Vomiting of bile and mucus (high obstruction) or fecal material (low obstruction). Obstipation develops. Obstipation early. Vomiting late if at all. Prior symptoms of underlying cause
Acute onset, persistent pain	Lying supine. Dyspnea if pleural effusions from capillary leak syndrome. Selected medications, high triglycerides may exacerbate	Leaning forward with trunk flexed	Nausea, vomiting, abdominal distention, fever. Often recurrent; 80% with a history of previous attacks and alcohol abuse or gallstones
Chronic or recurrent course	Alcohol, heavy or fatty meals	Possibly leaning forward with trunk flexed; often intractable	Symptoms of decreased pancreatic function may appear: diarrhea with fatty stools (*steatorrhea*) and diabetes mellitus.
Persistent pain; relentlessly progressive illness	Smoking, chronic pancreatitis		Painless jaundice, anorexia, weight loss. Glucose intolerance, depression
Pain is persistent, slowly progressive. Duration of pain is typically shorter than in peptic ulcer.	Often food. *H. pylori* infection	*Not* relieved by food or antacids	Anorexia, nausea, early satiety, weight loss, and sometimes bleeding. Most common in ages 50–70
Often a gradual onset			Fever, constipation. Nausea, vomiting, abdominal mass with rebound tenderness
Usually abrupt in onset, then persistent	Underlying cardiac disease		Vomiting, bloody stool, soft distended abdomen with peritoneal signs, shock; age >50

TABLE

16-2

Dysphagia

Process and Problem	Timing	Factors That Aggravate	Factors That Relieve	Associated Symptoms and Conditions
Oropharyngeal dysphagia (due to motor disorders affecting the pharyngeal muscles)	Acute or gradual onset and a variable course, depending on the underlying disorder	Attempts to start the swallowing process		Aspiration into the lungs or regurgitation into the nose with attempts to swallow. Neurologic evidence of stroke, bulbar palsy, or other neuromuscular conditions
Esophageal dysphagia				
Due to Mechanical Narrowing				
• Mucosal rings and webs	Intermittent	Solid foods	Regurgitation of the bolus of food	Usually none
• Esophageal stricture	Intermittent; may become slowly progressive	Solid foods	Regurgitation of the bolus of food	A long history of heartburn and regurgitation
• Esophageal cancer	May be intermittent at first; progressive over months	Solid foods, with progression to liquids	Regurgitation of the bolus of food	Pain in the chest and back and weight loss, especially late in the course of illness
Due to Motor Disorders				
• Diffuse esophageal spasm	Intermittent	Solids or liquids	Maneuvers described below; sometimes nitroglycerin	Chest pain that mimics angina pectoris or myocardial infarction and lasts minutes to hours; possibly heartburn
• Scleroderma or • Achalasia	Intermittent; may progress slowly	Solids or liquids	Repeated swallowing; movements such as straightening the back, raising the arms, or a Valsalva maneuver (straining down against a closed glottis)	Heartburn; other manifestations of scleroderma Regurgitation, often at night when lying down, with nocturnal cough; possibly chest pain precipitated by eating

TABLE 16-3 Constipation

Problem	Process	Associated Symptoms and Setting
Life Activities and Habits		
Inadequate time or setting for the defecation reflex	Ignoring the sensation of a full rectum inhibits the defecation reflex.	Hectic schedules, unfamiliar surroundings, bed rest
False expectations of bowel habits	Expectations of "regularity" or more frequent stools than a person's norm	Beliefs, treatments, and advertisements that promote the use of laxatives
Diet deficient in fiber	Decreased fecal bulk	Other factors such as debilitation and constipating drugs may contribute.
Irritable Bowel Syndrome[16]	Functional change in frequency or form of bowel movement without known pathology; possibly from change in intestinal bacteria	Three patterns: diarrhea-predominant, constipation-predominant, or mixed. Symptoms present ≥6 months and abdominal pain for ≥3 months plus at least two of three features (improvement with defecation; onset with change in stool frequency; onset with change in stool form and appearance)
Mechanical Obstruction		
Cancer of the rectum or sigmoid colon	Progressive narrowing of the bowel lumen	Change in bowel habits; often diarrhea, abdominal pain, and bleeding. In rectal cancer, tenesmus and pencil-shaped stools
Fecal impaction	A large, firm, immovable fecal mass, most often in the rectum	Rectal fullness, abdominal pain, and diarrhea around the impaction; common in debilitated, bedridden, and elderly patients
Other obstructing lesions (such as diverticulitis, volvulus, intussusception, or hernia)	Narrowing or complete obstruction of the bowel	Colicky abdominal pain, abdominal distention, and, in intussusception, often "currant jelly" stools (red blood and mucus)
Painful Anal Lesions	Pain may cause spasm of the external sphincter and voluntary inhibition of the defecation reflex	Anal fissures, painful hemorrhoids, perirectal abscesses
Drugs	A variety of mechanisms	Opiates, anticholinergics, antacids containing calcium or aluminum, and many others
Depression	A disorder of mood	Fatigue, anhedonia, sleep disturbance, weight loss
Neurologic Disorders	Interference with the autonomic innervation of the bowel	Spinal cord injuries, multiple sclerosis, Hirschsprung disease, and other conditions
Metabolic Conditions	Interference with bowel motility	Pregnancy, hypothyroidism, hypercalcemia

TABLE

16-4

Diarrhea

Problem	Process	Characteristics of Stool
Acute Diarrhea[77]		
Secretory infection (noninflammatory)	Infection by viruses, preformed bacterial toxins (such as *Staphylococcus aureus*, *Clostridium perfringens*, toxigenic *Escherichia coli*, *Vibrio cholerae*), cryptosporidium, *Giardia lamblia*, rotavirus	Watery, without blood, pus, or mucus
Inflammatory infection	Colonization or invasion of intestinal mucosa (nontyphoid *Salmonella*, *Shigella*, *Yersinia*, *Campylobacter*, enteropathic *E. coli*, *Entamoeba histolytica*, *C. difficile*)	Loose to watery, often with blood, pus, or mucus
Drug-Induced Diarrhea	Action of many drugs, such as magnesium-containing antacids, antibiotics, antineoplastic agents, and laxatives	Loose to watery
Chronic Diarrhea		
Diarrheal syndrome		
• Irritable bowel syndrome[12]	Change in frequency and form of bowel movements without chemical or structural abnormality	Loose; ~50% with mucus; small to moderate volume. Small, hard stools with constipation. May be mixed pattern
Cancer of the sigmoid colon	Partial obstruction by a malignant neoplasm	May be blood-streaked.
Inflammatory bowel disease		
• Ulcerative colitis	Mucosal inflammation typically extending proximally from the rectum (*proctitis*) to varying lengths of the colon (*colitis* to *pancolitis*), with microulcerations and if chronic, inflammatory polyps.	Frequent watery, often containing blood.
• Crohn disease of the small bowel (*regional enteritis*) or colon (*granulomatous colitis*)	Chronic transmural inflammation of the bowel wall, with skip pattern involving the terminal ileum and/or proximal colon (and rectal sparing). May cause strictures.	Small, soft to loose or watery with bleeding if *colitis*, obstructive symptoms if *enteritis*
Voluminous diarrhea		
• Malabsorption syndrome	Defective membrane transport or absorption of intestinal epithelium (*Crohn's*, *celiac disease*, *surgical resection*); impaired luminal digestion (*pancreatic insufficiency*); epithelial defects at brush border (*lactose intolerance*).	Typically bulky, soft, light yellow to gray, mushy, greasy or oily, and sometimes frothy; particularly foul-smelling; usually floats in the toilet (*steatorrhea*)
• Osmotic diarrhea		
–Lactose intolerance	Intestinal lactase deficiency	Watery diarrhea of large volume
–Abuse of osmotic purgatives	Laxative habit, often surreptitious	Watery diarrhea of large volume
• Secretory diarrhea	Variable: from bacterial infection, secreting villous adenoma, fat or bile salt malabsorption, hormone-mediated conditions (gastrin in Zollinger–Ellison syndrome, vasoactive intestinal peptide)	Watery diarrhea of large volume

Timing	Associated Symptoms	Setting, Persons at Risk
Duration of a few days, possibly longer. Lactase deficiency may lead to a longer course.	Nausea, vomiting, periumbilical cramping pain. Temperature normal or slightly elevated	Often travel, a common food source, or an epidemic
An acute illness of varying duration	Lower abdominal cramping pain and often rectal urgency, tenesmus; fever	Travel, contaminated food or water. Frequent anal intercourse.
Acute, recurrent, or chronic	Possibly nausea; usually little if any pain	Prescribed or over-the-counter medications
Worse in the morning; rarely at night.	Cramping lower abdominal pain, abdominal distention, flatulence, nausea. Urgency, pain relieved with defecation.	Young and middle-aged adults, especially women.
Variable	Change in usual bowel habits, cramping lower abdominal pain, constipation.	
Typically abrupt. Often recurrent, persisting, and may awaken at night.	Cramping, with urgency, tenesmus. Fever, fatigue, weakness. Abdominal pain if complicated by toxic megacolon. May include episcleritis, uveitis, arthritis, erythema nodosum.	Often young adults, Ashkenazi Jewish descendants. Linked to altered CD4+ T-cell Th2 response. Increases risk of colon cancer.
Cramping periumbilical or right lower quadrant (*enteritis*) or diffuse (*colitis*) pain, with a weight loss. Perianal or perirectal abscesses and fistulas. May cause small or large bowel obstruction	Cramping periumbilical or right lower quadrant (*enteritis*) or diffuse (*colitis*) pain, with a weight loss. Perianal or perirectal abscesses and fistulas. May cause small or large bowel obstruction.	Often teens or young adults. More common in Ashkenazi Jewish descendants. Increases risk of colon cancer
Onset of illness typically insidious	Anorexia, weight loss, fatigue, abdominal distention, often cramping lower abdominal pain. Symptoms of nutritional deficiencies such as bleeding (vitamin K), bone pain and fractures (vitamin D), glossitis (vitamin B), and edema (protein).	Variable, depending on cause
Follows the ingestion of milk and milk products; relieved by fasting	Cramping abdominal pain, abdominal distention, flatulence	In >50% of African Americans, Asians, Native Americans, Hispanics; in 5–20% of Caucasians
Variable	Often none	Persons with anorexia nervosa or bulimia nervosa
Variable	Weight loss, dehydration, nausea, vomiting, and cramping abdominal pain	Variable depending on cause.

TABLE 16-5   Black and Bloody Stools

Problem	Selected Causes	Associated Symptoms and Setting
Melena Refers to passage of black, tarry stools. Fecal blood tests are positive. Involves ≥60 mL of blood into the gastrointestinal tract (less in children), usually from the esophagus, stomach, or duodenum with transit time of 7–14 hours. Less commonly, if slow transit, blood loss originates in the jejunum, ileum, or ascending colon. In infants, melena may result from swallowing blood during the birth process.	Gastritis, GERD, peptic ulcer (gastric or duodenal)	Usually epigastric discomfort from heartburn, dysmotility; if peptic ulcer, pain after meals (delay of 2–3 hours if duodenal ulcer). May be asymptomatic.
	Gastritis or stress ulcers	Recent ingestion of alcohol, aspirin, or other anti-inflammatory drugs; recent body trauma, severe burns, surgery, or increased intracranial pressure
	Esophageal or gastric varices	Cirrhosis of the liver or other cause of portal hypertension
	Reflux esophagitis Mallory–Weiss tear, a mucosal tear in the esophagus due to retching and vomiting	Retching, vomiting, often recent ingestion of alcohol
Black stool Black stool from other causes with negative fecal blood tests. Stool change has no pathologic significance.	Ingestion of iron, bismuth salts, licorice, or even chocolate cookies	Asymptomatic
Stool with red blood (hematochezia) Usually originates in the colon, rectum, or anus, and much less frequently in the jejunum or ileum. Upper gastrointestinal hemorrhage may also cause red stool, usually with large blood loss ≥1 liter Rapid transit time through the intestinal tract leaves insufficient time for the blood to turn black.	Colon cancer	Often a change in bowel habits, weight loss
	Hyperplasia or adenomatous polyps	Often no other symptoms
	Diverticula of the colon	Often no other symptoms unless inflammation causes diverticulitis
	Inflammatory conditions of the colon and rectum	
	• Ulcerative colitis, Crohn's, disease • Infectious diarrhea • Proctitis (various causes) from frequent anal intercourse	See Table 16-4, Diarrhea, pp. 522–523. See Table 16-4, Diarrhea, pp. 522–523. Rectal urgency, tenesmus
	Ischemic colitis	Lower abdominal pain, sometimes fever or shock in older adults. Abdomen typically soft to palpation
	Hemorrhoids	Blood on the toilet paper, on the surface of the stool, or dripping into the toilet
	Anal fissure	Blood on the toilet paper or on the surface of the stool; anal pain
Reddish but nonbloody stools	Ingestion of beets	Pink urine, which usually precedes the reddish stool: from poor metabolism of betacyanin

TABLE
16-6

Frequency, Nocturia, and Polyuria

Problem	Mechanisms	Selected Causes	Associated Symptoms
Frequency	Decreased bladder capacity		
	• Increased bladder sensitivity to stretch because of inflammation	*Infection,* stones, tumor, or foreign body in the bladder	Burning on urination, urinary urgency, sometimes gross hematuria
	• Decreased elasticity of the bladder wall	Infiltration by scar tissue or tumor	Symptoms of associated inflammation (see above) are common.
	• Decreased cortical inhibition of bladder contractions	Motor disorders of the central nervous system, such as a stroke	Urinary urgency; neurologic symptoms such as weakness and paralysis
	Impaired bladder emptying with residual urine in the bladder		
	• Partial mechanical obstruction of the bladder neck or proximal urethra	Most commonly, benign prostatic hyperplasia; also urethral stricture and other obstructive lesions of the bladder or prostate	Prior obstructive symptoms: hesitancy in starting the urinary stream, straining to void, reduced size and force of the stream, and dribbling during or at the end of urination
	• Loss of S2–4 innervation to the bladder	Neurologic disease affecting the sacral nerves or nerve roots (e.g., diabetic neuropathy)	Weakness or sensory defects
Nocturia			
With high volumes	Most types of polyuria (see Chapter 16, p. 488)		
	Decreased concentrating ability of the kidney with loss of the normal decrease in nocturnal urinary output	Chronic renal insufficiency due to a number of diseases	Possibly other symptoms of renal insufficiency
	Excessive fluid intake before bedtime	Habit, especially involving alcohol and coffee	
	Fluid-retaining, edematous states. Daytime accumulation of dependent edema that is excreted at night when the patient is supine	Heart failure, nephrotic syndrome, hepatic cirrhosis with ascites, chronic venous insufficiency	Edema and other symptoms of the underlying disorder. Urinary output during the day may be reduced as fluid accumulates in the body.
With low volumes	Urinary frequency Voiding while up at night without a real urge, a "pseudo-frequency"	Insomnia	Variable
Polyuria	Deficiency of antidiuretic hormone (diabetes insipidus)	A disorder of the posterior pituitary and hypothalamus	Thirst and polydipsia, often severe and persistent; nocturia
	Renal unresponsiveness to antidiuretic hormone (nephrogenic diabetes insipidus)	A number of kidney diseases, including hypercalcemic and hypokalemic nephropathy; drug toxicity (e.g., from lithium)	
	Solute diuresis • Electrolytes, such as sodium salts	Large saline infusions, potent diuretics, certain kidney diseases	Variable
	• Nonelectrolytes, such as glucose	Uncontrolled diabetes mellitus	Thirst, polydipsia, and nocturia
	Excessive water intake	Primary polydipsia	Polydipsia tends to be episodic. Thirst may not be present. Nocturia is usually absent.

TABLE 16-7

Urinary Incontinence[a]

Problem	Mechanisms
Stress Incontinence The urethral sphincter is weakened so that transient increases in intra-abdominal pressure raise the bladder pressure to levels that exceed urethral resistance.	In women, pelvic floor weakness and inadequate muscular and ligamentous support of the bladder and proximal urethra change in the angle between the bladder and the urethra. Causes include childbirth and surgery. Local conditions affecting the internal urethral sphincter, such as postmenopausal atrophy of the mucosa and urethral infection, may also contribute. In men, stress incontinence may follow prostatic surgery.
Urge Incontinence Detrusor contractions are stronger than normal and overcome the normal urethral resistance. The bladder is typically *small*.	Decreased cortical inhibition of detrusor contractions from strokes, brain tumors, dementia, and lesions of the spinal cord above the sacral level Hyperexcitability of sensory pathways, as in bladder infections, tumors, and fecal impaction Deconditioning of voiding reflexes, as in frequent voluntary voiding at low bladder volumes
Overflow Incontinence Detrusor contractions are insufficient to overcome urethral resistance, causing urinary retention. The bladder is typically flaccid and *large*, even after an effort to void.	Obstruction of the bladder outlet, as in *benign prostatic hyperplasia* or tumor Weakness of the detrusor muscle associated with peripheral nerve disease at S2–4 level Impaired bladder sensation that interrupts the reflex arc, as in diabetic neuropathy
Functional Incontinence This is a functional inability to get to the toilet in time because of impaired health or environmental conditions.	Problems in mobility resulting from weakness, arthritis, poor vision, or other conditions. Environmental factors such as an unfamiliar setting, distant bathroom facilities, bed rails, or physical restraints
Incontinence Secondary to Medications Drugs may contribute to any type of incontinence listed.	Sedatives, tranquilizers, anticholinergics, sympathetic blockers, and potent diuretics

[a]Patients may have more than one kind of incontinence.

Symptoms	Physical Signs
Momentary leakage of small amounts of urine with coughing, laughing, and sneezing while the person is in an upright position. Urine loss is unrelated to a conscious urge to urinate.	Stress incontinence may be demonstrable, especially if the patient is examined before voiding and in a standing position. Atrophic vaginitis may be evident. Bladder distention is absent.
Involuntary urine loss preceded by an urge to void. The volume tends to be moderate. Urgency Frequency and nocturia with small to moderate volumes If acute inflammation is present, pain on urination Possibly "pseudo-stress incontinence"—voiding 10–20 seconds after stresses such as a change of position, going up or down stairs, and possibly coughing, laughing, or sneezing	The small bladder is not detectable on abdominal examination. When cortical inhibition is decreased, mental deficits or motor signs of central nervous system disease are often, present. When sensory pathways are hyperexcitable, signs of local pelvic problems or a fecal impaction may be present.
When intravesicular pressure overcomes urethral resistance, continuous dripping or dribbling incontinence ensues. Decreased force of the urinary stream Prior symptoms of partial urinary obstruction or other symptoms of peripheral nerve disease may be present.	Examination often reveals an enlarged, sometimes tender bladder. Other signs include prostate enlargement, motor signs of peripheral nerve disease, a decrease in sensation (including perineal sensation), and diminished to absent reflexes.
Incontinence on the way to the toilet or only in the early morning	The bladder is not detectable on physical examination. Look for physical or environmental clues to the likely cause.
Variable. A careful history and chart review are important.	Variable

TABLE
16-8

Localized Bulges in the Abdominal Wall

Localized bulges in the abdominal wall include *ventral hernias* (defects in the wall through which tissue protrudes) and subcutaneous tumors such as *lipomas*. The more common ventral hernias are umbilical, incisional, and epigastric. Hernias and a diastasis rectus usually become more evident when the patient is supine and raises the head and shoulders.

Umbilical Hernia
A protrusion through a defective umbilical ring is most common in infants but also occurs in adults. In infants, but not in adults, it usually closes spontaneously within 1 to 2 years.

Diastasis Recti
Separation of the two rectus abdominis muscles, through which abdominal contents form a midline ridge typically extending from the xiphoid to the umbilicus and seen only when the patient raises the head and shoulders. Often present in patients with repeated pregnancies, obesity, and chronic lung disease. It is clinically benign.

Ridge

Incisional Hernia
This is a protrusion through an operative scar. Palpate to detect the length and width of the defect in the abdominal wall. A small defect, through which a large hernia has passed, has a greater risk for complications than a large defect.

Epigastric Hernia
A small midline protrusion through a defect in the linea alba occurs between the xiphoid process and the umbilicus. With the patient coughing or performing a Valsalva maneuver, palpate by running your finger pad down the linea alba to feel it.

Lipoma
Common, benign, fatty tumors usually in the subcutaneous tissues almost anywhere in the body, including the abdominal wall. Small or large, they are usually soft and often lobulated. Press your finger down on the edge of a lipoma. The tumor typically slips out from under your finger and is well demarcated, nonreducible, and usually nontender.

TABLE
16-9

Protuberant Abdomens

Fat

Fat is the most common cause of a protuberant abdomen. Fat thickens the abdominal wall, the mesentery, and omentum. The umbilicus may appear sunken. A *pannus,* or apron of fatty tissue, may extend below the inguinal ligaments. Lift it to look for inflammation in the skin folds or even for a hidden hernia.

Gas

Gaseous distention may be localized or generalized. It causes a tympanitic percussion note. Selected foods may cause mild distention from increased intestinal gas production. More serious are intestinal obstruction and adynamic (paralytic) ileus. Note the location of the distention. Distention becomes more marked in obstruction in the colon than in the small bowel.

Tumor

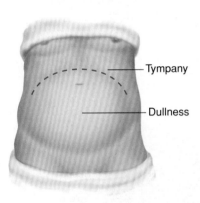

A large, solid tumor, usually rising out of the pelvis, is dull to percussion. Air-filled bowel is displaced to the periphery. Causes include ovarian tumors and uterine fibroids. Occasionally a markedly distended bladder may be mistaken for such a tumor.

Pregnancy

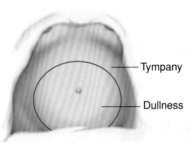

Pregnancy is a common cause of a pelvic "mass." Listen for the fetal heart.

Ascitic Fluid

Ascitic fluid seeks the lowest point in the abdomen, producing bulging flanks that are dull to percussion. The umbilicus may protrude. Turn the patient onto one side to detect the shift in position of the fluid level (shifting dullness). (See Chapter 16, pp. 506–507. for the assessment of ascites.)

TABLE
16-10

Sounds in the Abdomen

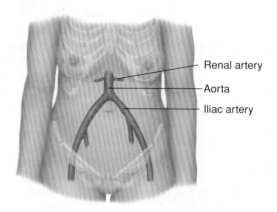

Bowel Sounds

Bowel sounds may be:

* Increased, as in diarrhea or early intestinal obstruction
* *Decreased,* then absent, as in *adynamic ileus* and *peritonitis.* Before deciding that bowel sounds are absent, sit down and listen where shown for 2 minutes or even longer.

High-pitched tinkling sounds suggest intestinal fluid and air under tension in a dilated bowel. *Rushes of high-pitched sounds* coinciding with an abdominal cramp indicate intestinal obstruction.

Bruits

A *hepatic bruit* suggests carcinoma of the liver or cirrhosis. *Arterial bruits* with both systolic and diastolic components suggest partial occlusion of the aorta or large arteries. Such bruits in the epigastrium are suspicious for *renal artery stenosis* or *renovascular hypertension.*

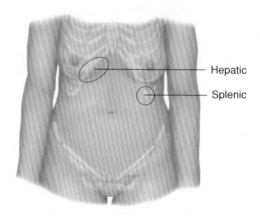

Venous Hum

A venous hum is rare. It is a soft humming noise with both systolic and diastolic components. It indicates increased collateral circulation between portal and systemic venous systems, as in *hepatic cirrhosis.*

Friction Rubs

Friction rubs are rare. They are grating sounds with respiratory variation. They indicate inflammation of the peritoneal surface of an organ, as in liver cancer, chlamydial or gonococcal perihepatitis, recent liver biopsy, or splenic infarct. When a systolic bruit accompanies a hepatic friction rub, suspect carcinoma of the liver.

TABLE

16-11

Liver Enlargement: Apparent and Real

A palpable liver does not necessarily indicate hepatomegaly (an enlarged liver), but more often results from a change in consistency—from the normal softness to an abnormal firmness or hardness, as in cirrhosis. Clinical estimates of liver size should be based on both percussion and palpation, although even these techniques are imperfect compared to ultrasound.

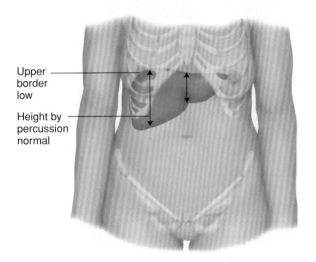

Upper border low

Height by percussion normal

Elongated right lobe

Downward Displacement of the Liver by a Low Diaphragm

This finding is common when the diaphragm is flattened and low, as in COPD. The liver edge may be palpable well below the costal margin. Percussion, however, reveals a low upper edge also, and the vertical span of the liver is normal.

Normal Variations in Liver Shape

In some individuals the right lobe of the liver may be elongated and easily palpable as it projects downward toward the iliac crest. Such an elongation, sometimes called *Riedel lobe,* represents a variation in shape, not an increase in liver volume or size.

Smooth Large Liver

Cirrhosis may produce an enlarged liver with a firm, *nontender* edge. The cirrhotic liver may also be scarred and contracted. Many other diseases may produce similar findings such as hemochromatosis, amyloidosis, and lymphoma. An enlarged liver with a smooth, *tender* edge suggests inflammation, as in hepatitis, or venous congestion, as in right-sided heart failure.

Irregular Large Liver

An enlarged liver that is firm or hard with an irregular edge or surface suggests *hepatocellular carcinoma.* There may be one or more nodules. The liver may or may not be tender.

TABLE
16-12

Tender Abdomen

Abdominal Wall Tenderness

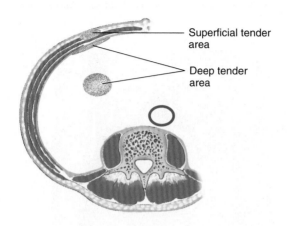

Superficial tender area

Deep tender area

Tenderness may originate in the abdominal wall. When the patient raises the head and shoulders, this tenderness persists, whereas tenderness from a deeper lesion (protected by the tightened muscles) decreases.

Visceral Tenderness

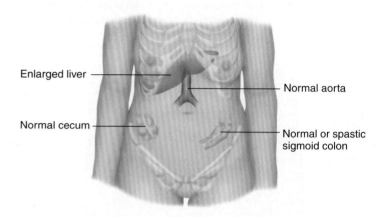

Enlarged liver

Normal aorta

Normal cecum

Normal or spastic sigmoid colon

The structures shown may be tender to deep palpation. Usually the discomfort is dull with no muscular rigidity or rebound tenderness. A reassuring explanation to the patient may prove helpful.

Tenderness From Disease in the Chest and Pelvis

Unilateral or bilateral, upper or lower abdomen

Acute Pleurisy

Abdominal pain and tenderness may result from acute pleural inflammation. When unilateral, it may mimic *acute cholecystitis* or *appendicitis*. Rebound tenderness and rigidity are less common; chest signs are usually present.

Acute Salpingitis

Frequently bilateral, the tenderness of acute salpingitis (inflammation of the fallopian tubes) is usually maximal just above the inguinal ligaments. Rebound tenderness and rigidity may be present. On pelvic examination, motion of the cervix and uterus causes pain.

Tenderness of Peritoneal Inflammation

Tenderness associated with peritoneal inflammation is more severe than visceral tenderness. Muscular rigidity and rebound tenderness are frequently but not necessarily present. Generalized peritonitis causes exquisite tenderness throughout the abdomen, together with board-like muscular rigidity. These signs on palpation, especially abdominal rigidity, double the likelihood of peritonitis.[30] Local causes of peritoneal inflammation include:

Acute Cholecystitis[73]

Signs are maximal in the right upper quadrant. Check for the Murphy sign (see Chapter 16, p. 503).

Acute Pancreatitis[74]

In acute pancreatitis, epigastric tenderness and rebound tenderness are usually present, but the abdominal wall may be soft.

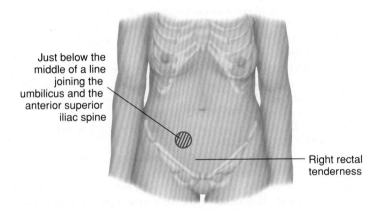

Just below the middle of a line joining the umbilicus and the anterior superior iliac spine

Right rectal tenderness

Acute Appendicitis[14,15]

Right lower quadrant signs are typical of acute appendicitis but may be absent early in the course. The typical area of tenderness, McBurney point, is illustrated. Examine other areas of the right lower quadrant as well as the right flank.

Acute Diverticulitis

Acute diverticulitis is a confined inflammatory process, usually in the left lower quadrant, that involves the sigmoid colon. If the sigmoid colon is redundant there may be suprapubic or right-sided pain. Look for localized peritoneal signs and a tender underlying mass. Microperforation, abscess, and obstruction may ensue.

BIBLIOGRAPHY

CITATIONS

1. National Institute of Diabetes and Digestive and Kidney Diseases (NIDDK). The urinary tract and how it works. Available at http://www.niddk.nih.gov/health-information/health-topics/Anatomy/urinary-tract-how-it-works/Pages/anatomy.aspx. Accessed October 27, 2015.

2. Talley NJ, Vakil NB, Moayyedi P, et al. American Gastroenterological Association technical review on the evaluation of dyspepsia. *Gastroenterology*. 2005;129:1756–1780.

3. Ranji SR, Goldman LE, Simel DL, et al. Do opiates affect the clinical evaluation of patients with acute abdominal pain? *JAMA*. 2006;296:1764.

4. Bates CM, Plevris JN. Clinical evaluation of abdominal pain in adults. *Medicine*. 2013;41(2):81–86.

5. Schneider L, Büchler MW, Werner J. Acute pancreatitis with an emphasis on infection. *Infect Dis Clin North Am*. 2010;24:921.

6. Fogel EL, Sherman S. ERCP for gallstone pancreatitis. *N Engl J Med*. 2014;370:150.

7. Guptak WB. In the clinic: acute pancreatitis. *Ann Intern Med*. 2010;153:ITC5-1.

8. Tack J, Talley NJ. Functional dyspepsia–symptoms, definitions and validity of the Rome III criteria. *Nat Rev Gastroenterol Hepatol*. 2013;10:134.

9. DeVault KR, Castell DO. Updated guidelines for the diagnosis and treatment of gastroesophageal reflux disease. *Am J Gastroenterol*. 2005;100:190.

10. Wilson JF. In the clinic. Alcohol use. *Ann Intern Med*. 2009;150:ITC3-1.

11. Shaheen NJ, Weinberg DS, Denberg TD. Upper endoscopy for gastroesophageal reflux disease: best practice advice from the clinical guidelines committee of the American College of Physicians. *Ann Intern Med*. 2012;157:808.

12. Spechler SJ, Souza RF. Barrett's esophagus. *N Engl J Med*. 2014;371:836.

13. Bao J, Lopez JA, Huerta S. Acute abdominal pain and abnormal CT findings. *JAMA*. 2013;310:848.

14. Howell JM, Eddy OL, Lukens TW, et al. Clinical policy: critical issues in the evaluation and management of emergency department patients with suspected appendicitis. *Ann Emerg Med*. 2010;55:71.

15. Andersson RE. The natural history and traditional management of appendicitis revisited: spontaneous resolution and predominance of prehospital perforations imply that a correct diagnosis is more important than an early diagnosis. *World J Surg*. 2007;31:86.

16. Camilleri M. Peripheral mechanisms in irritable bowel syndrome. *N Engl J Med*. 2012;367:1626.

17. Roden DF, Altman KW. Causes of dysphagia among different age groups: a systematic review of the literature. *Otolaryngol Clin North Am*. 2013;46:965.

18. Rome III Diagnostic Criteria for Functional Gastrointestinal Disorders—Appendix A. 2006;885–898. Available at http://www.romecriteria.org/criteria/. Accessed October 27, 2015.

19. Longstreth GF, Thompson WG, Chey WD, et al. Functional bowel disorders. *Gastroenterology*. 2006;130:1480.

20. Leffler DA, Lamont JT. Clostridium difficile infection. *N Engl J Med*. 2015;372:1539.

21. Shah BJ, Rughwani N, Rose S. Constipation. In the clinic: constipation. *Ann Intern Med*. 2015;162:ITC-1.

22. Gallegos-Orozco JF, Foxx-Orenstein AE, Sterler SM, et al. Chronic constipation in the elderly. *Am J Gastroenterol*. 2012;107:18.

23. Bradway C, Bixby MB, Hirschman KB, et al. Case study: transitional care for a patient with benign prostatic hyperplasia and recurrent urinary tract infections. *Urologic Nsg*. 2013;33:177–179, 200.

24. Robinson JP, Bradway CW, Bunting-Perry L, et al. Lower urinary tract symptoms in men with parkinson disease. *J Neurosci Nurs*. 2013;45:382–392.

25. Hooton TM. Uncomplicated urinary tract infection. *N Engl J Med*. 2012;366:1028.

26. Gupta K, Trautner B. In the clinic: urinary tract infection. *Ann Intern Med*. 2012;156:ITC3-1.

27. Dowling-Castronovo A, Specht JK. How to try this: assessment of transient urinary incontinence in older adults. *Am J Nurs*. 2009;109(2):62–71.

28. Doughty DB. *Urinary & Fecal Incontinence: Current Management Concepts*. Mosby, MO: St. Louis; 2009.

29. Dowling-Castronovo A, Bradway C. Urinary incontinence. In: Boltz M, Capezuti E, Fulmer T, et al., eds. *Geriatric Nursing Protocols for Best Practice*. 4th ed. New York, NY: Springer; 2012;18:393–387.

30. McGee S. *Evidence-Based Physical Diagnosis*. Philadelphia, PA: Saunders; 2012:428–453.

31. de Bruyn G, Graviss EA. A systematic review of the diagnostic accuracy of physical examination for the detection of cirrhosis. *BMC Med Inform Decis Mak*. 2001;1:6.

32. Naylor CD. Physical examination of the liver. *JAMA*. 1994;271:1859.

33. Zoli M, Magalotti D, Grimaldi M, et al. Physical examination of the liver: is it still worth it? *Am J Gastroenterol*. 1995;90:1428.

34. Grover SA, Barkun AN, Sackett DL. Does this patient have splenomegaly? *JAMA*. 1993;270:2218.

35. Kent KC. Clinical practice. Abdominal aortic aneurysms. *N Engl J Med*. 2014;371:2101.

36. Lederle F. In the clinic. Abdominal aortic aneurysm. *Ann Intern Med*. 2009;150:ITC5-1.

37. U.S. Preventive Services Task Force. Final Recommendation Statement. Abdominal Aortic Aneurysm: Screening, June 2014. Available at http://www.uspreventiveservicestaskforce.org/Page/Document/RecommendationStatementFinal/abdominal-aortic-aneurysm-screening. Accessed October 27, 2015.

38. Runyon BA, American Association for the Study of Liver Diseases. Introduction to the revised American association for the study of liver diseases practice guideline management of adult patients with ascites due to cirrhosis. *Hepatology*. 2013;57:1651.

39. Williams JW, Simel DL. Does this patient have ascites? How to divine fluid in the abdomen. *JAMA*. 1992;267:2645.

40. Hlibczuk V, Dattaro JA, Jin Z, et al. Diagnostic accuracy of noncontrast computed tomography for appendicitis in adults: a systematic review. *Ann Emerg Med*. 2010;55:51–59.

41. Substance Abuse and Mental Health Services Administration (SAMHSA). 2013 National Survey on Drug Use and Health

(NSDUH). Table 2.41B—Alcohol Use in Lifetime, Past Year, and Past Month among Persons Aged 18 or Older, by Demographic Characteristics: Percentages, 2012 and 2013. Available at http://www.samhsa.gov/data/sites/default/files/NSDUH-DetTabsPDFWHTML2013/Web/HTML/NSDUH-DetTabsSect2peTabs1to42–2013.htm#tab2.41b. Accessed October 27, 2015.

42. SAMHSA. 2013 National Survey on Drug Use and Health (NSDUH). Table 2.46B—Alcohol Use, Binge Alcohol Use, and Heavy Alcohol Use in the Past Month among Persons Aged 18 or Older, by Demographic Characteristics: Percentages, 2012 and 2013. Available at http://www.samhsa.gov/data/sites/default/files/NSDUH-DetTabsPDFWHTML2013/Web/HTML/NSDUH-DetTabsSect2peTabs43to84–2013.htm#tab2.46b. Accessed October 27, 2015.

43. Centers for Disease Control and Prevention. Fact Sheets—Alcohol Use and Your Health. 2014. Available at http://www.cdc.gov/alcohol/pdfs/alcoholyourhealth.pdf. Accessed October 27, 2015.

44. Moyer VA, U.S. Preventive Services Task Force. Screening and behavioral counseling interventions in primary care to reduce alcohol misuse: U.S. preventive services task force recommendation statement. *Ann Intern Med*. 2013;159:210.

45. Govier A, Rees C. Reducing alcohol-related health risks: the role of the nurse. *Nursing Standard*. 2013;27(50):42–46.

46. National Institute of Alcohol Abuse and Alcoholism. Alcohol Facts and Statistics. 2014. Available at http://pubs.niaaa.nih.gov/publications/AlcoholFacts&Stats/AlcoholFacts&Stats.pdf. Accessed October 25 2015.

47. Centers for Disease Control and Prevention. Hepatitis A. General information: U.S. Department of Health & Human Services; updated 2015. Available at http://www.cdc.gov/hepatitis/hav/pdfs/hepageneralfactsheet.pdf. Accessed October 25 2015.

48. Centers for Disease Control and Prevention. Viral Hepatitis Statistics & Surveillance. 2014. Available at http://www.cdc.gov/hepatitis/Statistics/2012Surveillance/Table2.3.htm. Accessed October 25 2015.

49. Fiore AE, Wasley A, Bell BP. Prevention of hepatitis A through active or passive immunization: recommendations of the Advisory Committee on Immunization Practices (ACIP). *MMWR Recomm Rep*. 2006;55:1.

50. Mast EE, Weinbaum CM, Fiore AE, et al. A comprehensive immunization strategy to eliminate transmission of hepatitis B virus infection in the United States: recommendations of the advisory committee on immunization practices (ACIP) part II: immunization of adults. *MMWR Recomm Rep*. 2006;55:1.

51. LeFevre ML. Screening for hepatitis B virus infection in nonpregnant adolescents and adults: U.S. Preventive Services Task Force recommendation statement. *Ann Intern Med*. 2014;161:58.

52. Centers for Disease Control and Prevention. Viral Hepatitis C. 2014. Available at http://www.cdc.gov/hepatitis/HCV/. Accessed October 25, 2015.

53. Chou R, Cottrell EB, Wasson N, et al. *Screening for Hepatitis C Virus Infection in Adults*. Rockville, MD; 2012. Available at http://www.ncbi.nlm.nih.gov/pubmed/23304739. Accessed October 25, 2015.

54. Rosen HR. Clinical practice. Chronic hepatitis C infection. *N Engl J Med*. 2011;364:2429.

55. El-Serag HB. Hepatocellular carcinoma. *N Engl J Med*. 2011;365:1118.

56. Moyer VA. Screening for hepatitis C virus infection in adults: U.S. Preventive Services Task Force recommendation statement. *Ann Intern Med*. 2013;159:349.

57. Howlader N, Noone AM, Krapcho M, et al., eds. *SEER Cancer Statistics Review, 1975–2012*. Bethesda, MD: National Cancer Institute; 2015. Accessed at http://seer.cancer.gov/csr/1975_2012/This link goes offsite. Click to read the external link disclaimer. Accessed October 27, 2015.

58. U.S. Preventive Services Task Force. Screening for colorectal cancer: U.S. Preventive Services Task Force recommendation statement. *Ann Intern Med*. 2008;149:627.

59. American Cancer Society. Colorectal Cancer Facts and Figures 2014–2015. Available at http://www.cancer.org/acs/groups/content/documents/document/acspc-042280.pdf. Accessed October 25, 2015.

60. Holme O, Bretthauer M, Fretheim A, et al. Flexible sigmoidoscopy versus faecal occult blood testing for colorectal cancer screening in asymptomatic individuals. *Cochrane Database Syst Rev*. 2013;9:CD009259.

61. Elmunzer BJ, Hayward RA, Schoenfeld PS, et al. Effect of flexible sigmoidoscopy-based screening on incidence and mortality of colorectal cancer: a systematic review and meta-analysis of randomized controlled trials. *PLoS Med*. 2012;9:e1001352.

62. Boyle T, Keegel T, Bull F, et al. Physical activity and risks of proximal and distal colon cancers: a systematic review and meta-analysis. *J Natl Cancer Inst*. 2012;104:1548.

63. Dube C, Rostom A, Lewin G, et al. The use of aspirin for primary prevention of colorectal cancer: a systematic review prepared for the U.S. Preventive Services Task Force. *Ann Intern Med*. 2007;146:365.

64. Rostom A, Dube C, Lewin G, et al. Nonsteroidal anti-inflammatory drugs and cyclooxygenase-2 inhibitors for primary prevention of colorectal cancer: a systematic review prepared for the U.S. Preventive Services Task Force. *Ann Intern Med*. 2007;146:376.

65. Chlebowski RT, Wactawski-Wende J, Ritenbaugh C, et al. Estrogen plus progestin and colorectal cancer in postmenopausal women. *N Engl J Med*. 2004;350:991.

66. U.S. Preventive Services Task Force. Routine aspirin or nonsteroidal anti-inflammatory drugs for the primary prevention of colorectal cancer: U.S. Preventive Services Task Force recommendation statement. *Ann Intern Med*. 2007;146:361.

67. Levin TR, Zhao W, Conell C, et al. Complications of colonoscopy in an integrated health care delivery system. *Ann Intern Med*. 2006;145:880.

68. Gorina Y, Schappert S, Bercovitz A, et al. Prevalence of incontinence among older Americans. National Center for Health Statistics. *Vital Health Stat*. 2014;3(36).

69. Sandvik H, Espuna M, Hunskaar S. Validity of the incontinence severity index: Comparison with pad-weighing tests. *Int Urogynecol J Pelvic Floor Dysfunct*. 2006;17(5):520–524.

70. Hensley D, Driscoll A, Bradway C, et al. *Urologic Nursing: Scope and Standards of Practice*. 2nd ed. Pitman, NJ: Jannetti; 2013.

71. Ryan DP, Hong TS, Bardeesy N. Pancreatic adenocarcinoma. *N Engl J Med*. 2014;371:1039.

72. Yadav D, Lowenfels AB. The epidemiology of pancreatitis and pancreatic cancer. *Gastroenterology*. 2013;144:1252.

73. Strasberg S. Acute calculus cholecystitis. *N Engl J Med*. 2008; 358:2804.

74. Katz LH, Guy DD, Lahat A, et al. Diverticulitis in the young is not more aggressive than in the elderly, but it tends to recur more often: systematic review and meta-analysis. *J Gastroenterol Hepatol*. 2013;28:1274.

75. Acosta S. Mesenteric ischemia. *Curr Opin Crit Care*. 2015; 21:171.

76. Sise MJ. Acute mesenteric ischemia. *Surg Clin North Am*. 2014;94:165.

77. DuPont HL. Acute infectious diarrhea in immunocompetent adults. *N Engl J Med*. 2014;370:1532.

The Breasts and Axillae

The student will:

1. Identify the structures and function of the breasts and axillae.

2. Elicit an accurate health history of the breasts and axillae.

3. Describe the physical examination techniques performed to evaluate the breasts and axillae.

4. Demonstrate how to perform a clinical breast examination.

5. Document a complete breast and axilla assessment using information from the health history and the physical examination.

6. Describe the measures for prevention or early detection of breast cancer.

Hormonal changes at puberty in women cause the breast tissue to enlarge and prepares the ductal system for lactation. Until puberty, the male and female breasts are similar.

ANATOMY AND PHYSIOLOGY

The Female Breast

The female breast lies against the anterior thoracic wall, extending from the 2nd rib down to the 6th rib, and from the sternum across to the midaxillary line. Its surface area is generally rectangular rather than round. The breast overlies the pectoralis major and, at its inferior margin, the serratus anterior.

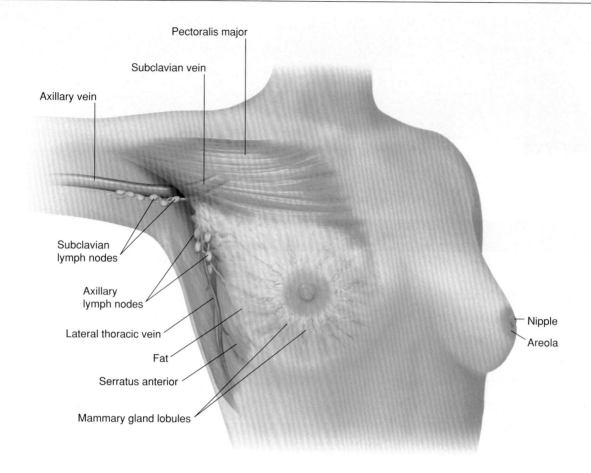

The breast is hormonally sensitive tissue, responsive to the changes of monthly menstrual cycles and aging. At the tip of the breast is an area called the areola and at the center is the nipple. About 15 to 20 lactiferous ducts empty into a depression at the top of the nipple. Each duct leads from the alveoli within the breast called lobules, where the milk is secreted. Along their length, the duct widens into areas that form reservoirs where milk can be stored. These ducts and lobules form the *glandular tissue*. *Fibrous connective tissue* provides structural support in the form of fibrous bands or suspensory ligaments connected to both the skin and the underlying fascia. *Adipose tissue*, or fat, surrounds the breast, predominantly in the superficial and peripheral areas. After menopause, there is a decreased number of lobules noted, glandular tissue atrophies and is replaced with fat. The proportions of these components vary with age, the general state of nutrition, pregnancy, exogenous hormone use, and other factors.

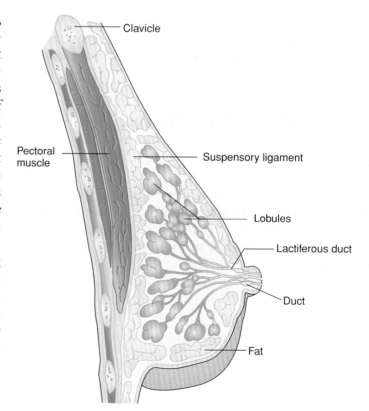

The surface of the areola has small, rounded elevations formed by sebaceous glands, sweat glands, and accessory areolar glands. A few hairs are often seen on the areola.

Both the nipple and the areola are well supplied with smooth muscle that contracts to express milk from the ductal system during breast-feeding. Rich sensory innervation, especially in the nipple, triggers "milk letdown" following neurohormonal stimulation from infant sucking. Tactile stimulation of the area, including the breast examination, makes the nipple smaller, firmer, and more erect, whereas the areola puckers and wrinkles. These smooth muscle reflexes are normal and should not be mistaken for signs of breast disease.

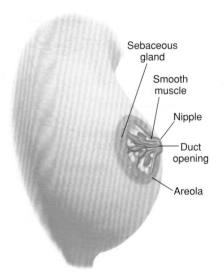

The adult breast may be soft, but it often feels granular, nodular, or lumpy. This uneven texture is normal and may be termed *physiologic nodularity* or fibrocystic breast. It is often bilateral. It may be evident throughout the breast or only in parts of it. The nodularity may increase before menses—a time when breasts often enlarge and become tender or even painful. For breast changes during adolescence go to p. 896.

Occasionally, one or more extra or supernumerary nipples are located along the "milk line" (see illustration). Only a small nipple and areola are usually present, often mistaken for a common mole. There may be underlying glandular tissue. An extra nipple has no pathologic significance.

The Male Breast

The male breast consists chiefly of a small nipple and areola. These overlie a thin disc of undeveloped breast tissue consisting primarily of ducts. Lacking estrogen and progesterone stimulation, ductal branching, and development of lobules are minimal.[1] It may be difficult to distinguish male breast tissue from the surrounding muscles of the chest wall. A firm button of breast tissue, 2 cm or more in diameter has been described in roughly one of three adult men.

Lymphatics

Lymphatics from most of the breast drain toward the axilla. Of the axillary lymph nodes, the *central nodes* are palpable most frequently. They lie along the chest wall, usually high in the axilla and midway between the anterior and posterior axillary folds. Channels from three other groups of lymph nodes drain into them and are seldom palpable. They include:

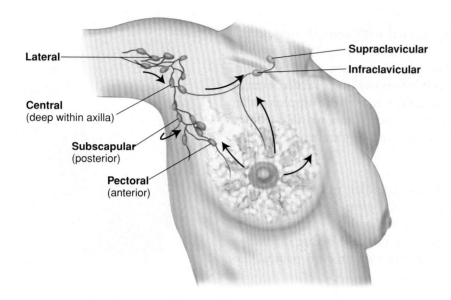

- *Pectoral nodes—anterior,* located along the lower border of the pectoralis major inside the anterior axillary fold. These nodes drain the anterior chest wall and much of the breast.

- *Subscapular nodes—posterior,* located along the lateral border of the scapula; palpated deep in the posterior axillary fold. They drain the posterior chest wall and a portion of the arm.

- *Lateral nodes*—located *along the upper humerus.* They drain most of the arm.

Lymph drains from the central axillary nodes to the *infraclavicular* and *supraclavicular* nodes.

Not all the lymphatics of the breast drain into the axilla. Malignant cells from a breast cancer may spread directly to the infraclavicular nodes or into deep channels within the chest.

THE HEALTH HISTORY

Common or Concerning Symptoms in Females or Males

- Breast lump or mass
- Breast pain or discomfort
- Change in shape
- Nipple discharge
- Edema
- Rashes
- Scaling
- Dimpling
- Retraction
- Gynecomastia (males)

During the breast examination, cultural considerations and sexual orientation and identity that were elicited during the health history should be taken into account. Once a rapport has developed, begin with an open-ended question, such as:

"Have you noticed any changes in your breast?"

If the patient does not have any comments, then more specific questions are necessary as they may trigger a memory, reveal another area that the patient thought was "nothing" or not worth mentioning. Patients may be too embarrassed to ask or answer questions regarding their breasts. In addition, if the patient does have a positive response then additional questions should be asked related to the finding.

Lump or Mass

Have you ever felt a lump in your breast or under your arm?
Below are sample questions to ask patients if there are positive findings:
Onset: When did you first notice the lump?
Location: In which breast is the lump? Where on the breast?
Duration: Does the lump remain at all times or does it come and go? If it comes and goes, when is it present and when does it disappear?
Characteristic Symptoms: What does the lump feel like?
Are there multiple lumps or one distinct lump?
Associated Manifestations: What else happens when the lump is present:
Pain?
Discharge?
During menstruation?
Relieving Factors: Does anything make it go away?
Hurt less if there is pain?
Treatment: Have you done anything about the lump to make it disappear?
Have you spoken to a health care provider?

Pain or Discomfort

Onset: Do you ever have breast pain/discomfort?
When do you have pain/discomfort?
Location: Where do you have pain/discomfort?
Duration: Does the pain/discomfort come and go or is it constant?
Characteristic Symptoms: Describe the pain/discomfort.
Associated Manifestations: What else happens with the pain/discomfort?
Relieving Factors: What have you done to make the pain/discomfort feel better?
Treatment: Have you done anything to treat the pain?
There are many questions related to the breast and use of the OLD CART mnemonic which ensures all areas of questioning are covered. Additional examples of questions continue for a variety of findings.

Lumps may be physiologic or pathologic, ranging from cysts and fibroadenomas to breast cancer. See Table 17-1, Common Breast Masses, p. 563 and Table 17-2, Visible Signs of Breast Cancer p. 564.

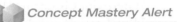 *Concept Mastery Alert*

When collecting the health history of a patient who reports a lump or swelling in the breast, the nurse must gather additional information to evaluate whether the lump is physiologic or pathologic. The priority question would be to first determine if the lumps change in size during the menstrual cycle. Women with fibrocystic breasts will often have lumpy areas in the breast that increase in size in the two weeks prior to the menstrual period and then decrease in size during the period and for the first two weeks after the period. Pain is often associated with these lumps, so a report of pain from the patient does not provide specific information about whether lump is physiologic or pathologic.

Change in Shape

Have you noticed any change in the *shape* of your breast?
  When did you notice the change in shape?
  Where is the change? Which breast?
  When did this occur?
  What else happened at this time?
  Can you associate anything else with this?
  How are you coping with the treatment?

Discharge

Have you ever had *nipple discharge*?
  When does the discharge occur?
  In which breast does it occur? Unilateral? Bilateral?
  How long does the discharge last?
  Can you describe the discharge? (Color, Consistency, Amount, Odor)
  What is associated with the discharge?
  How do you deal with this?

Galactorrhea, or the inappropriate discharge of milk-containing fluid, is abnormal if it occurs 6 or more months after childbirth or cessation of breast-feeding.

Edema

Have you noticed any breast *edema* (swelling)?
  When does the edema occur?
  Where does it occur? Which breast? Which quadrant?
  How long does it last?
  Is it painful?
  What is the color of the breast?
  What else occurs?
  What do you do to relieve the swelling?

Rashes or Scaling

Have you noticed any *rashes*? *Scaling*? (Scaling consists of thin flakes of keratinized epithelium.)
  When did this begin?
  Where did this begin?
  How long has it been going on?
  Besides the rash/scaling of the skin, what else is happening?
  Does it hurt?
  What do you do to relieve the rash/scaling?

Dimpling

Have you noticed *dimpling* (small indents) of the breast tissue?
  When did this begin?
  In which breast did this begin?
  How long has it been going on? Is it constant?

Are there any other symptoms occurring at this time?

Do you associate anything with this?

Are you treating this?

Retraction

Have you ever had nipple *retraction*?

When did the retraction occur?

Which nipple is retracted?

How long does it occur for? Does it evert at any time? When?

What happens when the nipple retracts?

Does anything else occur during the retraction?

Do you do anything to protract the nipple?

Nipple retraction is when the nipple is pulled inward. This is not an issue if the breast has had an inverted nipple since birth; however, it is noteworthy if this is a change as it could be an indicator of breast cancer or adhesions below the skin surface. (See Table 17-2, Visible Signs of Breast Cancer, p. 564).

Past History

What medications (menopausal replacement therapy [MRT], oral contraceptives [OC]) are you currently taking?

When did you begin taking the medication?

What is the medication name and dosage?

Are you having any side effects?

What other medications have you taken in the past?

When did you take them?

For how long did you take them?

Why did you stop?

Were there any side effects?

Have you ever been pregnant?

When?

How many live births? Abortions? Miscarriages?

How old were you when your first baby was delivered? Was it full term?

Did you breastfeed your child(ren)? For how long?

Menstrual history

How old were you at menarche (first menses)?

How old were you at menopause?

How many days in your cycle?

Previous history of breast cancer and/or reproductive cancer (e.g., ovarian)

When did you have breast cancer and/or reproductive cancer?

In which breast did you have cancer? Or where was the reproductive cancer?

How did you find the cancer? Was there a lump?

How was it treated?

Who was on your health care team?

Previous breast biopsy

Have you ever had a breast biopsy? If yes:

When? Where?

Results?

Breast self-examination (BSE)

How often do you perform BSE?

When do you perform BSE?

What technique do you use?

Have you ever palpated a lump or found any changes?

Clinical breast examination (CBE)

When was your last examination by a health care provider?

What were the results?

Mammogram or Magnetic Resonance Imaging (MRI)

When was your last mammogram or MRI?

What were the results?

What testing site do you use?

Has the site changed? Did you transfer previous mammograms or MRI results to this site?

Family History

Do you have a family history of breast cancer? Genetic information or testing?

Do you have a family history of reproductive cancer?

If yes: who in the family has had any of the above? (sisters, mother, daughters, maternal aunts, maternal grandmother)

Have you had BRCA testing?

Lifestyle Habits

How much alcohol do you drink each day/week?

What do you do for physical activity?

PHYSICAL EXAMINATION

The Female Breast

Clinical investigation has shown that examiner experience and technique significantly affect the efficacy of the clinical breast examination. Clinicians are advised to adopt a more standardized approach, especially for palpation, and to use a systemic up and down search pattern, varying palpation pressure, and a circular motion with the finger pads.[2-4] For screening examinations, the length of time spent on palpation is one of the most important factors in detecting suspicious changes, with highest sensitivity when examiners spend 5 to 10 minutes for the examination of both breasts.[5,6] When examination time falls, especially for clinicians in practice compared to trained examiners in clinical trials, sensitivity for detection of breast cancer drops from the 65% range to 28–35%, with the attendant hazards of high numbers of false positives.[3,5,7] Experts concur on the importance of the CBE for women with symptoms or a palpable mass, since mammography in women with self-reported or palpable masses may miss up to 13% of invasive cancers.[8]

As you begin the examination, adopt a courteous and gentle approach. Let the patient know that you are about to examine the breasts. This may be a good time to ask if the individual has noticed any lumps, other problems, and enhance her awareness of screening guidelines, including techniques

The most significant risk factors for breast cancer are age, BRCA status, and breast density on mammogram. Personal history of breast cancer, family history, and reproductive factors affecting duration of uninterrupted estrogen exposure are also important.[9] For numerous additional risk factors, see also the table on Breast Cancer in Women: Factors That Increase Relative Risk, p. 556.

See Patient Instructions for Breast Awareness and Self Examination, pp. 552–553.

for self-examination if requested. Because breasts tend to swell and become more nodular before menses from increasing estrogen stimulation, the best time for examination is 5 to 7 days *after* the onset of menstruation. Nodules appearing prior to menstruation should be reevaluated at this later time. See Patient Instructions for the Breast Self-Examination, pp. 552–553.

Draping the chest. Adequate inspection initially requires full exposure of the chest, but later in the examination, cover one breast while you are palpating the other.

Inspection

Inspect the breasts and nipples with the patient in the sitting position and disrobed to the waist. A thorough examination of the breast includes careful inspection for skin changes, symmetry, contours, and retraction in four views—arms at sides, arms over head, arms pressed against hips, and leaning forward. When examining an adolescent girl, assess her breast development according to Tanner sex maturity ratings described in Chapter 23, Assessing Children: Infancy Through Adolescence, p. 896.

Arms at Sides

Note the clinical features listed below.

- The appearance of the skin, including:

  - Color

- Thickening of the skin and unusually prominent pores, which may accompany lymphatic obstruction

- The *size and symmetry of the breasts*. Some difference in the size of the breasts, including the areolae, is common and is usually normal, as shown in the photograph below.

Redness in a light complexion or deeper pigmentation in a dark skin woman may be from local infection or inflammatory carcinoma.

Thickening and prominent pores suggest breast cancer.

- The *contour of the breasts*. Look for changes such as masses, dimpling, or flattening. Compare one side with the other.

Flattening of the normally convex breast suggests cancer. See Table 17-2, Visible Signs of Breast Cancer, p. 564.

- The *characteristics of the nipples*, including *size and shape*, *direction* in which they point, any *rashes or ulceration*, or any *discharge*

Asymmetry of directions in which nipples point suggests an underlying cancer. Rash or ulceration in Paget disease of the breast[10] (see Table 17-2, Visible Signs of Breast Cancer, p. 564).

Occasionally, the shape of the nipple is *inverted*, or depressed below the areolar surface. It may be enveloped by folds of areolar skin, as illustrated. Longstanding inversion is usually a normal variant of no clinical consequence, except for possible difficulty when breast-feeding.

Recent or fixed flattening or depression of the nipple suggests nipple retraction. A retracted nipple may also be broadened and thickened, suggesting an underlying cancer.

Arms Over Head; Hands Pressed Against Hips; Leaning Forward

To bring out dimpling or retraction that may otherwise be invisible, ask the patient to raise her arms over her head, and then press her hands against her hips to contract the pectoral muscles. Inspect the breast contours carefully in each position. If the breasts are large or pendulous, it may be useful to have the patient stand and lean forward, supported by the back of the chair.

ARMS OVER HEAD

Dimpling or retraction of the breasts in these positions suggests an underlying cancer. When a cancer or its associated fibrous strands are attached to both the skin and the fascia overlying the pectoral muscles, pectoral contraction can draw the skin inward, causing dimpling.

HANDS PRESSED AGAINST HIPS

Occasionally, these signs may be associated with benign lesions such as posttraumatic fat necrosis or mammary duct ectasia, but they must always be evaluated.

LEANING FORWARD

This position may reveal an asymmetry of the breast or nipple not otherwise visible. Retraction of the nipple and areola suggests an underlying cancer. See Table 17-2, Visible Signs of Breast Cancer, p. 564.

Palpation

The Breast

Palpation is best performed when the breast tissue is flattened. The patient should be supine. Plan to palpate a rectangular area extending from the clavicle to the inframammary fold or lower bra line, and from the midsternal line to the posterior axillary line and well into the axilla for the tail of the breast.

A thorough examination will take time and focus.

- While lying supine, have the patient reach behind their head, with their right hand when the right breast is examined (placing the hand behind the head will displace the breast tissue for easier palpation.)

- Use the finger pads of the 2nd, 3rd, and 4th fingers, keeping the fingers slightly flexed.

- The vertical stripping pattern is currently the best validated technique for detecting breast masses. It is important to be systematic.

- Palpate in small, dime-size, concentric circles at each examining point, if possible apply light, medium, and deep pressure. You will need to press more firmly to reach the deeper tissues of a large breast.

- Continue in vertical overlapping strips until your examination covers the entire breast, including the periphery, tail, and axilla.

- When you have completed all areas on the right breast, have the patient switch arms, placing the left hand behind the head to complete the assessment on the left side. Pay special attention to the upper outer quadrant and axilla, as 50% of breast lumps are found in the upper outer quadrant.

When pressing deeply on the breast, you may mistake a normal rib for a hard breast mass.

Examine the breast tissue carefully for:

- *Consistency* of the tissues. Normal consistency varies widely, depending in part on the relative proportions of firmer glandular tissue and soft fat. Physiologic nodularity may be present, increasing before menses. There may be a firm transverse ridge of compressed tissue along the lower margin of the breast, especially in large breasts. This is the normal inframammary ridge, not a tumor.

  > A lump near a clogged nipple may suggest *mammary duct ectasia*, a benign but sometimes painful condition of dilated ducts with surrounding inflammation, sometimes with associated masses.

- *Tenderness.* This may be premenstrual fullness.

- *Nodules.* Palpate carefully for any lump or mass that is different from the rest of the breast tissue. This is sometimes called a dominant mass and may reflect a pathologic change that requires evaluation by mammogram, MRI, aspiration, or biopsy.

  > See Table 17-1, Common Breast Masses, p. 563.

- Document the characteristics of any nodule:

  Location—which breast, the quadrant or clock site, centimeters from the nipple

  > Hard, irregular, poorly circumscribed nodules, fixed to the skin or underlying tissues, strongly suggest breast cancer.

  Size—in centimeters
  Shape—round or cystic, disc-like, or irregular in contour
  Consistency—soft, firm, or hard
  Delineation—well circumscribed or not
  Tenderness—tender or nontender

  > Cysts, inflamed areas; some cancers may be tender.

  Mobility—assess in relation to the skin, pectoral fascia, and chest wall. Gently move the breast near the mass and watch for dimpling.

- Next, try to move the mass itself while the patient relaxes her arm and then while she presses her hand against her hip.

  > A mobile mass that becomes fixed when the arm relaxes is attached to the ribs and intercostal muscles; if fixed when the hand is pressed against the hip, it is attached to the pectoral fascia.

If a lump is detected, documentation of the breast assessment is acceptable in either of two forms:

1. Divide the breast into four quadrants with a horizontal line and a vertical line crossing at the nipple, which would be the center point.

2. The breast is the face of a clock with 12 o'clock at the top, 6 o'clock at the bottom.

If an area needs to be specifically identified (e.g., to determine the exact site of a lump), the distance in centimeters from the nipple in the respective quadrant is charted. The area that extends laterally across the exterior fold is the tail of Spence.

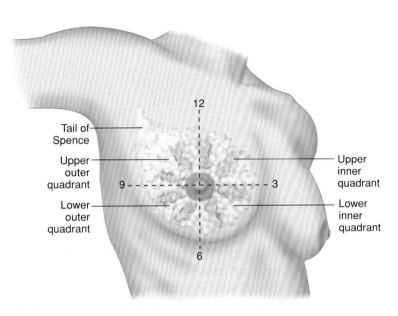

The Male Breast

Examination of the male breast may be brief but is important. *Inspect the nipple and areola* for nodules, swelling, or ulceration. *Palpate the areola and breast tissue* for nodules. If the breast appears enlarged, distinguish between the soft fatty enlargement of obesity and the firm disc of glandular enlargement caused by an imbalance of estrogen and testosterone, called *gynecomastia*. This can occur in one or both breasts, in newborns, adolescents, or older men, due to changes in hormone levels. In addition, certain diseases or medications, including anabolic steroids for athletic enhancement, can contribute to the swollen breast tissue or tenderness. Gynecomastia usually resolves without treatment.[11]

GYNECOMASTIA

A hard, irregular, eccentric, or ulcerating nodule suggests breast cancer.

Male breast cancer constitutes only 1% of breast cancer cases, peaking in frequency around age 71.[12,13]

The Axillae

Although the axillae may be examined with the patient lying down, a sitting position is preferable.

Inspection

Inspect the skin of each axilla, noting evidence of:

- Rash

- Infection

- Unusual pigmentation

Deodorant and other rashes

Sweat gland infection (*hidradenitis suppurativa*)

Deeply pigmented, velvety axillary skin suggests *acanthosis nigricans*—one form is associated with internal malignancy.

Palpation

To examine the left axilla, ask the patient to relax with the left arm down. Help by supporting the left wrist or hand with your left hand. Wearing a glove, cup together the fingers of your right hand and reach as high as you can toward the apex of the axilla. Warn the patient that this may feel uncomfortable. Your fingers should lie directly behind the pectoral muscles, pointing toward the midclavicle. Now press your fingers in toward the chest wall and slide them downward, trying to feel the central nodes against the chest wall. Of the axillary nodes, these are the most often palpable. One or more soft, small (<1 cm), nontender nodes are frequently felt.

Enlarged axillary nodes are from an infection of the hand or arm, recent immunizations or skin tests in the arm, or part of a generalized lymphadenopathy. Check the epitrochlear nodes and other groups of lymph nodes.

Nodes that are large (≥1 cm) and firm or hard, matted together, or fixed to the skin or to underlying tissues suggest malignant involvement.

Use your gloved left hand to examine the right axilla.

If the central nodes feel large, hard, or tender, or if there is a suspicious lesion in the drainage areas for the axillary nodes, feel for the other groups of axillary lymph nodes:

- *Pectoral nodes*—grasp the anterior axillary fold between your thumb and fingers, and with your fingers, palpate inside the border of the pectoral muscle.

- *Lateral nodes*—from high in the axilla, feel along the upper humerus.

- *Subscapular nodes*—step behind the patient and, with your fingers, feel inside the muscle of the posterior axillary fold.

Also, feel for infraclavicular nodes and reexamine the supraclavicular nodes.

SPECIAL TECHNIQUES

Assessment of Nipple Discharge

If there is a history of spontaneous nipple discharge, try to determine its origin by compressing the areola with your index finger, placed in radial positions around the nipple. Watch for discharge appearing through one of the duct openings on the nipple's surface. Note the color, consistency, and quantity of any discharge and the exact location where it appears. Discharge from the nipple is usually bilateral and the fluid is released when stimulated or compressed. The color alone is not indicative of the cause of the discharge.

Some findings include a milky discharge unrelated to a prior pregnancy and lactation, known as *nonpuerperal galactorrhea*. Causes include *hypothyroidism*, pituitary *prolactinoma*, and drugs that are dopamine agonists, including many psychotropic agents and phenothiazines.

Spontaneous unilateral bloody discharge from one or two ducts warrants further evaluation for intraductal *papilloma*, as shown; ductal carcinoma in situ (DCIS); or Paget disease of the breast.[10]

Examination of the Mastectomy or Breast Augmentation Patient

The woman with a mastectomy warrants special care on examination. Inspect the mastectomy scar and axilla carefully for any masses or unusual nodularity. Note any change in color or signs of inflammation. Lymphedema may be present in the axilla and upper arm from impaired lymph drainage after surgery. Palpate gently along the scar—these tissues may be unusually sensitive. Use a circular motion with two or three fingers. Note any enlargement of the lymph nodes or signs of inflammation or infection.

Masses, nodularity, and change in color or inflammation, especially in the incision line, suggest recurrence of breast cancer.

It is especially important to carefully palpate the breast tissue and incision lines or edges of the implant of women with breast augmentation or reconstruction.

Self-Awareness and Instructions for the Breast Self-Examination

If a woman chooses to perform BSE after reviewing the advantages and limitations, the nurse should take the opportunity to teach her the technique.

Breast masses can be detected by women examining their own breasts. Although BSE has not been shown to reduce breast cancer mortality, BSE is inexpensive and may promote stronger health awareness and more active self-care. For early detection of breast cancer, the BSE is an option for women and is most useful when coupled with regular breast examination by an experienced clinician and mammography or MRI. The BSE is an individual choice as research has shown that many lumps are randomly found and not during a monthly self-examination. If a woman chooses to practice BSE it is best timed, 5 to 7 days after the start of menses, when hormonal stimulation and breast tenderness is lower.

Breast Awareness and Self-Examination Instructions

Lying Supine

- Lie down and place your right arm behind your head. The examination is done while lying down, not standing up.
- Use the finger pads of the 3 middle fingers on your left hand to feel for lumps in the right breast. Use overlapping dime-sized circular motions of the finger pads to feel the breast tissue.
- Use 3 different levels of pressure to feel all the breast tissue. Light pressure is needed to feel the tissue closest to the skin; medium pressure to feel a little deeper; and firm pressure to feel the tissue closest to the chest and ribs. If you are not sure how hard to press, talk with your health care provider.

- Move in an up and down pattern. Be sure to check the entire breast.
- Repeat the examination on your left breast, putting your left arm behind your head and using the finger pads of your right hand to do the examination.

Standing

- Stand in front of a mirror with your hands pressing firmly on your hips, look for any changes of size, shape, contour, dimpling, redness or scaliness of the nipple or breast skin.
- Examine each underarm while sitting up or standing and with your arm only slightly raised so you can easily feel in this area.

http://www.cancer.org/cancer/breastcancer/moreinformation/breastcancerearlydetection/breast-cancer-early-detection-acs-recs-bse. Accessed May 6, 2015.

RECORDING YOUR FINDINGS

Recording the Physical Examination—Breasts and Axillae

"Breasts symmetric, color tan without pigment changes and smooth bilaterally; no masses, dimpling, lumps, edema, thickening, rashes, or ulcerations; nipples everted, equal in size, point outward; no discharge, no axillary adenopathy detected."

OR

"Breasts pendulous with diffuse fibrocystic changes. Single firm 1 × 1 cm mass, mobile and nontender, with overlying peau d'orange appearance in right breast, upper outer quadrant at 11 o'clock, 2 cm from the nipple, nipples everted, no discharge, no axillary adenopathy."

Suggests possible breast cancer

HEALTH PROMOTION AND COUNSELING

Important Topics for Health Promotion and Counseling

- Palpable masses of the breast
- Assessing risk of breast cancer
- Breast cancer screening

Women may experience a wide range of changes in breast tissue and sensation, from cyclic swelling and nodularity to a distinct lump or mass. The examination of the breast provides a meaningful opportunity for the nurse to explore concerns important to women's health—what to do if a lump or mass is detected, risk factors for breast cancer, and screening measures such as BSE, the CBE by a health care provider, mammography, and MRI. Women will frequently seek information during the clinical encounter. Men can also have breast cancer. If any noted changes or lumps are detected, men should also see their health care provider.

Palpable Masses of the Breast and Breast Symptoms

Breast cancer occurs in up to 4% of women with breast complaints, in approximately 5% of women reporting a nipple discharge, and in up to 11% of women specifically complaining of a breast lump or mass.[13] Breast masses show marked variation in etiology, from fibroadenomas and cysts seen in younger women, to abscess or mastitis, to primary breast cancer. On initial assessment, the woman's age and physical characteristics of the mass provide clues about its etiology. All breast masses require careful assessment. Nurses are patient advocates and help to navigate the complex health care system. Nurses assist patients to follow up on all breast irregularities for accurate diagnosis and treatment.

Assessing Risk of Breast Cancer

Women are increasingly interested in information about breast cancer. Nurses and the health care team should be familiar with the literature detailing the epidemiology of and risk factors for breast cancer that supports recommendations for screening. Key facts and figures are presented here, but further reading will enhance your counseling of patients.

Breast cancer continues to be the leading cancer diagnosed in all women today, excluding skin cancers. The total number of white women diagnosed with breast cancer over the past years remains constant, in addition, the black women diagnosed has been relatively stable, although there has been a 0.3% increase.

- *Declines in new cases of invasive breast cancer.* The number of new cases of invasive breast cancer has been falling since 2000, explained primarily by a decreased use of menopausal hormone therapy (MRT) in postmenopausal women since the Women's Health Initiative study was published showing the use of MRT increased breast cancer risk. In addition, decreased mammography screening, occurred during this same time frame, however the correlation was not related to a true decrease in disease incidence and led to under diagnosis or a delayed diagnosis rather than a true decrease in disease incidence.[13]

White women under age 60 are more likely to be diagnosed with breast cancer than African-American women. However, over age 60, black women surpass all other racial/ethnic groups in breast cancer incidence. The American Indian and Alaska native groups repeatedly have the lowest incidence throughout the lifespan.

A number of factors may contribute to the later diagnosis such as access to care with fewer black woman receiving mammograms, longer time periods between mammograms or follow up to health care providers. In addition, the presence of comorbidities, and there has also been data that suggest the tumors are more aggressive in black women.[14] Nurses and the health care team should advocate for access to care, educate this population on the importance of screening mammograms, and give prompt attention and follow up to any breast changes or lumps.

Breast cancer continues to be the second leading cause of cancer deaths in women. Overall, the numbers related to breast cancer deaths have continued to decrease especially for women under 50 years of age. These numbers have decreased, 3.2% per year for white women and 2.4% in black women. For women over 50 years old, the decrease has been 1.8% for white women and 1.1% for black women. These decreases in breast cancer deaths are thought to be the result of earlier detection and better treatment modalities.[13]

Assessing Risk Factors for Breast Cancer

Both *modifiable* and *nonmodifiable risk factors* for breast cancer have been identified, as listed in the table on the next page. Many risk factors cannot be readily altered, such as gender, age, family history, race, genetics, personal history of breast cancer, age at first full-term pregnancy, early menarche, late menopause, and breast density.[13] Others can be modified, although these tend to confer lower relative risk: postmenopausal obesity, use of estrogen–progesterone combination MRT, alcohol use, and physical inactivity. The table below summarizes the strengths of current risk factors. Although not included per se as a risk factor itself but lesbian, gay, and bisexual women may have a compilation of these risk factors, which includes not having children or having them later in life. This is of concern as it puts them at a higher risk for breast cancer.

Research on the health risks for breast cancer in transgender and transsexual individuals is limited at this time. Finding a health care provider who is responsive to the health care needs is important. Assessing the individual risks and necessary screening tools is instrumental based on the needs of each person.

Breast Cancer in Women: Factors That Increase Relative Risk	
Relative Risk	**Factor**
>4.0	• Female • Age (65+ vs. <65 years, although risk increases across all ages until age 80) • Certain inherited genetic mutations for breast cancer (BRCA1 and/or BRCA2) • Two or more first-degree relatives with breast cancer diagnosed at an early age • Personal history of breast cancer (<age 40) • Lobular carcinoma in situ • High breast tissue density on mammogram • Biopsy-confirmed atypical hyperplasia
2.1–4.0	• Personal history of breast cancer (≥age 40) • High endogenous estrogen or testosterone levels (postmenopausal) • One first-degree relative with breast cancer • High-dose radiation to chest
1.1–2.0	Late age at first full-term pregnancy (>30 years) • Early menarche (<12 years) • Late menopause (>55 years) • No full-term pregnancies • Never breast-fed a child • Recent oral contraceptive use • Recent and long-term use of hormone replacement therapy • Obesity (postmenopausal/adult weight gain) • Diethylstilbestrol (DES) exposure • Personal history of endometrium, ovary, or colon cancer • Alcohol consumption • Height (tall) • High socioeconomic status • Ashkenazi Jewish heritage

Source: American Cancer Society. Breast Cancer Facts & Figures 2013–2014. Atlanta: American Cancer Society, Inc. Available at: http://www.cancer.org/acs/groups/content/ @research/documents/document/acspc-042725.pdf. Accessed May 1, 2015.

Selected Risk Factors That Affect Screening Decisions

BRCA1 and 2 Mutations

Begin evaluating a woman's risk for breast cancer as early as her 20s. Women of all ages should be asked if there is a family history of breast, ovarian, tubal, or peritoneal cancer on either the maternal or paternal side. Approximately 5% to 10% of women have genetic risk of BRCA1 or BRCA2 gene mutation. These genes are autosomal dominant. Women with BRCA1 mutations and

BRCA2 mutations have an estimated 57% and 49% risk of developing breast cancer by age 70, respectively.[13] The United States Preventive Health Services Task Force (USPSTF) recommends screening women to determine if there is a high risk of a mutation of BRCA1 or BRCA2 genes. The screening should be considered for women with a positive family history and at least a 5% to 10% chance of a gene mutation. Those with positive results from the screening should receive genetic counseling. BRCA testing should not be done routinely but based on risk factors. There are a number of models available to determine risk. Each of these identifies different areas and may have variable results. The Gail Model focuses primarily on nonfamilial risk factors and the Claus Model highlights familial risk factors. The Tyrer–Cuzick Model takes into account family history, length of time for estrogen exposure, and atypical hyperplasia which addresses issues of other models. Currently, clinical trials continue using the Tyrer–Cuzick Model and takes into consideration mammography breast density to increase the prediction of those at risk for breast cancer.

Benign Breast Disorders

Mammograms are resulting in increasing numbers of breast biopsies, and clinicians should now understand the effects of benign breast disease on risk for later breast cancer. Within a decade of starting annual screening, 20% of women have had a breast biopsy.[15] Breast lesions are believed to evolve in somewhat linear fashion from usual ductal hyperplasia, or unfolded lobules, to atypical hyperplasia, to the pathologic stages of DCIS and invasive cancer. These disorders are now classified by degree of cellular proliferation on biopsy and degree of risk for breast cancer. Women with atypia are more likely to have strong family history of breast cancer (approximately 28% vs. 20%). Their risk increases when atypia is diagnosed at younger ages. Currently studies show no increased risk for women with *nonproliferative* findings and no family history of breast cancer.[16]

Risk of Breast Cancer and Histology of Benign Breast Lesions[1,17]	
• *No increased risk*, relative risk approximately 1.3	*Nonproliferative changes:* including cysts and ductal *ectasia*, mild *hyperplasia*, simple *fibroadenoma*, *mastitis*, *granuloma*, diabetic mastopathy
• *Small increased risk*, or relative risk 1.5–2.0	*Proliferative without atypia:* including usual ductal hyperplasia, complex fibroadenoma, papilloma
• *Moderate increased risk*, or relative risk >2.0 to approximately 4.2	*Proliferative with atypia:* including atypical ductal hyperplasia and atypical lobular hyperplasia

Breast Density

Mammographic breast density has been identified as "the most undervalued and underused risk factor" in studies of breast cancer.[18] It is a strong independent risk factor even after adjusting for the effects of other risk factors, and it has the important attribute of "being present in the tissue from which the cancer arises."[19] Stromal and epithelial tissues appear radiologically light and dense, reflecting higher proportions of stromal and glandular tissue and increased ductal and atypical ductal hyperplasia. A proposed mechanism is proliferation of breast epithelial cells and stromal fibrosis in response to growth factors induced by circulating sex hormones.

An analysis of studies quantifying breast density found that women with radiologic density in more than 60% to 75% of the breast are at four to six times greater risk of breast cancer than women with no breast density.[16] Breast density may account for up to 30% of the risk for breast cancer and has a strong inherited component.[18] It is not yet known if breast density is associated with the increased risk of breast cancer seen in women with elevated blood levels of estrogen, free estradiol, and testosterone, which metabolizes to estrone and estradiol.[20]

Breast density affects the sensitivity and specificity of mammograms, dropping from 88% and 96% in women with predominantly fatty breast tissue to 62% and 89% in women with breasts that are extremely dense, respectively.[16] Sensitivity and specificity appear lowest in younger women taking MRT, leading authors to recommend that mammography reports include statements about breast density that might influence decisions about use of MRT.

Recommendations for Breast Cancer Screening and Chemoprevention

Overview of Screening Recommendations

Mammography combined with the clinical breast examination (CBE) are the most common screening modalities, however recommendations from professional groups vary about how to screen, when to start screening, and screening intervals, as shown in the table below. The evidence and rationale for decisions about screening bear thoughtful review of the balance of benefits and risks. For mammography, experts commonly raise concerns about *overdiagnosis*, defined as detection of lesions on mammogram that would not otherwise be detected or pathologic during a woman's lifetime. Estimates of overdiagnosis range from 0% to 50%, although some claim that they mostly reflect variations in study follow-up time and adjustment for screening lead time and incidence trends.[21] In 2014 the Canadian National Breast Screening study reported the same 25-year cumulative mortality from breast cancer in a screening trial of almost 90,000 women ages 40 to 59 randomized to either CBE plus five annual mammography screens or CBE and no mammography, with overdiagnosis of 22%; although some have questioned the equivalence of the study and control groups.[22] Changes in the recommended guidelines underscore the need for clinicians to be well informed as they counsel individual patients, particularly as more evidence emerges to guide risk-based screening.

Mammography

Women 40 to 50 Years

Use of screening *mammography* for women in this age group has been controversial because of lower sensitivity and specificity, possibly related to breast density; increasing risk of false positives and subsequent biopsy; difficulty individualizing risks and benefits; and variation in individual values and preferences. Over the past years, there have been some differing opinions among the professional groups over the best recommendations; the American Cancer Society and the American Medical Association endorse mammography annually for women in their 40s.

The USPSTF supports individualized discussion of risks and benefits in this age group. *Shared decision making* is especially important for this group given the varying risks and benefits.[23,24]

Women 50 to 74 Years

Screening mammography reduces breast cancer mortality in women 50 to 74 years.[4] Mammography is most beneficial in this age group and detects 80% to 90% of breast cancers in asymptomatic women and has a specificity of 94% to 97%. The USPSTF recommends biennial screening mammography for women aged 50 to 74 years, believing this will reduce the exposure to routine mammograms. The American Cancer Society and American Medical Association support annual mammography. Digital mammography shows promise for even greater accuracy, especially for younger women and women with dense breasts.[25]

Women Over 75 Years

Screening should continue for women older than 74 years, taking life expectancy and health status into account. Inform women of the increased likelihood of recall for return examinations because of unclear findings and that abnormal findings may lead to biopsy.[26] The USPSTF and The American Cancer Society support individual decision making in regards to mammography, comorbidities, and life expectancy more than 5 years in length.

Clinical Breast Examination

The American Cancer Society recommends performing the *CBE* every 3 years in women 20 to 39 years, and annually after 40 years. Other professional groups find evidence of benefit insufficient to support a definitive recommendation.[4] CBE sensitivity and specificity are 54% and 94%, respectively, and depend on the technique of the examiner.[3] CBE has not been clearly shown to decrease mortality and should be performed in conjunction with mammography.

Breast Self-Examination

The American Cancer Society no longer recommends monthly BSE due to evidence that it does not reduce mortality and may lead to a higher rate of benign breast biopsies.[27] Although BSE does not improve detection of breast cancer, it does promote breast self-awareness. A nurse should instruct women interested in using BSE in proper technique and to report changes in breast appearance or texture promptly. Monthly BSE 5 to 7 days after the onset of menses can be taught to women as early as their 20s. It has been determined the technique for assessment is crucial and properly educated practitioners should be teaching patients. (See Patient Instructions for the BSE on pp. 552–553.)

Magnetic Resonance Imaging

Studies have investigated the use of screening *MRI* in women with a high risk for breast cancer of greater than 20% based on the risk assessment tools available (Gail, Claus, or Tyrer–Cuzick models), personally have a BRCA1 or BRCA2 gene mutation or a first-degree relative with a gene mutation, had chest radiation between the ages of 10 and 30 years old. In these groups, breast MRI has helped improve detection of multicentric or contralateral breast cancer prior to management decisions about breast conserving strategies or initiation of treatment regimens.[28–29] However, cost is high and specificity is 77%, resulting in more false positives, recalls, and biopsies.[4,28] Expertise in reading MRIs and MRI-guided biopsy is an important component to use of breast MRI. Currently the American Cancer Society recommends breast MRI for women at high lifetime risk, or risk of 20% or more.[4] Women at moderately increased lifetime risk, or risk of 15% to 20%, are encouraged to discuss benefits and drawbacks with their providers. Criteria for classifying risk are provided in the table. MRI should not be done in isolation but in conjunction with a mammogram. Each test may pick up cancers that the other could miss.

Criteria for Classifying Breast Cancer Risk and Referrals for Breast MRI	
High Risk, or 20–25%	**Moderate Risk, or 15–20%**
• Known BRCA1 or 2 mutation • Known first-degree relative, including father or brother, with BRCA1 or 2 mutation, but woman not tested • Lifetime risk 20–25% using assessment tools • History of chest radiation between ages 10 and 30 years • Has high-risk genetic syndrome or first-degree relative with high-risk syndrome	• History of breast cancer, ductal or lobular carcinoma in situ, atypical ductal or lobular hyperplasia • Extremely dense breasts or unevenly dense breasts on mammograms

Source: American Cancer Society. Breast Cancer Facts and Figures 2009–2010. p 16. Available at: http://www.cancer.org/acs/groups/content@nho/documents/document/ f861009final90809pdf.pdf. Accessed June 2, 2015.

Chemoprevention

The U.S. Preventive Services Task Force recommends discussion of chemoprevention with estrogen-receptor modulators in women at high risk for breast cancer and at low risk for adverse effects, but it recommends against routine use for primary prevention in women at low or average risk. The Task Force found substantial evidence that these modulators reduce the incidence of estrogen-receptor–positive breast cancer.[4,30,31] Clinicians are urged to review the literature on risks and benefits of these agents for women at high risk for developing breast cancer within 5 years. The Task Force notes that the balance of benefit and harm is more favorable for women in their 40s or 50s at increased risk and without predisposition to thromboembolic events, and for women in their 50s without a uterus. Further, key studies use the Gail model cut-off of 1.66 as high risk; however, the revised Gail model addresses prevention of invasive and noninvasive cancers, but it does not discriminate between risks of estrogen-receptor–positive versus estrogen-receptor–negative cancers.[30,32] *Prophylactic bilateral mastectomy* may also be advised in women at very high genetic risk.

Counseling Women About Breast Cancer

The Challenges of Communicating Risks and Benefits

As breast cancer screening and prevention options become more complex, nurses should consider how best to express statistics on risks and benefits in terms that patients can easily understand. Framing, or the effect of presenting the same information in terms of either increased benefit or decreased harm, is one of several ways of presenting data that can compromise informed consent. Elmore recommends, for example, that instead of reporting a Gail model risk of diagnosis of breast cancer in 5 years as 1.1%, explaining that only 11 out of 1,000 women would get such a diagnosis is easier for patients to grasp.[17] Likewise, for patients absolute risk might be preferable to relative risk. Instead of stating that 379 of 6,061 women with nonproliferative breast disease developed breast cancer, compared with an expected number of 298, giving a relative risk of 1.27, it is clearer to use absolute risk. In 100 women followed for 15 years, 6 in 100 with nonproliferative disease developed breast cancer, compared with 5 in the general population.

Websites for Breast Cancer Information

Encourage patients to pursue breast cancer–related information from recommended reputable sources to help make informed choices during shared decision making.[28]

Breast Cancer Websites

Calculation of the risk of a breast cancer diagnosis and death at the level of individual women:

http://bcra.nci.nih.gov/brc/start.htm (Gail model)

http://www.cancer.gov/types/breast/hp/breast-ovarian-genetics-pdq(Gail Model, Claus Model, and http://www.ems-trials.org/riskevaluator/Tyrer–Cuzick model that predicts the probability of carrying a *BRCA1* or *BRCA2* mutation)

National Guidelines for Breast Cancer Screening:

http://www.guidelines.gov

Randomized Clinical Trials of New Modalities in Breast Cancer Screening:

http://www.clinicaltrials.gov

Support:

http://www.cancer.org/Treatment/SupportProgramsServices/

Susan G. Komen: www.komen.org

The Mautner Project of Whitman-Walker Health: www.whitman-walker.org/mautnerproject

National LGBT Cancer Network: www.cancer-network.org

Kelly Rooney Foundation: kellyrooneyfoundation.org

TABLE
17-1

Common Breast Masses

The three most common kinds of breast masses are *fibroadenoma* (a benign tumor), *cysts,* and *breast cancer.* The clinical characteristics of these masses are listed below. However, any breast mass should be carefully evaluated and usually warrants further investigation by ultrasound, aspiration, mammography, or biopsy. The masses depicted below are large for purposes of illustration. Ideally, breast cancer should be identified early, when the mass is small. *Fibrocystic changes,* not illustrated, are also commonly palpable as nodular, rope-like densities in women ages 25–50. They may be tender or painful. They are considered benign and are not viewed as a risk factor for breast cancer.

	Fibroadenoma	Cysts	Cancer
Usual Age	15–25, usually puberty and young adulthood, but up to age 55	30–50, regress after menopause except with estrogen therapy	30–90, most common over age 50
Number	Usually single, may be multiple	Single or multiple	Usually single, although may coexist with other nodules
Shape	Round, disc-like, or lobular	Round	Irregular or stellate
Consistency	May be soft, usually firm	Soft to firm, usually elastic	Firm or hard
Delineation	Well delineated	Well delineated	Not clearly delineated from surrounding tissues
Mobility	Very mobile	Mobile	May be fixed to skin or underlying tissues
Tenderness	Usually nontender	Often tender	Usually nontender
Retraction Signs	Absent	Absent	May be present

TABLE

17-2

Visible Signs of Breast Cancer

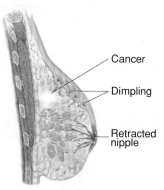

Cancer

Dimpling

Retracted nipple

Retraction Signs

As breast cancer advances, it causes fibrosis (scar tissue). Shortening of this tissue produces *dimpling, changes in contour,* and *retraction or deviation of the nipple.* Other causes of retraction include fat necrosis and mammary duct ectasia.

Nipple Retraction and Deviation

A retracted nipple is flattened or pulled inward, as illustrated here. It may also be broadened, and feels thickened. When involvement is radially asymmetric, the nipple may deviate or point in a different direction from its normal counterpart, typically toward the underlying cancer.

Skin Dimpling

Look for this sign with the patient's arm at rest, during special positioning, and on moving or compressing the breast, as illustrated here.

Abnormal Contours

Look for any variation in the normal convexity of each breast, and compare one side with the other. Special positioning may be useful. Shown here is marked flattening of the lower outer quadrant of the left breast.

Edema of the Skin

Edema of the skin is produced by lymphatic blockade. It appears as thickened skin with enlarged pores—the so-called *peau d'orange* (orange peel) *sign.* It is often seen first in the lower portion of the breast or areola.

Paget Disease of the Nipple

This uncommon form of breast cancer usually starts as a scaly, eczema-like lesion that may weep, crust, or erode. A breast mass may be present. Suspect Paget disease in any persisting dermatitis of the nipple and areola. Can present with invasive breast cancer or ductal carcinoma in situ.[3]

BIBLIOGRAPHY

CITATIONS

1. Harris J, Lipman M, Morrow M, et al. *Diseases of the Breast.* Philadelphia, PA: Wolters Kluwer Health; 2014.

2. Barton MB, Harris R, Fletcher SW. Does this patient have breast cancer? The screening clinical breast examination: should it be done? How? *JAMA.* 1999;282:1270.

3. Barton MB, Elmore JG. Pointing the way to informed medical decision making: test characteristics of clinical breast examination. *J Natl Cancer Inst.* 2009;101:1223.

4. U.S. Preventive Services Task Force. Screening for breast cancer: U.S. Preventive Services Task Force recommendation statement. *Ann Intern Med.* 2009;151:716.

5. Fenton JJ, Barton MB, Geiger AM, et al. Screening clinical breast examination: how often does it miss lethal breast cancer? *J Natl Cancer Inst Monogr.* 2005;(35):67.

6. Miller AB, Baines CJ. The role of clinical breast examination and breast self-examination. *Prev Med.* 2011;53:118.

7. Chiarelli AM, Majpruz V, Brown P, et al. The contribution of clinical breast examination to the accuracy of breast screening. *J Natl Cancer Inst.* 2009;101:1236.

8. Bryan T, Snyder E. The clinical breast exam: a skill that should not be abandoned. *J Gen Intern Med.* 2013;28:719.

9. American Cancer Society. *Breast Cancer Early Detection.* Available at: http://www.cancer.org/cancer/breastcancer/moreinformation/breastcancerearlydetection/breast-cancer-early-detection-acs-recs-bse. Accessed June 4, 2015.

10. Hoda S, Brogi E, Koerner F, et al. *Rosen's Breast Pathology.* Philadelphia, PA; Lippincott Williams & Wilkins; 2014.

11. Dickson G. Gynecomastia. *Am Fam Physician.* 2012;85:716.

12. Susan G. Komen. Breast Cancer Statistics. Available at: http://ww5.komen.org/BreastCancer/Statistics.html#st-hash.R026VqCu.dpuf. Accessed June 4, 2015.

13. American Cancer Society. Breast Cancer Facts and Figures 2009–2010. Available at: http://www.cancer.org/downloads/STT/BCFF-Final.pdf. Accessed June 4, 2015.

14. Howlader N, Noone AM, Krapcho M, et al., eds. *SEER Cancer Statistics Review, 1975–2012, National Cancer Institute.* Bethesda, MD. http://seer.cancer.gov/csr/1975_2012/, based on November 2014 SEER data submission, posted to the SEER web site, April 2015.

15. Yarbo CH, Wuicik D, Gobel BH. *Cancer Symptom Management.* Sunbury, MA: Jones & Bartlett Publishers; 2014.

16. Ripping TM, Hubbard RA, Otten JD, et al. Towards personalized screening: cumulative risk of breast cancer screening outcomes in women with and without a first degree relative with a history of breast cancer. Available at: ncbi.nlm.nih.gov/pubmed/26537645. Accessed on November 16, 2015.

17. Kiely D, Schwartz S. Assessing breast cancer risk in a primary care setting. *Nurse Pract.* 2014;39(10):49–53.

18. Vachon CM, Sellers TA, Carlson EE, et al. Strong evidence of a genetic determinant for mammographic density, a major risk factor for breast cancer. *Cancer Res.* 2007;67(17):8412–8418.

19. Kiyang LN, Labrecque M, Doualla-Bell F, et al. Family physicians' intention to support women in making informed decisions about breast cancer screening with mammography: a cross sectional survey. *BMC Res Notes.* 2015;8:663. Available at: ncbi.nlm.nih.gov/pubmed/26555569. Accessed on November 16, 2015.

20. Yager JD, Davidson NE. Estrogen carcinogenesis in breast cancer. *N Engl J Med.* 2006;354(3):270–282.

21. Loberg M, Lousdal ML, Bretthauer M, et al. Benefits and harms of mammography screening. *Breast Cancer Res.* 2015;17(1):63.

22. Miller AB, Wall C, Baines CJ, et al. Twenty five year follow-up for breast cancer incidence and mortality of the Canadian National Breast Screening Study: randomised screening trial. *BMJ.* 2014;348:366. DOI: 10.1136/bmj

23. Gutnik LA, Castro MC. Does spatial access to mammography have an effect on early stage of breast cancer diagnosis? A county level analysis for New York state. *Breast J.* Available at ncbi.nlm.nih.gov/pubmed/26549798. Accessed November 16, 2016.

24. Qaseem A, Snow V, Sherif K, et al. Screening mammography in women 40 to 49 years of age: a clinical practice guideline from the American College of Physicians. *Ann Intern Med.* 2007;146(7):511–515.

25. Chen W, Rosner B, Colditz G. Moving forward with breast cancer prevention. *Cancer.* 2007;109(12):2387–2391.

26. Pilewskie M, Hirsch A, Eaton A, et al. Breast cancer in the elderly: Is MRI helpful? *Breast J.* 2015;(6):651–657.

27. Nelson HD, Tyne K, Haik A, et al. Screening for breast cancer: an update for the U.S. Preventive Services Task Force. *Ann Intern Med.* 2009;151:727.

28. Amir E, Freedman OC, Seruga B, et al. Assessing women at high risk of breast cancer: a review of risk assessment models. *J Natl Cancer Inst.* 2010;102(10):680–691.

29. U.S. Preventive Services Task Force. *Chemoprevention of Breast Cancer: Summary of the Evidence.* Rockville, MD: Agency for Healthcare Research and Quality. Available at: www.uspreventiveservicestaskforce.org/uspstf/uspsbrpv.htm. Accessed June 8, 2015.

30. Vogel VG, Constantino JP, Wickerham DL, et al. Effects of tamoxifen vs raloxifene on the risk of developing invasive breast cancer and other disease outcomes. The NSABP study of tamoxifen and raloxifene (STAR) P-2 trial. *JAMA.* 2006;295(23):2727–2741.

31. Gail MH, Costantino JP. Validating and improving models for projecting the absolute risk of breast cancer. *J Natl Cancer Inst.* 2001;93(5):334–335.

32. Darabi H, Czene K, Zhao W, et al. Breast cancer risk prediction and individualized screening based on common genetic variation and breast density measurement. *Breast Cancer Res.* 2012;14:R25.

ADDITIONAL REFERENCES

Baglietto L, Krishnan K, Stone J, et al. Associations of mammographic dense and nondense areas and body mass index with risk of breast cancer. *Am J Epidemiol.* 2014; 179:475–483.

Béatrice SL, Scoccianti C, Loomis D, et al. Breast-cancer screening – viewpoint of the International Agency for Research working group on June 3, 2015. DOI: 10.1056/ NEJMsr1504363. Accessed June 8, 2015.

Harris JR, Morrow M, Bonadonna G. Cancer of the breast. In: DeVita VT, Lawrence TS, Rosenberg SA, eds. *DeVita, Hellman, and Rosenberg's Cancer: Principles & Practice of Oncology*. 8th ed. Philadelphia, PA: Lippincott Williams & Wilkins; 2008.

Quante AS, Whittemore AS, Shriver T, et al. Breast cancer risk assessment across the risk continuum: genetic and nongenetic risk factors contributing to differential model performance. *Breast Cancer Res.* 2012;14:R144.

White J, Kearins O, Dodwell D, et al. Male breast carcinoma: increased awareness needed. *Breast Can Res.* 2011; 12:219.

CHAPTER 18

The Musculoskeletal System

LEARNING OBJECTIVES

The student will:

1. Describe the structure and functions of the bones, muscles, and joints.
2. Identify the key landmarks of each joint.
3. Obtain an accurate history of the musculoskeletal system.
4. Appropriately prepare and position the patient for the musculoskeletal examination.
5. Identify the equipment necessary to perform a musculoskeletal examination.
6. Inspect and palpate the joints, bones, and muscles.
7. Assess the range of motion of the major joints.
8. Assess muscle strength using the muscle strength grading scale.
9. Correctly document the findings of the musculoskeletal assessment.
10. Discuss risk factors for osteoporosis.
11. Discuss risk factors for falls.
12. Discuss risk reduction and health promotion strategies to reduce musculoskeletal injuries and disease.

ASSESSING THE MUSCULOSKELETAL SYSTEM

Musculoskeletal complaints and disorders are leading causes of health care visits in clinical practice. Since the musculoskeletal system is enervated by the neurologic system, examinations of the two systems are closely aligned. Indeed, these systems may be examined at the same time. Careful questioning during the history and acute observations will help the nurse distinguish the cause of the patient's symptoms.

Because of the nature of the musculoskeletal assessment, the organization of this chapter is a different from the other body system chapters. Examination of joints requires both visualization and knowledge of surface landmarks and underlying anatomy. Therefore to help students pair their knowledge of joint structure and function with methods of examination, the anatomy and physiology and physical examination for specific joints *are combined*.

Joint Structure and Function

Begin by reviewing basic anatomic terminology.

- *Articular structures* include the joint capsule and articular cartilage, the synovium and synovial fluid, intra-articular ligaments, and juxta-articular bone.

Articular disease typically involves swelling and tenderness of the entire joint and limits both active and passive range of motion.

- *Extra-articular structures* include periarticular ligaments, tendons, bursae, muscle, fascia, bone, nerve, and overlying skin.

- *Ligaments* are rope-like bundles of collagen fibrils that connect bone to bone.

- *Tendons* are collagen fibers connecting muscle to bone.

- *Cartilage,* another form of collagen, overlies the articular surfaces of the bone ends and facilitates smooth painless movement of the joint.

- *Bursae* are pouches of synovial fluid that cushion the movement of tendons and muscles over bone or other joint structures.

Types of Joint Articulation

There are three types of joint articulation—synovial, cartilaginous, and fibrous—allowing varying degrees of joint movement.

Joints		
Type of Joint	Extent of Movement	Example
Synovial	Freely movable	Knee, shoulder
Cartilaginous	Slightly movable	Vertebral bodies of the spine
Fibrous	Immovable	Skull sutures

Synovial Joints

The bones do not touch each other, and the joint articulations are *freely movable*. The bone ends are covered by *articular cartilage* and separated by a *synovial cavity* that cushions joint movement. The *synovial membrane* lines the synovial cavity and secretes a small amount of viscous lubricating fluid—the *synovial fluid*. The membrane is attached at the margins of the articular cartilage and pouched to allow joint movement. Surrounding the synovial membrane is a fibrous *joint capsule,* which is strengthened by ligaments extending from bone to bone.

Bone
Ligament
Synovial membrane
Joint space
Joint capsule
Synovial cavity
Articular cartilage

SYNOVIAL

Cartilaginous Joints

These joints, such as those between vertebrae and the symphysis pubis, are *slightly movable*. Fibrocartilaginous discs separate the bony surfaces. At the center of each disc is the *nucleus pulposus,* fibrocartilaginous material that serves as a cushion or shock absorber between bony surfaces.

Vertebral body
Nucleus pulposus of the disc
Disc
Ligament

CARTILAGINOUS

Fibrous Joints

In these joints, such as the sutures of the skull, intervening layers of fibrous tissue or cartilage hold the bones together. The bones are almost in direct contact, which allows *no appreciable movement*.

FIBROUS

Structure of Synovial Joints

Many of the joints examined are *synovial,* or movable, *joints*. The shape of the articulating surfaces of synovial joints determines the direction and extent of joint motion.

- *Spheroidal joints* have a ball-and-socket configuration—a rounded, convex surface articulating with a cup-like cavity, allowing a wide range of rotatory movement, as in the shoulder and hip.

Synovial Joints			
Type of Joint	**Articular Shape**	**Movement**	**Example**
Spheroidal (ball and socket)	Convex surface in concave cavity	Wide-ranging flexion, extension, abduction, adduction, rotation, circumduction	Shoulder, hip
Hinge	Flat, planar	Motion in one plane; flexion, extension	Interphalangeal joints of hand and foot; elbow
Condylar	Convex or concave articulating surfaces	Movement of two articulating surfaces	Knee; temporomandibular joint

SPHEROIDAL JOINT (BALL AND SOCKET)

- *Hinge joints* are flat, planar, or slightly curved, allowing only a gliding motion in a single plane, as in flexion and extension of the digits.

- In *condylar joints,* such as the knee, the articulating surfaces are convex or concave, termed condyles. One articulating surface is convex and the matching surface is concave.

HINGE JOINT

Bursae

Easing joint action are *bursae,* disc-shaped synovial sacs that allow adjacent muscles or muscles and tendons to glide over each other during movement. They lie between the skin and the convex surface of a bone or joint (as in the prepatellar bursa of the knee, p. 616), or in areas where tendons or muscles rub against bone, ligaments, or other tendons or muscles (as in the subacromial bursa of the shoulder, p. 581).

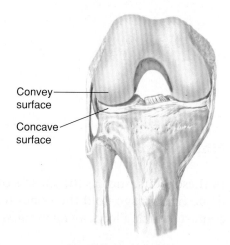

Convex surface

Concave surface

CONDYLAR JOINT

THE HEALTH HISTORY

Common or Concerning Symptoms
• Joint pain
• Joint pain associated with systemic symptoms, such as fever, chills, rash, weakness, and weight loss
• Low back pain
• Neck pain
• Bone pain
• Muscle pain or cramps
• Muscle weakness

Begin the history with a broad open-ended question:

"Do you have any pain in your joints, bones, or muscles?"

Joint pain is a leading complaint of patients seeking health care. Joint pain may also be *extra-articular*, involving bones, muscles, and tissues around the joint such as tendons, ligaments, bursae, or overlying skin.

May be due to sprains from stretching or tearing of ligaments, muscle or tendon strain, bursitis, or tendinitis

Generalized "aches and pains" are called *myalgias* if they occur in muscles, and *arthralgias* if there is pain in a joint but no evidence of arthritis.

The "OLD CART" mnemonic may be used to obtain more information.

O*nset:* When did the pain begin?
  Was the onset rapid or slow?
  Did the pain follow an injury? Describe the injury.
L*ocation:* Where is the pain located? Point to the site.
  Is the pain in one joint or multiple joints (or multiple muscles)?

Pain in one joint suggests trauma, monoarticular arthritis, possible tendinitis, or bursitis. Lateral hip pain near the greater trochanter suggests *trochanteric bursitis.*

  Does the pain migrate from joint to joint?
  Does the pain radiate (e.g., down a limb)?
D*uration:* How long have you had the pain?
  Does the pain come and go or is it constant?
  Is it worse at a particular time of day or night?

A migratory pattern of joint pain occurs in *rheumatic fever;* a progressive and symmetric joint involvement occurs in *rheumatoid arthritis*

C*haracteristic Symptoms:* Describe the pain. Is it sharp, dull, achy, or shooting? Use an appropriate pain scale to have the patient rate the pain.
A*ssociated Manifestations:* Do you have any other symptoms such as bruising, warmth, swelling, stiffness, deformity such as nodules, fever, chills, rash, muscle weakness, numbness, tingling, or burning?
  Is your motion limited?
  Does the limitation affect activities, such as walking, rising from a chair, holding objects, or other activities of daily living?
R*elieving/Exacerbating Factors:* Does anything relieve the pain or make it worse, such as a heating pad or cool compress?
T*reatment:* Have you taken any medication or tried other treatments to relieve the pain?

Extra-articular pain is seen with inflammation of bursae (*bursitis*), tendons (*tendinitis*), or tendon sheaths (*tenosynovitis*); and *sprains* from stretching or tearing of ligaments

Low Back Pain

Low back pain is the second most common reason for office visits. Using open-ended questions gives a clearer picture of the problem, especially the location of the pain.

See Table 18-1, Chapter 18, Low Back Pain, p. 636.

Low back pain has a lifetime prevalence of nearly 80% in the United States.[1]

Determine if the pain is *on the midline*, over the vertebrae, or *off the midline*.

Midline back pain, suggests a musculo-ligamentous injury, disc herniation, vertebra collapse, spinal cord metastases. *Pain off the midline*, suggests sacroiliitis, trochanteric bursitis, sciatica, or hip arthritis.

Is there radiation into the leg? If yes, is there any associated numbness or paresthesias?

Radiation of pain is seen in sciatica. Leg pain that resolves with rest and/or lumbar forward flexion suggests *spinal stenosis.*

Ask about associated bladder or bowel dysfunction?

Neck Pain

Neck pain is also common. Although usually self-limited, it is important to ask about radiation into the arm, arm or leg weakness or paresthesias, or change in bladder or bowel function. Persisting pain after blunt trauma or a motor vehicle accident warrants referral to a specialist.

See Table 18-2, Chapter 18, Pains in the Neck, p. 637.

Radicular pain (radiating along a dermatome) may be from spinal nerve compression, most commonly C7 followed by C6.

EXAMINATION OF JOINTS: ANATOMY AND PHYSIOLOGY AND PHYSICAL EXAMINATION

Important Areas of Examination for Each of the Major Joints

- Inspect joint symmetry, alignment, bony deformities

- Inspect and palpate surrounding tissues for skin changes, nodules, muscle atrophy, crepitus

- Perform range of motion maneuvers to test joint function and stability. Assess for signs of inflammation, swelling, warmth, tenderness, redness

- Assess muscle strength

During the history the patient's ability to carry out normal activities of daily living can be assessed. Keep these abilities in mind during the physical examination.

The detail needed for examination of the musculoskeletal system varies widely. This section presents examination techniques for both comprehensive and targeted assessment of joint function. Patients with extensive or severe musculoskeletal problems will require more time.

In the general survey of the patient, general appearance, body proportions, and ease of movement were assessed. The musculoskeletal examination should be systematic. It should include inspection and palpation of the bones and joints, assessment of range of motion, and muscle strength. There are two phases to *range of motion: active* (by the patient) and *passive* (by the examiner).

Equipment

- Tape measure
- Goniometer
- Skin marking pen

Tips for Successful Examination of the Musculoskeletal System

- During inspection, look for *symmetry*. Is there a symmetric change in joints on both sides of the body, one side or is the change only in one or two joints?

Acute involvement of only one joint suggests trauma, septic arthritis, gout. *Rheumatoid arthritis* typically involves several joints, symmetrically distributed.

Note any *joint deformities* or *malalignment of bones*.

Dupuytren contracture (see Table 18-6, Chapter 18, Swellings and Deformities of the Hands, p. 642), bowlegs, or knock-knees.

- Use inspection and palpation to assess the *surrounding tissues*, note skin changes, subcutaneous nodules, and muscle atrophy. Assess for *crepitus*, an audible or palpable crunching during movement of tendons or ligaments over bone.

Look for subcutaneous nodules in *rheumatoid arthritis* or *rheumatic fever;* effusions in trauma; crepitus over inflamed joints, in *osteoarthritis,* or in inflamed tendon sheaths

- Test range of motion and maneuvers (described for each joint) to demonstrate *limitations in range of motion* or joint instability from excess mobility of joint ligaments, called *ligamentous laxity*. During range of motion evaluation the angle of the joint can be measured with a *goniometer.* This is useful for documenting the degree of limitation.

Decreased range of motion in arthritis, inflammation of tissues around a joint, fibrosis in or around a joint, or bony fixation (*ankylosis*). Ligamentous laxity of the anterior cruciate ligament (ACL) in knee trauma.

- Finally, test *muscle strength*.

Muscle atrophy or weakness in *rheumatoid arthritis.*

Assess the Four Signs of Inflammation

- *Swelling*. Palpable swelling may involve (1) the synovial membrane, which can feel boggy or doughy; (2) effusion from excess synovial fluid within the joint space; or (3) soft-tissue structures such as bursae, tendons, and tendon sheaths.
- *Warmth*. Use the backs of your fingers to compare the involved joint with its unaffected contralateral joint, or with nearby tissues if both joints are involved.
- *Tenderness*. Try to identify the specific anatomic structure that is tender. Trauma may also cause tenderness.

- *Redness*. Redness of the overlying skin is the *least* common sign of inflammation near the joints.

Seen in arthritis, tendinitis, bursitis, *osteomyelitis*

Tenderness and warmth over a thickened synovium suggest arthritis or infection.

Redness over a tender joint suggests septic or gouty arthritis, or possibly *rheumatoid arthritis*.

Examination of the muscles includes muscle bulk, muscle tone and muscle strength.

Muscle Bulk

Begin the examination by inspecting the size and contours of muscles. Do the muscles look shrunken, flat or concave, suggesting atrophy? If so, is the atrophy unilateral or bilateral? Is it proximal or distal?

Muscular *atrophy* refers to a loss of muscle bulk, or wasting. It results from diseases of the peripheral nervous system such as diabetic neuropathy, as well as diseases of the muscles themselves. *Hypertrophy* is an increase in bulk with proportionate strength, whereas increased bulk with diminished strength is called *pseudohypertrophy* (seen in the *Duchenne form of muscular dystrophy*).

When looking for atrophy, pay particular attention to the hands, shoulders, and thighs. The thenar and hypothenar eminences should be full and convex, and the spaces between the metacarpals, where the dorsal interosseous muscles lie, should be full or only slightly depressed. Atrophy of hand muscles may occur with normal aging, however, as shown on the next page.

Flattening of the thenar and hypothenar eminences and furrowing between the metacarpals suggest atrophy. Localized atrophy of the thenar and hypothenar eminences occur in median and ulnar nerve damage, respectively.

Other causes of muscular atrophy include motor neuron diseases, and rheumatoid arthritis

Hand of a 44-year-old woman

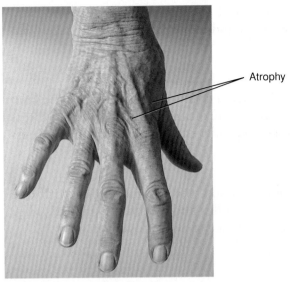

Hand of an 84-year-old woman

— Atrophy

Hand of a 44-year-old woman

Hand of an 84-year-old woman

— Hypothenar eminence

— Flattening of the thenar eminence due to mild atrophy

Look for fasciculations (fine tremors of the muscles), in atrophic muscles.

Muscle Tone

When a normal muscle with an intact nerve supply is relaxed voluntarily, it maintains a slight residual tension known as muscle tone. This can be assessed best by feeling the muscle's resistance to passive stretch. Persuade the patient to relax. Take one hand with yours and, while supporting the elbow, flex and extend the patient's fingers, wrist, and elbow, and put the shoulder through a moderate range of motion. With practice, these actions can be combined into a single smooth movement. On each side, note muscle tone—the resistance offered to your movements. Tense patients may show increased resistance. The feel of normal resistance is learned with repeated practice.

Fasciculations with atrophy and muscle weakness suggest disease of the peripheral motor unit.

Decreased resistance occurs with diseases of the peripheral nervous system, cerebellar disease, or the acute stages of spinal cord injury. See Table 20-12, Chapter 20, Disorders of Muscle Tone, p. 742.

If you suspect decreased resistance, hold the forearm and shake the hand loosely back and forth. Normally the hand moves back and forth freely but is not completely floppy.

Marked floppiness indicates muscle *hypotonia* or *flaccidity,* usually from a disorder of the peripheral motor system.

If resistance is increased, determine whether it varies as you move the limb or whether it persists throughout the range of movement and in both directions, for example, during both flexion and extension. Feel for any jerkiness in the resistance.

Spasticity is the increased resistance that worsens at the extremes of range. *Rigidity* is the increased resistance throughout the range of movement and in both directions.

To assess muscle tone in the legs, support the patient's thigh with one hand, grasp the foot with the other, and flex and extend the patient's knee and ankle on each side. Note the resistance to your movements.

Muscle Strength

People vary widely in their strength, and the assessment should allow for such variables as age, sex, and muscular training. A person's dominant side is usually slightly stronger than the other side. Keep this difference in mind when comparing sides.

Impaired strength is called weakness, or *paresis.* Absence of strength is called paralysis, or plegia. *Hemiparesis* refers to weakness of one half of the body; *hemiplegia is* paralysis of one half of the body. *Paraplegia* means paralysis of the legs; *quadriplegia* is paralysis of all four limbs.

Test muscle strength by asking the patient to flex and extend actively against your resistance or to resist your movement. A muscle is strongest when shortest, and weakest when longest.

See Table 20-1, Chapter 20, Disorders of the Central and Peripheral Nervous Systems, pp. 726–728.

If the muscles are too weak to overcome resistance, test them against gravity alone or with gravity eliminated. When the forearm rests in a pronated position, for example, dorsiflexion at the wrist can be tested against gravity alone. When the forearm is midway between pronation and supination, extension at the wrist can be tested with gravity eliminated. Finally, if the patient fails to move the body part, watch or feel for weak muscular contraction.

Scale for Grading Muscle Strength

Muscle strength is graded on a 0 to 5 scale:
0—No muscular contraction detected
1—A barely detectable flicker or trace of contraction
2—Active movement of the body part with gravity eliminated
3—Active movement against gravity
4—Active movement against gravity and some resistance
5—Active movement against full resistance without evident fatigue. This is normal muscle strength.

When documenting muscle strength, indicate the scale used (e.g., muscle strength 3 out of 5 or 3/5).

Methods for testing the major muscle groups are described in the next sections. The spinal root innervations and the muscles affected are shown in parentheses.

If the person has painful joints, move the person gently. Patients may move more comfortably by themselves. Let them show you how they manage. If joint trauma is present, ask the nurse practitioner or physician about an x-ray before attempting movement.

TEMPOROMANDIBULAR JOINT

Overview, Bony Structures, and Joints

The temporomandibular joint (TMJ) is the most active joint in the body, opening and closing up to 2,000 times a day. It is formed by the fossa and articular tubercle of the temporal bone and the condyle of the mandible. It lies midway between the external acoustic meatus and the zygomatic arch.

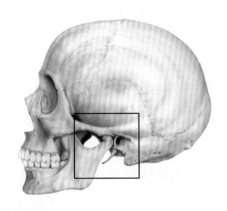

A fibrocartilaginous disc cushions the action of the condyle of the mandible against the synovial membrane and capsule of the articulating surfaces of the temporal bone. Hence, it is a condylar synovial joint.

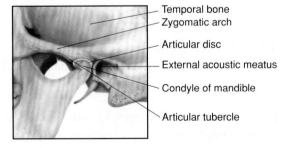

Temporal bone
Zygomatic arch
Articular disc
External acoustic meatus
Condyle of mandible
Articular tubercle

Muscle Groups and Additional Structures

The principal muscles opening the mouth are the *external pterygoids*. Closing the mouth are the muscles innervated by cranial nerve V, the trigeminal nerve (see Chapter 20, p. 671)—the *masseter*, the *temporalis*, and the *internal pterygoids*.

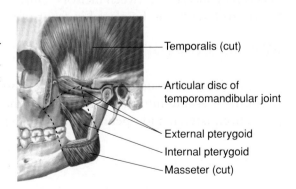

Temporalis (cut)
Articular disc of temporomandibular joint
External pterygoid
Internal pterygoid
Masseter (cut)

Physical Examination

Inspection and Palpation

Inspect the face for symmetry. Inspect the TMJ for swelling or redness. Swelling may appear as a rounded bulge approximately 0.5 cm anterior to the external auditory meatus.

Facial asymmetry associated with *TMJ syndrome.* Typical features are unilateral chronic pain with chewing, jaw clenching, or teeth grinding, often associated with stress (may also present as headache).

To locate and palpate the joint, place the tips of your index fingers just in front of the tragus of each ear and ask the patient to open his or her mouth. The fingertips should drop into the joint spaces as the mouth opens. Check for smooth range of motion; note any swelling or tenderness. Snapping or clicking may be felt or heard in normal people.

Dislocation of the TMJ may be seen in trauma.

Palpable crepitus or clicking occurs with poor occlusion, meniscus injury, or synovial swelling from trauma.

Palpate the muscles of mastication for tenderness:

- The *masseters,* externally at the angle of the mandible

Pain and tenderness on palpation in *TMJ syndrome*

- The *temporal muscles,* externally during clenching and relaxation of the jaw

Range of Motion and Maneuvers

The TMJ has glide and hinge motions in its upper and lower portions, respectively. Chewing consists primarily of gliding movements in the upper compartments.

Range of motion is threefold: ask the patient to demonstrate opening and closing, protrusion and retraction (by jutting the jaw forward), and lateral, or side-to-side, motion. Normally as the mouth is opened wide, three fingers can be inserted between incisors. During normal protrusion of the jaw, the bottom teeth can be placed in front of the upper teeth.

Muscle Strength

If the patient complains of difficulty chewing or jaw weakness, test muscle strength by asking him or her to perform the range-of-motion maneuvers, projection, lateral, and opening of mouth, against your resistance.

THE SHOULDER

Overview

The glenohumeral joint of the shoulder is distinguished by wide ranging movement in all directions. This joint is largely uninhibited by bony structure. The shoulder derives its mobility from a complex interconnected structure of four joints, three large bones, and three principal muscle groups, often referred to as the *shoulder girdle*.

Bony Structures

The bony structures of the shoulder include the humerus, the clavicle, and the scapula.

IMPORTANT BONES OF THE SHOULDER

Identify in the diagram the *manubrium*, the *sternoclavicular joint*, and the *clavicle*. Then identify the *tip of the acromion*, the *greater tubercle of the humerus*, and the *coracoid process*, which are important landmarks for shoulder anatomy.

Joints

Three joints articulate at the shoulder:

• The *glenohumeral joint*. In this joint, the head of the humerus articulates with the shallow glenoid fossa of the scapula. This joint is deeply situated and not normally palpable. It is a ball-and-socket joint, allowing the arm its wide arc of movement—flexion, extension, abduction (movement away from the trunk), adduction (movement toward the trunk), rotation, and circumduction.

- The *sternoclavicular joint.* The convex medial end of the clavicle articulates with the concave hollow in the upper sternum.

- The *acromioclavicular joint.* The lateral end of the clavicle articulates with the acromion process of the scapula.

Muscle Groups

Three groups of muscles attach at the shoulder:

The Scapulohumeral Group

This group extends from the scapula to the humerus and includes the muscles inserting directly on the humerus, known as *"SITS muscles"* of the *rotator cuff:*

- *Supraspinatus, Infraspinatus and Teres minor*

- *Subscapularis (not illustrated)*

Axioscapular group

Scapulohumeral group

Levator scapulae

Rhomboids

Trapezius

Supraspinatus

Infraspinatus

Deltoid

Teres minor

Latissimus dorsi

Posterior view

Axioscapular group (pulls shoulder backward)

Scapulohumeral group (rotates shoulder laterally; includes rotator cuff)

The Axioscapular Group

This group attaches the trunk to the scapula and includes the trapezius, rhomboids, serratus anterior, and levator scapulae. These muscles rotate the scapula and pull the shoulder posteriorly.

The Axiohumeral Group

This group attaches the trunk to the humerus and includes the pectoralis major and minor and the latissimus dorsi. These muscles produce internal rotation of the shoulder.

The biceps and triceps, which connect the scapula to the bones of the forearm, are also involved in shoulder movement, especially forward flexion (biceps) and extension (triceps).

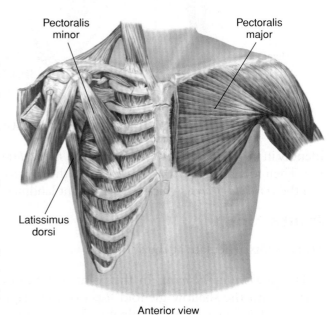

Pectoralis minor

Pectoralis major

Latissimus dorsi

Anterior view

Axiohumeral group (rotates shoulder internally)

Additional Structures

Surrounding the glenohumeral joint is a fibrous *articular capsule* formed by the tendon insertions of the rotator cuff and other capsular muscles.

The long head of the biceps tendon runs in the bicipital groove of the humerus between the greater and lesser tubercles. To locate this tendon, rotate your arm externally and find the tendinous cord that runs just medial to the greater tubercle. The tendon will roll under your fingers.

The principal bursa of the shoulder is the *subacromial bursa,* positioned between the acromion and the head of the humerus and overlying the supraspinatus tendon. Normally, the supraspinatus tendon and the subacromial bursa are not palpable.

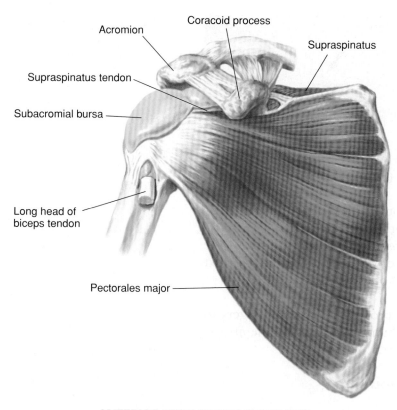

ANTERIOR VIEW OF THE SHOULDER

Physical Examination

Inspection

Observe the shoulder and shoulder girdle anteriorly, and inspect the scapulae and related muscles posteriorly.

Scoliosis may cause elevation of one shoulder. With *anterior dislocation of the shoulder,* the rounded lateral aspect of the shoulder appears flattened.[2]

Note any swelling, deformity, muscle atrophy or fasciculations or abnormal positioning.

Atrophy of supraspinatus and infraspinatus over posterior scapula with increased prominence of scapular spine indicate a *rotator cuff tear.*

Inspect the entire upper extremity for color change, skin alteration, or unusual bony contours.

Palpation

Begin by palpating the bony landmarks of the shoulder; then palpate any area of pain.

See Table 18-4, Chapter 18, Painful Shoulders, p. 640.

- Beginning medially, at the *sternoclavicular joint,* trace the clavicle laterally with your fingers.

- Now, from behind, follow the bony spine of the scapula laterally and upward until it becomes the acromion (**A**), the summit of the shoulder. Its upper surface is rough and slightly convex. Identify the anterior tip of the acromion.

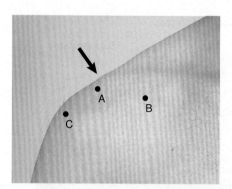

- With your index finger on top of the acromion, just behind its tip, press medially with your thumb to find the slightly elevated ridge that marks the distal end of the clavicle at the *acromioclavicular joint* (shown by the arrow). Move your thumb medially and down a short step to the next bony prominence, the *coracoid process* (**B**) of the scapula.

- Now, with your thumb on the coracoid process, allow your fingers to fall on and grasp the lateral aspect of the humerus to palpate the *greater tubercle* (**C**), where the SITS muscles insert.

Range of Motion and Special Maneuvers

Range of Motion

The six motions of the shoulder girdle are flexion, extension, abduction, adduction, and internal and external rotation.

Range of motion is restricted in *bursitis, capsulitis, rotator cuff tears* or *sprains,* or *tendinitis.*

Standing in front of the patient, watch for smooth fluid movement as the patient performs the range of motions listed in the table on pp. 583–584. Refer to the table for clear, simple instructions that prompt the patient and the muscles responsible for each movement.

Shoulder Movement	Patient Instructions	Principal Muscles Affecting Movement
Flexion	*"Raise your arms in front of you and overhead."*	Anterior deltoid, pectoralis major (clavicular head), coracobrachialis, biceps brachii (short head)
Hyperextension	*"Raise your arms behind you."*	Latissimus dorsi, teres major, posterior deltoid, triceps brachii (long head)
Abduction	*"Raise your arms out to the side and overhead."* Note that to test *pure glenohumeral motion,* the patient should raise the arms to shoulder level at 90 degrees, with palms facing down. To test *scapulothoracic motion,* the patient should turn the palms up and raise the arms an additional 60 degrees. The final 30 degrees tests combined glenohumeral and scapulothoracic motion.	Supraspinatus, middle deltoid, serratus anterior (via upward rotation of the scapula)

(continued)

Adduction	"Lower your arms to your sides, then bring them across your body."	Pectoralis major, coraco-brachialis, latissimus dorsi, teres major, subscapularis
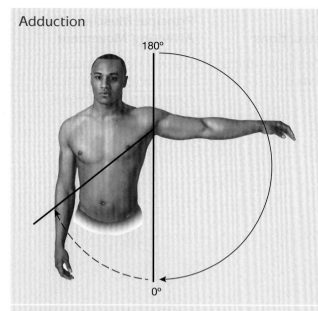		
Internal Rotation	"Place one hand behind your back and touch your shoulder blade." Identify the highest midline spinous process the patient is able to reach.	Subscapularis, anterior deltoid, pectoralis major, teres major, latissimus dorsi
External Rotation	"Raise your arm to shoulder level; bend your elbow and rotate your forearm toward the ceiling." or "Place one hand behind your neck or head as if you are brushing your hair."	Infraspinatus, teres minor, posterior deltoid

Maneuvers to Assess Shoulder Function

When the patient complains of shoulder pain or weakness, carry out the special maneuvers described below. If any of these common maneuvers are positive, the patient should be referred to a specialist for further testing and diagnosis.

The most common cause of shoulder pain involves the rotator cuff, usually the supraspinatus tendon.

Age 60 years or older and a positive dropped-arm test are the individual findings most likely to identify a rotator cuff tear.

Special Maneuvers for Examining the Shoulder

Structure	Technique	
Acromioclavicular Joint	Palpate and compare both joints for swelling or tenderness. Adduct the patient's arm across the chest, sometimes called the "crossover test."	See Table 18-4, Chapter 18, Painful Shoulders, p. 640. Pain with adduction is positive for a rotator cuff tear.
Overall Shoulder Rotation	Ask the patient to touch the opposite scapula using the two motions shown below (the Apley scratch test). Tests abduction and external rotation Tests adduction and internal rotation	Pain during these motions suggests rotator cuff disorder or adhesive capsulitis.

(continued)

Rotator Cuff	Test the *"drop-arm" sign*. Ask the patient to fully abduct the arm to shoulder level (or up to 90 degrees) and lower it slowly. (Note that abduction above shoulder level, from 90 degrees to 120 degrees, reflects action of the deltoid muscle.)		If the patient cannot hold the arm fully abducted at shoulder level, the test is *positive,* indicating a *rotator cuff tear*[3] or bicipital tendenitis.
Muscle Strength Tests	Test *supraspinatus strength* (sometimes called the "empty can test"). Elevate the arms to 90 degrees and internally rotate the arms with the thumbs pointing down, as if emptying a can. Ask the patient to resist as you place downward pressure on the arms.		Weakness during this maneuver is a *positive test* for a superspinatus *rotator cuff tear.*
	External rotation resistance test. Ask the patient to place arms at the side and flex the elbows to 90 degrees with the thumbs turned up. Provide resistance as the patient presses the forearms outward.		Pain or weakness during this maneuver is a positive test for an infraspinatus disorder. Limited external rotation points to glenohumeral disease or adhesive capsulitis.
Pain Provocation Test	Painful arc test. Fully adduct the patient's arm from 0 degree to 180 degrees.		Shoulder pain from 60 degrees to 120 degrees is a positive test for a subacromial impingement/rotator cuff tendinitis disorder.

THE ELBOW

Overview, Bony Structures, and Joints

The elbow helps position the hand in space and stabilizes the lever action of the forearm. The elbow joint is formed by the humerus and the two bones of the forearm, the radius, and the ulna. Identify the medial and lateral epicondyles of the humerus and the olecranon process of the ulna.

These bones have three articulations: the *humeroulnar joint*, the *radiohumeral joint*, and the *radioulnar joint*. All three share a large common articular cavity and an extensive synovial lining.

Muscle Groups and Additional Structures

Muscles traversing the elbow include the *biceps* and *brachioradialis* (flexion), the *triceps* (extension), the *pronator teres* (pronation), and the *supinator* (supination).

LEFT ANTERIOR ELBOW

Note the location of the *olecranon bursa* between the olecranon process and the skin. The bursa is not normally palpable but swells and becomes tender when inflamed. The *ulnar nerve* runs posteriorly in the ulnar groove between the medial epicondyle and the olecranon process. On the ventral forearm, the *median nerve* is just medial to the brachial artery.

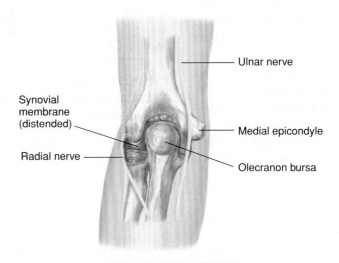

LEFT POSTERIOR ELBOW

Physical Examination

Inspection

Support the patient's forearm with your opposite hand so the elbow is flexed to about 70 degrees. Identify the medial and lateral epicondyles and the olecranon process of the ulna. Inspect the contours of the elbow, including the extensor surface of the ulna and the olecranon process. Note any nodules or swelling.

Swelling over the olecranon process occurs in olecranon bursitis; inflammation or synovial fluid in arthritis

Palpation

Palpate the olecranon process and press over the epicondyles for tenderness. Note any displacement of the olecranon.

Tenderness distal to the epicondyle occurs in *lateral epicondylitis* (tennis elbow) and less commonly in *medial epicondylitis* (pitcher's or golfer's elbow)

Palpate the grooves between the epicondyles and the olecranon, noting any tenderness, swelling, or thickening. The synovium is most accessible to examination between the olecranon and the epicondyles. (Normally neither synovium nor

POSTERIOR DISLOCATION OF THE ELBOW

SUPRACONDYLAR FRACTURE OF THE ELBOW

The olecranon is displaced posteriorly in *posterior dislocation of the elbow* and *supracondylar fracture.*

bursa is palpable.) The sensitive ulnar nerve can be felt posteriorly between the olecranon process and the medial epicondyle.

Range of Motion

Range of motion includes flexion and extension at the elbow and pronation and supination of the forearm. Refer to the table on the next page for clear, simple instructions that prompt the patient and the muscles responsible for each movement.

After injury, preservation of active range of motion and full elbow extension makes fracture unlikely.

Elbow Movement	Patient Instructions	Primary Muscles Affecting Movement
Flexion	*"Bend your elbow."*	Biceps brachii, brachialis, brachioradialis
Extension	*"Straighten your elbow."*	Triceps brachii, anconeus
Supination	*"Turn your palms up, as if carrying a bowl of soup."*	Biceps brachii, supinator
Pronation	*"Turn your palms down."*	Pronator teres, pronator quadratus

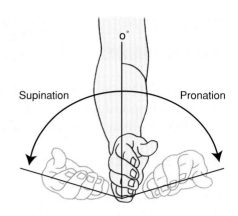

Muscle Strength Tests

Test flexion (C5, C6—biceps) *and extension* (C6, C7, C8—triceps) *at the elbow* by having the patient pull and push against your hand.

FLEXION AT ELBOW

EXTENSION AT ELBOW

THE WRIST AND HANDS

The wrist and hands form a complex unit of small, highly active joints used almost continuously during waking hours. There is little protection from overlying soft tissue, increasing vulnerability to trauma and disability.

Bony Structures

The wrist includes the distal radius and ulna and eight small carpal bones. At the wrist, identify the bony tips of the radius and the ulna.

The carpal bones lie distal to the wrist joint within each hand. Identify the carpal bones, each of the five metacarpals, and the proximal, middle, and distal phalanges. Note that the thumb lacks a middle phalanx.

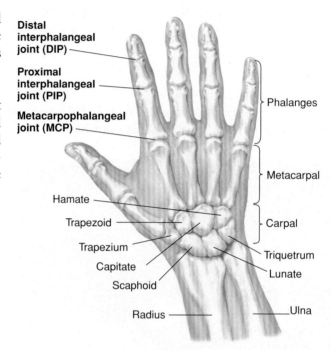

Joints

The numerous joints of the wrist and hand lend unusual dexterity to the hands.

- *Wrist joints.* The wrist joints include the *radiocarpal* or *wrist joint*, the *distal radioulnar joint*, and the *intercarpal joints*. The joint capsule, articular disc, and synovial membrane of the wrist join the radius to the ulna and to the proximal carpal bones. On the dorsum of the wrist, locate the groove of the *radiocarpal joint*, which provides most of the flexion and extension at the wrist because the ulna does not articulate directly with the carpal bones.

Metacarpo-
phalangeal
joint

- *Hand joints.* The joints of the hand include the *metacarpophalangeal (MCP) joints,* the *proximal interphalangeal (PIP) joints,* and the *distal interphalangeal (DIP) joints.* Flex the hand and find the groove marking the MCP joint of each finger. It is distal to the knuckle and is best felt on either side of the extensor tendon.

Muscle Groups

Wrist flexion arises from the two carpal muscles, located on the radial and ulnar surfaces. Two radial and one ulnar muscle provide wrist extension. Supination and pronation result from muscle contraction in the forearm.

The thumb is powered by three muscles that form the thenar eminence and provide flexion, abduction, and opposition. The muscles of extension are at the base of the thumb along the radial margin. Movement in the digits depends on action of the flexor and extensor tendons of muscles in the forearm and wrist.

The intrinsic muscles of the hand attaching to the metacarpal bones are involved in flexion (*lumbricals*), abduction (*dorsal interossei*), and adduction (*palmar interossei*) of the fingers.

Additional Structures

Soft-tissue structures, especially tendons and tendon sheaths, are especially important to movement of the wrist and hand. Six extensor tendons and two flexor tendons pass across the wrist and hand to insert on the fingers. Through much of their course these tendons travel in tunnel-like sheaths, generally palpable only when swollen or inflamed.

Understanding the structures in the *carpal tunnel* is important. It is a channel beneath the palmar surface of the wrist and proximal hand. The channel contains the sheath and flexor tendons of the forearm muscles and the *median nerve.*

Holding the tendons and tendon sheath in place is a transverse ligament, the *flexor retinaculum.* The median nerve lies between the flexor retinaculum and the tendon sheath. It provides sensation to the palm and the palmar surface of most of the thumb, the second and third digits, and half of the fourth digit. It also innervates the thumb muscles of flexion, abduction, and opposition.

Flexor retinaculum

Carpel tunnel

Median nerve

Physical Examination

Inspection

Observe the position of the hands in motion to see if movements are smooth and natural. At rest, the fingers should be slightly flexed and aligned almost in parallel.

Guarded movement suggests injury. Poor finger alignment is seen in flexor tendon damage.

Inspect the palmar and dorsal surfaces of the wrist and hand carefully for swelling over the joints.

Diffuse swelling is seen in arthritis or infection; local swelling from cystic ganglion. See Table 18-5, Chapter 18, Arthritis in the Hands, p. 641 and Table 18-6, Chapter 18, Swellings and Deformities of the Hands, p. 642.

Note any deformities of the wrist, hand, or finger bones, as well as any angulation from radial or ulnar deviation.

In *osteoarthritis,* Heberden nodes are seen at the DIP joints, and Bouchard nodes at the PIP joints. In *rheumatoid arthritis,* symmetric deformity in the PIP, MCP, and wrist joints, with ulnar deviation

Observe the contours of the palm, namely, the thenar and hypothenar eminences.

Thenar atrophy may be due to median nerve compression from *carpal tunnel syndrome;* hypothenar atrophy is seen in *ulnar nerve compression.*

Note any thickening of the flexor tendons or flexion contractures in the fingers.

Flexion contractures in the ring, 5th, and 3rd fingers, or *Dupuytren contractures,* arise from thickening of the palmar fascia (see p. 642).

Palpation

At the wrist, palpate the distal radius and ulna on the lateral and medial surfaces. Palpate the groove of each wrist joint with your thumbs on the dorsum of the wrist, your fingers beneath it. Note any swelling, bogginess, or tenderness.

Any tenderness or bony step-offs are suspicious for fracture.

Swelling and/or tenderness suggest *rheumatoid arthritis* if bilateral and of several weeks' duration.

Palpate the radial styloid bone and the *anatomic snuffbox,* a hollowed depression just distal to the radial styloid process formed by the abductor and extensor muscles of the thumb. The "snuffbox" becomes more visible with lateral extension of the thumb away from the hand.

Tenderness over the "snuffbox" occurs in *scaphoid fracture,* the most common injury of the carpal bones.

Palpate the eight carpal bones lying distal to the wrist joint, and then each of the five metacarpals and the proximal, middle, and distal phalanges.

Synovitis in the MCP joints is painful with this pressure—a point to remember when shaking hands.

Palpate any other area where you suspect an abnormality.

The MCP joints are often boggy or tender in *rheumatoid arthritis* (but rarely involved in osteoarthritis).

Compress the MCP joints by squeezing the hand from each side between the thumb and fingers. Alternatively, use your thumb to palpate each MCP joint just distal to and on each side of the knuckle as your index finger feels the head of the metacarpal in the palm. Note any swelling, bogginess, or tenderness.

Now examine the fingers and thumb. Palpate the medial and lateral aspects of each PIP joint between your thumb and index finger, again checking for swelling, bogginess, bony enlargement, or tenderness.

Bouchard nodes (bony enlargements) are seen in *osteoarthritis* at the PIP joints.

Using the same techniques, examine the DIP joints.

Hard dorsolateral nodules on the DIP joints, or *Heberden nodes,* common in osteoarthritis

HEBERDEN NODES AND BOUCHARD NODES IN THE SAME HANDS

In any area of swelling or inflammation, palpate along the tendons inserting on the thumb and fingers.

Wrists: Range of Motion and Maneuvers

Range of Motion

Refer to the table below for clear, simple instructions that prompt the patient and the muscles responsible for each movement.

Conditions that impair range of motion include *arthritis, tenosynovitis, Dupuytren contracture.* See Table 18-6, Chapter 18, Swellings and Deformities of the Hands, p. 642.

Wrist Movement	Patient Instructions	Primary Muscles Affecting Movement
Flexion	*"With palms down, point your fingers toward the floor."*	Flexor carpi radialis, flexor carpi ulnaris
Extension	*"With palms down, point your fingers toward the ceiling."*	Extensor carpi ulnaris, extensor carpi radialis longus, extensor carpiradialis brevis
Adduction (radial deviation)	*"With palms down, bring your fingers toward the midline."*	Flexor carpi ulnaris
Abduction (ulnar deviation)	*"With palms down, bring your fingers away from the midline."*	Flexor carpi radialis

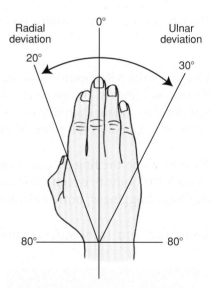

Muscle Strength Tests

Test extension at the wrist (C6, C7, C8, radial nerve—extensor carpi radialis longus and brevis). Ask the patient to make a fist; place your hand on top of the patient's fist; ask the patient to resist your effort to push down his fist. See photo at the top of the next page.

Weakness of extension is seen in peripheral nerve disease such as radial nerve damage and in central nervous system disease producing hemiplegia, as in *stroke* or *multiple sclerosis.*

EXTENSION AT WRIST

Test the grip (C7, C8, T1). Ask the patient to squeeze two of your fingers as hard as possible and not let them go. (To avoid getting hurt by hard squeezes, place your own middle finger on top of your index finger.) You should normally have difficulty removing your fingers from the patient's grip. Testing both grips simultaneously with arms extended or in the lap facilitates comparison.

A weak grip in cervical radiculopathy, *carpal tunnel syndrome,* arthritis, epicondylitis

TEST OF GRIP

(AP) Maneuvers to Test for Carpal Tunnel Syndrome

Several maneuvers useful for assessing common office complaints relating to the wrist are listed below. For complaints of dropping objects, inability to twist lids off jars, aching at the wrist or even the forearm, and numbness of the first three digits, use the tests for assessing *carpal tunnel syndrome*. Note the distribution of the median, radial, and ulnar nerve innervations of the wrist and hand below.

Onset of *carpal tunnel syndrome* is often related to repetitive motion with wrists flexed (as in keyboard use, mail sorting), pregnancy, rheumatoid arthritis, diabetes, hypothyroidism.

Thenar atrophy may also be present.

Decreased sensation in the median nerve distribution in *carpal tunnel syndrome*

DORSAL SURFACE

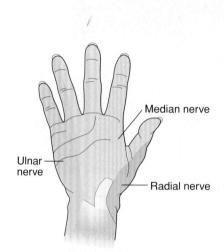

VOLAR SURFACE

Test sensation of:

* The index finger pad—median nerve

* The fifth finger pad—ulnar nerve

* Dorsal web space of the thumb and index finger—radial nerve

Test *thumb abduction* by asking the patient to raise the thumb straight up as you apply downward resistance.[4-6]

Weak thumb abduction and decreased sensation indicate carpal tunnel disease.

Test *Tinel sign* for median nerve compression by tapping lightly over the course of the median nerve in the carpal tunnel as shown.[4-6]

Aching and numbness in the median nerve distribution is a *positive test*.

Test *Phalen sign* for median nerve compression by asking the patient to hold the wrists in flexion for 60 seconds. Alternatively, ask the patient to press the backs of both hands together to form right angles. These maneuvers compress the median nerve.[4–6]

Numbness and tingling in the median nerve distribution within 60 seconds is a *positive test result.*

Fingers and Thumbs: Range of Motion

Range of Motion

Assess *flexion, extension, abduction,* and *adduction* of the fingers.

- *Flexion and extension.* For *flexion,* to test the finger flexor muscles, ask the patient to "*Make a tight fist with each hand, thumb across the knuckles.*" For *extension,* to test the finger extensor muscles, ask the patient to "*Extend and spread the fingers.*"

  The fingers should open and close easily.

FLEXION

Impaired hand movement in arthritis, trigger finger, Dupuytren contracture

- *Abduction and adduction.* Ask the patient to spread the fingers apart (abduction from dorsal interossei) and back together (adduction from palmar interossei). Check for smooth, coordinated movement.

ABDUCTION

Thumbs

At the *thumb,* assess *flexion, extension, abduction, adduction,* and *opposition.* Each of these movements is powered by a related muscle of the thumb. Ask the patient to move the thumb across the palm and touch the base of the fifth finger to test *flexion,* and then to move the thumb back across the palm and away from the fingers to test *extension.*

FLEXION   **EXTENSION**

Next, ask the patient to place the fingers and thumb in the neutral position with the palm up; then have the patient move the thumb anteriorly away from the palm to assess abduction and back down for adduction. To test opposition or movements of the thumb across the palm, ask the patient to touch the thumb to the base of the small finger.

ABDUCTION AND ADDUCTION   **OPPOSITION**

Finger Muscle Strength Tests

Test finger abduction (C8, T1, ulnar nerve). Position the patient's hand with palm down and fingers spread. Instructing the patient not to let you move the fingers, try to force them together.

Weak finger abduction in ulnar nerve disorders

FINGER ABDUCTION

Test opposition of the thumb (C8, T1, median nerve). The patient should try to touch the tip of the little finger with the thumb, against your resistance.

Weak opposition of the thumb in median nerve disorders such as *carpal tunnel syndrome*

OPPOSITION OF THE THUMB

THE SPINE

The vertebral column, or spine, is the central supporting structure of the trunk and back. Note the *concave curves* of the cervical and lumbar spine and the *convex curves* of the thoracic and sacrococcygeal spine. These curves help distribute upper body weight to the pelvis and lower extremities and cushion the concussive impact of walking or running.

The complex mechanics of the back reflect the coordinated action of:

- The vertebrae and intervertebral discs

- An interconnecting system of ligaments between anterior vertebrae and posterior vertebrae, ligaments between the spinous processes, and ligaments between the lamina of two adjacent vertebrae

- Large superficial muscles, deeper intrinsic muscles, and muscles of the abdominal wall

Bony Structures

The vertebral column contains 24 vertebrae stacked on the sacrum and coccyx. A typical vertebra contains sites for joint articulations, weight bearing, and muscle attachments, as well as foramina for the spinal nerve roots and peripheral nerves. Anteriorly, the *vertebral body* supports weight bearing. The posterior *vertebral arch* encloses the spinal cord. Review the location of the vertebral processes and foramina: Note:

- The *spinous process* projecting posteriorly in the midline and the two transverse processes. Muscles attach at these processes.

Representative Cervical and Lumbar Vertebrae

C4–C5 Coronal and Lateral Views

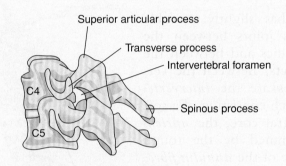

T12–L1 Coronal and Lateral Views

- The *articular processes*—two on each side of the vertebra, one facing up and one facing down, allow the vertebrae to articulate with each other, therefore often called *articular facets*.

- The *vertebral foramen*, which encloses the spinal cord, the *intervertebral foramen*, formed by the inferior and superior articulating process of adjacent vertebrae, creating a channel for the spinal nerve roots; and in the cervical vertebrae, the *transverse foramen* for the vertebral artery.

The proximity of the spinal cord and spinal nerve roots to their bony vertebral casing and the intervertebral discs makes them especially vulnerable to disc herniation, impingement from degenerative changes in the vertebrae, and trauma.

Joints

The spine has slightly movable cartilaginous joints between the vertebral bodies and between the articular facets. Between the vertebral bodies are the *intervertebral discs*, each consisting of a soft mucoid central core, the *nucleus pulposus*, rimmed by the tough fibrous tissue of the *annulus fibrosis*. The intervertebral discs cushion movement between vertebrae and allow the vertebral column to curve, flex, and bend.

Note that the vertebral column angles sharply posterior at the *lumbosacral junction* and becomes immovable. The mechanical stress at this angulation contributes to the risk for disc herniation and subluxation, or slippage, of L5 on S1.

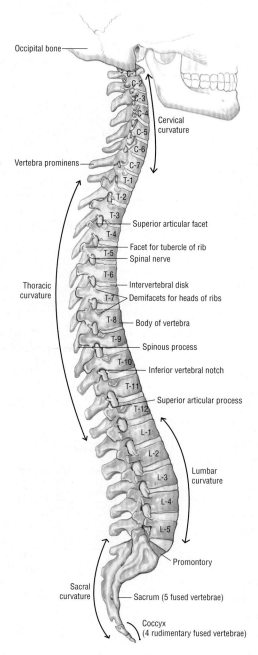

Occipital bone
C-1
C-2
C-3
C-4
Cervical curvature
C-5
C-6
Vertebra prominens
C-7
T-1
T-2
T-3
Superior articular facet
T-4
Facet for tubercle of rib
T-5
Spinal nerve
T-6
Intervertebral disk
Thoracic curvature
T-7
Demifacets for heads of ribs
T-8
Body of vertebra
T-9
Spinous process
T-10
Inferior vertebral notch
T-11
Superior articular process
T-12
L-1
L-2
L-3
Lumbar curvature
L-4
L-5
Promontory
Sacral curvature
Sacrum (5 fused vertebrae)
Coccyx (4 rudimentary fused vertebrae)

Muscle Groups

The *trapezius* and *latissimus dorsi* form the large outer layer of muscles attaching to each side of the spine. They overlie two deeper muscle layers—a layer attaching to the head, neck, and spinous processes (*splenius capitis, splenius cervicis,* and *sacrospinalis*) and a layer of smaller intrinsic muscles between vertebrae. Muscles attaching to the anterior surface of the vertebrae, including the *psoas* muscle and muscles of the abdominal wall, assist with flexion.

Muscles moving the neck and lower vertebral column are summarized in the table at the top of pp. 605–606.

Trapezius (neck extension; overlies small intrinsic neck muscles of neck extension and rotation)

Sternocleidomastoid (neck flexion, rotation)

Splenius capitis (neck extension)

Deltoid

Teres minor

Teres major

Spinous process T12

External abdominal oblique

Iliac crest

Gluteus maximus

Latissimus dorsi

Physical Examination

Inspection

Begin by observing the patient's posture, including the position of both the neck and trunk, when entering the room.

Assess the patient for erect position of the head; smooth, coordinated neck movement; and ease of gait.

Neck stiffness may signal arthritis, muscle strain, or other underlying pathology.

Drape or gown the patient to expose the entire back for complete inspection. If possible, the patient should be upright in the natural standing position—with feet together and arms hanging at the sides. The head should be midline in the same plane as the sacrum, and the shoulders and pelvis should be level.

Lateral deviation and rotation of the head suggest *torticollis*, from contraction of the sternocleidomastoid muscle.

Viewing the patient from behind, identify the following landmarks:

- Spinous processes of C7 and T1 are usually more prominent with forward neck flexion

- Paravertebral muscles on either side of the midline

- Iliac crests

- Posterior superior iliac spines, usually marked by skin dimples

Paravertebral muscles

Spinous process of L4

Iliac crest

Posterior superior iliac spine

Sciatic nerve

Sacroiliac joint

Ischial tuberosity and site of ischial bursa

A line drawn above the posterior iliac crests crosses the spinous process of L4.

Inspect the patient from the side and from behind. Evaluate the spinal curvatures and the features described in the table below.

Palpation

From a sitting or standing position, palpate the spinous processes of each vertebra with your thumb. Note any tenderness and/or whether any spinous process appears more forward or recessed from its neighbor.

Palpate over the *sacroiliac joint,* often identified by the dimple overlying the posterior superior iliac spine.

Tenderness suggests fracture or dislocation if preceded by trauma; if no trauma, suspect infection or arthritis.

Forward slippage of one of the lumbar vertebra may compress the spinal cord.

Tenderness over the sacroiliac joint in sacroiliitis[7]

Inspection of the Spine		
View of Patient	**Focus of Inspection**	
From the Side	Cervical, thoracic, and lumbar curves Kyphosis—increased thoracic curvature Lordosis—increased lumbar curvature	Cervical concavity Thoracic convexity Lumbar concavity

Increased *thoracic kyphosis* often occurs with aging. In children, a correctable structural deformity should be referred to an advanced practitioner.

From Behind

Upright spinal column (an imaginary line should fall straight from C7 through the gluteal cleft)

Alignment of the shoulders, the iliac crests, and the skin creases below the buttocks (gluteal folds)

Scoliosis—lateral curvature of the spine

If scoliosis is suspected, perform the Adam bend test and use a scoliometer to test for the degree of scoliosis. See further discussion in Chapter 23, Assessing Children: Infancy through Adolescence.

Note any skin markings, tags, or masses

In *scoliosis,* there is lateral and compensatory curvature of the spine to bring the head back to midline. Scoliosis often becomes evident during adolescence.

Unequal shoulder heights are seen in scoliosis.

Unequal heights of the iliac crests, or *pelvic tilt,* suggest scoliosis. Unequal leg lengths also cause pelvic tilt. The tilt will disappear when a block is placed under the short leg and foot.

Birthmarks, port-wine stains, hairy patches, and lipomas often overlie bony defects such as *spina bifida.*

Café-au-lait spots (discolored patches of skin), skin tags, and fibrous tumors are seen in *neurofibromatosis.*

Inspect and palpate the *paravertebral muscles* for tenderness and spasm. Muscles in spasm feel firm and knotted and may be visible.

With the hip flexed and the patient lying on the opposite side, palpate the *sciatic nerve,* the largest nerve in the body, consisting of nerve roots from L4, L5, S1, S2, and S3. The nerve lies midway between the greater

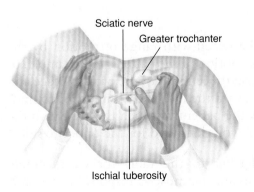

Sciatic nerve

Greater trochanter

Ischial tuberosity

Spasm occurs in degenerative and inflammatory processes of muscles, prolonged contraction from abnormal posture, or anxiety.

Sciatic nerve tenderness suggests a herniated disc or mass lesion impinging on the contributing nerve roots.

trochanter and the ischial tuberosity as it leaves the pelvis through the sciatic notch.

Herniated intervertebral discs, most common at L5–S1 or L4–L5, may produce tenderness of the spinous processes, the intervertebral joints, the paravertebral muscles, the sacrosciatic notch, and the sciatic nerve.

Palpate for tenderness in any other areas that are suggested by the patient's symptoms.

Rheumatoid arthritis may also cause tenderness of the intervertebral joints.

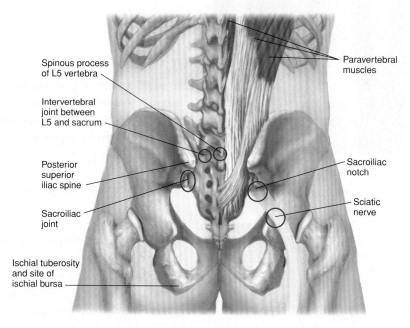

Spinous process of L5 vertebra

Intervertebral joint between L5 and sacrum

Posterior superior iliac spine

Sacroiliac joint

Ischial tuberosity and site of ischial bursa

Paravertebral muscles

Sacroiliac notch

Sciatic nerve

Remember that tenderness in the costovertebral angles may signify kidney infection rather than a musculoskeletal problem.

See Table 18-1, Chapter 18, Low Back Pain, p. 636.

Range of Motion and Maneuvers

Range of Motion: Neck

The neck is the most mobile portion of the spine, remarkable for its seven fragile vertebrae supporting the 10- to 15-lb head. *Flexion* and *extension* occur primarily between the skull and C1, the atlas; *rotation* at C1–C2; the axis, and *lateral bending* at C2–C7.

Limitations in range of motion can arise from stiffness from arthritis, pain from trauma, or muscle spasm such as *torticollis*.

Muscle Strength Test: Neck

Muscle strength of the neck may be tested with range of motion by the examiner placing a hand to resist the motion of the patient. For example, to test rotation, place your right hand on the left side of the patient's face and ask the patient to rotate the head toward the left, and then return to midline; then, to test lateral flexion, ask the patient to touch the left ear to the shoulder against your resistance. Use your left hand for the opposite side.

Assess neck range of motion referring to the table for clear, simple instructions that prompt the patient and the muscles responsible for each movement.

Neck, shoulder, or arm pain or numbness may indicate cervical cord or nerve root compression. See Table 18-2, Chapter 18, Pains in the Neck, p. 637.

Neck Movement	Patient Instructions	Primary Muscles Affecting Movement
Flexion	*"Bring your chin to your chest."*	Sternocleidomastoid, scalene, prevertebral muscles
Extension	*"Look up at the ceiling."*	Splenius capitis and cervicis, small intrinsic neck muscles
Rotation	*"Look over one shoulder, and then the other."*	Sternocleidomastoid, small intrinsic neck muscles
Lateral Flexion	*"Bring your ear to your shoulder."*	Scalenes and small intrinsic neck muscles

If the patient has tenderness, loss of sensation, muscle weakness or impaired movement, perform neurologic testing of the neck and upper extremities.

Range of Motion: Spinal Column

Next assess range of motion in the spinal column. Refer to the table for clear, simple instructions that prompt the patient and the muscles responsible for each movement, note the specific muscles responsible for each motion and clear, simple instructions that prompt the requested patient response.

Back Movement	Patient Instructions	Primary Muscles Affecting Movement
Flexion	*"Bend forward and try to touch your toes."* Note the smoothness and symmetry of movement, the range of motion, and the curve in the lumbar area. As flexion proceeds, the lumbar concavity should flatten out.	Psoas major, psoas minor, quadratus lumborum; abdominal muscles attaching to the anterior vertebrae, such as the internal and external obliques and rectus abdominis

10+ cm

5 cm

Normally increased by up to 4 cm

Deformity of the thorax on forward bending is seen in *scoliosis*.

Provide support to patient if unsteady while bending backward.

To measure flexion of the spine, mark the spine at the lumbosacral junction, then 10 cm above and 5 cm below the first mark. A 4-cm increase between the two upper marks is normal; the distance between the lower two marks should be unchanged.

Persistence of lumbar lordosis suggests muscle spasm or *ankylosing spondylitis*.

(continued)

Extension	"Bend back as far as possible."	Deep intrinsic muscles of the back, such as the erector spinae and transversospinalis groups	Decreased *spinal mobility* is seen in *osteoarthritis* and *ankylosing spondylitis*.
	Support the patient by placing your hand on the posterior superior iliac spine, with your fingers pointing toward the midline.		
Rotation	"Rotate from side to side."	Abdominal muscles, intrinsic muscles of the back	
	Stabilize the patient's pelvis by placing one hand on the patient's hip and the other on the opposite shoulder. Then rotate the trunk by pulling the shoulder and then the hip posteriorly. Repeat these maneuvers for the opposite side.		
Lateral Flexion	"Bend to the side from the waist."	Abdominal muscles, intrinsic muscles of the back	
	Stabilize the patient's pelvis by placing your hand on the patient's hip. Repeat for the opposite side.		

Muscle Strength Test: Spinal Column

Assessment of **muscle strength** of the spinal column may also be performed during the range-of-motion assessment by having the patient flex, extend, and flex laterally against resistance.

Pain or tenderness with these maneuvers, particularly with radiation into the leg, warrants neurologic testing of the lower extremities and referral to an advanced practitioner or physician.

See Chapter 20, The Nervous System.

May indicate cord or nerve root compression. Arthritis or infection in the hip, rectum, or pelvis may cause symptoms in the lumbar spine. See Table 18-1, Chapter 18, Low Back Pain, p. 636.

THE HIP

The hip joint is deeply embedded in the pelvis and is notable for its strength, stability, and wide range of motion. The stability of the hip joint, so essential for weight bearing, arises from the deep fit of the head of the femur into the *acetabulum*, its strong fibrous articular capsule, and the powerful muscles crossing the joint and inserting below the femoral head, providing leverage for movement of the femur.

Bony Structures and Joints

The hip joint lies below the middle third of the inguinal ligament but in a deeper plane. It is a ball-and-socket joint—note how the rounded head of the femur articulates with the cup-like cavity of the acetabulum. Because of its overlying muscles and depth, it is not readily palpable. Review the bones of the pelvis—the *acetabulum*, the *ilium*, and the *ischium*—and the connection inferiorly at the *symphysis pubis* and posteriorly with the sacroiliac bone.

On the *anterior surface of the hip,* locate the following bony landmarks:

- The iliac crest at the level of L4

- The iliac tubercle

- The anterior superior iliac spine

- The greater trochanter

- The pubic symphysis

Wing of ilium
Iliac tubercle
Greater trochanter (femur)
Iliac crest
Anterior superior iliac spine
Acetabulum
Psoas bursa
Trochanteric bursa
Ischial bursa
Ischium
Pubic symphysis

ANTERIOR VIEW

On the *posterior surface of the hip*, locate the following:

- The posterior superior iliac spine

- The greater trochanter

- The ischial tuberosity

- The sacroiliac joint

Note that an imaginary line between the posterior superior iliac spines crosses the joint at S2.

POSTERIOR VIEW

Muscle Groups

Four powerful muscle groups move the hip.

The *flexor group* lies anteriorly and flexes the thigh. The primary hip flexor is the *iliopsoas*, extending from above the iliac crest to the lesser trochanter. The *extensor group* lies posteriorly and extends the thigh. The *gluteus maximus* is the primary extensor of the hip. It forms a band crossing from its origin along the medial pelvis to its insertion below the trochanter.

Flexor Group

Extensor Group

The *adductor group* is medial and swings the thigh toward the body. The muscles in this group arise from the rami of the pubis and ischium and insert on the posteromedial aspect of the femur. The *abductor group* is lateral, extending from the iliac crest to the head of the femur, and moves the thigh away from the body. This group includes the *gluteus medius* and *minimus*. These muscles help stabilize the pelvis during the stance phase of gait.

Adductor Group

Abductor Group

Additional Structures

A strong, dense articular capsule, extending from the acetabulum to the femoral neck, encases and strengthens the hip joint, reinforced by three overlying ligaments and lined with synovial membrane. There are three principal bursae at the hip. Anterior to the joint is the *psoas* (also termed *iliopectineal* or *iliopsoas*) *bursa*, overlying the articular capsule and the psoas muscle. Find the bony prominence lateral to the hip joint—the *greater trochanter* of the femur. The large multilocular *trochanteric bursa* lies on its posterior surface. The *ischial* (or *ischiogluteal*) *bursa*—not always present—lies under the *ischial tuberosity*, on which a person sits. Note its proximity to the sciatic nerve, as shown on p. 604.

Physical Examination

Inspection

Inspection of the hip begins with careful observation of the patient's gait on entering the room. Observe the two phases of gait:

- *Stance*—when the foot is on the ground and bears weight (60% of the walking cycle)

Most problems appear during the weight-bearing stance phase.

| Heelstrike | Foot flat | Midstance | Push-off |

THE STANCE PHASE OF GAIT

- *Swing*—when the foot moves forward and does not bear weight (40% of the cycle)

Observe the gait for the width of the base (*distance between the feet*), the shift of the pelvis, and flexion of the knee. The width of the base should be 2 to 4 in from heel to heel. Normal gait has a smooth, continuous rhythm, The knee should be flexed throughout the stance phase, except when the heel strikes the ground to counteract motion at the ankle. The ankle should dorsiflex so the foot does not drag the ground during the swing phase.

2"–4"

A wide base suggests cerebellar disease or foot problems. Pain during weight bearing or examiner strike on the heel occurs in *femoral neck stress fractures*.[8,9]

Hip dislocation, arthritis, or abductor weakness can cause the pelvis to drop on the opposite side, producing a waddling gait.

Lack of knee flexion interrupts the smooth pattern of gait. The leg swings out to the side, as the patient walks (*circumduction*).

Inspect the lumbar portion of the spine for slight lordosis and, with the patient supine, assess the length of the legs for symmetry. (To measure leg length, see Special Techniques, p. 626.)

Lack of dorsiflexion may be due to footdrop. The patient will compensate by lifting the knee higher when walking.

Inspect the anterior and posterior surfaces of the hip for any areas of muscle atrophy or bruising.

Changes in leg length are seen in scoliosis. Leg shortening and external rotation suggest *hip fracture.*

Palpation

Bony Landmarks

Palpate the surface landmarks of the hip, identified on pp. 607–608. On the *anterior aspect* of the hips, palpate the key structures listed below.

- Identify the *iliac crest* at the upper margin of the pelvis at the level of L4.

- Follow the downward anterior curve and locate the *iliac tubercle,* marking the widest point of the crest, and continue tracking downward to the *anterior superior iliac spine.*

- Place your thumbs on the anterior superior spines and move your fingers downward from the iliac tubercles to the *greater trochanter* of the femur.

- Then move your thumbs medially and obliquely to the *pubic symphysis,* which lies at the same level as the greater trochanter.

On the *posterior aspect* of the hips, palpate the bony landmarks below.

- Palpate the *posterior superior iliac spine* directly underneath the visible dimples just above the buttocks.

Placing your left thumb and index finger over the posterior superior iliac spine, next locate the *greater trochanter* laterally with your fingers at the level of the gluteal fold, and place your thumb medially on the *ischial tuberosity.* The *sacroiliac joint* is not always palpable. Note that an imaginary line along the posterior superior iliac spines crosses the joint at S2.

Note any tenderness or deformity during palpation.

(AP) Inguinal Structures

With the patient supine, ask the patient to place the heel of the leg being examined on the opposite knee. Then palpate along the *inguinal ligament,* which extends from the anterior superior iliac spine to the pubic tubercle. The femoral nerve, artery, and vein bisect the overlying inguinal ligament; lymph nodes lie medially. The mnemonic **NAVEL** may help you remember the lateral-to-medial sequence of **N**erve—**A**rtery—**V**ein—**E**mpty space—**L**ymph node.

Inguinal ligament

Femoral **n**erve
Femoral **a**rtery
Femoral **v**ein

Bulges along the ligament may suggest an *inguinal hernia* or, on occasion, an *aneurysm.*

Enlarged lymph nodes suggest infection in the lower extremity or pelvis.

Tenderness in the groin area may be from *synovitis* of the hip joint, *bursitis.*

Range of Motion and Muscle Strength Testing

Active Range of Motion

Now assess hip range of motion, referring to the table below for clear, simple instructions that prompt the patient and the muscles responsible for each movement.

Hip Movement	Patient Instructions	Primary Muscles Affecting Movement
Flexion	*"Bend your knee to your chest and pull it against your abdomen."*	Iliopsoas
Hyperextension	*"Lie face down, and then bend your knee and lift it up."* Or *"Lying flat, move your lower leg away from the midline and down over the side of the table."*	Gluteus maximus
Abduction	*"Lying flat, move your lower leg away from the midline."*	Gluteus medius and minimus
Adduction	*"Lying flat, bend your knee and move your lower leg toward the midline."*	Adductor brevis, adductor longus, adductor magnus, pectineus, gracilis
External Rotation	*"Lying flat on your back, bend your knee and hip 90 degrees and turn your ankle and foot across your opposite leg."*	Internal and external obturators, quadratus femoris, superior and inferior gemelli
Internal Rotation	*"Lying flat on your back, bend your knee and hip 90 degrees and turn your lower ankle and foot away from your body."*	Gluteus medius and minimus

Active range of motion (AROM) is the amount of motion at a given joint when the patient moves the part voluntarily without assistance from another body part, person or device.

Passive range of motion (PROM) is the amount of motion at a given joint when the joint is moved by an external force or person.

Before performing range of motion on patients who have had hip replacement surgery, ascertain whether they have hip motion limitations. To prevent hip dislocation, patients may have limited range of motion, which is different for an anterior versus a posterior surgical approach.

Passive Range of Motion

If it is necessary to assist the patient with hip range of motion, follow the instructions on the next page for knee flexion, abduction, adduction, and external and internal rotation.

FLEXION. With the patient supine, place your hand under the patient's lumbar spine. Ask the patient to bend each knee one at a time up to the chest and pull it firmly against the abdomen. Note that the hip can flex further when the knee is flexed. When the back touches your hand, indicating normal flattening of the lumbar lordosis, further flexion arises from the hip joint itself.

If the patient is unable to keep the opposite leg extended, when one leg is flexed, it suggests a *flexion deformity of the opposite leg's hip,* as seen in the photo.

HIP FLEXION AND FLATTENING OF LUMBAR LORDOSIS

As the thigh is held against the abdomen, observe the degree of flexion at the hip and knee. Normally the anterior portion of the thigh can almost touch the chest wall. Note whether the opposite thigh remains fully extended, resting on the table.

Flexion deformity may be masked by an increase, rather than flattening, in lumbar lordosis and an anterior pelvic tilt.

EXTENSION. With the patient lying face down, extend the thigh toward you in a posterior direction. Alternatively, carefully position the supine patient near the edge of the table and extend the leg posteriorly.

ABDUCTION. Stabilize the pelvis by pressing down on the opposite anterior superior iliac spine with one hand. With the other hand, grasp the ankle and abduct the extended leg until you feel the iliac spine move. This movement marks the limit of hip abduction.

Restricted abduction is common in hip *osteoarthritis.*

Alternatively, stand at the foot of the table, grasp both ankles, and spread them maximally, abducting both extended legs at the hips. This method provides easy comparison of two sides when movements are restricted, but it is impractical when range of motion is full.

ADDUCTION. With the patient supine, stabilize the pelvis, hold one ankle, and move the leg medially across the body and over the opposite extremity.

EXTERNAL AND INTERNAL ROTATION. Flex the leg to 90 degrees at hip and knee, stabilize the thigh with one hand, grasp the ankle with the other, and swing the lower leg—medially for external rotation at the hip and laterally for internal rotation. Although confusing at first, it is the motion of the head of the femur in the acetabulum that identifies these movements.

Restrictions of internal and external rotation are indicators of hip disease such as arthritis.

Muscle Strength Tests

Flexion

Test muscle strength during flexion at the hip (L2, L3, L4—iliopsoas) by placing your hand on the patient's thigh and asking the patient to raise the leg against your hand.

FLEXION OF THE HIP

Extension

Test muscle strength during extension at the hips (S1—gluteus maximus) by having the supine patient push the posterior thigh down against your hand.

Abduction

Test muscle strength during abduction at the hips (L4, L5, S1—gluteus medius and minimus) by placing your hands firmly on the bed outside the patient's knees. Ask the patient to spread both legs against your hands.

Adduction

Test muscle strength during adduction at the hips (L2, L3, L4—adductors) by placing your hands firmly on the bed between the patient's knees. Ask the patient to bring both legs together.

Symmetric weakness of the proximal muscles suggests a *myopathy* or muscle disorder; symmetric weakness of distal muscles suggests a *polyneuropathy*, or disorder of peripheral nerves.

THE KNEE

The knee joint is the largest joint in the body. It is a hinge joint involving three bones: the femur, the tibia, and the patella (or knee cap), with three articular surfaces, two between the femur and the tibia and one between the femur and the patella. Note how the two rounded condyles of the femur rest on the relatively flat tibial plateau. There is no inherent stability in the knee joint itself, making it dependent on ligaments to hold its articulating bones in place. This feature, in addition to the lever action of the femur on the tibia and lack of padding from fat or muscle, makes the knee highly vulnerable to injury.

Femur

Adductor tubercle

Lateral epicondyle

Medial epicondyle

Lateral collateral ligament

Posterior cruciate ligament

Anterior cruciate ligament

Medial meniscus

Medial condyle of tibia

Lateral meniscus

Medial collateral ligament

Lateral condyle of tibia

Tibia

Head of fibula

Tibial tuberosity

Fibula

ANTERIOR ASPECT OF THE KNEE

Bony Structures

Review the bony landmarks in and around the knee before you examine the knee. On the *medial surface,* identify the *medial epicondyle* of the femur and the *medial condyle* of the tibia.

- On the *anterior surface,* identify the patella, which rests on the anterior articulating surface of the femur midway between the epicondyles, embedded in the tendon of the quadriceps muscle. This tendon continues below the knee joint as the *patellar tendon,* which inserts distally on the *tibial tuberosity.*

- On the *lateral surface,* find the *lateral epicondyle* of the femur and the *lateral condyle* of the tibia.

Joints

Two condylar *tibiofemoral joints* are formed by the convex curves of the medial and lateral condyles of the femur as they articulate with the concave condyles of the tibia. The third articular surface is the *patellofemoral joint.*

The patella slides on the groove of the anterior aspect of the distal femur, called the *trochlear groove,* during flexion and extension of the knee.

Muscle Groups

Powerful muscles move and support the knee. The *quadriceps femoris* extends the leg, covering the anterior, medial, and lateral aspects of the thigh. The *hamstring muscles* lie on the posterior aspect of the thigh and flex the knee.

Quadriceps femoris

Rectus femoris

Vastus lateralis

Vastus medialis

Hamstring muscles

Semimembranosus

Gracilis

Sartorius

Semitendinosus

ANTERIOR VIEW   **MEDIAL VIEW**

Additional Structures

The menisci and two important pairs of ligaments, the collaterals and the cruciates, are crucial to stability of the knee. Identify these structures on the illustrations on the right and on pp. 616, 618.

- The *medial and lateral menisci* cushion the action of the femur on the tibia. These crescent-shaped fibrocartilaginous discs add a cup-like surface to the otherwise flat tibial plateau.

- The *medial collateral ligament (MCL),* not easily palpable, is a broad, flat ligament connecting the medial femoral epicondyle to the medial condyle of the tibia. The medial portion of the MCL also attaches to the medial meniscus.

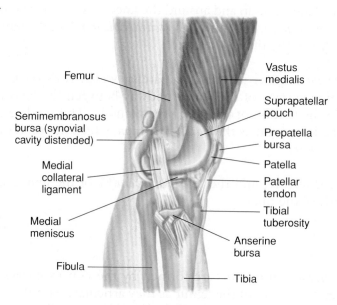

Femur

Semimembranosus bursa (synovial cavity distended)

Medial collateral ligament

Medial meniscus

Fibula

Vastus medialis

Suprapatellar pouch

Prepatella bursa

Patella

Patellar tendon

Tibial tuberosity

Anserine bursa

Tibia

LEFT KNEE—MEDIAL VIEW

- The *lateral collateral ligament (LCL)* connects the lateral femoral epicondyle and the head of the fibula. The MCL and LCL provide medial and lateral stability to the knee joint.

- The *anterior cruciate ligament (ACL)* crosses obliquely from the *anterior* medial tibia to the lateral femoral condyle, preventing the tibia from sliding forward on the femur.

- The *posterior cruciate ligament (PCL)* crosses from the *posterior* tibia and lateral meniscus to the medial femoral condyle, preventing the tibia from slipping backward on the femur. Because these ligaments lie within the knee joint, they are not palpable. They are nonetheless crucial to the anteroposterior stability of the knee.

Physical Examination

Inspection

Observe the gait for a smooth, rhythmic flow as the patient enters the room. The knee should be extended at heel strike and flexed at all other phases of swing and stance.

Check the alignment and contours of the knees. Observe any atrophy of the quadriceps muscles.

Look for loss of the normal hollows around the patella, a sign of swelling in the knee joint and suprapatellar pouch; note any other swelling in or around the knee.

Stumbling or pushing the knee into extension with the hand during heel strike suggests *quadriceps weakness*.

Bowlegs (*genu varum*) and knock-knees (*genu valgum*) can be observed; flexion contracture (inability to extend fully) occurs with limb paralysis.

Swelling over the patella suggests *prepatellar bursitis*. Swelling over the tibial tubercle suggests *infrapatellar* or, if more medial, *anserine bursitis*.

Palpation

Ask the patient to sit on the edge of the examining table with the knees in flexion. In this position, bony landmarks are more visible, and the muscles, tendons, and ligaments are more relaxed, making them easier to palpate.

Pay special attention to any areas of tenderness. Pain is a common complaint in knee problems, and localizing the structure causing pain is important for accurate evaluation.

Tibiofemoral Joint

Palpate the *tibiofemoral joint*. Facing the knee, place your thumbs in the soft-tissue depressions on either side of the *patellar tendon*. Identify the groove of the tibiofemoral joint. Note that the patella lies just above this joint line. As you press your thumbs downward, feel the edge of the tibial plateau. Follow it medially, then laterally, until you are stopped by the converging femur and tibia. By moving your thumbs upward toward the midline to the top of the patella, you can follow the articulating surface of the femur and identify the margins of the joint.

Note any irregular bony ridges along the joint margins.

Osteoarthritis is likely, when there are tender bony ridges along the joint margins, genu varum deformity, and stiffness lasting 30 minutes or less.[10,11] Crepitus may also be present.

Medial femoral condyle

Adductor tubercle

Medial femoral epicondyle

Medial collateral ligament

Anserine bursa

Patellar tendon

Medial tibial plateau

Tibial tuberosity

(AP) Now locate the *patella* and trace the *patellar tendon* distally until you palpate the *tibial tuberosity*. Ask the patient to extend the leg to make sure the patellar tendon is intact.

Tenderness over the tendon or inability to extend the leg suggests a partial or complete tear of the patellar tendon.

(AP) With the patient supine and the knee extended, compress the patella against the underlying femur. Ask the patient to tighten the quadriceps as the patella moves distally in the trochlear groove. Check for a smooth sliding motion (the *patellofemoral grinding test*).

Pain and crepitus suggest roughening of the patellar undersurface that articulates with the femur. Similar pain may occur with climbing stairs or getting up from a chair.

Pain with compression and with patellar movement during quadriceps contraction suggests *chondromalacia*, or degenerative patella (the *patellofemoral syndrome*).

ⓐ Suprapatellar Pouch, Prepatellar Bursa, and Anserine Bursa

Palpate for thickening or swelling in the *suprapatellar pouch* and along the margins of the patella. Start 10 cm above the superior border of the patella, well above the pouch, and feel the soft tissues between your thumb and fingers. Move your hand distally in progressive steps, trying to identify the pouch. Continue your palpation along the sides of the patella. Note any tenderness or warmth greater than in the surrounding tissues.

Swelling above and adjacent to the patella suggests synovial thickening or effusion in the knee joint.

Thickening, bogginess, or warmth in these areas indicates synovitis or nontender effusions from osteoarthritis.

Gastrocnemius and Soleus Muscles, Achilles Tendon

Palpate the *gastrocnemius* and *soleus muscles* on the posterior surface of the lower leg. Their common tendon, the Achilles, is palpable from about the lower third of the calf to its insertion on the calcaneus.

A defect in the muscles with tenderness and swelling occur in a *ruptured Achilles tendon;* tenderness and thickening of the tendon above the calcaneus, sometimes with a protuberant posterolateral bony process of the calcaneus in *Achilles tendinitis.*

ⓐ To test the integrity of the *Achilles tendon,* place the patient prone with the knee and ankle flexed at 90 degrees, or, alternatively, ask the patient to kneel on a chair. Squeeze the calf and watch for plantar flexion at the ankle.

Absence of plantar flexion is a positive test indicating rupture of the Achilles tendon.

Range of Motion

Now assess knee range of motion. Refer to the table on the next page for clear, simple instructions that prompt the patient through the motion and the specific muscles responsible for each movement. Be sure to examine both knees and compare findings.

Knee Movement	Patient Instructions	Primary Muscles Affecting Movement
Flexion	"Bend or flex your knee." Or "Squat down to the floor."	Hamstring group: biceps femoris, semitendinosus, and semimembranosus
Extension	"Straighten your leg." Or "After you squat down to the floor, stand up."	Quadriceps: rectus femoris, vastus medialis, lateralis, and intermedius
Internal Rotation	"While sitting, swing your lower leg toward the midline."	Sartorius, gracilis, semitendinosus, semimembranosus
External Rotation	"While sitting, swing your lower leg away the midline."	Biceps femoris

Crepitus with flexion and extension in osteoarthritis[10]

Muscle Strength Test

Test muscle strength during extension at the knee (L2, L3, L4—quadriceps). Support the knee in flexion and ask the patient to straighten the leg against your hand. The quadriceps is the strongest muscle in the body, so expect a forceful response.

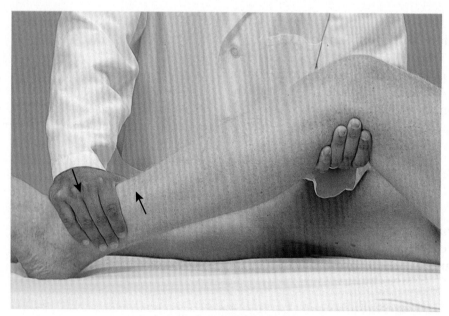

EXTENSION AT THE KNEE

Test flexion at the knee (L4, L5, S1, S2—hamstrings) as shown on the next page. Place the patient's leg so that the knee is flexed with the foot resting on the bed. Tell the patient to keep the foot down as you try to straighten the leg.

FLEXION AT THE KNEE

THE ANKLE AND FOOT

The total weight of the body is transmitted through the ankle to the foot. The ankle and foot must balance the body and absorb the impact of the heel strike and gait. Despite thick padding along the toes, sole, and heel and stabilizing ligaments at the ankles, the ankle and foot are frequent sites of sprain and bony injury.

Bony Structures and Joints

The ankle is a hinge joint formed by the *tibia*, the *fibula*, and the *talus*. The tibia and fibula act as a mortise, stabilizing the joint while bracing the talus like an inverted cup.

The principal joints of the ankle are the *tibiotalar joint*, between the tibia and the talus, and the *subtalar (talocalcaneal) joint*.

Note the principal landmarks of the ankle: the *medial malleolus*, the bony prominence at the distal end of the tibia, and the *lateral malleolus*, at the distal end of the fibula. Lodged under the talus and jutting posteriorly is the *calcaneus*, or heel.

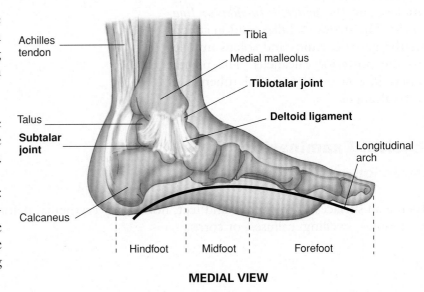

MEDIAL VIEW

An imaginary line, the *longitudinal arch*, spans the foot, extending from the calcaneus of the hind foot along the tarsal bones of the mid-foot (see cuneiforms, navicular, and cuboid bones below) to the fore-foot metatarsals and toes. The *heads of the metatarsals* are palpable in the ball of the foot. In the forefoot, identify the *metatarsophalangeal joints*, proximal to the webs of the toes, and the *PIP and DIP joints* of the toes.

Muscle Groups and Additional Structures

Movement at the tibiotalar ankle joint is limited to dorsiflexion and plantar flexion. *Plantar flexion* (*pointing the toe*) is powered by the gastrocnemius, the posterior tibial muscle, and the toe flexors. Their tendons run behind the malleoli. The *dorsiflexors* include the anterior tibial muscle and the toe extensors. They lie prominently on the anterior surface, or dorsum, of the ankle, anterior to the malleoli.

Ligaments extend from each malleolus onto the foot.

- Medially, the triangle-shaped *deltoid ligament* fans out from the inferior surface of the medial malleolus to the talus and proximal tarsal bones, protecting against stress from eversion (ankle bowing inward).

- Laterally, the three ligaments are less substantial, with higher risk for injury: the *anterior talofibular ligament*—most at risk in injury from inversion (ankle bows outward) injuries; the *calcaneofibular ligament*; and the *posterior talofibular ligament*. The strong Achilles tendon attaches the gastrocnemius and soleus muscles to the posterior calcaneus. The plantar fascia inserts on the medial tubercle of the calcaneus.

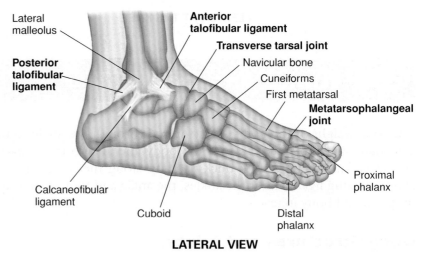

LATERAL VIEW

Physical Examination

Inspection

Observe all surfaces of the ankles and feet, noting any erythema, deformities, nodules, swelling, calluses, or corns.

See Tables 18-7, Chapter 18, Abnormalities of the Feet, p. 643 and Table 18-8, Chapter 18, Abnormalities of the Toes and Soles, p. 644.

Palpation

With your thumbs, palpate the anterior aspect of each *ankle joint,* noting any bogginess, swelling, or tenderness.

Feel along the *Achilles tendon* for nodules and tenderness.

Palpate the heel, especially the posterior and inferior calcaneus, and the plantar fascia for tenderness.

Localized tenderness is found in arthritis, ligamentous injury, or infection of the ankle.

Rheumatoid nodules; tenderness in Achilles is seen in tendinitis, bursitis, or partial tear from trauma.

Bone spurs may be present on the calcaneus. Focal heel pain on palpation of the plantar fascia suggests *plantar fasciitis;*[12] seen in prolonged standing or heel-strike exercise, also in *rheumatoid arthritis, gout.*

Palpate for tenderness over the medial and lateral malleolus, especially in cases of trauma.

After trauma, inability to bear weight after four steps and tenderness over the posterior aspects of either malleolus, especially the medial malleolus, is suspicious for ankle fracture.

Palpate the *metatarsophalangeal joints* for tenderness. Compress the forefoot between the thumb and fingers. Exert pressure just proximal to the heads of the 1st and 5th metatarsals.

Tenderness on compression is an early sign of *rheumatoid arthritis.* Acute inflammation of the first metatarsophalangeal joint is seen in *gout.*

Palpate the heads of the five metatarsals and the grooves between them with your thumb and index finger. Place your thumb on the dorsum of the foot and your index finger on the plantar surface.

Pain and tenderness, called *metatarsalgia,* occurs with trauma, arthritis, and vascular compromise.

Range of Motion and Muscle Strength Tests

Active Range of Motion

Assess flexion and extension at the tibiotalar (ankle) joint. In the foot, assess inversion and eversion at the subtalar and transverse tarsal joints. Ask the patient to to follow your directions according to the table below to assess ankle range of motion.

Ankle and Foot Movement	Patient Instructions	Primary Muscles Affecting Movement
Ankle Flexion (Plantar Flexion)	*"Point your foot toward the floor."*	Gastrocnemius, soleus, plantaris, tibialis posterior
Ankle Extension (Dorsiflexion)	*"Point your foot toward the ceiling."*	Tibialis anterior, extensor digitorum longus, and extensor hallucis longus
Inversion	*"Bend your heel inward."*	Tibialis posterior and anterior
Eversion	*"Bend your heel outward."*	Peroneus longus and brevis

Passive Range of Motion Maneuvers

If the patient cannot perform active range of motion, test for passive range of motion using the directions below.

- *The Ankle (Tibiotalar) Joint.* Dorsiflex and plantar flex the foot at the ankle.

Pain during movements of the ankle and the foot helps to localize possible arthritis.

DORSIFLEXION AT THE ANKLE

- *The Subtalar (Talocalcaneal) Joint.* Stabilize the ankle with one hand, grasp the heel with the other, and invert and evert the foot.

An arthritic joint is frequently painful when moved in any direction, whereas a ligamentous sprain produces maximal pain when the ligament is stretched. For example, in a common form of sprained ankle, inversion and plantar flexion of the foot cause pain, whereas eversion and plantar flexion are relatively pain free.

INVERSION

EVERSION

- *The Transverse Tarsal Joint.* Stabilize the heel and invert and evert the forefoot.

- *The Metatarsophalangeal Joints.* Flex the toes in relation to the feet.

INVERSION

EVERSION

Muscle Strength Tests

Test muscle strength during dorsiflexion (mainly L4, L5, tibialis anterior) and *plantar flexion* (mainly S1, gastrocnemius, soleus) at the ankle by asking the patient to pull up and push down against your hand.

Describing Limited Motion of a Joint

Although measurement of motion is seldom necessary, limitations can be described in degrees. Pocket goniometers are available for this purpose. In the two examples shown on the next page, the red lines indicate the limited range of the patient's movement, and the black lines suggest the normal range.

Observations may be described in several ways.

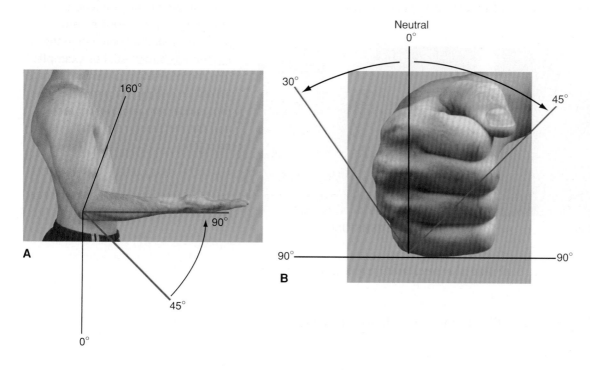

A. The elbow flexes from 45 to 90 degrees
   -or-
   The elbow flexion limited to 45 to 90 degrees

B. Supination at elbow limited to 30 degrees
   Pronation at elbow limited to 45 degrees

SPECIAL TECHNIQUES

Measuring the Length of Legs

If you suspect that the patient's legs are unequal in length, measure them. Have the patient relax in the supine position and symmetrically aligned with legs extended. With a tape, measure the distance between the anterior superior iliac spine and the medial malleolus. The tape should cross the knee on its medial side.

Unequal leg length may explain a scoliosis.

RECORDING YOUR FINDINGS

The examples below contain phrases appropriate for most write-ups. Note that use of the anatomic terms specific to the structure and function of individual joint problems makes your write-up of musculoskeletal findings more meaningful and informative.

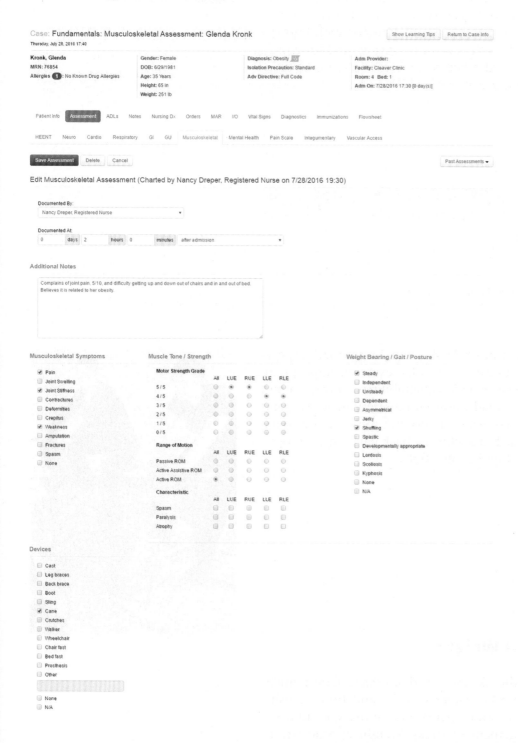

Recording the Examination—The Musculoskeletal System

"FROM (Full range of motion) in all joints with muscle strength 5/5. No erythema, warmth, swelling, or deformity."

OR

"FROM in all joints except hands, with inability to fully close fists. Heberden nodes noted at the DIP joints of hand, Bouchard nodes at PIP joints bilaterally; hand muscle strength 4/5 bilaterally; hand pain 4/10 with flexion of fingers. Hip Pain 2/10 bilaterally with flexion, extension, and rotation; hip muscle strength 5/5. FROM in the knees, with moderate crepitus; strength 5/5. Hallux valgus bilaterally at the first MTP joints."

Suggests osteoarthritis

HEALTH PROMOTION

Health Promotion Topics

- Nutrition, exercise, and weight
- Low back pain
- Fall prevention
- Osteoporosis screening and prevention

Maintaining the integrity of the musculoskeletal system brings many aspects of daily life into play—balanced nutrition, regular exercise, appropriate body weight. Each joint has its own specific vulnerabilities to trauma and wear. Care with lifting, avoidance of falls, household safety measures, and exercise help to protect and preserve well-functioning muscles and joints and prevent or delay the onset of arthritis, chronic back pain, and osteoporosis, all important targets for Healthy People 2020.[13]

Nutrition, Exercise, and Weight

Healthy habits directly benefit the skeleton and muscles. Good nutrition supplies calcium needed for bone mineralization and bone density. Exercise appears to maintain and possibly increase bone mass, in addition to improving outlook and management of stress. Weight appropriate to height and body frame reduces excess mechanical wear on weight-bearing joints such as hips and knees. Twenty percent to 30% of adult Americans report sedentary lifestyles The Healthy People 2020 objectives set goals for physical activity aimed at increasing the proportion of adults meeting guidelines for aerobic and muscle-strengthening physical activity.[14] These goals are based on the 2008 *Physical Activity Guidelines for Americans*[15] an evidence-based report that highlights the benefits of physical activity, including risk reduction for early death, cardiovascular disease, hypertension, type 2 diabetes, breast and colon cancer, obesity, osteoporosis, falls, and depression. Physical activity also helps improve sleep quality and cognitive function in older adults.

Physical Activity Guidelines for Americans

- At least 2 hours and 30 minutes a week of moderate-intensity, or 1 hour and 15 minutes a week of vigorous-intensity, *aerobic physical activity*, or an equivalent combination
- Moderate- or high-intensity *muscle-strengthening activity* that involves all major muscle groups on 2 or more days a week

The report includes guidelines to help sedentary people gradually build up their activity level, starting with 10 minutes of exercise a day. Guided exercise regimens help reduce sports and exercise injuries, which are a significant source of musculoskeletal disorders.

Low Back Pain Prevention

The estimated lifetime prevalence of low back pain in the U.S. population is over 80%.[16] Spinal disorders are among the most frequent reasons for adult outpatient visits.[17] Most patients with acute low back pain get better within 6 weeks. Overall, about 10% to 15% of patients with acute low back pain develop chronic symptoms, often associated with long-term disability.

See Table 18-1, Chapter 18, Low Back Pain, p. 636, for causes of low back pain.

Nurses should educate healthy patients on strategies[18] to prevent back pain. These include:

- Diet: to maintain a healthy weight as excess weight puts strain on the back. The diet should contain calcium and vitamin D to maintain bone strength. Osteoporosis in the spine can lead to back pain.

See chart with recommended Calcium and Vitamin D intake on p. 634.

- Exercise: Flexion, extension, stretching and aerobic exercise are recommended. Exercises such as tai chi and yoga or any weight-bearing exercise that challenges one's balance are helpful.

- Maintaining good posture and avoiding heavy lifting. Education on lifting strategies, posture, and the biomechanics of injury is prudent for people doing repetitive lifting such as: nurses, heavy-machinery operators, and construction workers.

Preventing Falls[19,20]

Among elderly people in the United States, *falls* exact a heavy toll in morbidity and mortality. They are the leading cause of nonfatal injuries and account for a dramatic rise in death rates after 65 years. One out of three older people fall each year and one out of five falls causes a serious injury such as broken bones or a head injury. More than 95% of hip fractures are caused by falling, usually by falling sideways. Each year at least 250,000 older people are hospitalized for hip fractures. For those living independently before a hip fracture, 15% to 25% will still be in long-term care institutions a year after their fracture. Falls are the most common cause of traumatic brain injuries (TBIs).

Fall risk factors are both cognitive and physiologic, including unstable gait, imbalanced posture, reduced strength, previous fall, impaired mobility, medications, incontinence, hypertension, cognitive loss as in dementia, altered mental status, deficits in vision and proprioception, and osteoporosis. Poor lighting, stairs, chairs at awkward heights, slippery or irregular surfaces, and ill-fitting shoes are environmental dangers that can often be corrected. Nurses should work with patients and families to help modify such risks whenever possible. Home health assessments have proven useful in reducing environmental hazards, as have exercise programs to improve patient balance and strength. Fall-risk assessment tools, such as the Morse, Hendrich II, St. Thomas, or Spartanburg, are helpful for identifying persons at risk for falling. (See Chapter 24, Assessing Older Adults, pp. 968–969.)

Osteoporosis

Screening and Prevention

Osteoporosis is a common U.S. health problem: 9% of adults over age 50 years have osteoporosis at the femoral neck or lumbar spine, including 16% of women and 4% of men.[21]

- Half of all postmenopausal women sustain an osteoporosis-related fracture during their lifetime; 25% develop vertebral deformities, and 15% suffer hip fractures that increase risk of chronic pain, disability, loss of independence, and increased mortality.[22]

- Although mortality rates are declining, about 3 in 10 patients die in the year following a hip fracture.[23]

- Men are also at risk: The lifetime risk for an osteoporotic fracture in men over age 50 years is one in four, and men are more likely than women to die in the year following a hip fracture.

- Nearly half of adults age ≥50 years have osteopenia, representing well over 30 million people, including about 12 million men.[21-24] The majority of fragility fractures actually occur among osteopenic adults.

Osteoporosis is a disease marked by reduced bone strength leading to an increased risk of fractures (broken bones). The Osteoporosis objectives for Healthy People 2020 track bone mineral density as a measure of the major risk factor for fractures, and hip fractures, the major and most serious of osteoporosis-related fractures.[25] *Bone strength* reflects both *bone density* and *bone quality*. *Bone density* is determined by the interaction of bone mass (highest in the second decade), new bone formation, and bone resorption or loss. *Bone quality* refers to "architecture, turnover, damage accumulation from microfractures, and mineralization." Osteoporosis typically arises from bone loss during aging, but reduced bone mass from suboptimal bone growth in childhood and adolescence can also cause osteoporosis.

Measuring Bone Density

Bone strength depends on bone quality, bone density, and overall bone size. Because there is no direct measurement of bone strength. Bone mineral density, which accounts for approximately 70% of bone strength, is used as a proxy measure. The World Health Organization uses bone density to define osteopenia and osteoporosis:

- *Osteopenia:* bone density T score between −2.5 and −1.0 (1.0–2.5 standard deviations below the young adult mean).

- *Osteoporosis:* T score less than −2.5 (bone density 2.5 or more standard deviations below the young adult mean).

Bone densitometry scoring also includes Z scores representing comparisons with age-matched controls. These measurements are useful for determining whether bone loss is caused by an underlying disease or condition.

Bone density is measured at the hip, femoral neck, Ward triangle at the femoral neck, greater trochanter, and total hip, which includes all the measurements. A 10% drop in bone density, equivalent to 1.0 standard deviation, is associated with a 20% increase in risk for fracture.

Bone density peaks by age 30 years. Bone loss from age-related declines in estrogen and testosterone is initially rapid, then slows and becomes continuous.

Screening Recommendations

The U.S. Preventive Services Task Force (USPSTF) gives a grade B recommendation supporting osteoporosis screening for women age ≥65 years and for younger women whose 10-year fracture risk equals or exceeds that of an average-risk 65-year-old white woman.[22] The USPSTF finds that evidence about risks and benefits for men is insufficient for recommending routine screening. However, the American College of Physicians recommends that clinicians periodically assess older men for osteoporosis risk and measure bone density for those at increased risk who are candidates for drug therapy.[26]

Risk Factors for Osteoporosis

- Postmenopausal status in women
- Age ≥50 years
- Low body mass index
- Low dietary calcium intake
- Vitamin D deficiency
- Prior fragility fracture
- Osteoporosis in a first-degree relative, especially with a prior fragility fracture
- Sedentary lifestyle or extended bed rest
- Tobacco and excessive alcohol use
- Inflammatory disorders of the musculoskeletal, pulmonary, or gastrointestinal systems, including celiac sprue, chronic renal disease, organ transplantation, diabetes, HIV hypogonadism, multiple myeloma, anorexia nervosa, and rheumatologic and autoimmune diseases
- Medications such as oral and high-dose inhaled corticosteroids, anticoagulants (long-term use), aromatase inhibitors for breast cancer, methotrexate, selected antiseizure medications, immunosuppressive agents, proton-pump inhibitors (long-term use) and antigonadal therapy for prostate cancer

The USPSTF recommends using WHO's Fracture Risk Assessment (FRAX) calculator. The FRAX calculator generates a 10-year osteoporotic fracture risk based on age; gender; weight; height; parental fracture history; use of glucocorticoids; presence of rheumatoid arthritis (RA) or conditions associated with secondary osteoporosis; tobacco and heavy

A previous low-impact fracture from standing height or less is the greatest risk factor for subsequent fracture.

FRAX has been validated for African American, Hispanic, and Asian women in the United States and has calculators that are continent and country-specific.

alcohol use; and, when available, femoral neck bone mass density (BMD). The FRAX calculator also provides a 10-year hip fracture risk.

The website for the FRAX Calculator for Assessing Fracture Risk for the United States is http://www.shef. ac.uk/FRAX/tool.jsp?country=9.

The USPSTF recommends using a *10-year osteoporotic fracture risk threshold of 9.3%* when considering bone density screening in women ages 50 to 64 years. Screening decisions for women in this age range should account for menopausal status, clinical judgment, and patient preferences and values.

Prevention and Treatment

The therapeutic uses of available agents and options for preventing and treating osteoporosis are briefly summarized here:

- Adequate **calcium intake** at all ages is necessary to prevent osteoporosis. By the time teens finish their growth spurt 90% of adult bone mass is established. Fewer than 1 in 10 girls and 1 in 4 boys ages 9 to 13 are at or above their adequate calcium intake.[27]

- For the older person, **increased calcium** intake reduces age-related hyperparathyroidism and increases mineralization of newly formed bone. The nurse should assess the calcium intake with the history.

There are two main forms of calcium supplements, calcium carbonate and calcium citrate. Supplements contain variable amounts of elemental calcium.[28] Patients can read these amounts on the Supplement Facts panel of the calcium containers. Calcium carbonate is less expensive and should be consumed with food. Calcium citrate is absorbed more easily in individuals with reduced levels of stomach acid and can be taken with or without food. Calcium absorption depends on the total amount consumed at one time—absorption diminishes at higher doses. Counsel patients to take doses of 500 mg at two separate times each day. Vitamin D supplements are available in two forms, D_2 (ergocalciferol) and D_3 (cholecalciferol); D_3 increases serum $25(OH)D$ levels more effectively than D_2.[29]

Patients on proton-pump inhibitor medicine have reduced stomach acid levels and should take calcium citrate supplements.

Recommended Calcium and Vitamin D Intakes

Life-Stage Group	Calcium (mg/day)	Vitamin D (IU/day)
Infants 0–6 months	200	400
Infants 6–12 months	260	400
1–3 years old	700	600
4–8 years old	1,000	600
9–13 years old	1,300	600
14–18 years old	1,300	600
19–30 years old	1,000	600
31–50 years old	1,000	600
51- to 70-year-old males	1,000	600
51- to 70-year-old females	1,200	600
>70 years old	1,200	800
14–18 years old, pregnant/lactating	1,300	600
19–50 years old, pregnant/lactating	1,000	600

mg, milligrams; IU, International units.
Source: *Food and Nutrition Board, Institute of Medicine, National Academy of Sciences, 2010.*
Available at http://www.niams.nih.gov/Health_Info/Bone/Osteoporosis/osteoporosis_ff.asp

- Up to two thirds of patients with hip fractures are deficient in **vitamin D**, essential for calcium absorption and muscle strength (National Institutes of Health. Office of Dietary Supplements).[30] Vitamin D is synthesized in the skin through exposure to sunlight. Many people obtain enough vitamin D naturally, by receiving 15 minutes of sunlight each day. Studies show that vitamin D production decreases in the elderly, in people who are housebound, and for most people during the winter. They may need vitamin D supplements to achieve the recommended daily intake. Food sources of vitamin D include egg yolks, saltwater fish, and liver.[30]

- **Antiresorptive agents** inhibit osteoclast activity and slow bone remodeling, allowing better mineralization of bone matrix and stabilization of the trabecular microarchitecture. These agents include bisphosphonates, selective estrogen-receptor modulators (SERMs), calcitonin, and postmenopausal estrogen, now in question because of associated risks of breast cancer and vascular problems.

Bisphosphonates have been linked to osteonecrosis of the jaw and atypical femur fractures. SERMs increase the risk for thromboembolic events. Postmenopausal estrogen replacement is linked to increased risk of breast cancer and venous thromboembolism (VTE).

- **Anabolic agents** such as parathyroid hormone stimulate bone formation by acting primarily on osteoblasts but require subcutaneous administration and monitoring for hypercalcemia. They are reserved for moderate to severe cases of osteoporosis (T scores <–3.5 or <–2.5 with a fragility fracture) or those who have failed or not tolerated other therapies.[31]

- **Regular exercise** that includes weight-bearing and resistance training can increase bone density and muscle strength but has not yet been shown to reduce fracture risk.[32] Multidisciplinary programs to improve strength, balance, and home and medication safety can help prevent falls.

- Alcohol prevents absorption of calcium. Women should limit alcohol to one drink per day and men to two drinks per day.

- Limit caffeine in the diet. Caffeine causes increased calcium excretion.

TABLE

18-1

Low Back Pain

Patterns	Possible Causes	Physical Signs
Mechanical Low Back Pain[1,16,33–35] Aching pain in the lumbosacral area; may radiate into lower leg, especially along L5 (lateral leg) or S1 (posterior leg) dermatomes. Refers to anatomic or functional abnormality in the absence of neoplastic, infectious, or inflammatory disease. Usually acute (<3 months), idiopathic, benign, and self-limiting; represents 97% of symptomatic low back pain. Commonly work-related and occurring in patients 30–50 years. Risk factors include heavy lifting, poor conditioning, and obesity.	Often arises from muscle and ligament injuries (~70%) or age-related intervertebral disc or facet disease (~4%).[2] Causes also include herniated disc (~4%), spinal stenosis (~3%), compression fractures (~4%), and spondylolisthesis (2%).	Paraspinal muscle or facet tenderness, pain with back movement, loss of normal lumbar lordosis, but no motor or sensory loss or reflex abnormalities. In osteoporosis, check for thoracic kyphosis, percussion tenderness over a spinous process, or fractures in the thoracic spine or hip.[46]
Sciatica (Radicular Low Back Pain)[1,5,34] Shooting pain below the knee, commonly into the lateral leg (L5) or posterior calf (S1); typically accompanies low back pain. Patients report associated paresthesias and weakness. Bending, sneezing, coughing, straining during bowel movements often worsen pain.	Sciatic pain very sensitive, ~95%, and specific, ~88%, for disc herniation. Usually from herniated intervertebral disc with compression or traction of nerve root(s) in people 50 years or older. Involves L5 and S1 roots in ~95% of disc herniations. Root or spinal cord compression from neoplastic conditions in fewer than 1% of cases. Tumor or midline disc herniation in bowel or bladder dysfunction, leg weakness from cauda equina syndrome (S2–S4).	Disc herniation most likely if calf wasting, weak ankle dorsiflexion, absent ankle jerk, positive crossed straight-leg raise (pain in affected leg when healthy leg tested); negative straight-leg raise makes diagnosis highly unlikely. Ipsilateral straight-leg raise sensitive, ~65–98%, but not specific, ~10–60%.
Chronic Back Stiffness[7,36]	*Ankylosing spondylitis,* an inflammatory poly-arthritis, most common in men younger than 40 years *Diffuse idiopathic hyperostosis (DISH)* affects men more than women, usually age ≥50 years.	
Pain Referred From the Abdomen or Pelvis Usually a deep, aching pain; the level varies with the source. Accounts for approximately 1% of low back pain.	Peptic ulcer, pancreatitis, pancreatic cancer, chronic prostatitis, endometriosis, dissecting aortic aneurysm, retroperitoneal tumor, and other causes.	Variable with the source. Local vertebral tenderness may be present. Spinal movements are not painful and range of motion is not affected. Look for signs of the primary disorder.

TABLE
18-2

Pains in the Neck[37,38]

Patterns	Possible Causes	Physical Signs
Mechanical Neck Pain Aching pain in the cervical paraspinal muscles and ligaments with associated muscle spasm, with associated stiffness and tightness in the upper back and shoulder, lasting up to 6 weeks. No associated radiation, paresthesias, or weakness. Headache may be present.	Mechanism poorly understood, possibly sustained muscle contraction. Associated with poor posture, stress, poor sleep, poor head position during activities such as computer use, watching television, driving.	Local muscle tenderness, pain on movement. No neurologic deficits. Possible trigger points in *fibromyalgia*. *Torticollis* if prolonged abnormal neck posture and muscle spasm.
Mechanical Neck Pain—Whiplash Also mechanical neck pain with aching paracervical pain and stiffness, often beginning the day after injury. Occipital headache, dizziness, malaise, and fatigue may be present. Chronic whiplash syndrome if symptoms last more than 6 months, present in 20–40% of injuries.	Musculoligamental sprain or strain from forced hyperflexion–hyperextension injury to the neck, as in rear-end collisions.	Localized paracervical tenderness, decreased neck range of motion, perceived weakness of the upper extremities. Causes of cervical cord compression such as fracture, herniation, head injury, or altered consciousness are excluded.
Cervical Radiculopathy—from nerve root compression Sharp burning or tingling pain in the neck and one arm, with associated paresthesias and weakness. Sensory symptoms often in myotomal pattern, deep in muscle, rather than dermatomal pattern.	Dysfunction of cervical spinal nerve, nerve roots, or both from foraminal encroachment of the spinal nerve (~75%), herniated cervical disc (~25%). Rarely from tumor, syrinx, multiple sclerosis. Mechanisms may involve hypoxia of the nerve root and dorsal ganglion, release of inflammatory mediators.	C7 nerve root affected most often (45–60%), with weakness in triceps and finger flexors and extensors. C6 nerve root involvement also common, with weakness in biceps, brachioradialis, wrist extensors.
Cervical Myelopathy—from cervical cord compression Neck pain with bilateral weakness and paresthesias in both upper and lower extremities, often with urinary frequency. Hand clumsiness, palmar paresthesias, and gait changes may be subtle. Neck flexion often exacerbates symptoms.	Usually from cervical *spondylosis*, defined as cervical degenerative disc disease from spurs, protrusion of ligamentum flavum, and/or disc herniation (~80%); also from cervical stenosis from osteophytes, ossification of ligamentum flavum. Large central or paracentral disc herniation may also compress cord.	Hyperreflexia; clonus at the wrist, knee, or ankle; extensor plantar reflexes (positive Babinski signs); and gait disturbances. May also see *Lhermitte sign:* neck flexion with resulting sensation of electrical shock radiating down the spine. Confirmation of cervical myelopathy warrants neck immobilization and neurosurgical evaluation.

TABLE
18-3

Patterns of Pain in and Around the Joints

Problem	Process	Common Locations	Pattern of Spread	Onset	Progression and Duration
Rheumatoid Arthritis[39-41]	Chronic inflammation of *synovial membranes* with secondary erosion of adjacent cartilage and bone, and damage to ligaments and tendons	Hands (proximal interphalangeal and metacarpophalangeal joints), feet (metatarsophalangeal joints), wrists, knees, elbows, ankles	Symmetrically additive: progresses to other joints while persisting in the initial ones	Usually insidious	Often chronic, with remissions and exacerbations
Osteoarthritis (degenerative joint disease)[42]	Degeneration and progressive loss of *cartilage* within the joints, damage to underlying bone, and formation of new bone at the margins of the cartilage	Knees, hips, hands (distal, sometimes proximal interphalangeal joints), cervical and lumbar spine, and wrists (first carpometacarpal joint); also joints previously injured or diseased	Additive; however, only one joint may be involved.	Usually insidious	Slowly progressive, with temporary exacerbations after periods of overuse
Gouty Arthritis[43,44] *Acute Gout*	An inflammatory reaction to microcrystals of sodium urate	Base of the big toe (the first metatarsophalangeal joint), the instep or dorsa of feet, the ankles, knees, and elbows	Early attacks usually confined to one joint	Sudden, often at night, often after injury, surgery, fasting, or excessive food or alcohol intake	Occasional isolated attacks lasting days up to 2 weeks; they may get more frequent and severe, with persisting symptoms.
Fibromyalgia Syndrome[45]	Widespread musculoskeletal pain and tender points. May accompany other diseases. Mechanisms unclear	"All over," but especially in the neck, shoulders, hands, low back, and knees	Usually insidious	Variable	Chronic, with "ups and downs"

The vagueness of these characteristics is in itself a clue to the fibromyalgia syndrome

Swelling	Redness, Warmth, and Tenderness	Stiffness	Limitation of Motion	Generalized Symptoms
Frequent swelling of synovial tissue in joints or tendon sheaths; also subcutaneous nodules	Tender, often warm, but seldom red	Prominent, often for an hour or more in the mornings, also after inactivity	Often develops	Weakness, fatigue, weight loss, and low fever are common.
Small effusions in the joints may be present, especially in the knees; also bony enlargement	Possibly tender, seldom warm, and rarely red	Frequent but brief (usually 5–10 minutes), in the morning and after inactivity	Often develops	Usually absent
Present, within and around the involved joint	Exquisitely tender, hot, and red	Not evident	Motion is limited primarily by pain.	Fever may be present.
None	Multiple specific and symmetric tender "trigger points," often not recognized until the examination	Present, especially in the morning	Absent, though stiffness is greater at the extremes of movement	A disturbance of sleep, usually associated with morning fatigue; overlaps with depression.

TABLE
18-4
Painful Shoulders

Rotator Cuff Tendinitis

Repeated shoulder motion, as in throwing or swimming, can cause edema and hemorrhage followed by inflammation, most commonly involving the supraspinatus tendon. Acute, recurrent, or chronic pain may result, often aggravated by activity. Patients report sharp catches of pain, grating, and weakness when lifting the arm overhead. When the supraspinatus tendon is involved, tenderness is maximal just below the tip of the acromion. In older adults, bone spurs on the undersurface of the acromion may contribute to symptoms. Patients are typically athletically active.

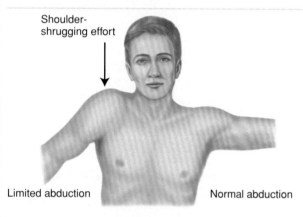

Shoulder-shrugging effort

Limited abduction   Normal abduction

Rotator Cuff Tears

The rotator cuff muscles and tendons keep the head of the humerus in place against the concave glenoid fossa and strengthen arm movement—the subscapularis is used with internal rotation, the supraspinatus with elevation, and the infraspinatus and teres minor with external rotation. Injury from a fall or repeated impingement of muscle or tendon against a bone may weaken the rotator cuff, causing a partial or complete tear, usually after age 40. Weakness, atrophy of the supraspinatus and infraspinatus muscles, pain, crepitus and tenderness may ensue. In a complete tear of the supraspinatus tendon (illustrated), active abduction and forward flexion at the glenohumeral joint are severely impaired, producing a characteristic shrugging of the shoulder and a positive "drop arm" sign (see p. 586).

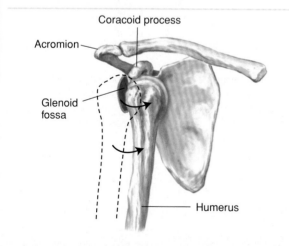

Coracoid process

Acromion

Glenoid fossa

Humerus

Anterior Dislocation of the Humerus

Shoulder instability from anterior dislocation of the humerus usually results from a fall or forceful throwing motion, then becomes recurrent. The shoulder seems to "slip out of the joint" when the arm is abducted and externally rotated, causing a *positive apprehension sign* for anterior instability when the examiner places the arm in this position. Any shoulder movement may cause pain, and patients hold the arm in a neutral position. The rounded lateral aspect of the shoulder appears flattened. Dislocations may also be inferior, posterior (relatively rare), and multidirectional.

TABLE 18-5	**Arthritis in the Hands**

Acute Rheumatoid Arthritis

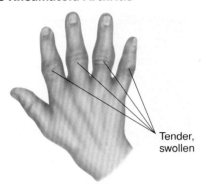

Tender, swollen

Tender, painful, stiff joints in *rheumatoid arthritis,* usually with *symmetric* involvement on both sides of the body. The proximal interphalangeal, metacarpophalangeal, and wrist joints are the most frequently affected. Note the fusiform or spindle-shaped swelling of the proximal interphalangeal joints in acute disease.

Chronic Rheumatoid Arthritis

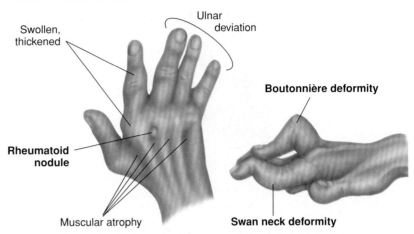

Swollen, thickened

Ulnar deviation

Boutonnière deformity

Rheumatoid nodule

Muscular atrophy

Swan neck deformity

In chronic disease, note the swelling and thickening of the metacarpophalangeal and proximal interphalangeal joints. Range of motion becomes limited, and fingers may deviate toward the ulnar side. The interosseous muscles atrophy. The fingers may show *"swan neck"* deformities (hyperextension of the proximal interphalangeal joints with fixed flexion of the distal interphalangeal joints). Less common is a *boutonnière deformity* (persistent flexion of the proximal interphalangeal joint with hyperextension of the distal interphalangeal joint). Rheumatoid nodules are seen in the acute or the chronic stage.

Osteoarthritis (*Degenerative Joint Disease*)

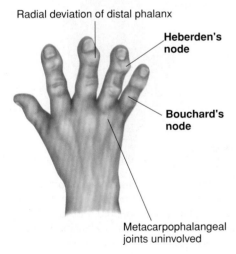

Radial deviation of distal phalanx

Heberden's node

Bouchard's node

Metacarpophalangeal joints uninvolved

Heberden nodes on the dorsolateral aspects of the distal interphalangeal joints from bony overgrowth of osteoarthritis. Usually hard and painless, they affect the middle-aged or elderly; often associated with arthritic changes in other joints. Flexion and deviation deformities may develop. *Bouchard nodes* on the proximal interphalangeal joints are less common. The metacarpophalangeal joints are spared.

Chronic Tophaceous Gout[39]

Swollen

Draining tophus

Knobby swelling

The deformities of long-standing chronic tophaceous gout can mimic rheumatoid arthritis and osteoarthritis. Joint involvement is usually not as symmetric as in rheumatoid arthritis. Acute inflammation may be present. Knobby swellings around the joints ulcerate and discharge white chalk-like urates.

TABLE

18-6

Swellings and Deformities of the Hands

Dupuytren Contracture

Flexion contraction

Cord

The first sign of a *Dupuytren contracture* is a thickened plaque overlying the flexor tendon of the ring finger and possibly the little finger at the level of the distal palmar crease. Subsequently, the skin in this area puckers, and a thickened fibrotic cord develops between palm and finger. Flexion contracture of the fingers may gradually develop.

Trigger Finger

Caused by a painless nodule in a flexor tendon in the palm, near the metacarpal head. The nodule is too big to enter easily into the tendon sheath during extension of the fingers from a flexed position. With extra effort or assistance, the finger extends and flexes with a palpable and audible snap as the nodule pops into the tendon sheath. Watch, listen, and palpate the nodule as the patient flexes and extends the fingers.

Thenar Atrophy

Normal hypothenar eminence

Flattened thenar eminence

Thenar atrophy suggests a *median nerve disorder* such as *carpal tunnel syndrome* (see Chapter 18, pp. 596–597). Hypothenar atrophy suggests an *ulnar nerve disorder.*

Ganglion

Cystic swelling

Ganglia are cystic, round, usually nontender swellings along tendon sheaths or joint capsules, frequently at the dorsum of the wrist. The cyst contains synovial fluid. Flexion of the wrist makes ganglia more prominent; extension tends to obscure them. Ganglia may also develop elsewhere on the hands, wrists, ankles, and feet. They can disappear spontaneously.

TABLE
18-7

Abnormalities of the Feet

Hot, red, tender, swollen

Acute Gouty Arthritis
The metatarsophalangeal joint of the great toe is the initial joint involved in 50% of episodes of *acute gouty arthritis*. It is characterized by a very painful and tender, hot, dusky red swelling that extends beyond the margin of the joint. It is easily mistaken for a cellulitis. Acute gout may also involve the dorsum of the foot.

Medial border becomes convex

Sole touches floor

Flat Feet
Signs of *flat feet* may be apparent only when the patient stands, or they may become permanent. The longitudinal arch flattens so that the sole approaches or touches the floor. The normal concavity on the medial side of the foot becomes convex. Tenderness may be present from the medial malleolus down along the medial-plantar surface of the foot. Swelling may develop anterior to the malleoli. Inspect the shoes for excess wear on the inner sides of the soles and heels.

Hallux Valgus
In *hallux valgus,* there is lateral deviation of the great toe and enlargement of the head oft eh first metatarsal on its medial side, forming a bursa or bunion. This bursa may become inflamed. Women are more likely to be affected than men.

Morton's
neuroma

Morton Neuroma
Tenderness is seen over the plantar surface, between the 3rd and 4th metatarsal heads, from perineural fibrosis of the common digital nerve due to irritation. (It is not a true neuroma.) Pain radiates to the toes, when you press on the plantar interspace while squeezing the toes with your other hand. Symptoms include hyperesthesia, numbness, aching, and burning from the metatarsal heads into the 3rd and 4th toes.

TABLE
18-8

Abnormalities of the Toes and Soles

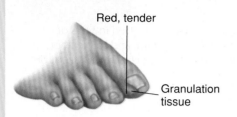

Red, tender

Granulation tissue

Ingrown Toenail

The sharp edge of a toenail may dig into and injure the lateral nail fold, resulting in inflammation and infection. A tender, reddened, overhanging nail fold, sometimes with granulation tissue and purulent discharge, results. The great toe is most often affected.

Hyperextended

Flexed

Hammer Toe

Most commonly involving the second toe, a hammer toe is characterized by hyperextension at the metatarsophalangeal joint with flexion at the proximal interphalangeal joint. A corn frequently develops at the pressure point over the proximal interphalangeal joint.

Red, thickened

Corn

A corn is a painful conical thickening of skin that results from recurrent pressure on normally thin skin. The apex of the cone points inward and causes pain. Corns characteristically occur over bony prominences such as the 5th toe. When located in moist areas such as pressure points between the 4th and 5th toes, they are called soft corns.

Callus

Like a corn, a callus is an area of greatly thickened skin that develops in a region of recurrent pressure. Unlike a corn, a callus involves skin that is normally thick, such as the sole, and is usually painless. If a callus is painful, suspect an underlying plantar wart.

Plantar Wart

A plantar wart is a common wart, caused by the *human papillomavirus*, located in the thickened skin of the sole. It may look like a callus or even be covered by one. Look for the characteristic small dark spots that give a stippled appearance to a wart. Normal skin lines stop at the wart's edge. It is tender if pinched from the side, whereas a callus is tender to direct pressure.

Neuropathic Ulcer

When pain sensation is diminished or absent, as in diabetic neuropathy, neuropathic ulcers may develop at pressure points on the feet. Although often deep, infected, and indolent, they are painless. Underlying osteomyelitis may develop.

BIBLIOGRAPHY

CITATIONS

1. Chou R. In the clinic. Low back pain. *Ann Intern Med.* 2014;160:ITC6–1.

2. McGee S. Examination of the musculoskeletal system: the shoulder. In: *Evidence-based Physical Diagnosis.* 3rd ed. St. Louise, MO: Elsevier Saunders; 2012:479.

3. McGee S. Examination of the musculoskeletal system: the shoulder. In: *Evidence-based Physical Diagnosis.* 3rd ed. St. Louise, MO: Elsevier Saunders; 2012:485.

4. Sauvé PS, Rhee PC, Shin AY, et al. Examination of the wrist: radial-sided wrist pain. *J Hand Surg Am.* 2014;39:2089.

5. McGee S. Peripheral nerve injury: diagnosis of carpal tunnel syndrome. In: *Evidenced-based Physical Diagnosis.* 3rd ed. St Louis, MO: Saunders; 2012:600,602–603.

6. D'Arcy CA, McGee S. Does this patient have carpal tunnel syndrome? The rational clinical examination. *JAMA.* 2000; 283:3110.

7. Raychaudhuri SP, Deodhar A. The classification and diagnostic criteria of ankylosing spondylitis. *J Autoimmun.* 2014;48:128.

8. Frank RM, Slabaugh MA, Grumet RC, et al. Hip pain in active patients: what you may be missing. *J Fam Pract.* 2012; 61:736.

9. Suarez JC, Ely EE, Mutnal AB, et al. Comprehensive approach to the evaluation of groin pain. *J Am Acad Orthop Surg.* 2013;21:558.

10. McGee S. Examination of the musculoskeletal system: the knee. In: *Evidence-based Physical Diagnosis.* 3rd ed. St. Louise, MO: Elsevier Saunders; 2012:499–500.

11. Cibere J, Bellamy N, Thorne A, et al. Reliability of the knee examination in osteoarthritis. *Arthritis Rheum.* 2004; 50(2):458–468.

12. Young C. In the clinic. Plantar fasciitis. *Ann Intern Med.* 2012; 156:ITC1–1.

13. U.S. Department of Health and Human Services. Office of Disease Prevention and Health Promotion. Healthy People 2020. *Arthritis, Osteoporosis, and Chronic Back Conditions.* Washington, DC. Available at http://www.healthypeople.gov/2020/topics objectives/topic/Arthritis-Osteoporosis-and-Chronic-Back-Conditions. Accessed December 28, 2015.

14. U.S. Department of Health and Human Services. Office of Disease Prevention and Health Promotion. Healthy People 2020. *Physical Activity Objectives.* Washington, DC. Available at http://www.healthypeople.gov/2020/topics-objectives/topic/physical-activity/objectives. Accessed January 3, 2016.

15. Office of Disease Prevention and Health Promotion. Physical Activity Guidelines for Americans Summary. 2008. Available at: http://health.gov/paguidelines/guidelines/summary.aspx. Accessed July 8, 2016.

16. Balague F, Mannion AF, Pellise F, et al. Non-specific low back pain. *Lancet.* 2012;379:482.

17. National Ambulatory Medical Care Survey. Factsheet. Outpatient Department. Centers for Disease Control and Prevention. National Center for Health Statistics. 2011. Available at http://www.cdc.gov/nchs/data/ahcd/NHAMCS_2011_opd_factsheet.pdf. Accessed December 31, 2015.

18. National Institute of Arthritis, Musculoskeletal and Skin Diseases. *Handout* on Health: Back Pain. March 2015. Available at http://www.niams.nih.gov/Health_Info/Back_Pain/default.asp. Accessed December 29, 2015.

19. CDC. Older Adult Falls. Hip Fractures among Older Adults. Available at http://www.cdc.gov/homeandrecreationalsafety/falls/adulthipfx.html. Accessed December 31, 2015.

20. American Geriatrics Society. Prevention of Falls in Older Persons: AGS and BGS Practice Guidelines. Available at http://www.medcats.com/FALLS/frameset.htm. Accessed December 31, 2015.

21. Looker AC, Borrud LG, Dawson-Hughes B, et al. Osteoporosior low bone mass at the femur neck or lumbar spine in older adults: United States, 2005–2008. *NCHS Data Brief.* 2012;(93):1–8.

22. U.S. Preventive Services Task Force. Screening for osteoporosis. U.S. preventive services task force recommendation statement. *Ann Intern Med.* 2011;154:356.

23. Brauer CA, Coca-Perraillon M, Cutler DM, et al. Incidence and mortality of hip fractures in the United States. *JAMA.* 2009;302:1573.

24. Looker AC, Melton LJ, 3rd, Harris TB, et al. Prevalence and trends in low femur bone density among older US adults: NHANES 2005–2006 compared with NHANES III. *J Bone Miner Res.* 2010;25:64.

25. U.S. Department of Health and Human Services. Office of Disease Prevention and Health Promotion. *Healthy People 2020: Arthritis, Osteoporosis, and Chronic Back Conditions.* Available at http://www.healthypeople.gov/2020/topics-objectives/topic/Arthritis-Osteoporosis-and-Chronic-Back-Conditions. Accessed January 1, 2016.

26. Qaseem A, Snow V, Shekelle P, et al. Screening for osteoporosis in men: a clinical practice guideline from the American College of Physicians. *Ann Intern Med.* 2008;148:680.

27. NIH.Eunice Kennedy Schriver National Institute of Children's Health and Human Development. Children's Bone Health and Calcium: Condition Information. Available at http://m.nichd.nih.gov/topics/bonehealth/conditioninfo/Pages/default.aspx. Accessed December 11, 2015.

28. National Institutes of Health. Office of Dietary Supplements. Calcium. Dietary Supplement Fact Sheet. 2013. Available at http://ods.od.nih.gov/factsheets/Calcium HealthProfessional/. Accessed June 19, 2015.

29. Tripkovic L, Lambert H, Hart K, et al. Comparison of vitamin D2 and vitamin D3 supplementation in raising serum 25-hydroxyvitamin D status: a systematic review and meta analysis. *Am J Clin Nutr.* 2012;95:1357.

30. National Institutes of Health. Office of Dietary Supplements. Vitamin D. Dietary Supplement Fact Sheet 2014. Available at https://ods.od.nih.gov/factsheets/VitaminD-HealthProfessional/ Accessed January 1, 2016.

31. Hodsman A, Papaioannou A, Ann C. Clinical practice guidelines for the use of parathyroid hormone in the treatment of osteoporosis. *CMAJ.* 2006;175:48.

32. National Institutes of Health Osteoporosis and Related Bone Disease National Resource Center. Osteoporosis overview: facts and figures. Available at http://www.niams.nih.gov/Health_Info/Bone/Osteoporosis/osteoporosis_ff.asp.

33. Rozenberg S, Foltz V, Fautrel B. Treatment strategy for chronic low back pain. *Joint Bone spine*. 2012;79:555.

34. Ropper AH, Zafonte RD. Sciatica. *N Engl J Med*. 2015; 372:1240.

35. Chou R, Shekelle P. Will this patient develop persistent disabling low back pain? *JAMA*. 2010;303:1295.

36. Assassi S, Weisman MH, Lee M, et al. New population-based reference values for spinal mobility measures based on the 2009–2010 National Health and Nutrition Examination Survey. *Arthritis Rheumatol*. 2014;66:2628.

37. Bono CM, Ghiselli G, Gilbert TJ, et al.; North American Spine Society. An evidence-based clinical guideline for the diagnosis and treatment of cervical radiculopathy from degenerative disorders. *Spine J*. 2011;11:64.

38. Onks CA, Billy G. Evaluation and treatment of cervical radiculopathy. *Prim Care*. 2013;40:837.

39. American College of Physicians. Approach to the Patient with Rheumatic Disease, in Rheumatology. In: Collier V, ed. *Medical Knowledge Self-Assessment Program (MKSAP) 16*. Philadelphia, PA: American College of Physicians; 2012.

40. Anderson J, Caplan L, Yazdany J, et al. Rheumatoid arthritis disease activity measures: American College of Rheumatology recommendations for use in clinical practice. *Arthritis Care Res (Hoboken)*. 2012;64:640.

41. Davis JM 3rd, Matteson EL; American College of Rheumatology; European League Against Rheumatism. My treatment approach to rheumatoid arthritis. *Mayo Clin Proc*. 2012;87:659.

42. Gelber AC. In the clinic. Osteoarthritis. *Ann Intern Med*. 2014;161:ITC1–1.

43. Mead T, Arabindoo K, Smith B. Managing gout: there's more we can do. *J Fam Pract*. 2014;63:707.

44. Neogi T. Gout. *New Engl J Med*. 2011;364;443.

45. Clauw DJ. Fibromyalgia: a clinical review. *JAMA*. 2014; 311:1547.

46. Golub AL, Laya MB. Osteoporosis: screening, prevention, and management. *Med Clin N Am*. 2015;99:587.

Mental Status

LEARNING OBJECTIVES

The student will:

1. Describe the areas assessed in the mental status examination.

2. Determine the symptoms and behaviors assessed in a mental health screening.

3. Obtain an accurate mental status history for a patient.

4. Perform a mental status examination.

5. Identify the screening and health promotion and counseling tools for depression, suicide, and substance use disorders.

6. Correctly document the findings of the mental status assessment.

As nurses, we are uniquely poised to screen, detect, and investigate clues to mental illness and harmful behavior and encourage health-promoting behaviors. Empathic listening and close observation offer a perspective to the patient's outlook, concerns, and habits. Nevertheless, health care providers, including nurses, often miss subtle clues of mental illness and harmful dysfunctional behaviors in patients. Recognizing mental illness is especially important given its significant prevalence and morbidity, the high likelihood that it is treatable, the shortage of psychiatrists, and the increasing importance of primary care clinicians as the first to encounter the patient's distress.[1] The prevalence of mental health disorders in U.S. adults in 2014 was 18.1%, affecting 43.6 million people.[2] Those receiving care were less than 50%, and of those individuals adherence to treatment guidelines in primary care offices is <50% and disproportionately lower for ethnic minorities.[3–5]

This chapter introduces:

- Common symptoms and behaviors suggestive of mental health disorders.

- Concepts that guide history taking and the general assessment of mental health.

- Priorities for mental health promotion and counseling.

- Components of the mental status examination, that should be conducted when behavioral problems are suspicious indicators of mental health disorders.

It is important for nurses to assess for both mental and physical changes. Mental health disorders are commonly masked by other clinical conditions, calling for sensitive and careful inquiry. Often patients have more than one mental disorder, with symptoms that mirror medical illnesses. The astute assessment and documentation of findings are crucial to formulate the best plan for each individual patient. The patient with depression or anxiety may also be dealing with substance or domestic abuse, and someone with substance or domestic abuse may have depression or anxiety. In addition, do not overlook patients with medical issues, such as a myocardial infarction, that could also trigger symptoms of mental illness, for example, depression. Further, it is increasingly important for nurses to recognize that "difficult patients" are frequently those with multiple unexplained symptoms and underlying psychiatric conditions or abuse that are amenable to therapy. Patient health, function, and quality of life are at risk without adequate assessment and treatment. All aspects must be treated for the patient to achieve optimal function.

SYMPTOMS AND BEHAVIOR

Understanding Symptoms: What Do They Mean?

For beginning nurses, the challenge is to sort out the array of symptoms encountered. Symptoms may be psychological, relating to mood change or an emotional state, or physical, relating to a body sensation such as pain, fatigue, or palpitations. Physical symptoms are often termed somatic in the mental health literature. Studies reveal that physical symptoms prompt more than 50% of U.S. office visits.[6] Common somatic complaints include: pain from headache, backache, or musculoskeletal conditions; gastrointestinal symptoms; sexual or reproductive symptoms; and neurologic symptoms such as dizziness or loss of balance.

Approximately 5% of somatic symptoms are acute, triggering immediate evaluation.[7] Another 70% to 75% are minor or self-limited and resolve in 6 weeks. Nevertheless, approximately 25% of patients have persisting and recurrent symptoms that elude assessment through the history and physical examination and fail to improve. Overall, 30% of symptoms are medically unexplained. Some of them involve single complaints that appear to persist longer than others—for example, back pain, headache, or musculoskeletal pain. Others occur in clusters presenting as functional syndromes, such as irritable bowel syndrome, fibromyalgia, chronic fatigue, temporomandibular joint disorder, or multiple chemical sensitivity.

Experts now propose that physical and psychological symptoms are interactive and represent "a varying mix of disease and nondisease input" that lies along a spectrum from medical to mental disorders.[7] Evidence shows that symptom etiology is often multifactorial, lacking a single cause; and often there are several related symptoms or symptom clusters rather than single complaints.

A physical symptom can be explained physically or medically or can be unexplained; a somatoform symptom lacks an adequate medical or physical explanation.

Unexplained Symptoms

Two thirds of patients with depression, for example, present with physical complaints, and half report multiple unexplained physical or somatic symptoms.[7]

Further, the functional syndromes have been shown to "frequently co-occur and share key symptoms and selected objective abnormalities."[6]

Failure to recognize the admixture of physical symptoms and functional syndromes with common mental health disorders—anxiety, depression, unexplained or somatoform physical symptoms, and substance abuse—adds to loss of the patient's quality of life and impaired treatment outcomes. Often these patients are "high users" of the health care system and have significant disability.

Patient Indicators for Mental Health Screening

Unexplained conditions lasting more than 6 weeks are increasingly recognized as chronic disorders that should prompt screening for depression, anxiety, or both. Because screening all patients is time-consuming and expensive, experts recommend a two-tier approach: brief screening questions with high sensitivity and specificity for patients at risk, followed by a referral for a more detailed investigation when indicated.

Patient Indicators for Mental Health Screening

- Medically unexplained physical symptoms—more than half have a depression or anxiety disorder
- Multiple physical or somatic symptoms or "high symptom count"
- High severity of the presenting somatic symptom
- Chronic pain
- Symptoms for more than 6 weeks
- Rating as a "difficult encounter"
- Recent stress
- Low self-rating of health
- High use of health care services
- Substance abuse

Chronic pain may be a spectrum disorder in patients with anxiety, depression, or somatic symptoms.

High-Yield Screening Questions for Patients (follow-up systems for diagnosis and treatment are needed)

Depression[8]
- Over the past 2 weeks, have you felt down, depressed, or hopeless?
- Over the past 2 weeks, have you felt little interest or pleasure in doing things (anhedonia)?

Anxiety[9–11]

- Anxiety disorders include generalized anxiety disorder, social phobia, panic disorder, post-traumatic stress disorder, and acute stress disorder.
- Over the past 2 weeks, have you been feeling nervous, anxious, or on edge?
- Over the past 2 weeks, have you been unable to stop or control worrying?
- Over the past 4 weeks, have you had an anxiety attack—suddenly feeling fear or panic?

Substance-Related and Addictive Disorders

- CAGE questions adapted for alcohol and drug abuse—see Chapter 4, The Health History, pp. 74–75.

THE HEALTH HISTORY

Common or Concerning Symptoms

- Changes in attention, mood, or speech
- Changes in insight, orientation, or memory
- Delirium or dementia

As with the General Survey, your assessment of mental status begins when you first meet with the patient. As you gather the health history, you will quickly observe the patient's level of alertness and orientation, mood, attention, and memory. As the history unfolds, you will learn about the patient's insight and judgment, as well as any recurring or unusual thoughts or perceptions. These and other components of mood and cognition will alert you to conditions that require more detailed follow-up, including a formal mental status examination and possible referral.

Many of the terms pertinent to the mental health history and the mental status examination are familiar to you from social conversation. It is important to learn their precise meanings in the context of formal evaluation of mental status, as detailed in the next table.

Terminology: The Mental Status Examination

Level of Consciousness	Alertness or State of Awareness of the Environment
Attention	The ability to focus or concentrate over time on one task or activity—an inattentive or distractible person with impaired consciousness has difficulty giving a history or responding to questions

Memory	The process of registering or recording information, tested by asking for immediate repetition of material, followed by storage or retention of information. Recent or short-term memory covers minutes, hours, or days; remote or long-term memory refers to intervals of years.
Orientation	Awareness of personal identity, place, and time; requires both memory and attention
Perceptions	Sensory awareness of objects in the environment and their interrelationships (external stimuli); also refers to internal stimuli such as dreams or hallucinations
Thought processes	The logic, coherence, and relevance of the patient's thought as it leads to selected goals, or how people think
Thought content	What the patient thinks about, including level of insight and judgment
Insight	Awareness that symptoms or disturbed behaviors are normal or abnormal; for example, distinguishing between daydreams and hallucinations that seem real
Judgment	Process of comparing and evaluating alternatives when deciding on a course of action; reflects values that may or may not be based on reality and social conventions or norms
Affect	An observable, usually episodic, feeling or tone expressed through voice, facial expression, and demeanor
Mood	A more sustained emotion that may color a person's view of the world (mood is to affect as climate is to weather)
Language	A complex symbolic system for expressing, receiving, and comprehending words; as with consciousness, attention, and memory, language is essential for assessing other mental functions.
Higher cognitive functions	Assessed by vocabulary, amount of information, abstract thinking, calculations, and construction of objects that have two or three dimensions

Attention, Mood, Speech; Insight, Orientation, Memory

Assess the patient's level of consciousness; general appearance; mood, including depression or mania; and ability to pay attention, remember, understand, and speak. Place the patient's vocabulary and general knowledge and

See Chapter 20, The Nervous System, Table 20-9, Disorders of Speech, p. 738.

information in the context of his or her cultural and educational background. The patient's account of illness and life circumstances often tell you about insight and judgment. If you suspect a problem in orientation and memory, you can ask, "Let's see, your last clinic appointment was when … ?" "And the date today?" Try to integrate your evaluation of mental status into the history, and it will seem less like an interrogation. The flow comes more easily with practice and interactions with a variety of patients.

Neurocognitive Disorders: Delirium, Major and Minor Neurocognitive Disorders

Delirium presents in varying states related to the metabolic or structural brain alteration in which there is a fluctuation of symptoms, such as in alertness or attention. Delirium is considered a separate classification of neurocognitive disorders.

Neurocognitive disorders, other than delirium, are divided into two categories, a major cognitive disorder, in which dementia is now classified, and a less severe level of cognitive impairment, now termed, mild neurocognitive disorder, which applies to younger individuals with impairment from traumatic brain injury or HIV infection. These varying levels and re-configurations have impacted clinicians on many levels from education of patients to reimbursement for care.

The term *dementia* is to be documented in parenthesis due to widespread clinical usage.

Major cognitive disorder (dementia)

A wide range of patients in clinical practice warrant assessment of mental status: patients with a brain injury, psychiatric symptoms, or reports from family members of vague or changed behavior, patients with subtle behavioral changes, difficulty taking medications as prescribed, problems attending to household chores or paying bills, or loss of interest in their usual activities. Other patients may have changes related to the hospitalization or medications and behave differently or have a change in orientation after surgery or during an acute illness. Each change should be identified and assessed as expeditiously as possible. The nurse is the patient advocate, and the person who with prompt assessment alleviates unexpected problems that can impact the patient and family on many levels (relationships, financial).

See Table 24-1, Delirium and Dementia, p. 975.

May be signs of depression or dementia

PHYSICAL EXAMINATION

Important Areas of the Mental Status Examination

The assessment of mental status is challenging and complex. Changes in mental status warrant careful evaluation for underlying pathologic and pharmacologic causes. The patient's personality, psychodynamics, family and life experiences, and cultural background all factor into the mental status assessment. The nervous system, mental status, and brain structure and function are intimately intertwined. The assessment of mental status is an integral component of the assessment of the nervous system, and the first segment of the nervous system write-up. With practice, you will learn to describe the patient's mood, speech, behavior, and cognition and relate these findings to your examination of the cranial nerves, motor and sensory systems, and reflexes.

Novice nurses may feel reluctant to perform mental status examinations, wondering if it will upset patients or invade their privacy. Such concerns are understandable. An insensitive examination may alarm a patient, and even a skillful examination may bring to conscious awareness a deficit that the patient is trying to ignore. Discuss concerns with your instructor or other experienced nurses. Remember that patients appreciate an understanding listener.

The mental status examination consists of five components:

- Appearance and behavior

- Speech and language

- Mood

- Thoughts and perceptions

- Cognitive function, which includes orientation, memory, attention, and higher cognitive functions such as information and vocabulary, calculations, abstract thinking, and constructional ability

The format should help to organize your observations, but it is not intended as a step-by-step guide. When a full examination is indicated, be flexible in approach but thorough. In some situations, however, sequence is important. If, during the initial interview, the patient's consciousness, attention, comprehension of words or ability to speak seems impaired, assess this attribute promptly. If a patient cannot give a reliable history, testing most of the other mental functions will be difficult and warrants an evaluation for acute causes.

Appearance and Behavior

Utilize all the relevant observations made throughout the course of the history and examination. Include these areas:

Level of Consciousness

Is the patient awake and alert? Does the patient seem to understand the questions and respond appropriately and reasonably quickly, or is there a tendency to lose track of the topic and fall silent or even asleep?

If the patient does not respond to your questions, escalate the stimulus in steps:

- Speak to the patient by name and in a loud voice.

Lethargic patients are drowsy but open their eyes and look at you, respond to questions, and then fall asleep.

- Shake the patient gently, as if awakening a sleeper.

Obtunded patients open their eyes and look at you, but respond slowly and are somewhat confused.

- If there is no response to these stimuli, promptly assess the patient for stupor or coma—severe reductions in level of consciousness.

Stuporous patients are unaware of surroundings and are totally or almost totally immobile and unresponsive, even to painful stimuli.

Comatose patients are unconscious and do not respond to painful stimuli or voice and do not open their eyes.

Posture and Motor Behavior

Does the patient sit or lie quietly or prefer to walk around? Observe the patient's posture and ability to relax. Note the pace, range, and type of movement. Are the movements voluntary, spontaneous, and fluid? Are any limbs immobile, flaccid, or fixed in position? Are posture and motor activity affected by topics under discussion, type of activity, or who is in the room?

Look for tense posture, restlessness, and anxious fidgeting; the crying, pacing, and hand wringing of agitated depression; the hopeless, slumped posture, and slowed movements of depression; the agitated and expansive movements of a manic episode

Dress, Grooming, and Personal Hygiene

How is the patient dressed? Is the clothing clean and appropriate for patient's age and the weather? Note the grooming of the patient's hair, nails, teeth, skin, and, if present, beard. How does the grooming and hygiene compare with peers of comparable age, lifestyle, culture, and socioeconomic group? Compare one side of the body with the other.

Grooming and personal hygiene may deteriorate in depression, schizophrenia, and dementia. Excessive fastidiousness may be seen in obsessive–compulsive disorder. One-sided neglect may result from a lesion in the opposite parietal cortex, usually the nondominant side.

Facial Expression

Observe the face, both at rest and when communicating with others. Watch for variations in expression with topics under discussion. Are they appropriate for the topics being discussed? Or is the face relatively immobile throughout?

Note expressions of anxiety, depression, apathy, anger, elation; facial immobility as seen in Parkinson disease.

Look for the anger, hostility, suspiciousness, or evasiveness of patients with paranoia; the elation and euphoria of mania; the flat affect and remoteness of schizophrenia; the apathy (dulled affect with detachment and indifference) of dementia; and anxiety or depression.

Manner, Affect, and Relationship to People and Things

Using your observations of facial expressions, voice, and body movements, assess the patient's affect, or external expression of the inner emotional state. Does it vary appropriately with topics under discussion, or is the affect labile, blunted, or flat? Does it seem inappropriate or extreme at certain points? If so, how? Note the patient's openness, approachability, and reactions to others and to the surroundings. Does the patient seem to hear or see things that you do not or seem to be conversing with someone who is not there?

Speech and Language

Throughout the interview, note the characteristics of the patient's speech, including the following:

Quantity

Is the patient talkative or silent? Is this a change? Is this related to cultural background? Are comments spontaneous or limited to direct questions?

Rate

Is speech fast or slow?

Loudness

Is speech loud or soft?

Note the slow speech of depression; the accelerated, louder speech of mania

Articulation of Words

Are the words clear and distinct? Does the speech have a nasal quality? Dysarthria refers to defective articulation. Aphasia is a disorder of language. Dysphonia results from impaired volume, quality, or pitch of the voice. See Chapter 20, The Nervous System, Table 20-9, Disorders of Speech, p. 738.

Fluency

Fluency reflects the rate, flow, and melody of speech and the content and use of words. Watch for abnormalities of spontaneous speech such as:

- Hesitancies and gaps in the flow and rhythm of words

- Disturbed inflections, such as a monotone

- Circumlocutions, in which phrases or sentences are substituted for a word the person cannot think of, such as "what you write with" for "pen"

- Paraphasias, in which words are malformed ("I write with a den"), wrong ("I write with a bar"), or invented ("I write with a dar")

These abnormalities suggest aphasia from cerebrovascular infarction. Aphasia may be receptive (impaired comprehension with fluent speech) or expressive (with preserved comprehension and slow nonfluent speech). If the patient's speech lacks meaning or fluency, proceed with further testing as outlined in the following table.

Testing for Aphasia	
Word Comprehension	Ask the patient to follow a one-stage command, such as "Point to your nose." Try a two-stage command: "Point to your mouth, then your knee."
Repetition	Ask the patient to repeat a phrase of one-syllable words (the most difficult repetition task): "No ifs, ands, or buts."
Naming	Ask the patient to name the parts of a watch.
Reading Comprehension	Ask the patient to read a paragraph aloud.
Writing	Ask the patient to write a sentence.

These questions help identify the type of aphasia. Check for deficits in vision, hearing, intelligence, and education which may affect responses. Two common kinds of aphasia—receptive (Wernicke's) and expressive (Broca's)—are compared in Table 20-9, Disorders of Speech, p. 738.

A person who can write a correct sentence does not have aphasia.

Mood

Ask the person to describe his or her mood, including usual mood level and how it has varied with life events. "How did you feel about that?," for example, or, more generally, "How is your overall mood?" The reports of relatives and friends may be of great value.

Moods include sadness and deep melancholy; contentment, joy, euphoria, and elation; anger and rage; anxiety and worry; and detachment and indifference.

Has the mood been intense and unchanging, or labile? How long has it lasted? Is it appropriate to the patient's circumstances or situation? If depressed, have there been episodes of an elevated mood, suggesting a bipolar disorder?

If you suspect depression, assess its severity and any risk of suicide. The following series of questions is useful, proceeding as far as the patient's positive answers warrant:

- Do you feel discouraged (or depressed or blue)?

- How low do you feel?

- What do you see for yourself in the future?

- Do you ever feel that life isn't worth living? Or that you want to be dead?

- Have you ever thought of killing yourself?

- How did (do) you think you would do it? Do you have a plan?

- What do you think would happen after you were dead?

Asking about suicidal thoughts does not implant the idea in the patient's mind, and it may be the only way to get the information. Although you may feel uneasy about direct questions, most patients discuss their thoughts and feelings freely, sometimes with considerable relief. By open discussion, you demonstrate your interest and concern for a possibly life-threatening problem. It is your responsibility to ask directly about suicidal thoughts. This may be the only way to uncover suicidal ideation and plans that launch immediate intervention and treatment.

Thought and Perceptions

Thought Processes

Assess the logic, relevance, organization, and coherence of the patient's thought processes throughout the interview. Does speech progress logically toward a goal? Listen for patterns of speech that suggest disorders of thought processes, as outlined in the table below.

Variations and Abnormalities in Thought Processes		
Circumstantiality	Speech with unnecessary detail, indirection, and delay in reaching the point. Some topics may have a meaningful connection. People without mental disorders may have circumstantial speech.	This occurs in people with obsessions.
Blocking	Sudden interruption of speech in midsentence or before the idea is completed, attributed to "losing the thought." Blocking occurs in normal people.	Seen in schizophrenia, manic episodes, and other psychotic disorders.
Flight of Ideas	An almost continuous flow of accelerated speech with abrupt changes from one topic to the next. Changes are based on understandable associations, plays on words, or distracting stimuli, but ideas are not well connected.	Most frequently noted in manic episodes.
Confabulation	Fabrication of facts or events in response to questions, to fill in the gaps from impaired memory.	Observed dementia, in schizophrenia, psychotic disorders, and aphasia.
Incoherence	Speech that is incomprehensible and illogic, with lack of meaningful connections, abrupt changes in topic, or disordered grammar or word use. Flight of ideas, when severe, may produce incoherence.	Observed in severe psychotic disturbances (usually schizophrenia).
Derailment (loosening of associations)	"Tangential" speech with shifting topics that are loosely connected or unrelated. The patient is unaware of the lack of association.	Derailment may be striking in schizophrenia.

(continued)

Neologisms	Invented or distorted words, or words with new and highly idiosyncratic meanings	Seen in Korsakoff syndrome from alcoholism.
Perseveration	Persistent repetition of words or ideas	Occurs in schizophrenia and other psychotic disorders.
Echolalia	Repetition of the words and phrases of others	Occurs in manic episodes and schizophrenia.
Clanging	Speech with choice of words based on sound rather than meaning, as in rhyming and punning. For example, "Look at my eyes and nose, wise eyes and rosy nose. Two to one, the ayes have it!"	Occurs in schizophrenia and manic episodes.

Thought Content

Thought content is what the person is thinking and is assessed during the interaction. To assess thought content, follow appropriate leads as they occur rather than asking scripted lists of specific questions. For example, "You mentioned that a neighbor was responsible for your entire illness. Can you tell me more about that?" Or, in another situation, "What do you think about at times like these?"

For more focused inquiries, be tactful and accepting. "When people are upset like this, sometimes they can't keep certain thoughts out of their minds," or "... things seem unreal. Have you experienced anything like this?"

Perceptions

Inquire about false perceptions in a manner similar to that used for thought content. For example, "When you heard the voice speaking to you, what did it say? How did it make you feel?" Or, "After you've been drinking a lot, do you ever see things that aren't really there?" Or, "Sometimes after major surgery like this, people hear peculiar or frightening things. Has anything like this ever happened to you?" In these ways, find out about abnormal perceptions.

Abnormalities of Perception[12]		
Illusions	Misinterpretations of real external stimuli, such as mistaking rustling leaves for the sound of voices	Illusions may occur in grief reactions, delirium, acute and posttraumatic stress disorders, and schizophrenia.
Hallucinations	Perception-like experiences that seem real, but unlike illusions, lack actual external stimulation. The person may or may not recognize the experiences as false. Hallucinations may be auditory, visual, olfactory, gustatory, tactile, or somatic. False perceptions associated with dreaming, falling asleep, and awakening are not classified as hallucinations.	Hallucinations may occur in delirium, dementia (less commonly), posttraumatic stress disorder, schizophrenia, and alcoholism.

Insight and Judgment

Insight is the ability to understand a situation and is often intuitive. Judgement is the ability to make a good decision after careful thought. These attributes are usually best assessed during the interview.

Insight

Some of the first interview questions to the patient often yield important information about insight: "What brings you to the hospital?" "What seems to be the trouble?" "What do you think is wrong?" Note whether the patient is aware that a particular mood, thought, or perception is abnormal or part of an illness.

Patients with psychotic disorders often lack insight into their illness. Denial of impairment may accompany some neurologic disorders.

Judgment

Assess judgment by noting the patient's responses to family situations, jobs, use of money, and interpersonal conflicts. "How do you plan to get the help you'll need after leaving the hospital?" "How are you going to manage if you lose your job?" "If your husband starts to abuse you again, what will you do?" "Who will attend to your financial affairs while you are in the nursing home?"

Judgment may be poor in delirium, dementia, intellectual disabilities, and psychotic states. Anxiety, mood disorders, intelligence, education, income, and cultural values also influence judgment.

Note whether decisions and actions are based on reality or impulse, wish fulfillment, or disordered thought content. What insights and values seem to underlie the patient's decisions and behavior? Allowing for cultural variations, how do these compare with mature adult standards? Because judgment reflects maturity, it may be variable and unpredictable during adolescence.

Poor judgment may occur when memory or attention is impaired, as in delirium.

Cognitive Functions

Orientation

The patient's orientation can usually be determined in the context of the interview. For example, you can naturally ask for clarification about specific dates and times, the patient's address and telephone number, the names of family members, or the route taken or why they are in the hospital. At times, direct questions are necessary to determine if the person is oriented to all four components as described below.

- Person—the patient's own name, and the names of relatives and professional personnel

  "Can you tell me your name?"

- Place—the patient's residence, city, and state

  "What is your address?"

- Time—the time of day, day of the week, month, season, date and year, duration of hospitalization

  "Can you tell me what time it is now? ... and what day it is?"

- Situation—what just happened/is happening (frequently used after an accident or anesthesia)

  "Can you tell me what just happened?"

- When choosing the questions, be sure you know the correct answer or be able to validate the answer. Otherwise, the person may answer appropriately; however, it may or may not be correct.

Attention

These tests of attention are commonly used:

Digit Span

Explain that you would like to test the patient's ability to concentrate, perhaps adding that this can be difficult if the patient is in pain, or ill. Recite a series of numbers, starting with two at a time and speaking each number clearly at a rate of about one per second. Ask the patient to repeat the numbers back to you. If this repetition is accurate, try a series of three numbers, then four, as long as the patient responds correctly. Jot down the numbers as you say them to ensure your own accuracy. If the patient makes a mistake, try once more with another series of the same length. Stop after a second failure in a single series.

When choosing digits you may use street numbers, zip codes, telephone numbers, and other numerical sequences that are familiar to you, but avoid consecutive numbers, easily recognized dates, and sequences that possibly are familiar to the patient.

Now, starting again with a series of two, ask the patient to repeat the numbers to you backward.

Normally, a person should be able to repeat correctly at least five numbers forward and four backward.

Causes of poor performance include delirium, dementia, intellectual disability, and performance anxiety.

Serial 7s

Instruct the patient, "Starting from a hundred, subtract 7, and keep subtracting 7...." Note the effort required and the speed and accuracy of the responses. After five correct answers, the patient has a positive serial 7 response. Writing down the answers helps you keep up with the arithmetic. Normally, a person can complete serial 7s in 1½ minutes, with fewer than four errors. If the patient cannot do serial 7s, try 3s or counting backward.

Poor performance may result from delirium, the late stage of dementia, intellectual disability, loss of calculating ability, anxiety, or depression. Also consider educational level.

Spelling Backward

This can substitute for serial 7s. Say a five-letter word, spell it, for example, W-O-R-L-D, and ask the patient to spell it backward.

Remote Memory

Inquire about birthdays, anniversaries, social security number, names of schools attended, jobs held, or past historical events such as wars relevant to the patient's past.

Remote memory may be impaired in the late stage of dementia.

Recent Memory

This can involve the events of the day. Ask questions with answers you can check against other sources to see if the patient is confabulating or making up facts to compensate for a defective memory. These might include the day's weather, today's appointment time, and medications or laboratory tests taken during the day. Asking what the patient had for breakfast may be a waste of time unless you can check the accuracy of the answer.

Recent memory is impaired in dementia and delirium. Amnestic disorders impair memory or new learning ability significantly and reduce a person's social or occupational functioning, but they do not have the global features of delirium or dementia. Anxiety, depression, and intellectual disability may also impair recent memory.

New Learning Ability

Give the patient three or four words such as "table, flower, purple, and hamburger." Ask the patient to repeat them so that you know that the information has been heard and registered. This step, like digit span, tests retention of information and immediate recall. Then proceed to other parts of the examination. After about 3 to 5 minutes, ask the patient to repeat the words. Note the accuracy of the response, awareness of whether it is correct, and any tendency to confabulate. Normally, a person should be able to remember the words.

Higher Cognitive Functions

Information and Vocabulary

If observed clinically in the context of cultural and educational background, information and vocabulary provide a rough estimate of the patient's baseline abilities. Begin assessing the patient's knowledge and vocabulary, during the interview. Ask about work, hobbies, reading, favorite television programs, or current events. Start with simple questions, then to more difficult questions. Note the person's grasp of information, the complexity of the ideas, and choice of vocabulary.

Information and vocabulary are relatively unaffected by psychiatric disorders except in the most severe cases. Testing may help distinguish adults with life-long intellectual impairment (whose information and vocabulary are limited) from those with mild or moderate dementia (whose information and vocabulary are fairly well preserved).

More directly, you can ask about specific facts such as:

- The name of the president, vice president, or governor

- The names of the last four or five presidents

- The names of five large cities in the country

Calculating Ability

Test the patient's ability to do arithmetic calculations, starting at the rote level with simple addition ("What is 4 + 3? ... 8 + 7?") and multiplication ("What is 5 × 6? ... 9 × 7?"). Proceed to more difficult tasks by using two-digit numbers ("15 + 12" or "25 × 6") or longer, written examples.

Poor performance suggests dementia or aphasia, but measured against knowledge and education. Alternatively, pose practical and functionally important questions, such as "If something costs 78 cents and you give the clerk a dollar bill, how much money should you get back?"

Abstract Thinking

Test the capacity to think abstractly in two ways.

Proverbs

Ask the patient what the following proverbs mean:

> People who live in glass houses should not throw stones.
> Don't count your chickens before they're hatched.
> A rolling stone gathers no moss.
> The squeaky wheel gets the grease.

Concrete responses are often given by people with an intellectual disability, delirium, or dementia but may also be a function of limited education, culture, or exposure. Patients with schizophrenia may respond concretely or with personal, bizarre interpretations.

Note the relevance of the answers and their degree of concreteness or abstractness. For example, "Don't throw stones at glass or it will break" is concrete, whereas "Someone who repeatedly does something (e.g., is late) should not criticize someone else when they are late" is abstract. Average patients should give abstract or semiabstract responses.

Similarities

Ask the patient to tell you how the following are alike:

> An orange and an apple   A church and a theater
> A cat and a mouse   A piano and a violin
> A child and a dwarf   Wood and coal

Note the accuracy and relevance of the answers and their degree of concreteness or abstractness. For example, "A cat and a mouse are both animals" is abstract, "They both have tails" is concrete, and "A cat chases a mouse" is not relevant.

Constructional Ability

The task here is to copy figures of increasing complexity onto a piece of blank unlined paper. Show each figure one at a time and ask the patient to copy it as well as possible.

The three diamonds below are rated poor, fair, and good (but not excellent).[13]

In another approach, ask the patient to draw a clock face complete with numbers and hands. The example below is rated excellent.

These three clocks are poor, fair, and good.[13]

If vision and motor ability are intact, poor constructional ability suggests dementia or parietal lobe damage. Cognitive disability may also impair performance.

SPECIAL TECHNIQUES

Mini-Mental State Examination (MMSE)

The Mini-Mental State Examination is a brief questionnaire which has been widely used to screen patients for cognitive dysfunction or dementia. Patients are asked a series of questions in regard to orientation, registration, attention and calculation, recall, language and the ability to follow simple instructions. The MMSE follows mental ability/decline over time and can be used in patients who are fluent in English and have a minimum of at an 8th grade education. The maximum score is 30 points and as cognition declines so does the score. A person with 0 to 17 points would have severe cognitive impairment.[14]

Although several versions are available on the internet, copyright permission for use and reproduction is required. More detailed information regarding the MMSE can be found through a variety of sources online (http://www4.parinc.com/Products/Product.aspx?ProductID= MMSE and http://www.dementiatoday.com/wp-content/uploads/ 2012/06/MiniMentalStateExamination.pdf).

RECORDING YOUR FINDINGS

Recording Behavior and Mental Status

"Mental Status: Alert and Oriented to person, place, time, and situation, well groomed, cheerful. Speech fluent, words clear. Thought processes coherent, insight intact. Serial 7s accurate; recent and remote memory intact. Calculations intact."

OR

"Mental Status: O × 2 (person and place). Appears sad, fatigued; clothes wrinkled. Speech slow, words mumbled. Thought processes coherent but insight into current life problems is limited. Digit span, serial 7s, and calculations accurate but responses delayed. Clock drawing appropriate."

Alert and Oriented to person, place, time, and situation can be abbreviated: A&O×4

Suggests depression

HEALTH PROMOTION AND COUNSELING

Important Topics for Health Promotion and Counseling

- Screening for depression
- Screening for suicide risk
- Screening for substance use disorders, including alcohol and prescription drugs

All screening tools need to be age appropriate.

Mental health disorders impose a significant burden of suffering. About 1 in 5 U.S. adults (43.6 million) experience mental illness in a given year, with about 1 in 25 (9.8 million) experiencing serious mental illness (schizophrenia, major depression, or bipolar disorder). Depression and anxiety disorders are a common cause of hospitalization in the United States, and mental illness is associated with increased risks for chronic medical conditions, decreased life expectancy, disability, substance abuse, and suicide.[2]

The graph depicts mental, behavioral, or emotional disorders (excluding developmental and substance use disorders).[15]

See Chapter 4, The Health History, p. 83.

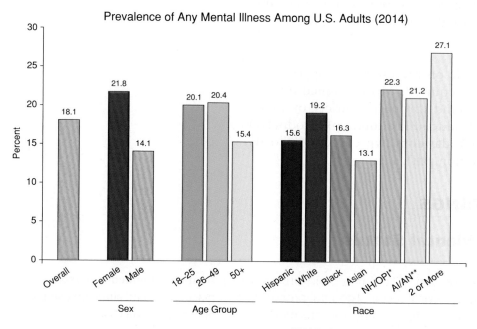

Prevalence of Any Mental Illness Among U.S. Adults (2014)

*NH/OPI = Native Hawaiian/Other Pacific Islander
**AI/AN = American Indian/Alaska Native

Depression

About 16 million adult Americans, or almost 7%, have major depression, often with coexisting anxiety disorders and substance abuse. Depression is nearly twice as common in women as men; the prevalence of postpartum

depression is 7% to 13%.[2] Depression frequently accompanies chronic medical illness. High-risk patients may have subtle early signs of depression, including low self-esteem, loss of pleasure in daily activities (anhedonia), sleep disorders, and difficulty concentrating or making decisions. Look carefully for symptoms of depression in vulnerable patients, especially those who are young, female, single, divorced or separated, seriously or chronically ill, bereaved, or have other psychiatric disorders, including substance abuse. A personal or family history of depression also places patients at risk.

The U.S. Preventive Services Task Force is under review and the latest draft recommends screening in clinical settings that can provide accurate diagnosis, treatment, and follow-up.[16] A positive test response has a sensitivity of 83% and a specificity of 92% for detecting major depression.[17] All positive screening tests warrant full diagnostic interviews. Failure to diagnose depression can have fatal consequences—the presence of an affective disorder is associated with an 11-fold increased risk for suicide.[17]

Suicide

Preventing suicide is a national public health initiative. Suicide now ranks as the 10th leading cause of death in the United States, accounting for nearly 40,000 deaths. Annually, there are almost 13 completed suicides per 100,000 population.[18] Suicide is the second leading cause of death among 15 to 24 year olds. Suicide rates are highest among those aged 45 to 54 years, followed by elderly adults 85 years of age or older. Men have suicide success rates nearly four times higher than women, though women are three times more likely to attempt suicide. Men are most likely to use firearms to commit suicide, while women are most likely to use poison. Overall, suicides in non-Hispanic whites account for about 90% of all suicides, though American Indian/Alaska Native women ages 15 to 24 years old have the highest suicide rates of any racial/ethnic group. An estimated 25 attempts are made for each death by suicide, with ratios of 100 to 1 to 200 to 1 among young adults. In 2013, nearly 17% of U.S. high school students reported that they had seriously considered attempting suicide in the previous year. Nurses are often the first in contact with a person contemplating suicide. Pursue any clinical suspicion of suicide by asking patients directly about suicidal ideation and plans. Refer at-risk patients immediately for psychiatric care.[19,20]

Substance Use Disorders, Including Alcohol and Prescription Drugs

The interactions and comorbidity of alcohol and substance use disorders and suicide are both extensive and profound. Alcohol, tobacco, and illicit drugs account for more illness, deaths, and disabilities than any other preventable condition. The 2014 National Survey on Drug Use and Health showed that 139.7 million people over the age of 12 in the United States drank in the past month, 60.9 million people admitted to binge drinking, and 16.3 million were heavy drinkers.[2]

Over 27 million Americans reported use of an illicit drug during the month before the survey, including nearly 22 million marijuana users, followed by 4.3 million users of prescription drugs for nonmedicinal indications as the second leading used illicit drug.[2] Nearly 22 million persons aged 12 or older were classified as having a substance use disorder based on Diagnostic and Statistical Manual of Mental Disorders (DSM-IV) criteria. Only about 2.5 million of these individuals received treatment at a specialty facility for an illicit drug or alcohol problem. Rates of drug-induced deaths continue to increase and are highest among whites and American Indian/Alaska Natives. The Centers for Disease Control and Prevention reports that prescription drugs have replaced illicit drugs as a leading cause of drug-induced deaths.[21] Every patient should be asked about alcohol use, substance abuse, and misuse of prescription drugs.

See Chapter 4, The Health History, Alcohol and Illicit Drugs, pp. 74–75. See also Chapter 16, The Gastrointestinal System and Renal Systems, Screening for Alcohol Abuse, pp. 510–512.

BIBLIOGRAPHY

CITATIONS

1. Olfson M, Kroenke K, Wang S. Trends in office-based mental health care provided by psychiatrists and primary care physicians. *J Clin Psychiatry.* 2014;75:247.

2. Center for Behavioral Health Statistics and Quality. Behavioral health trends in the United States: Results from the 2014 National Survey on Drug Use and Health. Health and Human Services SMA 15–4927, NSDUH Series H-50. Available at http://www.samhsa.gov/data. Accessed December 10, 2015.

3. Hepner KA, Rowe M, Rost K, et al. The effect of adherence to practice guidelines on depression outcomes. *Ann Int Med.* 2007;147:320.

4. Gonzalez HM, Vega WA, Williams DR, et al. Depression care in the United States: too little for too few. *Arch Gen Psychiatry.* 2010;67:37.

5. Williams DR, González HM, Neighbors H. Prevalence and distribution of major depressive disorder in African Americans, Caribbean blacks, and non-Hispanic whites: results from the National Survey of American Life. *Arch Gen Psychiatry.* 2007;64:305.

6. Kroenke K. Unburdening the difficult clinical encounter. *Arch Intern Med.* 2009;169:333.

7. Kroenke K. A practical and evidence-based approach to common symptoms: a narrative review. *Ann Intern Med.* 2014;161:579.

8. U.S. Preventive Services Task Force. Screening for depression: recommendations and rationale. December 2009. Available at http://www.uspreventiveservicestaskforce.org/Page/Document/RecommendationStatementFinal/depression-in-adults-screening. Accessed December 9, 2015.

9. Kroenke K, Spitzer RL, Williams JB, et al. An ultra-brief screening scale for anxiety and depression: the PHQ-4. *Psychosomatics.* 2009;50:613.

10. Spitzer RL, Kroenke K, Williams JB, et al. A brief measure for assessing generalized anxiety disorder: the GAD 7. *Arch Int Med.* 2006;166:1092.

11. Kroenke K, Spitzer RL, Williams JB, et al. Anxiety disorders in primary care: prevalence, impairment, comorbidity, and detection. *Ann Int Med.* 2007;146:317.

12. American Psychiatric Association. *Diagnostic and Statistical Manual of Mental Disorders.* 5th Ed. Washington, DC: American Psychiatric Press; 2013.

13. Louis ED, Mayer SA, Rowland LP. *Merritt's Neurology.* 13th ed. Philadelphia, PA: Wolters Kluwer; 2015.

14. Folstein MF, Folstein SE, McHugh PR. "'Mini-mental state'. A practical method for grading the cognitive state of patients for the clinician." *J Psychiatr Res.* 1975;12(3):189–198.

15. National Institutes of Mental Health. *Any Mood Disorder Among Adult.* Available at http://www.nimh.nih.gov/health/statistics/prevalence/any-mental-illness-ami-among-us-adults.shtml. Accessed March 11, 2016.

16. U.S. Preventive Services Task Force. Screening for depression in adults: draft recommendations. August 2015. Available at http://www.uspreventiveservicestaskforce.org/Page/Document/UpdateSummaryDraft/depression-in-adults-screening1. Accessed December 10, 2015.

17. Kroenke K, Spitzer RL, Williams JB. The PHQ-9 Validity of Brief Depression Severity Measure. *J Gen Intern Med.* 2001;16(9):606–613.

18. Maurer DM. Screening for Depression. *Am Fam Physician.* 2012;85(2):139–144. Available at http://www.cdc.gov/nchs/fastats/leading-causes-of-death.htm. Accessed December 10, 2015.

19. Bolster C, Holliday C, Oneal G, et al. Suicide assessment and nurses: what does the evidence show?. *Online J Issues Nurs.* 2015;20(1):2.

20. Bethel J. Assessment of suicidal intent in emergency care. *Nurs Stand.* 2013;28(4):52–58.

21. Center for Disease Control. Prescription painkiller use in the US. Available at http://www.cdc.gov/vitalsigns/Painkiller-Overdoses/index.html. Accessed December 10, 2015.

The Nervous System

The student will:

1. Describe the structure and function of the nervous system.
2. Obtain an accurate history of the neurologic system.
3. Identify the cranial nerves and the motor and sensory functions.
4. Perform a screening neurologic examination.
5. Describe the use of the Glasgow Coma Scale in an unresponsive patient.
6. Document the finding of the nervous system examination.
7. Discuss risk reduction and health promotion strategies to reduce strokes.

Evaluation of the cranial nerves, the motor system, the sensory system, and the reflexes is the focus of this chapter. The complex anatomy and physiology of the nervous system make examination and assessment especially challenging but attainable with practice and dedication. For many of the body systems, the history provides the essential clues to diagnosis. While this is true for the nervous system, the neurologic examination allows you to assess the involvement of all levels of the nervous system.[1]

ANATOMY AND PHYSIOLOGY

Central Nervous System

The Brain

The brain has four regions: the cerebrum, the diencephalon, the brainstem, and the cerebellum. Each cerebral hemisphere is subdivided into frontal, parietal, temporal, and occipital lobes, as shown on the next page.

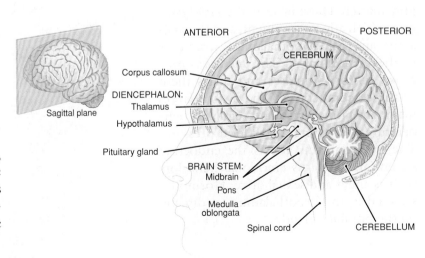

ANTERIOR   POSTERIOR

CEREBRUM

Corpus callosum

DIENCEPHALON:
  Thalamus
  Hypothalamus

Sagittal plane

Pituitary gland

BRAIN STEM:
  Midbrain
  Pons
  Medulla oblongata

Spinal cord   CEREBELLUM

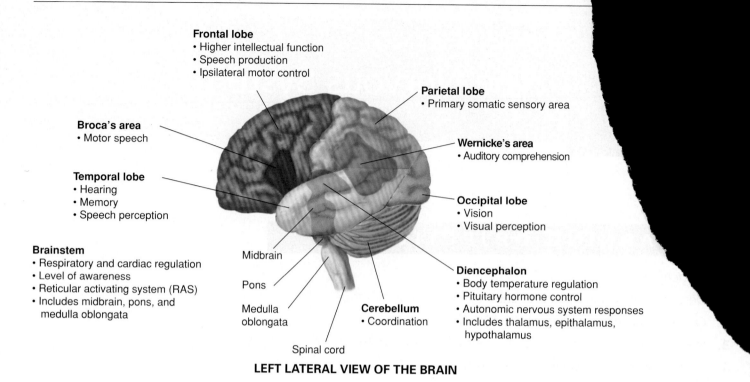

Frontal lobe
• Higher intellectual function
• Speech production
• Ipsilateral motor control

Parietal lobe
• Primary somatic sensory area

Broca's area
• Motor speech

Wernicke's area
• Auditory comprehension

Temporal lobe
• Hearing
• Memory
• Speech perception

Occipital lobe
• Vision
• Visual perception

Brainstem
• Respiratory and cardiac regulation
• Level of awareness
• Reticular activating system (RAS)
• Includes midbrain, pons, and medulla oblongata

Midbrain

Pons

Medulla oblongata

Cerebellum
• Coordination

Diencephalon
• Body temperature regulation
• Pituitary hormone control
• Autonomic nervous system responses
• Includes thalamus, epithalamus, hypothalamus

Spinal cord

LEFT LATERAL VIEW OF THE BRAIN

The central nervous system (CNS) of the brain is a vast network of interconnecting nerve cells, or *neurons,* consisting of cell bodies and their *axons*—single long fibers that conduct impulses to other parts of the nervous system.

Brain tissue may be gray or white. *Gray matter* consists of aggregations of neuronal cell bodies. It rims the surfaces of the cerebral hemispheres, forming the cerebral cortex. *White matter* consists of neuronal axons that are coated with myelin. The myelin sheaths, which create the white color, allow nerve impulses to travel more rapidly.

Deep in the brain lie additional clusters of gray matter. These include the *basal ganglia,* which affect movement, and the thalamus and the hypothalamus, structures in the diencephalon. The *thalamus* processes sensory impulses and relays them to the cerebral cortex. The *hypothalamus* maintains homeostasis and regulates temperature, heart rate, and blood pressure. The hypothalamus affects the endocrine system and governs emotional behaviors such as anger and sexual drive. Hormones secreted in the hypothalamus act directly on the pituitary gland.

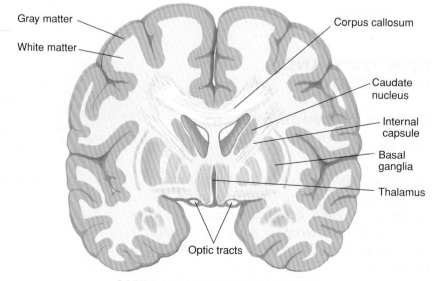

Gray matter

White matter

Corpus callosum

Caudate nucleus

Internal capsule

Basal ganglia

Thalamus

Optic tracts

CORONAL SECTION OF THE BRAIN

The *internal capsule* is a white-matter structure where myelinated fibers converge from all parts of the cerebral cortex and descend into the brainstem. The *brainstem*, which connects the upper part of the brain with the spinal cord, has three sections: the midbrain, the pons, and the medulla.

Consciousness depends on the interaction between intact cerebral hemispheres and an important structure in the diencephalon and upper brainstem, the *reticular activating (arousal) system*.

The *cerebellum*, which lies at the base of the brain, coordinates all movements and helps maintain the body upright in space.

The Spinal Cord

Below the medulla, the CNS extends itself as the elongated *spinal cord*, encased within the bony vertebral column and terminating at the first or second lumbar vertebra. The cord provides a series of segmental relays with the periphery, serving as a conduit for information flow to and from the brain. The motor and sensory nerve pathways relay neural signals that enter and exit the cord through posterior and anterior nerve roots through the spinal and peripheral nerves.

The spinal cord is divided into five segments: cervical, from C1 to C8; thoracic, from T1 to T12; lumbar, from L1 to L5; sacral, from S1 to S5; and coccygeal. The cervical spinal cord contains nerve tracts to and from both the upper and lower extremities. Note that the spinal cord is not as long as the vertebral canal. The lumbar and sacral roots travel the longest intraspinal distance and fan out like a horse's tail at L1–2, giving rise to the term *cauda equina*. To avoid injury to the spinal cord, most lumbar punctures are performed at the L3–4 or L4–5 vertebral interspaces.[2,3]

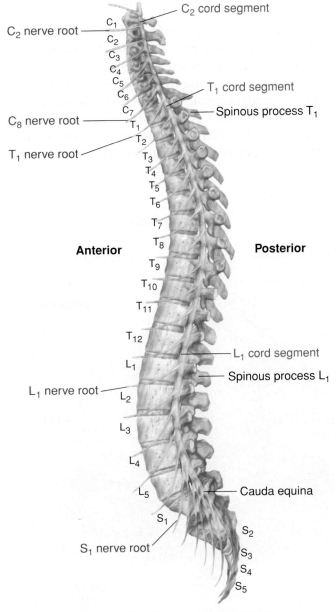

THE SPINAL CORD, LATERAL VIEW

Peripheral Nervous System

The *peripheral nervous system* (PNS) consists of both cranial nerves and peripheral nerves that supply nerve stimulus to the heart, visceral organs, skin, and limbs. It controls the *somatic nervous system,* which regulates muscle movements and response to the sensations of touch and pain, and the *autonomic nervous system* that connects to internal organs and generates autonomic reflex responses. The autonomic nervous system consists of the *sympathetic nervous system,* which "mobilizes organs and their functions during times of stress and arousal," and the *parasympathetic nervous system,* which "conserves energy and resources during times of rest and relaxation."[4]

The Cranial Nerves

Twelve pairs of special nerves called *cranial nerves* emerge from within the cranial vault through skull foramina and canals to structures in the head and neck. They are numbered sequentially with Roman numerals. Cranial nerves I and II are fiber tracts emerging from the brain. Cranial nerves III through XII arise from the diencephalon and the brainstem, as illustrated. Some cranial nerves are limited to general motor or sensory functions, whereas others are specialized and have both motor and sensory functions. Cranial nerves relevant to physical examination are summarized on the next pages.

INFERIOR SURFACE OF THE BRAIN

The Peripheral Nerves

The PNS includes spinal and peripheral nerves that carry impulses to and from the spinal cord. Thirty-one pairs of nerves attach to the spinal cord: 8 cervical, 12 thoracic, 5 lumbar, 5 sacral, and 1 coccygeal. Each nerve has an anterior (ventral) root containing motor fibers, and a posterior (dorsal) root containing sensory fibers. The anterior and posterior roots merge to form a short *spinal nerve*, less than 5 mm long. Spinal nerve fibers mix with similar fibers from other levels in plexuses outside the cord, from which *peripheral nerves emerge*. Most peripheral nerves contain both *sensory* (afferent) and *motor* (efferent) fibers.

Cranial Nerves

Number	Name	Function	Type of Impulse
I	**Olfactory**	Sense of smell	Sensory
II	**Optic**	Vision	Sensory
III	**Oculomotor**	Pupillary constriction, opening the eye (lid elevation), and most extraocular (outside the eye) movements	Motor
IV	**Trochlear**	Downward, internal rotation of the eye	Motor
V	**Trigeminal**	*Motor*—temporal and masseter muscles (jaw clenching), lateral pterygoids (lateral jaw movement) *Sensory*—facial. The nerve has three divisions: (1) ophthalmic, (2) maxillary, and (3) mandibular.	Both (motor, sensory)
VI	**Abducens**	Lateral deviation of the eye	Motor
VII	**Facial**	*Motor*—facial movements, including those of facial expression, closing the eye, and closing the mouth *Sensory*—taste for salty, sweet, sour, and bitter substances on the anterior two thirds of the tongue	Both (motor, sensory)

RIGHT EYE (CN III, IV, VI)

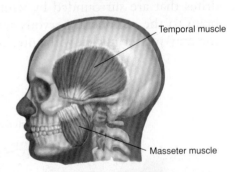

Temporal muscle

Masseter muscle

CN V—MOTOR

(1)

(2)

(3)

C2

CN V—SENSORY

(continued)

VIII	**Acoustic**	Hearing (cochlear division) and balance (vestibular division)	Sensory
IX	**Glossopharyngeal**	*Motor*—pharynx *Sensory*—posterior portions of the eardrum and ear canal, the pharynx, and the posterior tongue, including taste (salty, sweet, sour, bitter)	Both (motor, sensory)
X	**Vagus**	*Motor*—palate, pharynx, and larynx *Sensory*—pharynx and larynx	Both (motor, sensory)
XI	**Spinal accessory**	*Motor*—the sternomastoid and upper portion of the trapezius	Motor
XII	**Hypoglossal**	*Motor*—tongue	Motor

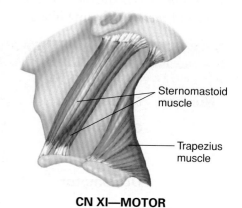

CN XI—MOTOR

Like the brain, the spinal cord contains both gray matter and white matter. The gray matter consists of an aggregation of nerve cell nuclei and dendrites that are surrounded by white tracts of nerve fibers connecting the brain to the peripheral nervous system. Note the butterfly appearance of the gray-matter nuclei, with anterior and posterior horns.

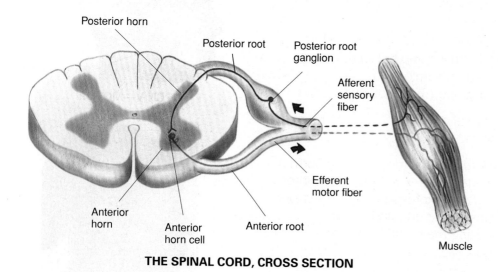

THE SPINAL CORD, CROSS SECTION

Motor Pathways

Motor pathways are complex avenues extending from *upper motor* neurons through long white-matter tracts, to synapses with lower motor neurons, and into the periphery (outward regions) through peripheral nerve structures. *Upper motor neurons* or nerve cell bodies, lie in the motor strip of the cerebral cortex and in several brainstem nuclei; their axons synapse with motor nuclei in the brainstem (for cranial nerves) and in the spinal cord (for peripheral nerves). *Lower motor neurons* have cell bodies in the spinal cord, called anterior horn cells; their axons transmit impulses through the anterior roots and spinal nerves into peripheral nerves, terminating at the neuromuscular junction.

Three kinds of motor pathways impinge on the anterior horn cells: the corticospinal tract, the basal ganglia system, and the cerebellar system. Additional pathways originating in the brainstem control flexor and extensor tone in limb movement and posture, most notably in coma (see Table 20-10, Abnormal Postures in Comatose Patients, p. 793).

The Principal Motor Pathways

- The **corticospinal (pyramidal) tract.** The corticospinal tracts control voluntary movement and integrate skilled, complicated, or delicate movements by stimulating selected muscular actions and inhibiting others. They also carry impulses that inhibit *muscle tone,* the slight tension maintained by normal muscle even when it is relaxed. The corticospinal tracts originate in the motor cortex of the brain. Motor fibers travel down into the lower medulla, where they form an anatomic structure resembling a pyramid. There, most of these fibers cross to the opposite or *contralateral* side of the medulla, continue downward, and synapse with anterior horn cells or with intermediate neurons. Tracts synapsing in the brainstem with motor nuclei of the cranial nerves are termed *corticobulbar.*
- The **basal ganglia system.** This very complex system includes motor pathways between the cerebral cortex, basal ganglia, brainstem, and spinal cord. It helps to maintain muscle tone and to control body movements, especially automatic movements such as walking.
- The **cerebellar system.** The cerebellum receives both sensory and motor input and coordinates motor activity, maintains equilibrium, and helps to control posture.

All of these higher motor pathways affect movement only through the lower motor neuron systems, sometimes called the "final common pathway." Any movement, whether initiated voluntarily in the cortex, "automatically" in the basal ganglia, or reflexively in the sensory receptors, must ultimately be translated into action via the anterior horn cells. A lesion in any of these areas will affect movement or reflex activity.

When the corticospinal tract is damaged or destroyed, its functions are reduced or lost below the level of injury. When upper motor neuron systems are damaged above the crossover of its tracts in the medulla, motor impairment develops on the opposite (or contralateral) side. In damage below the crossover, motor impairment occurs on the same (or ipsilateral) side of the body. The affected limb becomes weak or paralyzed, and skilled, complicated, or delicate movements are performed especially poorly when compared with large movements.

When there is an upper motor neuron lesion, muscle tone is increased and deep tendon reflexes are exaggerated. Damage to the lower motor neuron systems causes ipsilateral weakness and paralysis, but in this case, muscle tone and reflexes are decreased or absent.

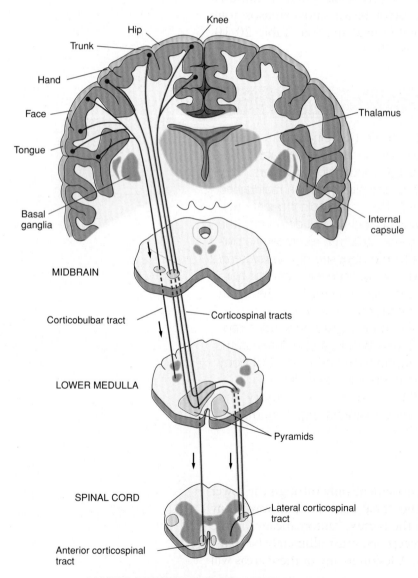

**MOTOR PATHWAYS: CORTICOSPINAL AND
CORTICOBULBAR TRACTS**

Disease of the basal ganglia system or cerebellar system does not cause paralysis but can be disabling. Damage to the basal ganglia system produces changes in muscle tone (most often an increase), disturbances in posture and gait, a slowness or lack of spontaneous and automatic movements termed *bradykinesia,* and various involuntary movements. Cerebellar damage impairs coordination, gait, and equilibrium and decreases muscle tone.

Sensory Pathways

Sensory impulses participate not only in reflex activity, as previously described, but also give rise to conscious sensation, calibrate body position in space, and help regulate internal autonomic functions like blood pressure, heart rate, and respiration.

**SENSORY PATHWAYS: SPINOTHALAMIC TRACT
AND POSTERIOR COLUMNS**

A complex system of sensory receptors relays impulses from skin, mucous membranes, muscles, tendons, and viscera that travel through peripheral projections into the posterior root ganglia, where a second projection of the ganglia directs impulses centrally into the spinal cord. Sensory impulses then travel to the sensory cortex of the brain via one of two pathways: the *spinothalamic tract,* consisting of smaller sensory neurons with unmyelinated or thinly myelinated axons, and the *posterior columns,* which have larger neurons with heavily myelinated axons.[4]

The peripheral component of the small fiber *spinothalamic tract* arises in free nerve endings in the skin that register *pain, temperature,* and *crude touch.* Within one or two spinal segments from their entry into the cord, these fibers pass into the posterior horn and synapse with secondary sensory neurons. The secondary neurons then cross to the opposite side and pass upward into the thalamus.

In the *posterior column* system, the peripheral large fiber projections of the dorsal root ganglia transmit the sensations of *vibration, proprioception, kinesthesia, pressure,* and *fine touch* from skin and joint position receptors to the dorsal root ganglia, where they travel through central projections in the posterior columns to second-order sensory neurons in the medulla. Fibers projecting from secondary neurons cross to the opposite side at the medullary level and continue on to the thalamus.

At the *thalamic level,* the general quality of sensation is perceived (e.g., pain, cold, pleasant, unpleasant), but fine distinctions are not made. For full perception, a third group of sensory neurons sends impulses from the thalamus to the *sensory cortex* of the brain. Here stimuli are localized and higher-order discriminations are made.

Lesions at different points in the sensory pathways produce different kinds of sensory loss. Patterns of sensory loss, together with their associated motor findings, help identify where the lesions might be that are causing the loss. A lesion in the sensory cortex may not impair the perception of pain, touch, and position, for example, but does impair finer discrimination. A patient with this lesion cannot appreciate the size, shape, or texture of an object by feeling it and therefore cannot identify the object. Loss of position and vibration sense with preservation of other sensations points to disease of the posterior columns, whereas loss of all sensations from the waist down, together with paralysis and hyperactive reflexes in the legs, indicates transection of the spinal cord (see Table 20-8, Metabolic and Structural Coma, p. 737). Crude and light touch are often preserved despite partial damage to the cord, because impulses originating on one side of the body travel up both sides of the cord.

Myelin is a mixture of proteins and phospholipids which form a sheath around nerve fibers and increases the conduction of nerve impulses.

Proprioception is a sense of position of parts of the body and the strength necessary to move.

Kinesthesia means movement sense.

Patients with diabetes with small fiber neuropathy report sharp, burning, or shooting foot pain, whereas those with large fiber neuropathy experience numbness and tingling or even no sensation at all.[5,6]

Dermatomes

A *dermatome* is the band of skin innervated (receiving nerve impulse) by the sensory root of a single spinal nerve. Knowledge and testing of dermatomes help identify which specific spinal cord segment has the lesion. The dermatome "maps" are on pp. 702–703.

Spinal Reflexes: The Muscle Stretch Reflex and Deep Tendon Reflex

The muscle stretch reflex is a monosynaptic reflex which is a simple reflex that relays information from a sensory neuron to a motor neuron across a single synapse. The monosynaptic reflex regulates muscle length via nerve stimulation at the muscle spindles. The alpha motor neurons cause the contraction to resist stretching and the gamma motor neurons control the tension and sensitivity. The effect of the stretch reflex is muscle contraction in response to increased length/stretch of the muscle. Muscle stretch reflexes are common in skeletal muscle and important for both balance and posture.

The patella reflex is the most common muscle stretch reflex or monosynaptic reflex.

The deep tendon reflex, or Golgi tendon reflex, is polysynaptic and relays information from a sensory neuron to a motor neuron across two or more synapses inducing muscle relaxation/lengthening in response to increased tension in the muscle. The reflex controls muscle tension through relaxation so that the muscle force or contraction does not become so strong that the tendon is torn. This protection from tissue damage is instrumental, as is the precision and control of motor activity that the deep tendon reflexes provide.

The muscle stretch reflex and the deep tendon reflex can be elicited by a brisk tap to the area of a partially stretched muscle/tendon. For the reflex to fire, all components of the reflex arc must be intact: sensory nerve fibers, spinal cord synapse, motor nerve fibers, neuromuscular junction, and muscle fibers. Tapping activates special sensory fibers in the partially stretched muscle/tendon, triggering a sensory impulse that travels to the spinal cord via a peripheral nerve. The stimulated sensory fiber synapses directly with the anterior horn cell innervating the same muscle. When the impulse crosses the neuromuscular junction, the muscle suddenly contracts, completing the reflex arc.

Because each deep tendon reflex involves specific spinal segments, together with their sensory and motor fibers, an abnormal reflex can help locate a pathologic lesion. Learn the segmental levels of the deep tendon reflexes. They can be remembered by their numerical sequence in ascending order from ankle to triceps: S1–L2, 3, 4–C5, 6, 7.

Often, all reflexes are referred to as deep tendon reflexes (DTRs).

Deep Tendon Reflexes (DTRs)/Muscle Stretch Reflexes	
Ankle reflex (Achilles)	Sacral 1 primarily
Knee reflex (patellar)	Lumbar 2, 3, 4
Supinator (brachioradialis) reflex	Cervical 5, 6
Biceps reflex	Cervical 5, 6
Triceps reflex	Cervical 6, 7

Reflexes may be initiated by stimulating skin as well as muscle. Stroking the skin of the abdomen, for example, produces a localized muscular twitch. Superficial (cutaneous) reflexes and their corresponding spinal segments include the following:

Cutaneous Stimulation Reflexes	
Abdominal reflexes—upper	Thoracic 8, 9, 10
Abdominal reflexes–lower	Thoracic 10, 11, 12
Cremasteric reflex	Lumbar 1, 2
Plantar responses	Lumbar 5, sacral 1
Anal reflex	Sacral 2, 3, 4

THE HEALTH HISTORY

Common or Concerning Symptoms

- Headache
- Head injury
- Dizziness or vertigo
- Weakness (generalized, proximal, or distal weakness)
- Numbness, abnormal or loss of sensations
- Fainting and blacking out (near-syncope and syncope)
- Seizures
- Tremors or involuntary movements

Two of the most common symptoms in neurologic disorders are *headache* and *dizziness*. Review the health history pertinent to headaches.

Headache

Headaches have many causes, ranging from benign to life threatening, and always warrant thorough assessment. Neurologic causes such as subarachnoid hemorrhage, meningitis, or mass lesions are especially ominous. Pay close attention to the headache history and your examination findings.

See Table 10-1, Primary Headaches, p. 229 and Table 10-2, Secondary Headaches, pp. 230–231.

Primary headaches include migraine, tension, cluster, and trigeminal autonomic *cephalagias; secondary headaches* arise from underlying structural, systemic, or infectious causes and may be life threatening.[7]

Ask about the severity of the headache and its onset, location, duration, and any associated symptoms such as double vision, visual changes, weakness, or loss of sensation.[8] Does the headache get worse with coughing, sneezing, or sudden head movements, which can alter intracranial pressure? Is there fever, stiff neck, or an ear, sinus, or throat infection that may signal meningitis?[9]

Subarachnoid hemorrhage classically presents as "the worst headache of my life" with instantaneous onset.[10-12] Severe headache and stiff neck accompany *meningitis*.[13-15]

Dull headache increased by coughing and sneezing, especially when reoccurring in the same location, occurs in mass lesions such as *brain* tumors or *abscess*.[16,17]

An atypical (not usual) presentation of the patient's usual migraine may be suspicious for stroke, especially in women using hormonal contraceptives.[18-20]

Migraine headache is often preceded by an aura or prodrome, and is highly likely if three of the five "POUND" features are present: **P**ulsatile or throbbing; **O**ne-day duration, or lasts 4 to 72 hours if untreated; **U**nilateral; **N**ausea or vomiting; **D**isabling or intensity causing interruption of daily activity.[21,22]

Always look for unusual headache warning signs, such as sudden onset "like a thunderclap," onset after age 50 years, and associated symptoms such as fever and stiff neck. Examine for papilledema and focal neurologic signs.

Dizziness or Vertigo

Dizziness and *lightheadedness* are common yet vague complaints that can have many meanings. You will need to elicit the patient's experience through a specific history and neurologic examination.[23]

Does the patient feel faint or about to fall or pass out (*presyncope*)? Or unsteady and off balance (*disequilibrium* or *ataxia*)? Or is there *true vertigo*, a spinning sensation within the patient or of the surroundings? If there is true vertigo, establish the time course of symptoms, which helps distinguish among the different types of peripheral vestibular disorders.

Feeling light-headed, weak in the legs, or about to faint points to *presyncope* from vasovagal stimulation, orthostatic hypotension, arrhythmia, or side effects from blood pressure and other medications.

Vertigo often reflects vestibular disease, usually from peripheral causes in the inner ear such as *benign positional vertigo, labyrinthitis,* or *Ménière disease.*[23]

See Table 12-1, Dizziness and Vertigo, p. 310.

Formulating subjective questions is important to differentiate whether the patient is experiencing dizziness or vertigo. Begin with an open-ended question: "Tell me about the dizziness." When eliciting additional information regarding a sign or symptom, use the "OLD CART" mnemonic to focus on specific questions so that the sequence of events will become clearer.

O*nset:* When did this feeling of "dizziness" begin?
L*ocation:* Does it seem to occur on one side of the head or the other?
D*uration:* How often does the dizziness occur?
   How long does it last?
   Does it go away?
   Does it come and go?
C*haracteristic Symptoms:* What does it feel like?
   Is the room spinning?
   Are you spinning?
   Is the room rotating?
   Are you light-headed?
   Do you feel faint?
A*ssociated Manifestations:* Does anything else occur when you feel dizzy?
   Do you have double vision (diplopia)?

If there are localizing symptoms or signs like double vision (*diplopia*), diffi-culty forming words (*dysarthria*), or problems with gait or balance (*ataxia*), investigate the central causes of vertigo.

Diplopia, dysarthria, ataxia in vertebrobasilar *transient ischemic attack* (TIA) or *stroke.*[18–22] See Table 20-2, Types of Stroke, pp. 729–730.

   Do you feel nauseous?
   Do you experience difficulty forming words (dysarthria)?
   Are there times when you have difficulty with balance or walking (ataxia)?
   Have you taken any new medications? Prescribed? Over the counter?
R*elieving Factors:* Does anything make the dizziness go away? Decrease?
   What makes it feel better?
T*reatment:* Have you taken any medications to relieve the dizziness?
   Have you used any therapies to help treat the dizziness? Aromatherapy?
      Chiropractor? Acupuncture? Any others?
   Have you talked to your health care provider previously about the dizziness?

Weakness

Weakness is another common symptom with many causes that bears careful investigation. It is important to clarify what the patient means by "weakness": fatigue, apathy, drowsiness, or actual loss of strength. True motor weakness can arise from the central nervous system, a peripheral nerve, the neuromus-cular junction, or a muscle. Time course and location are especially relevant. Is the onset sudden, gradual, or chronic, over a long period of time?

Abrupt onset of motor and sensory deficits occurs in *TIA* and *stroke.*[24–29] Progressive onset of lower extremity weakness suggests *Guillain–Barré syndrome.*[30] Chronic more gradual onset of lower extremity weakness occurs in primary and metastatic spinal cord tumors.

Focal or asymmetric weakness has both central (ischemic, vascular, or mass lesions) and peripheral causes ranging from neuromuscular junction disorders to myopathies.

O*nset:* When did the weakness begin?
   Did it start slowly or suddenly?
L*ocation:* What areas of the body are involved?
   Does the weakness affect one or both sides?
   What movements are affected?
D*uration:* Has it progressed? How so?
   How long does it last?
   Does it go away?
   Does it come and go?

For weakness without lightheadedness, try to distinguish between proximal and distal weakness.

Proximal—in the shoulder and/or hip girdle, for example
Distal—in the hands and/or feet
Symmetric—in the same areas on both sides of the body
Asymmetric—types of weakness include focal, in a portion of the face or extremity; monoparesis, in an extremity; paraparesis, in both lower extremities; and hemiparesis, in one side of the body

Proximal limb weakness, when symmetric with intact sensation, occurs in myopathies from alcohol, drugs like glucocorticoids, and inflammatory muscle disorders like *polymyositis* and *dermatomyositis*. In the neuromuscular junction disorder *myasthenia gravis,* there is proximal typically asymmetric weakness that gets worse with effort (fatigability), often with associated *bulbar symptoms* such as diplopia, ptosis, dysarthria, and dysphagia.[31,32]

Characteristic Symptoms
   If assessing for proximal weakness:
      Are you able to reach something on a high shelf?
      Do you have difficulty getting out of a chair?
      How does it feel when you brush your hair?
      Are you able to walk up steps? How many?
      Does the weakness increase with repeated effort?
      Does it improve with rest?
   If assessing for distal weakness in the arms:
      Have you noticed any changes in hand movements?
      Do you have any difficulty opening jars or cans?
      Has it become more cumbersome to use scissors, screwdrivers, or pliers?
   If assessing for distal weakness in the legs:
      Have you noticed yourself tripping?
Associated Manifestations: Are there any sensations you experience when the weakness occurs?
   Have you noticed that there are some activities that you are not able to participate in any longer? Or need assistance completing?
   Do you experience any other symptoms when the weakness occurs:
      Nausea/vomiting?
      Headaches?
      Double vision?
      Difficulty swallowing?
      Slurred speech?
      Rash?
      Have you recently changed medications?
Relieving Factors: Does anything relieve the weakness?
   What makes the weakness better:
      Rest?
      Caffeine?
      Exercise?
   Have you noticed you are sleeping or resting more?
Treatment: Have you taken any medications to relieve the weakness?
   Have you talked to your health care provider previously about the weakness?

Change or Loss of Sensation

In a patient who reports numbness, ask the patient to be more precise. Is there tingling like "pins and needles," which are altered sensations called *paresthesias*. These commonly occur when an arm or leg "goes to sleep" following compression of a nerve, and may be described as tingling, prickling, or feelings of warmth, coldness, or pressure. *Dysesthesias* are distorted sensations in response to a stimulus and may last longer than the stimulus itself. For example, a person may perceive a light touch or pinprick as a burning or tingling sensation that is irritating or unpleasant. *Pain* may arise from neurologic causes but is usually reported with symptoms of other body systems, such as the head and neck or the musculoskeletal system.

Sensory changes can arise at several levels: local nerve compression or "entrapment," seen in hand numbness in distributions specific to the median, ulnar, or radial nerve; nerve root compression with dermatomal sensory loss from vertebral bone spurs or herniated discs; or central lesions from *stroke* or *multiple sclerosis*.

Burning pain occurs in painful *sensory neuropathies* from conditions like diabetes.[33,34]

See Table 18-1, Lower Back Pain, p. 636 and Table 18-2, Pains in the Neck, p. 637.

Have you noticed any change in sensation?

O*nset:* When did this begin?
L*ocation:* What part(s) of the body experience this change/loss in sensation?
D*uration:* How long does it last? Is it continuous? Does it come and go?
C*haracteristic Symptoms:* Describe what it feels like (pins and needles, goes to sleep, tingling, prickling, pressure, warmth, cold, burning, irritating).
A*ssociated Manifestations:* Have you noticed any other changes (vision changes, difficulty eating)?
R*elieving Factors:* Does anything make it feel better?
T*reatment:* What treatments or medications have you tried? What were the results?

Fainting and Blacking Out (Near Syncope and Syncope)

Patient reports of fainting or "passing out" are common and warrant a meticulous history to guide management and possible hospital admission.[35] Begin by finding out whether the patient has experienced syncope or near syncope. In syncope the patient has actually lost consciousness and postural tone from transient global hypoperfusion of the brain. While in near syncope the patient feels light-headed or weak, but fails to actually lose consciousness. True syncope is a more serious symptom.

Get as complete and unbiased a description of the event as possible.

What brought on the episode?

Were there any warning symptoms?

Was the patient standing, sitting, or lying down when the episode began?

How long did it last?

Could voices be heard while passing out and coming to?

How rapidly did the patient recover?

In retrospect, were onset and offset slow or fast?

Causes include seizures, "neurocardiogenic" conditions such as *vasovagal syncope,* *postural orthostatic tachycardia syndrome (POTS), carotid sinus syncope,* and *orthostatic hypotension,* and cardiac disease causing arrhythmias, especially ventricular tachycardia and bradyarrhythmias.[36] Stroke and subarachnoid hemorrhage are unlikely causes of syncope unless both hemispheres are affected.

Also ask if anyone observed the episode.

If so, what did the patient look like before losing consciousness, during the episode, and afterward?

Was there any seizure-like movement of the arms or legs?

Any incontinence of the bladder or bowel?

Any drowsiness or impaired memory after the episode ended?

In *vasovagal syncope,* the most common cause of syncope, look for the prodrome of nausea, diaphoresis, and pallor triggered by a fearful or unpleasant event, then vagally mediated hypotension, often with slow onset and offset. In syncope from arrhythmias, onset and offset are often sudden, reflecting loss and recovery of cerebral perfusion.

Seizures

A *seizure* is a paroxysmal disorder caused by sudden excessive electrical discharge in the cerebral cortex or its underlying structures. Seizures can be of several types. Depending on the type, there may or may not be loss of consciousness. With some types of seizures, there may be abnormal feelings, thought processes, and sensations, including smells, as well as abnormal movements. Asking "Have you ever had any seizures? or 'spells'?" and "Any fits? or convulsions?" can open the discussion.

Common causes of *acute symptomatic seizures* include: epilepsy; head trauma; alcohol, cocaine, and other drugs; withdrawal from alcohol, benzodiazepines, and barbiturates; metabolic insults from low or high glucose or low calcium or sodium; acute stroke; and meningitis or encephalitis.

See Table 20-7, Seizure Disorders, pp. 735–736.

Tonic–clonic motor activity, bladder or bowel incontinence, and *postictal state* suggest a generalized *seizure.* Unlike syncope, injury such as tongue biting or bruising of limbs may occur.[37]

O*nset:* At what age did the seizures begin?

When was the last seizure?

Has there been a change in frequency?

L*ocation:* Do you lose consciousness when you have a seizure?

Does it affect your entire body?

D*uration:* How often do the seizures occur?

How long do the seizures last?

C*haracteristic Symptoms:* What are the precipitating circumstances or warnings prior to a seizure?

What are the behaviors and feelings that occur during the seizure?

What occurs after the seizure? How do you feel?

Associated Manifestations: What is causing the seizures?

Is there a history of a head injury or other condition that may be related to the seizures?

Relieving Factors: What can be done to relieve the actual seizure?

What is instrumental in relieving the symptoms associated with the actual seizure or postseizure period?

Treatment: What medications are currently being administered?

What has been used previously?

Who is monitoring your medications and condition?

Tremors

Tremors and other *involuntary movements* occur with or without additional neurologic manifestations. Ask about any trembling, shakiness, or body movements that the patient seems unable to control.

See Table 20-11, Tremors and Involuntary Movements, pp. 740–741.

Low-frequency unilateral resting tremor, rigidity, and bradykinesia are seen in *Parkinson disease*.[38–40] *Essential tremors* are high-frequency, bilateral, upper extremity tremors that occur with both limb movement and sustained posture and subside when the limb is relaxed; head, voice, and leg tremor may also be present.[39]

Distinct from these symptoms is *restless leg syndrome*, present in 6% to 12% of the U.S. population, described as an unpleasant sensation in the legs, especially at night, that gets worse with rest and improves with movement of the symptomatic limb(s).[41]

Reversible causes of restless legs syndrome include pregnancy, renal disease, and iron deficiency.[42]

PHYSICAL EXAMINATION

Assessment of the nervous system calls for many complex skills of examination and clinical reasoning. You have already learned the principles and techniques for assessing mental status, a critical component of the nervous system examination. As you saw in Chapter 19, Mental Status, often the patient's mental status offers clues about delirium, memory disorders, and other neurologic conditions. As you study this chapter, let three important questions guide the approach to this challenging clinical area:

• Is mental status intact?

• Are right-sided and left-sided examination findings symmetric?

• If the findings are asymmetric or otherwise abnormal, does the lesion lie in the *central nervous system,* consisting of the brain and spinal cord, or in the *peripheral nervous system,* consisting of the 12 pairs of cranial nerves and the spinal and peripheral nerves?

Patient symptoms or signs point to the affected area of the nervous system.

Equipment

Cranial Nerve Examination
Penlight
Snellen chart
Newspaper or hand-held news print
Ophthalmoscope
Cotton swab
Tongue depressor
Gloves
Scents for olfactory (e.g., vanilla, cinnamon, coffee, lemon juice, or soap)
Tuning fork

Sensory Examination
Objects to feel (e.g., coin, paper clip)
Tuning fork
Hot and cold water in test tubes/glass
Cotton swab

Muscle Stretch Response/Deep Tendon Reflexes
Reflex hammer
Tongue blade

Important Areas of Examination

- Mental status, as in Chapter 19
- Cranial nerves I through XII
- Motor system: coordination, gait, and stance. Also, muscle strength, bulk, and tone, as in Chapter 18, Musculoskeletal System.
- Sensory system: pain and temperature, position and vibration, light touch, discrimination
- Deep tendon, abdominal, and plantar reflexes

This section presents the techniques you need for a practical and reasonably comprehensive examination of the nervous system aligned with recommendations of the American Academy of Neurology.[43-45] It is important to master the techniques for a thorough examination. Be active in your learning and ask your instructors to review your skills.

The amount of detail in an appropriate neurologic examination varies widely. In healthy patients, the examination will be relatively brief. If abnormal findings are detected, the examination will become more comprehensive. Be aware that neurologists may use many other techniques in specific situations. Whether you conduct a comprehensive or screening examination, organize your thinking into five categories: (1) mental status, speech, and language; (2) cranial nerves; (3) the motor system; (4) the sensory system; and (5) reflexes. If your findings are abnormal, begin to group them into patterns of central or peripheral disorders.

For efficiency, integrate the neurologic assessment with other parts of the examination. Survey the patient's mental status and speech during the interview, even though further testing may be necessary during the neurologic examination. Assess the cranial nerves as you examine the head and neck, and any neurologic abnormalities in the arms and legs as you evaluate the peripheral vascular and musculoskeletal systems. Chapter 22 provides an outline of an integrated approach. Think about and describe your findings, however, in terms of the nervous system as a unit.

Guidelines for a Screening Neurologic Examination from the American Academy of Neurology[43]

Perform a screening neurologic examination in all patients, even those without neurologic complaints, that is sufficient for detection of significant neurologic disease. Although the exact sequence of such screening may vary, it should cover the major components of the full examination-mental status, cranial nerves, motor system (strength, gait, and coordination), sensation, and reflexes. One example of a screening examination is given here.

Mental Status
- Level of alertness
- Appropriateness of responses
- Orientation to date and place

Cranial Nerves
- Vision—visual fields, funduscopic examination
- Pupillary light reflex
- Eye movements
- Hearing
- Facial strength—smile, eye closure

Motor System
- Muscle strength—shoulder abduction, elbow extension, wrist extension, finger abduction, hip flexion, knee flexion, ankle dorsiflexion
- Muscle bulk and Tone
- Gait—casual, heel walk, toe walk, tandem walk
- Coordination—fine finger movements, finger-to-nose, heel to shin

Sensory System
- Light touch
- Pain/Temperature
- Proprioception

Reflexes
- Muscle stretch response/deep tendon reflexes
- Plantar responses

Note: If there is reason to suspect neurologic disease based on the patient's history or the results of any components of the screening examination, a more complete neurologic examination is necessary.

Source: Adapted from the American Academy of Neurology. Available at https://www.aan.com/uploadedFiles/4CME_and_Training/2Training/3Fellowship_Resources/5Core_Curricula/skilz.pdf. Accessed January 6, 2016.

The Cranial Nerves

The examination of the cranial nerves (abbreviated as CN) can be summarized as follows.

Summary: Cranial Nerves I–XII	
I	Smell
II	Visual acuity, visual fields, and ocular fundi
II, III	Pupillary reactions
III, IV, VI	Extraocular movements
V	Corneal reflexes, facial sensation, and jaw movements
VII	Facial movements
VIII	Hearing
IX, X	Swallowing and rise of the palate, gag reflex
V, VII, X, XII	Voice and speech
XI	Shoulder and neck movements
XII	Tongue symmetry and position

Cranial Nerve I—Olfactory

Test the *sense of smell* by presenting the patient with familiar and nonirritating odors. First, make sure that each nasal passage is patent by compressing one side of the nose and asking the patient to sniff through the other. Then ask the patient to close both eyes. Occlude one nostril and test smell in the other side with substances such as cloves, coffee, soap, or vanilla. Avoid noxious odors like ammonia that might stimulate CN V. Ask the patient to identify the odor. Test smell on the other side with a different odor. Normally a patient perceives odors on each side and identifies them correctly.

Loss of smell may occur in sinus conditions, head trauma, smoking, aging, use of cocaine or in *Parkinson disease.*

Cranial Nerve II—Optic

Test *visual acuity* (see pp. 246–247).

Inspect the *optic fundi* with your ophthalmoscope, paying special attention to the optic discs (see pp. 256–259).

Inspect each disc carefully for bulging and blurred margins (*papilledema*); pallor (*optic atrophy*); and cup enlargement (*glaucoma*).

Test the visual fields by confrontation (see pp. 248–249). Test each eye separately, and both eyes together. Occasionally, in stroke patients, for example, patients will complain of partial loss of vision, and testing of both eyes reveals a *visual field defect,* an abnormality in peripheral vision, such as *homonymous hemianopsia.* Testing one eye would not confirm the finding.

See Table 11-2, Visual Field Defects, p. 265. Check for prechiasmal, or anterior defects found in *glaucoma, retinal emboli, optic neuritis* (visual acuity poor), bitemporal hemianopsias from defects at the optic chiasm, usually from *pituitary tumor* or homonymous hemianopsias or quadrantanopsia in postchiasmal lesions, usually in the *parietal lobe,* with associated findings of stroke (visual acuity normal).[46]

Cranial Nerves II and III—Optic and Oculomotor

Inspect the size and shape of the pupils, and compare one side with the other. *Anisocoria,* or a difference of >0.4 mm in the diameter of one pupil compared to the other, is seen in up to 38% of healthy individuals. Test the *pupillary reactions to light.*

See Table 11-6, Pupillary Abnormalities, p. 269. If the large pupil reacts poorly to light or anisocoria worsens in light, the large pupil has abnormal pupillary constriction, seen in *CN III palsy.* If ptosis and *ophthalmoplegia* (eyes not aligned) are also present, consider *intracranial aneurysm* if the patient is awake, and *transtentorial herniation* if the patient is comatose.

Also check the *near response* or accommodation (p. 241), which tests pupillary constriction (pupillary constrictor muscle), convergence (medial rectus muscles), and accommodation of the lens (ciliary muscle).

If both pupils react to light and anisocoria worsens in darkness, the small pupil has abnormal pupillary dilation, seen in *Horner syndrome* and *simple anisocoria.*[47]

Cranial Nerves III, IV, and VI—Oculomotor, Trochlear, and Abducens

Test the *extraocular movements* in the six cardinal directions of gaze, and look for loss of conjugate movements in any of the six directions, which causes *diplopia.* Ask the patient which direction makes the diplopia worse and inspect the eye closely for asymmetric deviation of movement. Determine if the diplopia is *monocular* or *binocular* by asking the patient to cover one eye, or perform the cover–uncover test (see Table 11-7, Dysconjugate Gaze, p. 270).

See Table 11-7, Dysconjugate Gaze, p. 270. Monocular diplopia in local problems with glasses or contact lenses; cataracts; astigmatism; ptosis. Binocular diplopia in *CN III, IV, VI* neuropathy (40% of patients), eye muscle disease from *myasthenia gravis, trauma, thyroid ophthalmopathy, internuclear ophthalmoplegia.*[48]

Check convergence of the eyes. Identify any *nystagmus,* an involuntary jerking movement of the eyes with quick and slow components. Note the direction of gaze in which it appears, the plane of the nystagmus (horizontal, vertical, rotary, or mixed), and the direction of the quick and slow components (see p. 254). *Nystagmus is named for the direction of the quick component.* Ask the patient to fix his or her vision on a distant object and observe if the nystagmus increases or decreases.

See Table 20-6, Nystagmus, p. 734. Nystagmus in *cerebellar disease,* especially with gait ataxia and dysarthria (increases with retinal fixation) and *vestibular disorders* (decreases with retinal fixation)

Look for *ptosis* (drooping of the upper eyelids). A slight difference in the width of the palpebral fissures may be a normal variation in approximately one third of all people.

Ptosis in *third nerve palsy* (CN III), *Horner syndrome* (ptosis, meiosis, anhidrosis), or *myasthenia gravis.*

Cranial Nerve V—Trigeminal
Motor

While palpating the temporal and then the masseter muscles, ask the patient to clench the teeth. Note the strength of the muscle contraction. Ask the patient to move the jaw side to side.

Difficulty clenching the jaw or moving it to the opposite side in masseter and lateral pterygoid muscle weakness, respectively. Jaw deviation during opening points to weakness on the deviating side.

Look for unilateral weakness in CN V lesions in the pons; bilateral weakness in cerebral hemispheric disease because of bilateral cortical innervation.

CNS patterns from stroke include facial and body sensory loss on the same side (ipsilateral) but from contralateral cortical or thalamic lesion; ipsilateral face but contralateral body sensory loss in brainstem lesions.

PALPATING TEMPORAL MUSCLES

PALPATING MASSETER MUSCLES

Sensory

Sensation is tested on the forehead, cheeks, and chin on each side for *pain sensation,* as shown in the circled areas in the figure below. The patient's eyes should be closed during the actual test however prior to the examination, demonstrate what sharp and dull each feels like. Use an appropriate sharp object, such as a sharp wood splinter by breaking or twisting a cotton swab or tongue depressor for the sharp sensation and the use end of a cotton swab as a dull stimulus. Ask the patient to report whether it is "sharp" or "dull" and to compare sides.

Isolated facial sensory loss in peripheral nerve disorders including lesions of the *trigeminal neuralgia.*

If you detect sensory loss, confirm it by testing *temperature sensation*. Two test tubes, filled with hot and ice-cold water, are the traditional stimuli. A tuning fork may also be used. It usually feels cool. If you are near running water, the fork is easily made colder or warm. Dry it before use. Touch the skin and ask the patient to identify "hot" or "cold."

Then test for *light touch,* using a fine wisp of cotton. Ask the patient to respond whenever you touch the skin.

Corneal Reflex

Test the *corneal reflex.* Ask the patient to look up and away from you and approach from the opposite side, out of the patient's line of vision. Avoiding the eyelashes, lightly touch the cornea (not just the conjunctiva) with a fine wisp of cotton. If the patient is apprehensive, touching the conjunctiva first may be helpful.

Inspect for blinking of the eyes, the normal reaction to this stimulus. The sensory limb of this reflex is carried in CN V, and the motor response, in CN VII. Use of contact lenses frequently diminishes or abolishes this reflex and therefore it is not used as frequently.

Blinking is absent in both eyes in CN V lesions and on the side of weakness in lesions of CN VII. Absent blinking and sensorineural hearing loss in *acoustic neuroma.*

Cranial Nerve VII—Facial

Inspect the face, both at rest and during conversation with the patient. Note any asymmetry (e.g., of the nasolabial folds), and observe any tics or other abnormal movements.

Flattening of the nasolabial fold and drooping of the lower eyelid suggest facial weakness.

A peripheral injury to CN VII, as seen in *Bell palsy,* affects both the upper and lower face; a central lesion affects mainly the lower face. Loss of taste, *hyperacusis,* increased or decreased tearing also in *Bell palsy.*[49] See Table 20-5, Types of Facial Paralysis, p. 733.

Ask the patient to:

1. Raise both eyebrows.

2. Frown.

3. Close both eyes tightly so that you cannot open them. Test muscular strength by trying to open them, as illustrated.

4. Show both upper and lower teeth.

5. Smile.

6. Puff out both cheeks.

In unilateral facial paralysis, the mouth droops on the paralyzed side when the patient smiles or grimaces.

Cranial Nerve VIII—Acoustic

Assess hearing with the whispered voice test. Ask the patient to repeat numbers whispered into one ear while blocking or rubbing your fingers next to the contralateral ear.

The whispered voice test is both sensitive (>90%) and specific (>80%) when assessing presence or absence of hearing loss.[50]

If hearing loss is present, determine if the loss is *conductive*, from impaired "air through ear" transmission, or *sensorineural*, from damage to the cochlear branch of CN VIII. Test for *air and bone conduction*, using the Rinne test, and *lateralization*, using the Weber test.

See techniques for Weber and Rinne test and Table 12-4, Patterns of Hearing Loss, p. 314.

Excess cerumen, otosclerosis, *otitis media* in conductive hearing loss; *presbycusis* from aging, most commonly in sensorineural hearing loss.

Specific tests of the vestibular function of CN VIII are rarely included in the typical neurologic examination.

Vertigo with hearing loss and nystagmus in *Ménière disease*—see Table 12-1, Dizziness and Vertigo, p. 310 and Table 20-6, Nystagmus, p. 734.

Cranial Nerves IX and X—Glossopharyngeal and Vagus

Listen to the patient's *voice*. Is it hoarse, or does it have a nasal quality?

Hoarseness in vocal cord paralysis; nasal voice in paralysis of the palate.

Is there difficulty in swallowing?

Difficulty swallowing suggests pharyngeal or palatal weakness.

Ask the patient to say "ah" or to yawn as you watch the *movements of the soft palate and the pharynx*. The soft palate normally rises symmetrically, the uvula remains in the midline, and each side of the posterior pharynx moves medially, like a curtain. The slightly curved uvula seen occasionally as a normal variation should not be mistaken for a uvula deviated by a lesion of CN IX or X.

The palate fails to rise with a bilateral lesion of CN X. In unilateral paralysis, one side of the palate fails to rise and, together with the uvula, is pulled toward the normal side (see p. 304).

Warn the patient when testing the *gag reflex*, which consists of elevation of the tongue and soft palate and constriction of the pharyngeal muscles. Stimulate the back of the throat lightly on each side in turn and note the gag reflex. It may be symmetrically diminished or absent in some normal people. If a patient is healthy and swallowing is intact, then checking a gag reflex is not necessary.

Unilateral absence of this reflex suggests a lesion of CN IX, and perhaps CN X.

Cranial Nerve XI—Spinal Accessory

Look for atrophy or *fasciculations* in the trapezius muscles, and compare one side with the other when standing behind the patient. Fasciculations are fine flickering irregular movements in small groups of muscle fibers. Ask the patient to shrug both shoulders upward against your hands. Note the strength and contraction of the trapezii. (See picture on the next page.)

Trapezius weakness with atrophy and fasciculations indicates a peripheral nerve disorder. In trapezius muscle paralysis, the shoulder droops, and the scapula is displaced downward and laterally.

Ask the patient to turn the head to each side against your hand. Observe the contraction of the opposite sternomastoid and note the force of the movement against your hand.

A supine patient with bilateral weakness of the sternomastoids has difficulty raising the head off the pillow.

Cranial Nerve XII— Hypoglossal

Listen to the articulation of the patient's words. This depends on cranial nerves V, VII, IX, and X as well as XII. Inspect the patient's tongue as it lies on the floor of the mouth. Look for any atrophy or *fasciculations.* Some coarser restless movements are often seen in a normal tongue. Then, with the patient's tongue protruded, look for asymmetry, atrophy, or deviation from the midline. Ask the patient to move the tongue from side to side, and note the symmetry of the movement. In ambiguous cases, ask the patient to push the tongue against the inside of each cheek in turn as you palpate externally for strength.

For poor articulation, or *dysarthria,* see Table 20-3, Disorders of Speech, p. 731. Tongue atrophy and fasciculations in *amyotrophic lateral sclerosis* and a history of *polio* in the past.

In a unilateral cortical lesion, the protruded tongue deviates away from the side of the cortical lesion. In CN XII lesions, the tongue deviates to the weak side.

The Motor System

As you assess the motor system, focus on body position, involuntary movements, characteristics of the muscles (bulk, tone, and strength), and coordination. You can use this sequence for assessing overall motor function, or check each component in the arms, legs, and trunk. If you detect an abnormality, identify the muscle(s) involved and if it originates centrally or peripherally. Know which nerves innervate the major muscle groups.

Body Position

Observe the patient's body position during movement and at rest.

Abnormal positions alert you to conditions such as mono- or hemiparesis from stroke.

Involuntary Movements

Watch for involuntary movements such as tremors, tics, chorea, or fasciculations. Note their location, quality, rate, rhythm, and amplitude, and their relation to posture, activity, fatigue, emotion, and other factors.

See Table 20-11, Tremors and Involuntary Movements, pp. 740–741.

Muscle Bulk, Muscle Tone, and Muscle Strength

Muscle bulk, tone, and strength are detailed in Chapter 18, Musculoskeletal System.

Coordination

Coordination of muscle movement requires that four areas of the nervous system function in an integrated way:

- The motor system, for muscle strength

- The cerebellar system (also part of the motor system), for rhythmic movement and steady posture

In cerebellar disease look for nystagmus, dysarthria, hypotonia, and ataxia.

- The vestibular system, for balance and for coordinating eye, head, and body movements.

- The sensory system, for position sense.

To assess coordination, observe the patient performing:

- Rapid alternating movements

- Point-to-point movements

- Gait and other related body movements

- Standing in specified ways

Rapid Alternating Movements

ARMS. Show the patient how to strike one hand on the thigh, raise the hand, turn it over, and then strike the back of the hand down on the same place. Urge the patient to repeat these alternating movements as rapidly as possible.

Observe the speed, rhythm, and smoothness of the movements. Repeat with the other hand. The nondominant hand often performs somewhat less well.

In cerebellar disease, instead of alternating quickly, these movements are slow, irregular, and clumsy, an abnormality called *dysdiadochokinesis.* Upper motor neuron weakness and basal ganglia disease may also impair rapid alternating movements, but not in the same manner.

Show the patient how to tap the distal joint of the thumb with the tip of the index finger, again as rapidly as possible. Again, observe the speed, rhythm, and smoothness of the movements. The nondominant side often performs less well.

LEGS. Ask the patient to tap your hand or the floor as quickly as possible with the ball of each foot in turn. Note any slowness or awkwardness. Normally the feet do not perform as well as the hands.

Point-to-Point Movements

ARMS: FINGER-TO-NOSE TEST. Ask the patient to touch your index finger and then his or her nose alternately several times. Move your finger about so that the patient has to alter directions. Observe the accuracy and smoothness of movements and watch for any tremor. Normally the patient's movements are smooth and accurate.

In cerebellar disease, movements are clumsy, unsteady, and inappropriately variable in their speed, force, and direction. In *dysmetria,* the patient's finger may initially overshoot the mark, but then reach it fairly well. An *intention tremor* may appear toward the end of the movement. See Table 20-11, Tremors and Involuntary Movements, p. 740–741.

Now hold your finger in one place so that the patient can touch it with one arm and finger outstretched. Ask the patient to raise his or her arm overhead and lower it again to touch your finger. After several repeats, ask the patient to close both eyes and try several more times. Repeat on the other side. Normally a person can touch the examiner's finger successfully with eyes open or closed. These maneuvers test position sense and the functions of both the labyrinth of the inner ear and the cerebellum.

LEGS: HEEL-TO-SHIN TEST. Ask the patient to place one heel on the opposite knee, and then run it down the shin to the big toe. Observe the smoothness and accuracy of the movements. Repetition with the patient's eyes closed tests for position sense. Repeat on the other side.

In cerebellar disease incoordination modestly worsens with eyes closed, indicating loss of position sense. Consistent deviation to one side which worsens with the eyes closed, referred to as *past pointing,* suggests cerebellar or vestibular disease.

In cerebellar disease, the heel may overshoot the knee and then oscillate from side to side down the shin. If position sense is absent, the heel lifts too high and the patient tries to look. With eyes closed, performance is poor.

Gait

Ask the patient to:

- *Walk across the room* or down the hall, then turn, and come back. Observe posture, balance, swinging of the arms, and movements of the legs. Normally balance is easy, the arms swing at the sides, and turns are accomplished smoothly.

- *Walk heel-to-toe* in a straight line—a pattern called *tandem walking.*

- *Walk on the toes,* then *on the heels*—sensitive tests, respectively, for plantar flexion and dorsiflexion of the ankles, as well as for balance.

Abnormalities of gait increase risk of falls.

A gait that lacks coordination, with reeling and instability, is called *ataxic.* Ataxia may be due to cerebellar disease, loss of position sense, or intoxication. See Table 20-4, Abnormalities of Gait and Posture, p. 732.

Tandem walking may reveal an ataxia not previously obvious.

Walking on toes and heels may reveal distal muscular weakness in the legs. Inability to heel-walk is a sensitive test for corticospinal tract damage.

- *Hop in place* on each foot in turn (if the patient is not too ill). Hopping involves the proximal muscles of the legs as well as the distal ones and requires both good position sense and normal cerebellar function.

Difficulty with hopping may be due to weakness, lack of position sense, or cerebellar dysfunction.

- *Do a shallow knee bend,* first on one leg, then on the other. Support the patient's elbow if you think the patient is in danger of falling.

Difficulty here suggests proximal weakness (extensors of the hip), weakness of the quadriceps (the extensor of the knee), or both.

- *Rising from a sitting position* without arm support and *stepping up* on a sturdy stool are more suitable tests than hopping or knee bends if patients are unsteady, neurologically impaired, or frail.

Proximal muscle weakness involving the pelvic girdle and legs causes difficulty with both of these activities.

Stance

The following two tests can often be performed concurrently. They differ only in the patient's arm position and in what is assessed. In each case, stand close enough to the patient to prevent a fall.

THE ROMBERG TEST. This is mainly a test of position sense. The patient should first stand with feet together and eyes open and then close both eyes for 30 to 60 seconds without support. The nurse should stand next to the patient without touching him or her, in case of loss of balance, with arms in front and back of the patient. Note the patient's ability to maintain an upright posture. Normally only minimal swaying occurs.

In ataxia from dorsal column disease and loss of position sense, vision compensates for the sensory loss. The patient stands fairly well with eyes open but loses balance when they are closed, a *positive Romberg sign.* In *cerebellar ataxia,* the patient has difficulty standing with feet together whether the eyes are open or closed.

TEST FOR PRONATOR DRIFT. The patient should stand for 20 to 30 seconds with both arms straightforward, palms up, and eyes closed. A person who cannot stand may be tested for a pronator drift in the sitting position. In either case, a normal person can hold this arm position well.

Pronator drift is the pronation of one forearm. It is both sensitive and specific for a corticospinal tract lesion originating in the contralateral hemisphere. Downward drift of the arm with flexion of fingers and elbow may also occur.[51–53]

Now, instructing the patient to keep the arms up and eyes shut, as shown, *tap the arms briskly downward*. The arms normally return smoothly to the horizontal position. This response requires muscular strength, coordination, and a good sense of position.

In *loss of position sense* the arms drift sideward or upward, sometimes with writhing movements of the hands; the patient may not recognize the displacement and when asked, corrects it poorly. In *cerebellar incoordination,* the arm returns to its original position but overshoots and bounces.

The Sensory System

To evaluate the sensory system, you will test several kinds of sensation:

- Pain and temperature (spinothalamic tracts)

- Position and vibration (posterior columns)

- Light touch (both spinothalamic and posterior)

- Discriminative sensations, which depend on some of the above sensations but also involve the cortex

When abnormal findings are detected, correlate them with motor and reflex activity. Assess the patient carefully as the following questions are considered:

See Table 20-1, Disorders of the Central and Peripheral Nervous System, pp. 726–728.

> Is the underlying lesion central or peripheral?
> Is the sensory loss bilateral or unilateral?
> Does it have a pattern suggesting a dermatomal distribution, a polyneuropathy, or a spinal cord syndrome?
> Is there a loss of pain and temperature sensation? Intact touch and vibration?

Refer to specialty textbooks for discussion of *spinal cord syndromes* with crossed sensory findings, both ipsilateral and contralateral to the cord injury.

Patterns of Testing

Because sensory testing quickly fatigues many patients and can produce unreliable results, conduct the examination as efficiently as possible. Focus on areas that have numbness or pain, motor or reflex abnormalities suggesting a lesion of the spinal cord or peripheral nervous system, and trophic changes such as absent or excessive sweating, atrophic skin, or cutaneous ulceration. You will often need to retest at another time to confirm abnormalities.

Meticulous sensory mapping helps to establish the level of a spinal cord lesion and to determine whether a more peripheral lesion is in a nerve root, a major peripheral nerve, or one of its branches.

The following patterns of testing help you to identify sensory deficits accurately and efficiently.

Tips for Detecting Sensory Deficits

- *Compare symmetric areas* on the two sides of the body, including the arms, legs, and trunk.
- For pain, temperature, and touch sensation, *compare the distal to the proximal areas* of the extremities. Scatter the stimuli to sample most of the dermatomes and major peripheral nerves (see pp. 702–703). One suggested pattern is to include:
  - both shoulders (C4)
  - the inner and outer aspects of the forearms (C6 and T1)
  - the thumbs and little fingers (C6 and C8)
  - fronts of both thighs (L2)
  - the medial and lateral aspects of both calves (L4 and L5)
  - the little toes (S1)
  - the medial aspect of each buttock (S3).
- For vibration and position sensation, test the fingers and toes first. If these are normal, it is safe to assume that more proximal areas will also be normal.
- *Vary the pace of your testing so* the patient does not merely respond to the repetitive rhythm.
- When you detect an area of sensory loss or hypersensitivity, *map out its boundaries* in detail. Stimulate first at a point of reduced sensation, then in progressive steps until the patient reports a change to normal sensation.

Hemisensory loss pattern suggests a lesion in the contralateral cerebral hemisphere; a *sensory level* (when one or more sensory modalities are reduced below a dermatome on one or both sides) suggests a *spinal cord lesion.*

Symmetric distal sensory loss suggests a diabetic *polyneuropathy.* This finding may be missed unless the distal and proximal areas are compared.

Here all sensation in the hand is lost. Repetitive testing in a proximal direction reveals a gradual return to normal sensation at the wrist. This pattern does not fit either a peripheral nerve damage or dermatomal loss—see pp. 702–703. If bilateral, it suggests the "glove" of the "stocking-glove" sensory loss of a *polyneuropathy,* often seen in *alcoholism and diabetes.*

Before each of the following tests, show the patient what you plan to do and explain how you would like the patient to respond. The patient's eyes should be closed during actual testing.

Pain

Use a broken tongue blade/cotton swab or other suitable tool. Occasionally, substitute the blunt end for the point.

Ask the patient, "Is this sharp or is this dull?" or, when making comparisons, "Does this feel the same as this?" by touching the patient. Apply the lightest pressure needed for the stimulus to feel sharp, and do not draw blood.

Analgesia refers to absence of pain sensation, *hypalgesia* to decreased sensitivity to pain, and *hyperalgesia* to increased sensitivity.

Temperature

Testing is often omitted if pain sensation is normal. If there are sensory deficits, use two test tubes, filled with hot and cold water, or a tuning fork heated or cooled by running water. Touch the skin and ask the patient to identify "hot" or "cold."

Light Touch

With a fine wisp of cotton, touch the skin lightly, avoiding pressure. Ask the patient to respond whenever a touch is felt, and to compare one area with another. Avoid testing calloused skin, which is normally relatively insensitive.

Anesthesia is absence of touch sensation, *hypesthesia* is decreased sensitivity, and *hyperesthesia* is increased sensitivity.

Vibration

Use a relatively low-pitched tuning fork of 128 Hz. Tap it on the heel of your hand and place it firmly over a distal interphalangeal joint of the patient's finger, and test over the interphalangeal joint of the big toe. Ask what the patient feels. If you are uncertain whether it is pressure or vibration, ask the patient to tell you when the vibration stops, and then touch the fork to stop it. If vibration sense is impaired, proceed to more proximal bony prominences (e.g., wrist, elbow, medial malleolus, patella, anterior superior iliac spine, spinous processes, and clavicles).

Vibration sense is often the first sensation to be lost in a peripheral neuropathy. Common causes include *diabetes* or *alcoholism*. Vibration sense is also lost in posterior column disease, as in *tertiary syphilis* or *vitamin B$_{12}$ deficiency*.[54]

Testing vibration sense in the trunk may be useful in estimating the level of a cord lesion.

Proprioception (Joint Position Sense)

Grasp the patient's big toe, holding it by its sides between the thumb and index finger, and then pull it away from the other toes. This prevents extraneous tactile stimuli from affecting testing. Demonstrate "up" and "down" as you move the patient's toe clearly upward and downward. Then, with the patient's eyes closed, ask for a response of "up" or "down" when moving the large toe in a small arc.

Loss of position sense, like loss of vibration sense, in *tabes dorsalis, multiple sclerosis,* or B_{12} *deficiency* from posterior column disease; and in diabetic neuropathy.

Repeat the test several times on each side, avoiding simple alternation of the stimuli. If position sense is impaired, move proximally to test the ankle joint. In a similar fashion, test position in the fingers, moving proximally if indicated to the metacarpophalangeal joints, wrist, and elbow.

Discriminative Sensations

Several additional techniques test the ability of the sensory cortex to correlate, analyze, and interpret sensations. Because discriminative sensations depend on touch and position sense, they are useful only when these sensations are either intact or only slightly impaired.

If touch and position sense are normal, decreased or absent discriminative sensation indicates a lesion in the sensory cortex. Stereognosis, number identification, and two-point discrimination are also impaired in posterior column disease.

Screen a patient with *stereognosis,* and proceed to other methods if indicated. The patient's eyes should be closed during all these tests.

- *Stereognosis.* Stereognosis refers to the ability to identify an object by feeling it. Place a familiar object such as a coin, paper clip, key, pencil, or cotton ball, in the patient's hand, and ask the patient to tell you what it is. Normally a patient will manipulate it skillfully and identify it correctly within 5 seconds. Asking the patient to distinguish "heads" from "tails" on a coin is a sensitive test of stereognosis.

Astereognosis refers to the inability to recognize objects placed in the hand.

- *Number identification (graphesthesia)*. If arthritis or other conditions prevent the patient from manipulating an object well enough to identify it, test the ability to identify numbers. With the blunt end of a pen or pencil, draw a large number in the patient's palm. A person generally can identify most such numbers.

The inability to recognize numbers, or *graphanesthesia,* indicates a lesion in the sensory cortex.

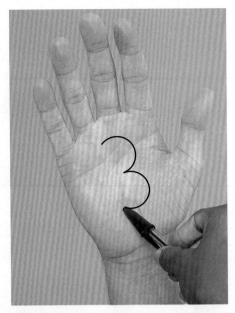

- *Two-point discrimination*. Using the two ends of an opened paper clip, touch a finger pad in two places simultaneously. Alternate the double stimulus irregularly with a one-point touch. Be careful not to cause pain.

- Find the minimal distance at which the patient can discriminate one from two points (normally <5 mm on the finger pads). This test may be used on other parts of the body, but normal distances vary widely from one body region to another.

Lesions of the sensory cortex increase the distance between two recognizable points.

- *Point localization*. Briefly touch a point on the patient's skin. Then ask the patient to open both eyes and point to the place touched. Generally a person can do so accurately. This test, together with the test for extinction, is especially useful on the trunk and the legs.

Lesions of the sensory cortex impair the ability to localize points accurately.

- *Extinction*. Simultaneously stimulate corresponding areas on both sides of the body. Ask where the patient feels your touch. Normally both stimuli are felt.

With lesions of the sensory cortex, only one stimulus may be recognized. The stimulus on the side opposite the damaged cortex is extinguished.

Dermatomes

Knowledge of dermatomes helps you localize neurologic lesions to a specific level of the spinal cord, particularly in spinal cord injury. *A dermatome is the band of skin innervated by the sensory root of a single spinal nerve.* Dermatome and peripheral nerve patterns are illustrated in the following figures, which reflect the international standard recommended by the American Spinal Injury Association.[55] Dermatome levels are more variable than these diagrams suggest. They overlap at their upper and lower margins and also slightly across the midline.

In spinal cord injury, the sensory level may be several segments *lower* than the spinal lesion, for reasons that are not well understood. Percussing for the level of vertebral pain may be helpful.[56]

Radial nerve

Ulnar nerve

Median nerve

Lateral cutaneous nerve of thigh

Anterior femoral cutaneous nerve

Lateral cutaneous nerve of calf

Superficial peroneal nerve

Cutaneous branches of saphenous nerve

CN V

C2

C3 Front of neck

C3

C4

T2

T3

C5

C5

T4

T4 Nipples

T5

T6

T7

T8

C6

T9

C6

T1

T10

T1

T10 Umbilicus

T11

T12

L1 Inguinal

L1

L2

L2

C8

C8

C7

C7

S2,3

L3

L3

C8 Ring and little fingers

L4

L4

L4 Knee

L5

L5

S1

S1

L5 Anterior ankle and foot

AREAS INNERVATED BY PERIPHERAL NERVES

DERMATOMES INNERVATED BY POSTERIOR ROOTS

Do not try to memorize all the dermatomes. Instead, focus on learning selected dermatomes such as those specifically named on the diagrams. The distribution of a few key peripheral nerves is shown in the inserts on the left.

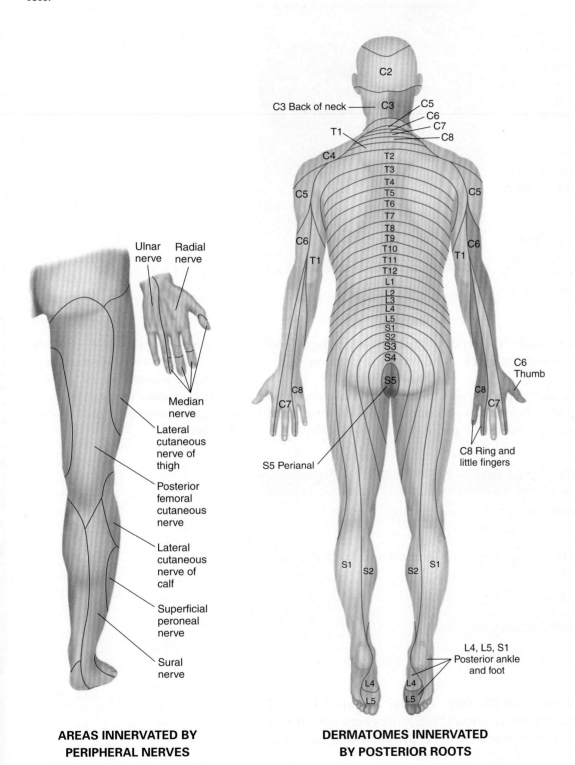

**AREAS INNERVATED BY
PERIPHERAL NERVES**

**DERMATOMES INNERVATED
BY POSTERIOR ROOTS**

Muscle Stretch Reflexes (Deep Tendon Reflexes)

Eliciting the *muscle stretch reflexes* requires special handling of the reflex hammer. Select a properly weighted reflex hammer and learn the different uses of the pointed end and the flat end. For example, the pointed end is useful for striking small areas, such as your finger as it overlies the biceps tendon. Test the reflexes as follows:

- Encourage the patient to relax, then position the limbs properly and symmetrically.

- Hold the reflex hammer loosely between your thumb and index finger so that it swings freely in an arc within the limits set by your palm and other fingers.

- With your wrist relaxed, strike the tendon briskly using a rapid wrist movement. Your strike should be quick and direct, not glancing.

- Note the speed, force, and amplitude of the reflex response and grade the response using the scale below. Always compare the response of one side with the other. Reflexes are usually graded on a 0 to 4 scale.[57]

Hyperactive reflexes (hyperreflexia) in CNS lesions along the descending corticospinal tract. Look for associated upper motor neuron findings of weakness, spasticity, or a Babinski sign.

Scale for Grading Reflexes	
4+	Very brisk, hyperactive, with *clonus* (rhythmic oscillations between flexion and extension)
3+	Brisker than average; possibly but not necessarily indicative of disease
2+	Average; normal
1+	Somewhat diminished; low normal
0	No response

Reflex response depends partly on the force of your stimulus. Use only enough force to provoke a definite response. Differences between sides are usually easier to assess than symmetric changes. Symmetrically increased, diminished, or even absent reflexes can be normal.

Reinforcement

If the patient's reflexes are symmetrically diminished or absent, use *reinforcement,* a technique involving isometric contraction of other muscles for up to 10 seconds that may increase reflex activity. In testing arm reflexes, for example, ask the patient to clench his or her teeth or to squeeze one thigh with the opposite hand. If leg reflexes are diminished or absent, reinforce them by asking the patient to lock fingers and pull one hand against the other. Tell the patient to pull just before you strike the tendon.

USING REINFORCEMENT

The Biceps Reflex (C5, C6)

The patient's elbow should be partially flexed and the forearm pronated with palm down. Place your thumb or finger firmly on the biceps tendon. Aim the strike with the reflex hammer directly through your digit toward the biceps tendon.

PATIENT SITTING

PATIENT LYING DOWN

Observe flexion at the elbow, and watch for and feel the contraction of the biceps muscle.

The Triceps Reflex (C6, C7)

The patient may be sitting or supine. Flex the patient's arm at the elbow, with palm toward the body, and pull it slightly across the chest. Strike the triceps tendon with a direct blow directly behind and just above the elbow. Watch for contraction of the triceps muscle and extension at the elbow.

If you have difficulty getting the patient to relax, try supporting the upper arm. Ask the patient to let the arm go limp, as if it were "hung up to dry." Then strike the triceps tendon.

The Brachioradialis Reflex (C5, C6)

The patient's hand should rest on the abdomen or the lap, with the forearm partly pronated. Strike the radius with the point or flat edge of the reflex hammer, about 1 to 2 in above the wrist. Watch for flexion and supination of the forearm.

The Quadriceps (Patellar) Reflex (L2, L3, L4)

The patient may be either sitting or lying down as long as the knee is flexed. Briskly tap the patellar tendon just below the patella. Note contraction of the quadriceps with extension at the knee. Place your hand on the patient's anterior thigh to feel this reflex.

PATIENT SITTING

There are two options for examining the supine patient. Supporting both knees at once, allows you to assess small differences between quadricep's reflexes by repeatedly testing one reflex and then the other. If supporting both legs is uncomfortable for you or the patient, you can place your supporting arm under the patient's leg. Some patients find it easier to relax with this method.

The Achilles (Ankle) Reflex (Primarily S1)

If the patient is sitting, partially dorsiflex the foot at the ankle. Persuade the patient to relax. Strike the Achilles tendon and watch and feel for plantar flexion at the ankle. Also note the speed of relaxation after muscular contraction.

The slowed relaxation phase of reflexes in *hypothyroidism* is often best detected during the ankle reflex.

PATIENT SITTING

When the patient is lying down, flex one leg at both hip and knee and rotate it externally so that the lower leg rests across the opposite shin. Then dorsiflex the foot at the ankle and strike the Achilles tendon.

PATIENT LYING DOWN

Clonus

If the reflexes seem hyperactive, test for *ankle clonus*. Support the knee in a partly flexed position. With your other hand, dorsiflex and plantar flex the foot a few times while encouraging the patient to relax, and then sharply dorsiflex the foot and maintain it in dorsiflexion. Look and feel for rhythmic oscillations between dorsiflexion and plantar flexion. Normally the ankle does not react to this stimulus. There may be a few clonic beats if the patient is tense or has exercised.

Clonus may also be elicited at other joints. A sharp downward displacement of the patella, for example, may elicit patellar clonus in the extended knee.

Sustained clonus indicates CNS disease. The ankle plantar flexes and dorsiflexes repetitively and rhythmically. Clonus must be present for a reflex to be graded 4.

Cutaneous or Superficial Stimulation Reflexes

The Abdominal Reflexes

Test the abdominal reflexes by lightly but briskly stroking each side of the abdomen, above (T8, T9, T10) and below (T10, T11, T12) the umbilicus, in the directions illustrated. Use a key, the wooden end of a cotton-tipped applicator, or a tongue blade twisted and split longitudinally. Note the contraction of the abdominal muscles and deviation of the umbilicus toward the stimulus. Obesity may mask an abdominal reflex. In this situation, use your finger to retract the patient's umbilicus away from the side to be stimulated. Feel with your retracting finger for the muscular contraction.

Abdominal reflexes may be absent in both central and peripheral nerve disorders.

The Plantar Response (L5, S1)

With a key, the wooden end of an applicator stick or the end of a tongue blade, stroke from the heel moving up toward the small toe to the ball of the foot, curving medially across the ball. Use the lightest stimulus that will provoke a response, but increase firmness if necessary. Closely observe movement of the big toe, normally plantar flexion with the toes curving down and inward. Dorsiflexion of the big toe and fanning of the other toes, is a *"present" Babinski response*, arising from a CNS lesion affecting the corticospinal tract. The Babinski response can be transiently found in unconscious states from drug or alcohol intoxication and during the post-ictal period following a seizure.

A Babinski response is either present or not present although often documented as positive or negative.

Some patients withdraw from this stimulus by flexing the hip and the knee. Hold the ankle, if necessary, to complete your observation. It is sometimes difficult to distinguish withdrawal from a Babinski response.[58]

A marked Babinski response is occasionally accompanied by reflex flexion at hip and knee.

As you proceed to the *general physical examination*, include the following assessments. Check for unusual odors.

Consider alcohol, liver failure, or uremia.

- Look for abnormalities of the skin, including color, moisture, evidence of bleeding disorders, needle marks, and other lesions.

Note any jaundice, cyanosis, or the cherry red color of carbon monoxide poisoning.

- Inspect the scalp and skull for signs of trauma.

  Check for bruises, lacerations, or swelling.

- Examine the fundi carefully.

  Examine closely for *hypertensive retinopathy* and *papilledema,* an important sign of elevated intracranial pressure.

- Test the corneal reflexes to make sure they are intact. Remember that contact lenses may abolish these reflexes.

  Corneal reflex loss occurs in coma and lesions affecting CN V or CN VII.

- Inspect the ears and nose, and examine the mouth and throat.

  Blood or cerebrospinal fluid in the nose or the ears suggests a skull fracture; otitis media suggests a possible brain abscess.

  Tongue injury suggests a seizure.

- Be sure to evaluate the heart, lungs, and abdomen.

Further Examination

As you complete the neurologic examination, check for facial asymmetry and asymmetries in motor, sensory, and reflex function. Test for meningeal signs if indicated.

Meningeal signs are suspicious for *meningitis or subarachnoid hemorrhage.*[59]

SPECIAL TECHNIQUES

Assessment for Stuporous or Comatose Patient

Coma is a state of impaired arousal and awareness, signals a potentially life-threatening event affecting the two hemispheres, the brainstem, or both. Accurate assessment is critical.[60–65] Although the arousal and awareness functions are interrelated, "a change in one is not always associated with a similar change in the other."[60] Arousal occurs in the ascending reticular activating system of the brainstem which projects through the thalamus to several areas of the cortex, which "processes, integrates, and gives context to the information provided to it thus generating awareness. Injury to any of these areas or their connections can result in impaired consciousness." The usual sequence of history, physical examination, and laboratory evaluation does not apply. Instead, you must:

See Table 20-8, Metabolic and Structural Coma, p. 737.

- First assess and stabilize the ABCs (airway, breathing, and circulation)

- Establish the patient's level of consciousness

- Perform the neurologic examination. Identify any focal or asymmetric findings and determine if the cause of impaired consciousness is structural or metabolic.

- Interview the relatives, friends, or witnesses to establish the speed of onset and duration of unconsciousness. The warning symptoms, precipitating factors, or previous episodes; and the prior appearance and behavior of the patient are helpful. Any history of past medical and psychiatric illnesses is also useful.

During the examination, remember two cardinal DON'Ts:

"Dont's" When Assessing the Comatose Patient

- *Don't* dilate the pupils, the single most important clue to the underlying cause of coma (structural vs. metabolic), and
- *Don't* flex the neck if there is any question of trauma to the head or neck. Immobilize the cervical spine and get an x-ray first to rule out fractures of the cervical vertebrae that could compress and damage the spinal cord.

Airway, Breathing, and Circulation

Quickly check the patient's color and pattern of breathing. Inspect the posterior pharynx and listen over the trachea for stridor to make sure the airway is clear. If respirations are slowed or shallow, or if the airway is obstructed by secretions, consider intubating the patient as soon as possible while stabilizing the cervical spine.

Assess the remaining vital signs: pulse, blood pressure, and *rectal* temperature. If hypotension or hemorrhage is present, establish intravenous access and begin intravenous fluids. (Further emergency management and laboratory studies are beyond the scope of this text.)

Level of Consciousness

Level of consciousness primarily reflects the patient's capacity for arousal, or wakefulness. Testing these targets is at the level of activity that the patient can be aroused to perform in response to escalating stimuli from the examiner.

Five clinical levels of consciousness are described in the table below, with related techniques for examination. Increase your stimuli in a stepwise manner, depending on the patient's response.

When you examine patients with an altered level of consciousness, describe and record exactly what you see and hear. Imprecise use of terms such as lethargy, obtunded, stupor, or coma may mislead other examiners.

Level of Consciousness (Arousal): Techniques and Patient Response

Level	Technique	Abnormal Responses
Alertness	Speak to the patient in a normal tone of voice. An alert patient opens the eyes, looks at you, and responds fully and appropriately to stimuli (arousal intact).	
Lethargy	Speak to the patient in a loud voice. For example, call the patient's name or ask, "How are you?"	A lethargic patient appears drowsy but opens the eyes and looks at you, responds to questions, and then falls asleep.
Obtunded	Shake the patient gently as if awakening a sleeper.	An obtunded patient opens the eyes and looks at you, but responds slowly and is somewhat confused. Alertness and interest in the environment are decreased.
Stupor	Apply a painful stimulus. For example, pinch a tendon, rub the sternum, or roll a pencil across a nail bed. (No stronger stimuli needed!)	A stuporous patient arouses from sleep only after painful stimuli. Verbal responses are slow or even absent. The patient lapses into an unresponsive state when the stimulus ceases. There is minimal awareness of self or the environment.
Coma	Apply repeated painful stimuli.	A comatose patient remains unarousable with eyes closed. There is no evident response to inner need or external stimuli.

The Glasgow Coma Scale

Because imprecise terms may mislead other examiners, the Glasgow Coma Scale (GCS), a standardized tool for objective assessment of patients, should be used. There is a numeric value assigned to three different components: eye opening, motor response, and verbal response. Each area receives a score and all the scores are then added together to determine the level of brain function.

Using the Glasgow Coma Scale

The points associated with the Glasgow Coma Scale are determined to assess levels of consciousness and coma. Points are allotted for each of the three areas: eye opening, verbal response and motor responses per the grid below:

Activity		Score
Eye Opening		
None	1 = Even to supraorbital pressure	
To pain	2 = Pain from sternum/limb/ supraorbital pressure	
To speech	3 = Nonspecific response, not necessarily to command	
Spontaneous	4 = Eyes open, not necessarily aware	_____
Motor Response		
None	1 = To any pain; limbs remain flaccid	
Extension	2 = Shoulder adducted and shoulder and forearm internally rotated	
Flexor response	3 = Withdrawal response or assumption of hemiplegic posture	
Withdrawal	4 = Arm withdraws to pain, shoulder abducts	
Localizes pain	5 = Arm attempts to remove supraorbital/chest pressure	
Obeys commands	6 = Follows simple commands	_____
Verbal Response		
None	1 = No verbalization of any type	
Incomprehensible	2 = Moans/groans, no speech	
Inappropriate	3 = Intelligible, no sustained sentences	
Confused	4 = Converses but confused, disoriented	
Oriented	5 = Converses and is oriented	_____
		TOTAL (3–15)[a]

[a]**Interpretation:** Patients with scores of 3–8 usually are considered to be in a coma. A score of 15 is a fully alert and functioning person. A score of 3 is the lowest possible score and denotes "no response" in any of the 3 areas assessed.[66]

Neurologic Evaluation

RESPIRATIONS. Observe the rate, rhythm, and pattern of respirations. Because neural structures that govern breathing in the cortex and brainstem overlap those that govern consciousness, abnormalities of respiration often occur in coma.

See Table 20-8, Metabolic and Structural Coma, p. 737 and Chapter 13, Abnormalities in Rate and Rhythm of Breathing, p. 365.

PUPILS. Observe the size and equality of the pupils and test their reaction to light. The presence or absence of the light reaction is one of the most important signs distinguishing structural from metabolic causes of coma. The light reaction often remains intact in metabolic coma.

See Table 20-9, Pupils in Comatose Patients, p. 738.

Structural lesions from stroke, bleeding, abscess, or tumor mass may lead to asymmetric pupils and loss of light reaction due to pressure on the cranial nerves.

OCULAR MOVEMENT. Observe the position of the eyes and eyelids at rest. Check for horizontal deviation of the eyes to one side (*gaze preference*). When the oculomotor pathways are intact, the eyes look straight ahead.

In structural hemispheric lesions, the eyes "look at the lesion" in the affected hemisphere.

In irritative lesions from epilepsy or early cerebral hemorrhage, the eyes "look away" from the affected hemisphere.

This reflex helps to assess brainstem function in a comatose patient. Holding open the upper eyelids so that you can see the eyes, turn the head quickly, first to one side and then to the other. Make sure the patient has no neck injury before performing this test.

In a comatose patient with absence of doll's eye movements, the ability to move both eyes to one side is lost, suggesting a lesion of the midbrain or pons.

In a comatose patient with an intact brainstem, as the head is turned, the eyes move toward the opposite side (the doll's eye movements). In the photo, for example, the patient's head has been turned to the right; her eyes have moved to the left. Her eyes still seem to gaze at the camera. The doll's eye movements are intact.

POSTURE AND MUSCLE TONE. Observe the patient's posture. If there is no spontaneous movement, you may need to apply a painful stimulus (see p. 713). Classify the resulting pattern of movement as:

See Table 20-10, Abnormal Postures in Comatose Patients, p. 739.

- *Normal–avoidant*—the patient pushes the stimulus away or withdraws.

- *Stereotypic*—the stimulus evokes abnormal postural responses of the trunk and extremities.

- *Flaccid paralysis or no response*

Test muscle tone by grasping each forearm near the wrist and raising it to a vertical position. Note the position of the hand, which is usually only slightly flexed at the wrist.

The hemiplegia of sudden cerebral accidents is usually flaccid at first. The limp hand drops to form a right angle with the wrist.

Then lower the arm to about 12 or 18 in off the bed and drop it. Watch how it falls. A normal arm drops somewhat slowly.

A flaccid arm drops rapidly, like a rock.

Support the patient's flexed knees. Then extend one leg at a time at the knee and let it fall (see below). Compare the speed with which each leg falls.

In *acute hemiplegia*, the flaccid leg falls more rapidly.

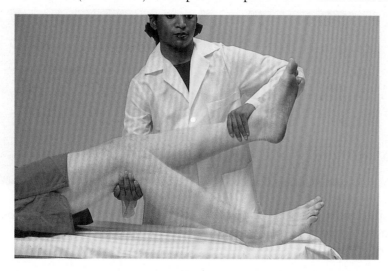

Flex both legs so that the heels rest on the bed and then release them. The normal leg returns slowly to its original extended position.

In acute hemiplegia, the flaccid leg falls rapidly into extension, with external rotation at the hip.

Meningeal Signs

Test for these important signs whenever you suspect meningeal inflammation from meningitis or subarachnoid hemorrhage.

Neck Mobility/Nuchal Rigidity

First make sure there is no injury or fracture to the cervical vertebrae or cervical cord. In trauma settings, this often requires radiologic evaluation. Then, with the patient supine, place your hands behind the patient's head and flex the neck forward, if possible, until the chin touches the chest. Normally the neck is supple, and the patient can easily bend the head and neck forward.

Neck stiffness and resistance to flexion in 84% of patients with *acute bacterial meningitis* and in 21% to 86% with *subarachnoid hemorrhage*.[67]

Brudzinski Sign

As you flex the neck, watch the hips and knees in reaction to your maneuver. Normally they should remain relaxed and motionless.

Flexion of the hips and knees is a *positive Brudzinski sign* and suggests meningeal inflammation.[68]

Kernig Sign

Flex the patient's leg at both the hip and the knee, and then straighten the knee. Discomfort behind the knee during full extension occurs in many normal people, but this maneuver should not produce pain.

Pain and increased resistance to extending the knee are *positive Kernig signs.* When bilateral, it suggests meningeal irritation.[68,69]

Compression of a lumbosacral nerve root may also cause resistance, together with pain in the low back and the posterior thigh. Only one leg is usually involved.

Reducing Risk of Diabetic Peripheral Neuropathy

Diabetes causes several types of peripheral neuropathy.[70] Maintaining optimal glycemic control can prevent or delay the onset of neuropathy, particularly from type 1 diabetes.

- *Distal symmetric sensorimotor polyneuropathy.* This is the most common type of diabetic neuropathy. It is slowly progressive, often asymptomatic, and a risk factor for ulcerations, arthropathy, and amputation. Symptomatic patients report burning electrical pain in the lower extremities, usually at night.

- *Autonomic dysfunction, mononeuropathies,* and *polyradiculopathies,* including *diabetic amyotrophy,* which initially causes unilateral thigh pain and proximal lower extremity weakness.

Patients with diabetes should have their feet examined regularly for neuropathy, including testing pinprick sensation, ankle reflexes, vibration perception (with a 128-Hz tuning fork) and plantar light touch sensation (with a Semmes–Weinstein monofilament), as well as checking for skin breakdown, poor circulation, and musculoskeletal abnormalities.[71]

The Lower Extremity Amputation Prevention (LEAP)/ Semmes–Weinstein test detects the loss of protective sensation using a 5.07 monofilament nylon wire with 10 g of force on designated sites on the plantar surface of the feet. The test is positive for diabetic neuropathy, if the patient cannot feel the monofilament.

Steps for the Monofilament (LEAP) Examination

1. Explain the rationale for the examination.
2. Patient's shoes and socks removed.
3. Demonstrate what the monofilament feels like on the patient's hand/arm.
4. Ask the patient to respond "yes" each time they feel the pressure of the monofilament.
5. Have the patient close his/her eyes and hold the monofilament perpendicular to the patient's foot.
6. Press the monofilament until it bends in a "C" shape on the designated areas (the patient should sense the monofilament by the time it bows).
7. Hold the monofilament in place for 1 to 2 seconds. Press so that it buckles one of two times and say "time one" or "time two." The patient identifies which time the foot was touched.
8. Randomize the site sequence.
9. Test both feet on plantar surface of the distal hallux and third toe, and the first, third, and fifth metatarsal heads. Avoid ulcers, calluses, or corns.

RECORDING YOUR FINDINGS

Recording the Examination—The Nervous System

Note that initially you may use sentences to describe your findings; later you will use phrases. The style below contains phrases appropriate for most write-ups. Note the five components of the examination and write-up of the nervous system.

"**Mental Status:** Alert, relaxed, and cooperative. Thought process coherent. O×4 (person, place, time, and situation). Detailed cognitive testing deferred. **Cranial Nerves:** I—not tested; II through XII intact. **Motor:** Good muscle bulk and tone. Strength 5/5 throughout. Cerebellar—Rapid alternating movements (RAMs), finger-to-nose, heel-to-shin intact bilaterally. Gait rhythmic, with smooth alternating arm swing and stable base. Romberg—maintains balance with eyes closed. No pronator drift. **Sensory:** Sharp/dull, light touch, position, and vibration intact bilaterally. **Reflexes** (biceps, triceps, brachioradialis, knee, ankle): 2+ and symmetric with bilateral plantar responses."

OR

"**Mental Status:** Patient alert and tries to answer questions but has difficulty finding words. **Cranial Nerves:** I—not tested; II—visual acuity intact, visual fields full; III, IV, VI—extraocular movements intact; V motor—temporal and masseter strength intact; VII motor—prominent right facial droop and flattening of right nasolabial fold, left facial movements intact, sensory—taste not tested; VIII—hearing intact bilaterally to whispered voice; IX, X—gag intact; XI—strength of sternomastoid and trapezius muscles 5/5; XII—tongue midline. **Motor:** strength in right biceps, triceps, iliopsoas, gluteals, quadriceps, hamstring, and ankle flexor and extensor muscles 3/5 with good bulk but increased tone and spasticity; strength in comparable muscle groups on the left 5/5 with good bulk and tone. Gait—unable to test. Cerebellar—unable to test on right due to right arm and leg weakness; RAMs, Finger → Nose, Heel → Shin intact on left, unable to perform on the right. Romberg—unable to test due to right leg weakness. Right pronator drift present. **Sensory:** decreased sensation to sharp over right face, arm, and leg; intact on the left. Stereognosis and two-point discrimination not tested. **Reflexes** per table:

	Biceps	Triceps	Brach	Knee	Ankle	Plantar
RT	4+	4+	4+	4+	4+	↑
LT	2+	2+	2+	2+	1+	↓

Suggests left hemispheric cerebrovascular accident in distribution of the left middle cerebral artery, with right sided hemiparesis.

HEALTH PROMOTION AND COUNSELING

Important Topics for Health Promotion and Counseling

* Preventing stroke or TIA

Preventing Stroke and Transient Ischemic Attack (TIA)

A *stroke* is a sudden neurologic deficit caused by cerebrovascular ischemia (87%) or hemorrhage (13%). *Hemorrhagic strokes* may be intracerebral (10% of all strokes) or subarachnoid (3% of all strokes). Strokes are the fifth

See Table 20-2, Types of Strokes, pp. 729–730.

leading cause of death in the United States and a leading cause of long-term disability.[72]

The American Heart Association (AHA) and the American Stroke Association (ASA) have established tissue-based definitions for ischemic stroke and TIA that have important implications for assessing and preventing strokes.[73] These definitions encourage early neurodiagnostic imaging following a TIA and risk stratification for subsequent stroke.

- *Ischemic stroke* is "an infarction of CNS tissue" that may be symptomatic or silent. "Symptomatic ischemic strokes are manifest by clinical signs of focal or global cerebral, spinal, or retinal dysfunction caused by CNS infarction. A silent stroke is a documented CNS infarction that was asymptomatic."

- *TIA* is now defined as "a transient episode of neurologic dysfunction caused by focal brain, spinal cord, or retinal ischemia, without acute infarction." The AHA/ASA guidelines recommend neurodiagnostic imaging within 24 hours of symptom onset and routine noninvasive imaging of the carotid and intracranial vessels.[74]

The AHA/ASA report cites the well-validated *ABCD2 scoring system* for predicting ischemic stroke within 2, 7, and 90 days after TIA: **A**ge ≥60 years; initial **B**lood pressure ≥140/90 mm Hg; **C**linical features of focal weakness or impaired speech without focal weakness; **D**uration 10 to 59 minutes or ≥60 minutes; and **D**iabetes.[73]

- TIAs are a major risk factor for stroke, which occurs in 3% to 10% of patients within 2 days and in 9% to 17% within 90 days.[47] Short-term stroke risk is highest in those with age 60 years and older, diabetes, focal symptoms of weakness or impaired speech, and a TIA lasting more than 10 minutes. One population-based study found a combined risk for recurrent TIA/stroke/and death of 25% within the 3 months following a TIA.[74]

Stroke at a Glance

Key Facts for Prevention and Patient Education[72,75,76]
- Stroke affects nearly 800,000 Americans each year, including more than 600,000 suffering a first stroke, and accounts for about 1 in every 20 deaths.
- The total annual costs associated with stroke are estimated to be about $34 billion.
- Stroke prevalence and mortality are disproportionately higher in *African Americans* compared to whites:
  - Prevalence, black vs. white men: 4.2% vs. 2.2%; black vs. white women: 4.7% vs. 2.5%
  - Mortality per 100,000, black vs. white men: 55 vs. 36; black vs. white women: 47 vs. 36
- Although younger and middle-aged women have lower age-specific stroke incidence rates than men, rates increase with age so that women, who on average live longer than men, have an overall higher lifetime

Cardiovascular causes of death, including stroke, are the greatest contributors to the 5-year disparity in life expectancy for African American men compared to white men and the 4-year racial disparity for women.[77] However, the racial gap in life expectancy has recently been declining.

risk for stroke. Risk factors for women include autoimmune collagen vascular disease and history of preeclampsia, gestational diabetes, and pregnancy-induced hypertension.

- The prevalence of silent stroke, estimated to range from 6% to 28%, increases with age.
- Individuals with TIA have a 1-year mortality of ~12%; 10-year risks for stroke and death from cardiovascular disease are 19% and 43%, respectively.
- Only 51% of the U.S. population is aware of the five stroke warning signs and would call 9-1-1 if they thought someone was having a stroke.
- Stroke outcomes improve significantly when thrombolytic therapy is given within 3 to 4.5 hours of symptom onset; however, only a minority of those suffering a stroke reaches an emergency room within this time window.

Symptoms and signs of stroke depend on the vascular territory affected in the brain. The most common cause of ischemic symptoms is occlusion of the *middle cerebral artery*, which causes *visual field cuts* and *contralateral hemiparesis and sensory deficits*. Occlusion of the *left middle cerebral artery* often produces *aphasia;* and occlusion of the right middle cerebral artery, *neglect* or *inattention* to the opposite side of the body.

See Table 20-2, Types of Strokes, pp. 729–730.

See Table 20-3, Disorders of Speech, p. 731 for discussion of *aphasia*.

Stroke Warning Signs

The AHA and the ASA urge patients to seek immediate care for any of the warning signs. It is important to teach these to your patients.

AHA/ASA Stroke Warning Signs and Symptoms[78]

F Face Drooping—Does one side of the face droop or is it numb? Ask the person to smile. Is the person's smile uneven?

A Arm Weakness—Is one arm weak or numb? Ask the person to raise both arms. Does one arm drift downward?

S Speech Difficulty—Is speech slurred? Is the person unable to speak or hard to understand? Ask the person to repeat a simple sentence, like "The sky is blue." Is the sentence repeated correctly?

T Time to call 9-1-1—If someone shows any of these symptoms, even if the symptoms go away, call 9-1-1 and get the person to the hospital immediately. Check the time so you'll know when the first symptoms appeared

Beyond FAST: Other important symptoms

Sudden numbness or weakness of the leg, arm, or face

Sudden confusion or trouble understanding

Sudden trouble seeing in one or both eyes

Sudden trouble walking, dizziness, loss of balance, or coordination

Sudden severe headache with no known cause

Stroke Risk Factors—Primary Prevention

Recognizing that stroke and coronary heart disease share common cardiovascular risk factors and threats to health, in Healthy People 2020 and the AHA presented a new concept of "cardiovascular health" that encompasses seven health behaviors and health factors, and a new set of combined impact goals for the coming decade:

By 2020, to improve the cardiovascular health of all Americans by 20%, while reducing deaths from cardiovascular disease and stroke by 20%.[79]

For primary prevention, target documented modifiable risk factors, detailed in the box. Learn the indications for using aspirin in healthy and diabetic individuals.[80,81]

Optimal blood pressure control is essential for preventing *hemorrhagic stroke*. Additional risk factors for the most common cause of hemorrhagic stroke—ruptured aneurysms in the circle of Willis—include smoking, alcohol use, oral contraceptives, and family history in a first-degree relative.

Stroke Risk Factors—Primary Prevention for Ischemic Stoke	
Hypertension	Hypertension is the leading determinant of risk for both ischemic and hemorrhagic strokes. Pharmacologic reduction of blood pressure of blood pressure significantly reduces stroke risk, particularly among African Americans and older adults.[82]
Smoking	Smoking is associated with doubling the risk of ischemic stroke and a 2- to 4-fold increased risk of subarachnoid hemorrhage. Smoking cessation rapidly reduces the risk of stroke, but never to the level of never smokers.
Dyslipidemia	Statin treatment reduce the risk of all strokes.
Diabetes	Stroke risk is doubled with diabetes and 20% of diabetic patients will die of stroke. Good blood pressure control and statin therapy reduce stroke risk in diabetic patients.
Weight	Obesity doubles risk of ischemic stroke by 64%.
Diet and nutrition	Dietary factors affect stroke risk primarily by elevating blood pressure. Decreasing salt and saturated fat intake and diets emphasizing fruits, vegetables, nuts, and low-fat dairy products may reduce stroke risk.

(continued)

Physical inactivity	Moderate exercise, like brisk walking for 150 minutes a week or 30 minutes on most days, improves cardiovascular health.
Alcohol use	Alcohol use has a direct dose-dependent effect on the risk of hemorrhagic stroke. Heavy alcohol use increases the risk for all types of stroke due to effects on hypertension, hypercoagulable states, cardiac arrhythmias, and reduced cerebral blood flow.

Disease-Specific Risk Factors

Atrial fibrillation	Valvular (rheumatic) and nonvalvular atrial fibrillation increases risk of stroke between 2- to 7-fold and 17-fold, respectively, compared to the general population. Antiplatelet agents and anticoagulants can reduce the risk for ischemic stroke. When considering antithrombotic therapy, experts recommend individual risk stratification into high-, moderate-, and low-risk groups to balance risk of stroke against risk of bleeding. $CHADS_2$ is a commonly used scoring system based on **C**ongestive heart failure, **H**ypertension, **A**ge ≥75 years, **D**iabetes, and prior **S**troke/TIA. The CHA_2DS_2-VASc, which adds an age category of 65 to 74 years, female sex, and vascular disease to the scoring system, improves risk stratification for individuals estimated as low or moderate risk with $CHADS_2$.[72]
Carotid artery disease	The estimated prevalence of clinically important carotid artery stenosis in the U.S. population over age 65 is 1%. Medical therapy, including statins, antiplatelet agents, treatment of diabetes and hypertension, and smoking cessation, has reduced the risk of stroke in individuals with asymptomatic carotid artery stenosis to less than 2% annually. Experts recommend carotid endarterectomy for selected asymptomatic patients with carotid artery stenosis >60%—provided that the surgeon and center have very low perioperative risks for stroke and mortality.[79]
Obstructive sleep apnea	Sleep apnea is an independent risk factor for stroke, particularly in men. Stroke risk increases with increasing sleep apnea severity as measured by the number of respiratory events (cessation or air flow reduction) per hour. Sleep apnea is usually treated with continuous positive airway pressure (CPAP), though its effectiveness for reducing stroke risk is unknown.

TIA and Stroke—Secondary Prevention

For the patient who has already suffered a TIA or stroke, focus on: identifying the underlying cause including noncardiac emboli, cardiac emboli, and carotid artery stenosis; reducing cardiovascular risk factors, including inactivity, hyperlipidemia, poorly controlled diabetes or hypertension, smoking, and heavy alcohol consumption; and identifying the most appropriate interventions for secondary prevention, including antiplatelet agents, anticoagulants, and carotid revascularization.[82] Strokes in young adults often have a different set of causes—patent foramen ovale and less commonly, carotid or vertebral/basilar artery dissection, hypercoagulable states, or cocaine and illicit drug use.[83]

TABLE
20-1

Disorders of the Central and Peripheral Nervous Systems

Central Nervous System Disorders

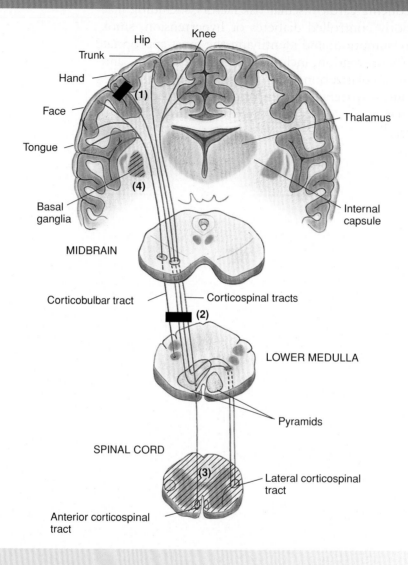

- Hip
- Knee
- Trunk
- Hand
- (1)
- Face
- Thalamus
- Tongue
- (4)
- Basal ganglia
- Internal capsule
- **MIDBRAIN**
- Corticobulbar tract
- Corticospinal tracts
- (2)
- **LOWER MEDULLA**
- Pyramids
- **SPINAL CORD**
- (3)
- Lateral corticospinal tract
- Anterior corticospinal tract

	Typical Findings			
Location of Lesion	Motor	Sensory	Deep Tendon Reflexes	Examples of Cause
Cerebral Cortex (1)	Chronic contralateral corticospinal-type weakness and spasticity. Flexion is stronger than extension in the arm, plantar flexion is stronger than dorsiflexion in the foot, and the leg is externally rotated at the hip.	Contralateral sensory loss in the limbs and trunk on the same side as the motor deficits	Increased	Cortical stroke
Brainstem (2)	Weakness and spasticity as above, plus cranial nerve deficits such as diplopia (from weakness of the extraocular muscles) and dysarthria	Variable; no typical sensory findings	Increased	Brainstem stroke, acoustic neuroma
Spinal Cord (3)	Weakness and spasticity as above, but often affecting both sides (when cord damage is bilateral), causing paraplegia or quadriplegia depending on the level of injury	Dermatomal sensory deficit on the trunk bilaterally at the level of the lesion, and sensory loss from tract damage below the level of the lesion	increased	Trauma, causing cord compression
Subcortical Gray Matter: Basal Ganglia (4)	Slowness of movement (bradykinesia), rigidity, and tremor	Sensation not affected	Normal or decreased	Parkinsonism
Cerebellar (not illustrated)	Hypotonia, ataxia, and other abnormal movements, including nystagmus, dysdiadochokinesis, and dysmetria	Sensation not affected	Normal or decreased	Cerebellar stroke, brain tumor

(table continues on page 728)

TABLE
20-1

Disorders of the Central and Peripheral Nervous Systems (continued)

Peripheral Nervous System Disorders

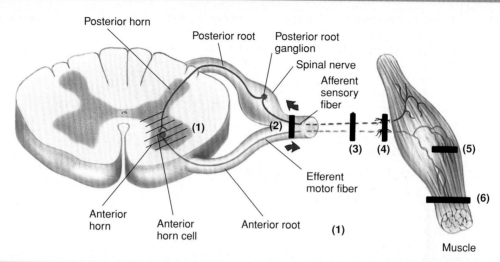

Posterior horn · Posterior root · Posterior root ganglion · Spinal nerve · Afferent sensory fiber · Anterior horn · Anterior horn cell · Anterior root · Efferent motor fiber · Muscle

Location of Lesion	Typical Findings			
	Motor	Sensory	Deep Tendon Reflexes/ Muscle Stretch Reflex	Examples of Cause
Anterior Horn Cell (1)	Weakness and atrophy in a segmental or focal pattern; fasciculations	Weakness and atrophy in a segmental or focal pattern; fasciculations	Decreased	Polio, amyotrophic lateral sclerosis
Spinal Roots and Nerves (2)	Weakness and atrophy in a root-innervated pattern; sometimes with fasciculations	Weakness and atrophy in a root-innervated pattern; sometimes with fasciculations	Decreased	Herniated cervical or lumbar disc
Peripheral Nerve— Mononeuropathy (3)	Weakness and atrophy in a peripheral nerve distribution; sometimes with fasciculations	Weakness and atrophy in a peripheral nerve distribution; sometimes with fasciculations	Decreased	Trauma
Peripheral Nerve— Polyneuropathy (4)	Weakness and atrophy more distal than proximal; sometimes with fasciculations	Weakness and atrophy more distal than proximal; sometimes with fasciculations	Decreased	Peripheral polyneuropathy of alcoholism, diabetes
Neuromuscular Junction (5)	Fatigability more than weakness	Fatigability more than weakness	Normal	Myasthenia gravis
Muscle (6)	Weakness usually more proximal than distal; fasciculations rare	Weakness usually more proximal than distal; fasciculations rare	Normal or decreased	Muscular dystrophy

TABLE

20-2

Types of Stroke

Assessment of stroke requires careful history-taking and a detailed physical examination, and should focus on three fundamental questions: *What brain area and related vascular territory explain the patient's findings? Is the stroke ischemic or hemorrhagic? If ischemic, is the mechanism thrombus or embolus?* Stroke is a medical emergency, and timing is of the essence. Answers to these questions are critical to patient outcomes and use of antithrombotic therapies in acute ischemic stroke.

In *acute ischemic stroke,* ischemic brain injury begins with a central core of very low perfusion and often irreversible cell death. This core is surrounded by an *ischemic penumbra* of metabolically disturbed cells that are still potentially viable, depending on restoration of blood flow and duration of ischemia. Because most irreversible damage occurs in the first 3–6 hours after onset of symptoms, therapies targeted to the 3-hour window achieve the best outcomes, with recovery in up to 50% of patients in some studies.[79]

Clinical Features and Vascular Territories of Stroke		
Clinical Finding	**Vascular Territory**	**Additional Comments**
Contralateral leg weakness	*Anterior circulation*—anterior cerebral artery (ACA)	Includes stem of circle of Willis connecting internal carotid artery to ACA, and the segment distal to ACA and its anterior choroidal branch
Contralateral face, arm > leg weakness, sensory loss, vision field cut, aphasia (left MCA) or neglect, apraxia (right MCA)	*Anterior circulation*—middle cerebral artery (MCA)	Largest vascular bed for stroke
Contralateral motor or sensory deficit without cortical signs	*Subcortical circulation*—lenticulostriate deep penetrating branches of MCA	Small vessel subcortical *lacunar infarcts* in internal capsule, thalamus, or brainstem. Four common syndromes: pure motor hemiparesis; pure sensory hemianesthesia; ataxic hemiparesis; clumsy hand–dysarthria syndrome
Contralateral field cut	*Posterior circulation*—posterior cerebral artery (PCA)	Includes paired vertebral and basilar artery, paired posterior cerebral arteries. Bilateral PCA infarction causes cortical blindness but preserved pupillary light reaction.
Dysphagia, dysarthria, tongue/palate deviation and/or ataxia with crossed sensory/motor deficits (= ipsilateral face with contralateral body)	*Posterior circulation*—brainstem, vertebral, or basilar artery branches	
Oculomotor deficits and/or ataxia with crossed sensory/motor deficits	*Posterior circulation*—basilar artery	Complete basilar artery occlusion—"locked-in syndrome" with intact consciousness but with inability to speak and quadriplegia

(table continues on page 730)

TABLE
20-2

Types of Stroke (continued)

Anterior cerebral artery

Anterior choroidal artery

Middle cerebral artery

Posterior cerebral artery

Lateral ventrical

Body of caudate

Internal capsule

Putamen

Globus pallidus

Thalamus

Uncus

Prefrontal area

Premotor area

Primary motor cortex

Motor speech (Broca's) area

Primary somatic sensory cortex

Somatic sensory association area

Taste area

Primary auditory cortex

Auditory association area

Sensory speech (Wernike's) area

Reading comprehension area

Visual association area

Visual cortex

- One can differentiate cortical from subcortical involvement. *Subcortical or lacunar syndromes* do not affect higher cognitive function, language, or visual fields.

Source: Adapted from American College of Physicians. *Stroke, in Neurology. Medical Knowledge Self-Assessment Program* (MKSAP) 14. Philadelphia, PA: American College of Physicians; 2012.

TABLE
20-3

Disorders of Speech

Disorders of speech fall into three groups: those affecting (1) phonation of the voice, (2) the articulation of words, and (3) the production and comprehension of language.

Aphonia. Refers to a loss of voice that accompanies disease affecting the larynx or its nerve supply. *Dysphonia* refers to less severe impairment in the volume, quality, or pitch of the voice. For example, a person may be hoarse or only able to speak in a whisper. Causes include laryngitis, laryngeal tumors, and a unilateral vocal cord paralysis (cranial nerve X).

Dysarthria. Refers to a defect in the muscular control of the speech apparatus (lips, tongue, palate, or pharynx). Words may be nasal, slurred, or indistinct, but the central symbolic aspect of language remains intact. Causes include motor lesions of the central or peripheral nervous system, parkinsonism, and cerebellar disease.

Aphasia. Refers to a disorder in producing or understanding language. It is often caused by lesions in the dominant cerebral hemisphere, usually the left.

Compared below are two common types of aphasia: (1) Wernicke, a fluent (receptive) aphasia, and (2) Broca, a nonfluent (or expressive) aphasia. There are other less common kinds of aphasia, which are distinguished by differing responses on the specific tests listed. Neurologic consultation is usually indicated.

	Wernicke Aphasia (Receptive)	Broca Aphasia (Expressive)
Qualities of Spontaneous Speech	Fluent; often rapid, voluble, and effortless. Inflection and articulation are good, but sentences lack meaning and words are malformed (paraphasias) or invented (neologisms). Speech may be totally incomprehensible.	Nonfluent; slow, with few words and laborious effort. Inflection and articulation are impaired but words are meaningful, with nouns, transitive verbs, and important adjectives. Small grammatical words are often dropped.
Word Comprehension	Impaired	Fair to good
Repetition	Impaired	Impaired
Naming	Impaired	Impaired, though the patient recognizes objects
Reading Comprehension	Impaired	Fair to good
Writing	Impaired	Impaired
Location of Lesion	Posterior superior temporal lobe	Posterior inferior frontal lobe

Although it is important to recognize aphasia early in the encounter with a patient, its full diagnostic meaning does not become clear until integrated with the neurologic examination.

TABLE
20-4
Abnormalities of Gait and Posture

Spastic Hemiparesis

Seen in corticospinal tract lesion in stroke, causing poor control of flexor muscles during swing phase. Affected arm is flexed, immobile, and held close to the side, with elbow, wrists, and interphalangeal joints flexed. Affected leg extensors spastic; ankle plantar flexed and inverted. Patients may drag toe, circle leg stiffly outward and forward (*circumduction*), or lean trunk to contralateral side to clear affected leg during walking.

Scissors Gait

Seen in spinal cord disease causing bilateral lower extremity spasticity, including adductor spasm, and abnormal proprioception. Gait is stiff. Patients advance each leg slowly, and the thighs tend to cross forward on each other at each step. Steps are short. Patients appear to be walking through water.

Steppage Gait

Seen in foot drop, usually secondary to peripheral motor unit disease. Patients either drag the feet or lift them high, with knees flexed, and bring them down with a slap onto the floor, thus appearing to be walking up stairs. They cannot walk on their heels. The steppage gait may involve one or both legs. Tibialis anterior and toe extensors are weak.

Parkinsonian Gait

Seen in the basal ganglia defects of Parkinson disease. Posture is stooped, with flexion of head, arms, hips, and knees. Patients are slow getting started. Steps are short and shuffling, with involuntary hastening (*festination*). Arm swings are decreased, and patients turn around stiffly—"all in one piece." Postural control is poor (*anteropulsion* or *retropulsion*).

← Eyes opened

Cerebellar Ataxia

Seen in disease of the cerebellum or associated tracts. Gait is staggering, unsteady, and wide based, with exaggerated difficulty on turns. Patients cannot stand steadily with feet together, whether eyes are open or closed. Other cerebellar signs are present such as dysmetria, nystagmus, and intention tremor.

← Eyes closed

Sensory Ataxia

Seen in loss of position sense in the legs (with polyneuropathy or posterior column damage). Gait is unsteady and wide based (with feet wide apart). Patients throw their feet forward and outward and bring them down, first on the heels and then on the toes, with a double tapping sound. They watch the ground for guidance when walking. With eyes closed, they cannot stand steadily with feet together (positive Romberg sign), and the staggering gait worsens.

TABLE
20-5

Types of Facial Paralysis

Facial weakness or paralysis may result either (1) from a peripheral lesion of CN VII, the facial nerve, anywhere from its origin in the pons to its periphery in the face, or (2) from a central lesion involving the upper motor neuron system between the cortex and the pons. A peripheral lesion of CN VII, exemplified here by a Bell palsy, is compared with a central lesion, exemplified by a left hemispheric cerebrovascular accident. These can be distinguished by their different effects on the upper part of the face.

The lower part of the face normally is controlled by upper motor neurons located on only one side of the cortex—the opposite side. *Left-sided damage to these pathways, as in a stroke, paralyzes the right lower face.* The upper face, however, is controlled by pathways from both sides of the cortex. Even though the upper motor neurons on the left are destroyed, others on the right remain, and the right upper face continues to function fairly well.

CN VII—Peripheral Lesion	CN VII—Central Lesion

Peripheral nerve damage to CN VII paralyzes the entire right side of the face, including the forehead.

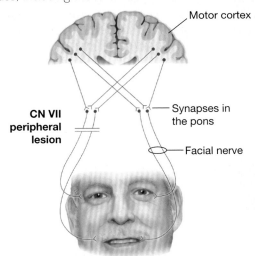

Motor cortex

CN VII peripheral lesion

Synapses in the pons

Facial nerve

Motor cortex

CN VII central lesion

Synapses in the pons

Facial nerve

Closing Eyes

Eye does not close; eyeball rolls up

Flat nasolabial fold

Closing Eyes

Eye closes; perhaps with slight weakness

Flat nasolabial fold

Raising Eyebrows
Forehead not wrinkled; eyebrow not raised

Smiling
Paralysis of lower face

Raising Eyebrows
Forehead wrinkled; eyebrow raised

Smiling
Paralysis of lower face

TABLE
20-6

Nystagmus

Nystagmus is a rhythmic oscillation of the eyes, analogous to a tremor in other parts of the body. Its causes are multiple, including impairment of vision in early life, disorders of the labyrinth and the cerebellar system, and drug toxicity. Nystagmus occurs normally when a person watches a rapidly moving object (e.g., a passing train). Study the characteristics of nystagmus described in this table to correctly identify the type of nystagmus.

Direction of Gaze in Which Nystagmus Appears

Example: Nystagmus on Right Lateral Gaze

Nystagmus Present (Right Lateral Gaze)

Although nystagmus may be present in all directions of gaze, it may appear or become accentuated only on deviation of the eyes (e.g., to the side or upward). On extreme lateral gaze, the normal person may show a few beats resembling nystagmus. Avoid making assessments in such extreme positions, and *observe for nystagmus only within the field of full binocular vision.*

Nystagmus Not Present (Left Lateral Gaze)

Direction of the Quick and Slow Components

Example: Left-Beating Nystagmus—a Quick Jerk to the Left in Each Eye, Then a Slow Drift to the Right

Nystagmus usually has both slow and fast movements, but *is defined by its fast phase.* For example, if the eyes jerk quickly to the patient's left and drift back slowly to the right, the patient is said to have *left-beating nystagmus.* Occasionally, nystagmus consists only of coarse oscillations without quick and slow components. It is then said to be *pendular.*

TABLE 20-7 Seizure Disorders[11]

Seizures were reclassified in 2010 into focal and generalized to better reflect current scientific advances. Underlying causes should be identified as genetic, structural/metabolic, or unknown. The complexities of the reclassification scheme are best explored by turning to the report of the ILAE Commission on Classification and Terminology, 2005–2009, cited below, and to more detailed references. This table presents only basic concepts from this report.

Focal Seizures
Focal seizures "are conceptualized as originating within networks limited to one hemisphere. They may be discretely localized or more widely distributed. Focal seizures may originate in subcortical structures. For each seizure type, ictal onset is consistent from one seizure to another, with preferential propagation patterns that can involve the contralateral hemisphere. In some cases, however, there is more than one network, and more than one seizure type, but each individual seizure type has a consistent site of onset. Focal seizures do not fall into any recognized set of natural causes." The distinction between simple partial and partial complex is eliminated, but clinicians are urged to recognize and describe "impairment of consciousness/awareness or other dyscognitive features, localization, and progression of ictal events."

Problem	Clinical Manifestations	Postictal State
Focal Seizures Without Impairment of Consciousness or Awareness		
• With observable motor and autonomic symptoms		
Jacksonian	Tonic and then clonic movements that start unilaterally in the hand, foot, or face and spread to other body parts on the same side	Normal consciousness
Other motor	Turning of the head and eyes to one side, or tonic and clonic movements of an arm or leg without the jacksonian spread	Normal consciousness
With autonomic symptoms	A "funny feeling" in the epigastrium, nausea, pallor, flushing, lightheadedness	Normal consciousness
• With subjective sensory or psychic phenomena	Numbness, tingling; simple visual, auditory, or olfactory hallucinations such as flashing lights, buzzing, or odors	Normal consciousness
	Anxiety or fear; feelings of familiarity (déjà vu) or unreality; dreamy states; fear or rage; flashback experiences; more complex hallucinations	Normal consciousness
Focal Seizures With Impairment of Consciousness	The seizure may or may not start with the autonomic or psychic symptoms outlined above. Consciousness is impaired, and the person appears confused. Automatisms include automatic motor behaviors such as chewing, smacking the lips, walking about, and unbuttoning clothes; also more complicated and skilled behaviors such as driving a car.	The patient may remember initial autonomic or psychic symptoms (which are then termed an *aura*), but is amnesic for the rest of the seizure. Temporary confusion and headache may occur.
Focal Seizures That Become Generalized	Partial seizures that become generalized resemble tonic–clonic seizures (see next page). Unfortunately, the patient may not recall the focal onset, and observers may overlook it.	As in a tonic–clonic seizure, described on the next page. Two attributes indicate a partial seizure that has become generalized: (1) the recollection of an *aura,* and (2) a *unilateral* neurologic deficit during the postictal period.

(table continues on page 736)

TABLE

20-7

Seizure Disorders[11] (continued)

Generalized Seizures and Pseudoseizures

Generalized seizures "are conceptualized as originating as some point within, and rapidly engaging, bilaterally distributed networks... that include cortical and subcortical structures, but do not necessarily include the entire cortex... the location and lateralization are not consistent from one seizure to another. Generalized seizures can be asymmetric." They may begin with body movements, impaired consciousness, or both. When tonic–clonic seizures begin after age 30, suspect either a partial seizure that has become generalized or a general seizure caused by a toxic or metabolic disorder. Toxic and metabolic causes include withdrawal from alcohol or other sedative drugs, uremia, hypoglycemia, hyperglycemia, hyponatremia, and bacterial meningitis.

Problem	Clinical Manifestations	Postictal (*Postseizure*) State
Generalized Seizures **Tonic–Clonic (grand mal)***[a]*	The person loses consciousness suddenly, sometimes with a cry, and the body stiffens into tonic extensor rigidity. Breathing stops, and the person becomes cyanotic. A clonic phase of rhythmic muscular contraction follows. Breathing resumes and is often noisy, with excessive salivation. Injury, tongue biting, and urinary incontinence may occur.	Confusion, drowsiness, fatigue, headache, muscular aching, and sometimes the temporary persistence of bilateral neurologic deficits such as hyperactive reflexes and Babinski responses. The person has amnesia for the seizure and recalls no aura.
Absence	A sudden brief lapse of consciousness, with momentary blinking, staring, or movements of the lips and hands but no falling. Two subtypes are recognized. *Typical absences* last less than 10 second and stop abruptly. *Atypical absences* may last more than 10 second.	No aura recalled. In petit mal absences, a prompt return to normal; in atypical absences, some postictal confusion
Myoclonic	Sudden, brief, rapid jerks, involving the trunk or limbs. Associated with a variety of disorders	Variable
Myoclonic Atonic (drop attack)	Sudden loss of consciousness with falling but no movements. Injury may occur.	Either a prompt return to normal or a brief period of confusion
Pseudoseizures May mimic seizures but are due to a conversion reaction (a psychological disorder)	The movements may have personally symbolic significance and often do not follow a neuroanatomic pattern. Injury is uncommon.	Variable

[a]Febrile convulsions that resemble brief tonic–clonic seizures may occur in infants and young children. They are usually benign but occasionally may be the first manifestation of a seizure disorder.

Source: Commission on Classification and Terminology of the International League Against Epilepsy. A proposed diagnostic scheme for people with epileptic seizures and with epilepsy: report of the ILAE Task Force on Classification and Terminology. Available at http://www.ilae-epilepsy.org/Visitors/Centre/ctf/overview.cfm#2. Accessed July 15, 2011. See also Berg AT, Berkovic SF, Brodie MJ et al. Revised terminology and concepts for organization of seizures and epilepsies: Report of the ILAE Commission on Classification and Terminology, 2005–2009. *Epilepsia*. 2010;51:676–685.

TABLE

20-8

Metabolic and Structural Coma

Although there are many causes of coma, most can be classified as either *structural* or *metabolic*. Findings vary widely in individual patients; the features listed are general guidelines rather than strict diagnostic criteria. Remember that psychiatric disorders may mimic coma.

	Toxic–Metabolic	Structural
Pathophysiology	Arousal centers poisoned or critical substrates depleted	Lesion destroys or compresses brainstem arousal areas, either directly or secondary to more distant expanding mass lesions.
Clinical Features		
• Respiratory pattern	If regular, may be normal or hyperventilation. If irregular, usually Cheyne–Stokes	Irregular, especially Cheyne–Stokes or ataxic breathing. Also with selected stereotypical patterns like "apneustic" respiration (peak inspiratory arrest) or central hyperventilation
• Pupillary size and reaction	Equal, reactive to light. If *pinpoint* from opiates or cholinergics, you may need a magnifying glass to see the reaction. May be unreactive if *fixed and dilated* from anticholinergics or hypothermia	Unequal or unreactive to light (fixed) *Midposition, fixed*—suggests midbrain compression *Dilated, fixed*—suggests *compression* of CN III from herniation
• Level of consciousness	Changes *after* pupils change	Changes *before* pupils change
Examples of Cause	Uremia, hyperglycemia Alcohol, drugs, liver failure Hypothyroidism, hypoglycemia Anoxia, ischemia Meningitis, encephalitis Hyperthermia, hypothermia	Epidural, subdural, or intracerebral hemorrhage Cerebral infarct or embolus Tumor, abscess Brainstem infarct, tumor, or hemorrhage Cerebellar infarct, hemorrhage, tumor, or abscess

TABLE

20-9

Pupils in Comatose Patients

Pupillary size, equality, and light reactions help in assessing the cause of coma and in determining the region of the brain that is impaired. Remember that unrelated pupillary abnormalities, including miotic drops for glaucoma or mydriatic drops for a better view of the ocular fundi, may have preceded the coma.

Small or Pinpoint Pupils

Bilaterally small pupils (1–2.5 mm) suggest (1) damage to the sympathetic pathways in the hypothalamus or (2) metabolic encephalopathy (a diffuse failure of cerebral function that has many causes, including drugs). Light reactions are usually normal.

Pinpoint pupils (<1 mm) suggest (1) a hemorrhage in the pons or (2) the effects of morphine, heroin, or other narcotics. The light reactions may be seen with a magnifying glass.

Large Pupils

Bilaterally fixed and dilated pupils may be due to severe anoxia and its sympathomimetic effects, as seen after cardiac arrest. They may also result from atropine-like agents, phenothiazines, or tricyclic antidepressants.

Bilaterally large reactive pupils may be due to cocaine, amphetamine, LSD, or other sympathetic nervous system agonists.

Midposition Fixed Pupils

Pupils that are in the *midposition or slightly dilated* (4–6 mm) and are *fixed to light* suggest structural damage in the midbrain.

One Large Pupil

A pupil that is *fixed and dilated* warns of herniation of the temporal lobe, causing compression of the oculomotor nerve and midbrain. A single large pupil is commonly seen in diabetic patients with infarction of CN III. Diabetic CN III palsy often spares pupillary function.

TABLE
20-10

Abnormal Postures in Comatose Patients

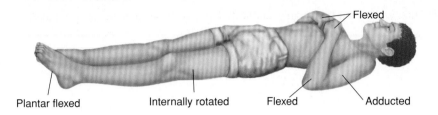

Flexed

Plantar flexed   Internally rotated   Flexed   Adducted

Decorticate Rigidity (Abnormal Flexor Response)

In *decorticate rigidity,* the upper arms are flexed tight to the sides with elbows, wrists, and fingers flexed. The legs are extended and internally rotated. The feet are plantar flexed. This posture implies a destructive lesion of the corticospinal tracts within or very near the cerebral hemispheres. When unilateral, this is the posture of chronic spastic hemiplegia.

Externally rotated   Flaccid

Hemiplegia (Early)

Sudden unilateral brain damage involving the corticospinal tract may produce a *hemiplegia* (one-sided paralysis), which early in its course is flaccid. Spasticity will develop later. The paralyzed arm and leg are slack. They fall loosely and without tone when raised and dropped to the bed. Spontaneous movements or responses to noxious stimuli are limited to the opposite side. The leg may lie externally rotated. One side of the lower face may be paralyzed, and that cheek puffs out on expiration. Both eyes may be turned away from the paralyzed side.

Plantar flexed   Flexed   Pronated   Extended   Adducted

Decerebrate Rigidity (Abnormal Extensor Response)

In *decerebrate rigidity,* the jaws are clenched and the neck is extended. The arms are adducted and stiffly extended at the elbows, with forearms pronated, wrists and fingers flexed. The legs are stiffly *extended at the knees,* with the feet plantar flexed. This posture may occur spontaneously or only in response to external stimuli such as light, noise, or pain. It is caused by a lesion in the diencephalon, midbrain, or pons, although may also arise from severe metabolic disorders such as hypoxia or hypoglycemia.

TABLE
20-11
Tremors and Involuntary Movements[38-40]

Tremors: Tremors are rhythmic oscillatory movements, which may be roughly subdivided into three groups: resting (or static) tremors, postural tremors, and intention tremors.

Resting (Static) Tremors

These tremors are most prominent at rest, and may decrease or disappear with voluntary movement. Illustrated is the common, relatively slow, fine, pill-rolling tremor of Parkinsonism, about 5 per second.

Postural (Action) Tremors

These tremors appear when the affected part is actively maintaining a posture. Examples include the fine rapid tremor of hyperthyroidism, the tremors of anxiety and fatigue, and benign essential (and sometimes familial) tremor. Tremor may worsen somewhat with intention.

Intention Tremors

Intention tremors, absent at rest, appear with activity and often get worse as the target is neared. Causes include disorders of cerebellar pathways, as in multiple sclerosis.

Oral–Facial Dyskinesias

Oral–facial dyskinesias are rhythmic, repetitive, bizarre movements that chiefly involve the face, mouth, jaw, and tongue: grimacing, pursing of the lips, protrusions of the tongue, opening and closing of the mouth, and deviations of the jaw. The limbs and trunk are involved less often. These movements may be a late complication of psychotropic drugs such as phenothiazines, termed *tardive* (late) dyskinesias. They also occur in long-standing psychoses, in some elderly individuals, and in some edentulous persons (without teeth).

Tics

Tics are brief, repetitive, stereotyped, coordinated movements occurring at irregular intervals. Examples include repetitive winking, grimacing, and shoulder shrugging. Causes include Tourette syndrome and drugs such as phenothiazines and amphetamines.

Dystonia

Dystonic movements are similar to athetoid movements, but often involve larger portions of the body, including the trunk. Grotesque, twisted postures may result. Causes include drugs such as phenothiazines, primary torsion dystonia, and as illustrated, spasmodic torticollis.

Athetosis

Athetoid movements are slower and more twisting and writhing than choreiform movements, and have larger amplitude. They most commonly involve the face and the distal extremities. Athetosis is often associated with spasticity. Causes include cerebral palsy.

Chorea

Choreiform movements are brief, rapid, jerky, irregular, and unpredictable. They occur at rest or interrupt normal coordinated movements. Unlike tics, they seldom repeat themselves. The face, head, lower arms, and hands are often involved. Causes include Sydenham chorea (with rheumatic fever) and Huntington disease.

TABLE

20-12

Disorders of Muscle Tone

	Spasticity	Rigidity	Flaccidity	Paratonia
Location of Lesion	Upper motor neuron of the corticospinal tract at any point from the cortex to the spinal cord	Basal ganglia system	Lower motor neuron system at any point from the anterior horn cell to the peripheral nerves	Both hemispheres, usually in the frontal lobes
Description	A form of muscular hypertonicity with increased resistance to stretch	Condition of hardness, stiffness, or inflexibility	Loss of muscle tone (*hypotonia*), causing the limb to be loose or floppy. The affected limbs may be hyperextensible or even flail-like. Flaccid muscles are also weak.	Sudden changes in tone with passive range of motion. Sudden loss of tone that increases the ease of motion is called *mitgehen* (moving with). Sudden increase in tone making motion more difficult is called *gegenhalten* (holding against).
Common Cause	Stroke, especially late or chronic stage	Parkinsonism	Guillain–Barré syndrome; also initial phase of spinal cord injury (spinal shock) or stroke	Dementia

BIBLIOGRAPHY

CITATIONS

1. Campbell WW. *DeJong's The Neurologic Examination.* 7th ed. Philadelphia, PA: Lippincott Williams & Wilkins; 2013.

2. Wright BL, Lai JT, Sinclair AJ. Cerebrospinal fluid and lumbar puncture: a practical review. *J Neurol.* 2012;259:1530.

3. National Institute of Neurologic Disorders and Stroke, National Institutes of Health. Spinal cord injury: hope through research. Updated February 23, 2015. Available at http://www.ninds.nih.gov/disorders/sci/detail_sci.htm. Accessed January 23, 2016.

4. Chad DA, Stone JH, Gupta R. Case 14–2011: A woman with asymmetric sensory loss and paresthesias. *N Engl J Med.* 2011;364:1856.

5. Dyck PJ, Herrmann DN, Staff NP, et al. Assessing decreased sensation and increased sensory phenomena in diabetic polyneuropathies. *Diabetes.* 2013;62:3677.

6. Anastasi JK, Capili B, Chang M. HIV peripheral neuropathy and foot care management: a review of assessment and relevant guidelines. *Am J Nurs.* 2013;113(12):34–40.

7. International Headache Society. *The International Classification of Headache Disorders.* 3rd ed. (beta version). *Cephalalgia.* 2013;33:629.

8. Veenstra P, Kollen BJ, deJong G, et al. Nurses improve migraine management in primary care. *Cephalalgia.* 2015;0333102415612767.

9. De Luca GC, Bartleson JD. When and how to investigate the patient with headache. *Semin Neurol.* 2010;30:131.

10. D'Souza S. Aneurysmal subarachnoid hemorrhage. *J Neurosurg Anesthesiol.* 2015;27:222.

11. Mortimer AM, Bradley MD, Stoodley NG, et al. Thunderclap headache: diagnostic considerations and neuroimaging features. *Clin Radiol.* 2013;68:e101.

12. Dill E. Thunderclap headache. *Curr Neurol Neurosci Rep.* 2014;14:437.

13. Bhimraj A. Acute community-acquired bacterial meningitis in adults: an evidence-based review. *Cleve Clin J Med.* 2012;79:393.

14. Brouwer MC, Tunkel AR, van de Beek D. Epidemiology, diagnosis, and antimicrobial treatment of acute bacterial meningitis. *Clin Microbiol Rev.* 2010;23:467.

15. Logan SA, MacMahon E. Viral meningitis. *BMJ.* 2008;336(7634):36.

16. Omuro A, DeAngelis LM. Glioblastoma and other malignant gliomas. *JAMA.* 2013;310:1842.

17. Brouwer MC, Tunkel AR, McKhann GM, et al. Brain abscess. *N Engl J Med.* 2014;371:447.

18. Bushnell C, McCullough L. Stroke prevention in women: synopsis of the 2014 American Heart Association/American Stroke Association guideline. *Ann Intern Med.* 2012;160:853.

19. Sacco S, Ornello R, Ripa P, et al. Migraine and hemorrhagic stroke: a meta-analysis. *Stroke.* 2012;44:3032.

20. Sacco S, Ricci S, Degan D, et al. Migraine in women: the role of hormones and their impact on vascular diseases. *J Headache Pain.* 2012;13:177.

21. McGregor EA. In the clinic: migraine. *Ann Intern Med.* 2013;159:ITC5–1.

22. Detsky ME, McDonald DR, Baerlocher MO, et al. Does this patient with headache have a migraine or need neuroimaging? *JAMA.* 2006;296:1274.

23. Wipperman J. Dizziness and vertigo. *Prim Care.* 2014;41:115.

24. Siket MS, Edlow JA. Transient ischemic attack: reviewing the evolution of the definition, diagnosis, risk stratification, and management for the emergency physician. *Emerg Med Clin North Am.* 2012;30:745.

25. Cucchiara B, Kasner SE. In the clinic. Transient ischemic attack. *Ann Intern Med.* 2011;154:ITC-1.

26. Karras C, Aitchison R, Aitchison P, et al. Adult stroke summary. *Dis Mon.* 2013;59:210.

27. Nouh A, Remke J, Ruland S. Ischemic posterior circulation stroke: a review of anatomy, clinical presentations, diagnosis, and current management. *Front Neurol.* 2014;5:30.

28. Ishiyama G, Ishiyama A. Vertebrobasilar infarcts and ischemia. *Otolaryngol Clin North Am.* 2011;44:415.

29. Runchey S, McGee S. Does this patient have a hemorrhagic stroke? Clinical findings distinguishing hemorrhagic stroke from ischemic stroke. *JAMA.* 2010;303:2280.

30. Yuki N, Hartung HP. Guillain-Barré Syndrome. *N Engl J Med.* 2012;366:2294.

31. Baggi F, Andreetta F, Maggi L, et al. Complete stable remission and autoantibody specificity in myasthenia gravis. *Neurology.* 2013;80:188.

32. Spillane J, Higham E, Kullmann DM. Myasthenia gravis. *BMJ.* 2012;345:e8497.

33. Yoo M, Sharma N, Pasnoor M, et al. Painful diabetic peripheral neuropathy: presentations, mechanisms, and exercise therapy. *J Diabetes Metab.* 2013;Suppl 10:005.

34. Gilron I, Baron R, Jensen T. Neuropathic pain: principles of diagnosis and treatment. *Mayo Clin Proc.* 2015;90:532.

35. Benditt DG, Adkisson WO. Approach to the patient with syncope: venues, presentations, diagnoses. *Cardiol Clin.* 2013;31:9.

36. Low PA, Tomalia VA. Orthostatic hypotension: mechanisms, causes, management. *J Clin Neurol.* 2015;11:220.

37. Alguire PC. American College of Physicians. Epilepsy syndromes and their diagnosis. In: *Neurology, Medical Knowledge Self-Assessment Program (MKSAP) 15.* Philadelphia, PA: American College of Physicians; 2016:74.

38. Elias WJ, Shah BB. Tremor. *JAMA.* 2014;311:948.

39. Benito-Leon J. Essential tremor: a neurodegenerative disease? *Tremor Other Hyperkinet Mov (NY).* 2014;4:252.

40. Connolly BS, Lang AE. Pharmacological treatment of Parkinson disease, a review. *JAMA.* 2014;311:1670.

41. Wijemanne S, Jankovic J. Restless legs syndrome: clinical presentation diagnosis and treatment. *Sleep Med.* 2015;16:678.

42. Silber MH, Becker PM, Earley C, et al. Willis-Ekbom Disease Foundation revised consensus statement on the management of restless legs syndrome. *Mayo Clin Proc.* 2013;88:977.

43. American Academy of Neurology. Neurology clerkship core curriculum guidelines. See also Appendix 2: Guidelines for a Screening Neurologic Examination, p. 7. Available at https://www.aan.com/uploadedFiles/4CME_and_Training/2Training/3Fellowship_Resources/5Core_Curricula/skilz.pdf. Accessed July 23, 2015.

44. Gelb DJ, Gunderson CH, Henry KA, et al. The neurology clerkship core curriculum. *Neurology.* 2002;58:849.

45. Moore FG, Chalk C. The essential neurologic examination. *Neurology.* 2009;72:2020.

46. McGee S. Chapter 56: Visual field testing. In: *Evidence-Based Physical Diagnosis.* 3rd ed. Philadelphia, PA: Elsevier Saunders; 2012:513–520.

47. McGee S. Chapter 20: The pupils In: *Evidence-Based Physical Diagnosis.* 3rd ed. Philadelphia, PA: Elsevier Saunders; 2012:176–178.

48. McGee S. Chapter 57: Nerves of the eye muscles. In: *Evidence-Based Physical Diagnosis.* 3rd ed. Philadelphia, PA: Elsevier Saunders; 2012:521–531.

49. Zandian A, Osiro S, Hudson R, et al. The neurologist's dilemma: a comprehensive clinical review of Bell's palsy, with emphasis on current management trends. *Med Sci Monit.* 2014;20:83.

50. McGee S. Chapter 22: Hearing. In: *Evidence-Based Physical Diagnosis.* 3rd ed. Philadelphia, PA: Elsevier Saunders; 2012:190.

51. Darcy P, Moughty AM. Pronator drift. *N Engl J Med.* 2013;369:320.

52. Daum C, Aybek S. Validity of the "drift without pronation" sign in conversion disorder. *BMC Neurol.* 2013;13:31.

53. Stone J, Carson A, Sharpe M. Functional symptoms and signs in neurology: assessment and diagnosis. *J Neurol Neurosurg Psychiatry.* 2005;76(Suppl 1):i2.

54. Stabler SP. Clinical practice. Vitamin B_{12} deficiency. *N Engl J Med.* 2013;368:149.

55. Kirshblum SC, Burns SP, Biering-Sorensen F, et al. International Standards for Neurological Classification of Spinal Cord Injury (Revised 2011). *J Spinal Cord Med.* 2011;34:535.

56. Stone J, Carson A, Duncan R, et al. Which neurological diseases are most likely to be associated with "symptoms unexplained by organic disease." *J Neurol.* 2012;259:33.

57. Hallett M. NINDS myotatic reflex scale. *Neurology.* 1993; 43:2723.

58. Isaza Jaramillo SP, Uribe Uribe CS, García Jimenez FA, et al. Accuracy of the Babinski sign in the identification of pyramidal tract dysfunction. *J Neurol Sci.* 2014;343:66.

59. McGee S. Chapter 24: Meninges. In: *Evidence-Based Physical Diagnosis.* 3rd ed. Philadelphia, PA: Elsevier Saunders; 2012:210–214.

60. Edlow JA, Rabinstein A, Traub SJ, et al. Diagnosis of reversible causes of coma. *Lancet.* 2014;384(9959):2064.

61. Moore SA, Wijdicks EF. The acutely comatose patient: clinical approach and diagnosis. *Semin Neurol.* 2013;33:110.

62. Wijdicks EFM. *The Comatose Patient.* 2nd ed. New York, NY: Oxford University Press; 2014.

63. Henry TR, Ezzeddine MA. Approach to the patient with transient alteration of consciousness. *Neurol Clin Pract.* 2012; 2:179.

64. Pope JV, Edlow JA. Avoiding misdiagnosis in patients with neurological emergencies. *Emerg Med Int.* 2012;2012:949275.

65. Brown EN, Lydic R, Schiff ND. General anesthesia, sleep, and coma. *N Engl J Med.* 2010;363:2638.

66. Teasdale G, Jennett B. Assessment of coma and impaired consciousness. A practical scale. *Lancet.* 1974;304(7872):81.

67. McGee S. Chapter 24: Meninges. In: *Evidence-Based Physical Diagnosis.* 3rd ed. Philadelphia, PA: Elsevier Saunders; 2012:210–214.

68. Thomas KE, Hasbun R, Jekel J, et al. The diagnostic accuracy of Kernig's sign, Brudzinski's sign, and nuchal rigidity in adults with suspected meningitis. *Clin Infect Dis.* 2002;35:46.

69. Ward MA, Greenwood TM, Kumar DR, et al. Josef Brudzinski and Vladimir Mikhailovich Kernig: signs for diagnosing meningitis. *Clin Med Res.* 2010;8:13.

70. Tesfaye S, Boulton AJ, Dyck PJ, et al. Diabetic neuropathies: update on definitions, diagnostic criteria, estimation of severity, and treatments. *Diabetes Care.* 2010;33:2285.

71. American Diabetes Association. Microvascular complications and foot care. *Diabetes Care.* 2015;38 Suppl:S58.

72. Mozaffarian D, Benjamin EJ, Go AS, et al. Heart disease and stroke statistics—2015 update: a report from the American Heart Association. *Circulation.* 2015;131:e29.

73. Easton JD, Saver JL, Albers GW, et al. Definition and evaluation of transient ischemic attack: a scientific statement for healthcare professionals from the American Heart Association/American Stroke Association Stroke Council; Council on Cardiovascular Surgery and Anesthesia; Council on Cardiovascular Radiology and Intervention; Council on Cardiovascular Nursing; and the Interdisciplinary Council on Peripheral Vascular Disease. The American Academy of Neurology affirms the value of this statement as an educational tool for neurologists. *Stroke.* 2009;40:2276.

74. Kleindorfer D, Panagos P, Pancioli A, et al. Incidence and short-term prognosis of transient ischemic attack in a population-based study. *Stroke.* 2005;36:720.

75. Bushnell C, McCullough LD, Awad IA, et al. Guidelines for the prevention of stroke in women: a statement for healthcare professionals from the American Heart Association/American Stroke Association. *Stroke.* 2014;45:1545.

76. Meschia JF, Bushnell C, Boden-Albala B, et al. Guidelines for the primary prevention of stroke: a statement for healthcare professionals from the American Heart Association/American Stroke Association. *Stroke.* 2014;45:3754.

77. Jauch EC, Saver JL, Adams HP Jr, et al. Guidelines for the early management of patients with acute ischemic stroke: a guideline for healthcare professionals from the American Heart Association/American Stroke Association. *Stroke.* 2013;44:870.

78. Harper S, Rushani D, Kaufman JS. Trends in the black-white life expectancy gap, 2003–2008. *JAMA.* 2012;307:2257.

79. American Heart Association, American Stroke Association. Stroke warning signs and symptoms. Available at http://www.strokeassociation.org/STROKEORG/WarningSigns/Stroke-Warning-Signs-and-Symptoms_UCM_308528_SubHomePage.jsp. Accessed January 23, 2016.

80. U.S. Department of Health and Human Services, Office of Disease Prevention and Health Promotion. Healthy People 2020—Heart disease and stroke, objectives. Available at http://www.healthypeople.gov/2020/topics-objectives/topic/heart-disease-and-stroke/objectives. Accessed January 23, 2016.

81. Wolff T, Miller T, Ko S. Aspirin for the primary prevention of cardiovascular events: an update of the evidence for the U.S. Preventive Services Task Force. *Ann Intern Med.* 2009;150:405.

82. Kernan WN, Ovbiagele B, Black HR, et al. Guidelines for the prevention of stroke in patients with stroke and transient ischemic attack: a guideline for healthcare professionals from the American Heart Association/American Stroke Association. *Stroke.* 2014;45:2160.

83. American College of Physicians. *Stroke, in Neurology. Medical Knowledge Self-Assessment Program (MKSAP) 14.* Philadelphia, PA: American College of Physicians; 2012.

ADDITIONAL REFERENCE

Jonas DE, Feltner C, Amick HR, et al. Screening for asymptomatic carotid artery stenosis: a systematic review and meta-analysis for the U.S. Preventive Services Task Force. *Ann Intern Med.* 2014;161:336.

Reproductive Systems

LEARNING OBJECTIVES

The student will:

1. Describe the anatomy and physiology of the female and male reproductive systems.

2. Obtain an accurate history of the reproductive system.

3. Explain appropriate technique in examining external reproductive structures.

4. Discuss developmental, psychosocial, cultural, and environmental factors that affect the reproductive systems.

5. Differentiate between normal and abnormal findings in the reproductive system.

6. Accurately document subjective and objective findings related to the reproductive system using the appropriate terminology.

The reproductive system is intimately intertwined with a person's self-concept. Cultural and religious beliefs and attitudes also influence a person's reproductive knowledge and health care. Sensitive care by all nurses is important. Although internal pelvic and rectal examinations are not within the role of the generalist nurse, it is important for the nurse to explain the anatomy and physiology of the reproductive systems to patients; interview a patient for a thorough system history; and recognize normal and abnormal external genitalia. This knowledge will allow the nurse to educate patients about their reproductive systems in order to promote optimal health and function; assist with family planning; prevent the spread of sexually transmitted infections; and promote early recognition of problems for referral to an advanced practice nurse or physician. It is not uncommon for a hospital or clinic patient who has developed a relationship with the nurse to feel more comfortable discussing intimate concerns with the nurse rather than family or the physician. For example, an adolescent may be uncomfortable discussing reproductive function with his or her parents. This chapter will provide the generalist nurse with the ability to carry out this role. The chapter is organized into the female reproductive system and the male reproductive system for ease of reading.

FEMALE REPRODUCTIVE SYSTEM

ANATOMY AND PHYSIOLOGY

The anatomy of the external female genitalia, or *vulva*, includes the *mons pubis*, a hair-covered fat pad overlying the symphysis pubis; the *labia majora*, rounded folds of adipose tissue; the *labia minora*, thinner pinkish-red folds that extend anteriorly to form the *prepuce;* and the *clitoris*. The *vestibule* is the boat-shaped channel, or fossa, between the labia minora. In its posterior portion lies the vaginal opening, the *introitus*, which in a woman who has never had intercourse may be hidden by the *hymen*. The term *perineum*, as commonly used clinically, refers to the tissue between the introitus and the anus.

Mons pubis

Prepuce

Clitoris

Urethral meatus

Opening of
paraurethral
(Skene's) gland

Vestibule

Introitus

Perineum

Labium majus

Labium minus

Hymen

Vagina

Opening of
Bartholin's gland

Anus

The *urethral meatus* opens into the vestibule between the clitoris and the vagina. Just posterior to the meatus on either side are the openings of the *para urethral* (Skene) *glands*.

The openings of *Bartholin glands* are located posteriorly on both sides of the vaginal opening but are not usually visible. Bartholin glands themselves are situated more deeply. Both the Skene glands and the Bartholin glands provide lubrication during sexual intercourse.

The *vagina* is a musculomembranous tube extending upward and posteriorly between the urethra and the rectum. The vaginal mucosa lies in transverse folds, or rugae.

Location of
Bartholin's glands

The vagina lies almost at a right angle to the *uterus,* a thick-walled fibromuscular structure shaped like an inverted pear. Its convex upper surface is the uterine *fundus.* The body of the uterus, or *corpus,* and the cylindrical *cervix* inferiorly are joined at the *isthmus.* The uterine walls contain three layers: the *perimetrium,* with its serosal coating from the perineum; the *myometrium* of distensible smooth muscle; and the *endometrium,* the adherent inner coating. The distal cervix protrudes into the vagina, dividing the upper vagina into three recesses, the *anterior, posterior,* and *lateral fornices.*

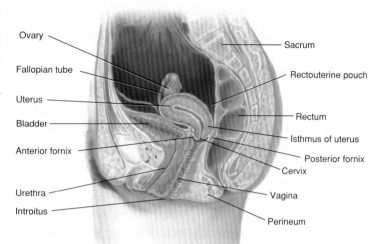

The vaginal surface of the cervix, the *ectocervix,* is seen easily with the help of a speculum. At its center is a round, oval, or slit-like depression, the *external os* of the cervix, which marks the opening into the endocervical canal. The ectocervix is covered by the plushy, red *columnar epithelium* that surrounds the os and lines the endocervical canal, and by a shiny pink *squamous epithelium* continuous with the vaginal lining. The *squamocolumnar junction* forms the boundary between these two types of epithelium. The squamocolumnar junction migrates toward the os, creating the *transformation zone.* This is the area at risk for later dysplasia and cancer, which is sampled by the Papanicolaou, or Pap smear.

CERVICAL EPITHELIA AND TRANSFORMATION ZONE

A *fallopian tube* with a fan-like tip, the fimbria, extends from the ovary to each side of the uterus and conducts the oocyte from the peri-ovarian peritoneal cavity to the uterine cavity. The two ovaries are almond-shaped glands that vary considerably in size but average approximately 3.5 by 2 by 1.5 cm from adulthood through menopause. The ovaries are palpable on pelvic examination in roughly half of women during the reproductive years. Normally, fallopian tubes are not palpable. The term *adnexa,* a plural Latin word meaning appendages, refers to the ovaries, tubes, and supporting tissues.

The ovaries have two primary functions: the production of oocytes and the secretion of hormones, including estrogen, progesterone, and testosterone. Increased hormonal secretion during puberty stimulates the growth of the uterus and its endometrial lining, enlargement of the vagina, and thickening of the vaginal epithelium and the development of secondary sex characteristics, including the breasts and pubic hair.

The pelvic organs are supported by a sling of tissues composed of muscle, ligaments, and endopelvic fascia, called the *pelvic floor,* which helps support the pelvic organs. The urethra, vagina, and rectum all pass through the pelvic floor. Pelvic floor muscles also aid in sexual function (orgasm), urinary and fecal continence, and stabilization of connecting joints.

Assessment of sexual maturity in girls, as classified by Tanner, depends not on internal examination, but on the growth of pubic hair and the development of breasts. Tanner stages, or sexual maturity ratings as they relate to pubic hair and breasts are shown in Chapter 23, Assessing Children: Infancy Through Adolescence, p. 896.

In most women, pubic hair spreads downward in a triangular pattern, pointing toward the vagina. In 10% of women, it may form an inverted triangle, pointing toward the umbilicus. This growth is usually not completed until the middle 20s or later.

Just before menarche, there is a physiologic increase in vaginal secretions—a normal change that sometimes causes concern in a girl or her mother. As menses become more regular, these increased secretions (*leukorrhea*) coincide with ovulation. They also accompany sexual arousal. These normal kinds of discharges must be differentiated from those of infectious processes.

Lymphatics

Lymph from the vulva and lower vagina drains into the inguinal nodes. Lymph from the internal genitalia, including the upper vagina, flows into the pelvic and abdominal lymph nodes, which are not palpable.

THE HEALTH HISTORY

Common Concerns

- Menarche, menstruation, menopause, postmenopausal bleeding
- Dysmenorrhea
- Pregnancy
- Contraception
- Vulvovaginal symptoms
- Sexual preference and sexual response
- Sexually transmitted infections

Weakness of the pelvic floor muscles may cause pain, urinary incontinence, fecal incontinence, and prolapse of the pelvic organs that can produce a *cystocele, rectocele,* or *enterocele.* Risk factors are advancing age, prior pelvic surgery or trauma, number of pregnancies and childbirth, medical conditions (diabetes, multiple sclerosis, Parkinson disease), medications (anticholinergics, alpha adrenergic blockers), and chronically increased intra-abdominal pressure from chronic obstructive pulmonary disease (COPD), chronic constipation, or obesity.[1]

There are three parts to a woman's reproductive history: menstrual history, obstetric history, and sexual history. It is usually more comfortable for the patient if the nurse begins with the menstrual and obstetric history and saves the sexual history questions for last. However, if the woman comes to you with a sexual problem, it is appropriate to follow her lead with questions relating to the issue.

There are five phases of a woman's reproductive health: prepuberty (pre-menstruation), puberty (menarche), childbearing (menstruation), peri-menopausal, and menopausal. The nurse must incorporate the needs of each phase into the assessment process as appropriate for the individual.

When a woman reports a problem in the reproductive system, the OLD CART mnemonic may be used to elicit a full history of the problem. If no problem is reported, obtain a baseline reproductive history starting with the menstrual history.

Menstrual History

Menarche, Menstruation, Menopause

Describe menstrual patterns using the terms below.

The Menstrual History—Helpful Definitions

1. Menses—monthly flow of bloody fluid from the uterus.
   * *Menarche*—age at onset of menses
   * *Menopause*—absence of menses for 12 consecutive months, usually occurring between 48 and 55 years
   * *Perimenopause*—period of years during which a woman transitions to menopause
   * *Postmenopausal bleeding*—bleeding occurring 6 months or more after cessation of menses
   * *Amenorrhea*—absence of menses
   * *Dysmenorrhea*—pain with menses, often with bearing down, aching, or cramping sensation in the lower abdomen or pelvis
   * *Premenstrual syndrome (PMS)*—a cluster of emotional, behavioral, and physical symptoms occurring 5 days before menses for three consecutive cycles
   * *Abnormal uterine bleeding*—bleeding between menses; or infrequent, excessive, prolonged, or postmenopausal bleeding
2. Frequency—measured from the first day of one menses to the first day of the next menses. The interval between periods ranges roughly from 24 to 32 days.
3. Duration—number of days the flow lasts, usually 3 to 7 days.

Questions about *menarche, menstruation,* and *menopause* often provide the nurse an opportunity to explore the patient's concerns and attitude about her body. When talking with an adolescent girl, for example, opening questions might include: "How did you first learn about monthly periods? How did you feel when they started?" Many girls worry when their periods are not regular or come late. "Has anything like that bothered you?" You can explain that girls in the United States usually begin to menstruate between the ages of 9 and 16 years, and often it takes 1 year or more before menstrual cycles settle into a regular pattern. Age at menarche is variable, depending on genetic endowment, socioeconomic status, and nutrition.

For the menstrual history, ask the patient:

> How old were you when your menstrual periods began (age at *menarche*)?
> When did your last period start? If possible, the one before that?
> How often do you have periods?
> How long do they last?

The dates of previous periods can signal possible pregnancy or menstrual irregularities.

> What color is the flow?
> How heavy is the flow?

Unlike the normal dark red menstrual discharge, excessive flow tends to be bright red and may include "clots" (not true fibrin clots).

Flow can be assessed roughly by the number of pads or tampons used daily. Because women vary in their practices for sanitary measures, however, ask the patient whether she usually soaks a pad or tampon, spots it lightly, etc. Further, does she use more than one at a time? Does she have any bleeding between periods? Any bleeding after intercourse?

Up to 50% of women report ***dysmenorrhea***, or pain with menses. Ask the patient:

> Do you have any discomfort or pain before or during your periods?
> If so, what is it like? How long does it last, and does it interfere with usual activities?
> Are there other associated symptoms?
> Dysmenorrhea may be *primary*, without an organic cause, or *secondary*, with an organic cause.

Primary dysmenorrhea results from increased prostaglandin production during the luteal phase of the menstrual cycle, when estrogen and progesterone levels decline.

Causes of *secondary dysmenorrhea* include endometriosis, adenomyosis (endometriosis in the muscular layers of the uterus), pelvic inflammatory disease, and endometrial polyps.

Premenstrual syndrome (PMS) includes emotional and behavioral symptoms such as depression, angry outbursts, irritability, anxiety, confusion, crying spells, sleep disturbance, poor concentration, and/or social withdrawal.[2] Ask about signs such as bloating and weight gain, swelling of the hands and feet, and generalized aches and pains. Criteria for diagnosis are symptoms and signs in the 5 days prior to menses for at least three consecutive cycles, cessation of symptoms and signs within 4 days after the onset of menses, and interference with daily activities.

Amenorrhea refers to the absence of periods. Failure of periods to initiate is called *primary amenorrhea,* whereas the cessation of periods after they have been established is termed *secondary amenorrhea.* Pregnancy, lactation, and menopause are physiologic causes of secondary amenorrhea.

Other causes of *secondary amenorrhea* include low body weight from any cause, including malnutrition, anorexia nervosa, stress, chronic illness, or hypothalamic–pituitary–ovarian dysfunction.

Abnormal bleeding ask about any abnormal bleeding. The term *abnormal uterine bleeding* encompasses several patterns:

- *Polymenorrhea,* or intervals of fewer than 21 days between menses

- *Oligomenorrhea,* or infrequent bleeding

- *Menorrhagia,* or excessive flow

- *Metrorrhagia,* or intermenstrual bleeding

- Postcoital bleeding

Causes vary by age group and include pregnancy, cervical or vaginal infection, cancer, cervical or endometrial polyps or hyperplasia, fibroids, bleeding disorders, hormonal contraception, or replacement therapy. *Postcoital bleeding* suggests cervical polyps or cancer, or in an older woman, atrophic vaginitis.

Menopause usually occurs between 48 and 55 years. It is defined retrospectively as cessation of menses for 12 months, progressing through several stages of erratic cyclical bleeding. These stages of variable cycle length, often with vasomotor symptoms like hot flashes, flushing, and sweating, represent *perimenopause.* The ovaries stop producing estradiol or progesterone and estrogen levels drop significantly, although some testosterone synthesis persists.[3] If the patient is *perimenopausal,* ask about such vasomotor symptoms as hot flashes, flushing, and sweating. Sleep disturbances are also common. After menopause, there may be vaginal dryness and *dyspareunia* (painful intercourse); hair loss; and mild hirsutism as the androgen-to-estrogen ratio increases. Urinary symptoms may also occur in the absence of infection because of atrophy of the urethra and urinary trigone.

Women may ask about many alternative compounds and botanicals for relief of menopause-related symptoms. Most are poorly studied and not proven to be beneficial. Estrogen replacement relieves symptoms but poses other health risks.[4]

Ask a middle-aged or older woman:

> Have you stopped menstruating? When?
> Did you have any symptoms at that time?
> Have you had any bleeding since?

Ask:

> How do (did) you feel about not having your period anymore?
> Has it affected your life in any way?
> Have you had any bleeding or spotting since menopause?

Postmenopausal bleeding may occur in endometrial cancer, hormone replacement therapy, uterine and cervical polyps.

Obstetric History

Pregnancy

Questions relating to pregnancy include:

Have you ever been pregnant? How many times?
What years did you give birth (or miscarry)?
How many living children do you have?
Did you have any difficulties during pregnancy?
Have you ever had a miscarriage? An abortion?
    When did this occur?
    What were the circumstances around the miscarriage or abortion?
How did you cope with these losses?

> The term *abortion* is used by health care providers to mean either a spontaneous or an induced termination of a pregnancy before the fetus is viable. *Miscarriage* is a lay term for the spontaneous loss of a pregnancy. Be sure to clarify whether an abortion is spontaneous or therapeutic (i.e., induced).

Obstetricians commonly record the pregnancy history using the "gravida-para" system.

The Gravida-Para Notation

- G = gravida, or total number of pregnancies.
- P = para, or outcomes of pregnancies. After P, you will often see the notations F (full-term), P (premature), A (abortion), and L (living child).

If amenorrhea suggests a *current pregnancy,* inquire about the date of last intercourse and *common early symptoms:* tenderness, tingling, or increased size of the breasts; urinary frequency; nausea and vomiting; easy fatigability; and sensations that the baby is moving, usually present at about 20 weeks. Be considerate of the patient's feelings about discussing these topics and explore them when the patient has special concerns.

> Amenorrhea followed by heavy bleeding suggests a *threatened abortion* or *dysfunctional uterine bleeding* related to lack of ovulation.

Contraception

Inquire about methods of contraception used by the patient and her partner. Is the patient satisfied with the method chosen? Are there any questions about the options available?

Vulvovaginal Symptoms

The most common vulvovaginal symptoms are *vaginal discharge* and local *itching.* Use the OLD CART approach to obtain a thorough history. If the patient reports a discharge, inquire about its amount, color, consistency, and odor. Ask about any local *sores* or *lumps* in the vulvar area. Are they painful or not? Because patients vary in their understanding of anatomic terms, be prepared to try alternative phrasing such as "Any itching (or other symptoms) near your vagina? ... between your legs? ... where you urinate?"

> See Table 21-1, Lesions of the Vulva, p. 780 and Table 21-2, Vaginal Discharge, p. 781.

Sexual Health

Sexual health plays an important and natural role in overall well-being. Patients immediately sense your receptiveness to their concerns in this sensitive and vital area. Maintaining a neutral nonjudgmental tone helps your patients feel safe and trust you with their concerns. Many patients have strong beliefs about sexual behavior related to their upbringing, faith, ethnicity, educational level, and past experiences. Reassure them that sex in a mature consensual relationship is healthy, and that you explore sexual health with all your patients. Be aware of your own body language, facial expressions, and tone of voice, so that you create an open environment for discussion. In younger patients and adolescents, consider asking the parents to leave the room so the patients feel free to answer questions without fear of parental disapproval or repercussions, especially when discussing possible sexual abuse.

Review the Tips for Taking the Sexual History below. Using neutral and nonjudgmental questions, ask about your patient's relationship status. If they are living (or have lived) with someone, ask what their relationship is to that person, then follow up using the patient's language. (Loss of a partner can sometimes be determined by asking about whom they have lived with in the past.)

Tips for Taking the Sexual History

- Explain why you are taking the sexual history.
- Note that you realize this information is highly personal, and encourage the patient to be open and direct.
- Relate that you gather this history on all your patients.
- Affirm that your conversation is confidential.

For example, you can begin with a general statement such as:

"To provide good care I need to review your sexual health and see if you are at risk for any sexually transmitted infections. I know this is a sensitive area. Any information you share is confidential."

Sexual Orientation and Gender Identity

Direct questions about sexual orientation may be difficult to answer. Patients with same-sex partners (or who have been in same-sex relationships) may be more anxious or fearful during clinical encounters because of past experiences. A reassuring manner will help them express concerns about their sexual health and activity.

As you talk with patients, begin with neutral questions about *sexual orientation* and *gender identity*, listed below.[5]

- Are you currently dating? sexually active? or in a relationship? How would you identify your sexual orientation?

The range of responses includes heterosexual or straight, lesbian, gay, women who have sex with women, men who have sex with men (MSM), bisexual, transexual, and questioning, among others.

- "How would you describe your gender identity?" Responses include male, female, transsexual, transgendered, intersex, female-to-male, male-to-female, unsure or questioning, or even "prefer not to answer."

- Do you have sex with men, women, or both?

- Do you use birth control? What method?

- Do you use protection against sexually transmitted diseases? What method?

- Has anyone ever tried to touch or have sex with you without your consent?

Continue with general questions such as:

How is sex for you?
Are you having any problems with sex?
Are you satisfied with your sex life as it is now?
Has there been any significant change in the last few years?
Are you satisfied with your ability to perform sexually?
How satisfied do you think your partner is?
Do you feel that your partner is satisfied with the frequency of sexual activity?
Are you comfortable with your partner's sexual practices?

Sexual Response

If the patient has concerns about sexual activity; ask her to tell you about them. Direct questions help you assess each phase of the sexual response: desire, arousal, and orgasm:

"Do you have an interest in (appetite for) sex?" This question inquires about the desire phase.

For the arousal phase:

Do you get sexually aroused?
Do you lubricate easily (get wet or slippery)?
Do you stay too dry?

For the orgasmic phase:

Are you able to reach climax (reach an orgasm or "come")?
Is it important for you to reach climax?

Ask also about *dyspareunia* (pain or discomfort during intercourse). If present, try to localize the symptom. Is it near the outside, occurring at the start of intercourse, or does she feel it farther in, when her partner is pushing deeper? *Vaginismus* refers to an involuntary spasm of the muscles surrounding the vaginal orifice that makes penetration during intercourse painful or impossible.

Sexual dysfunction is classified by the phase of sexual response. A woman may lack desire, she may fail to become aroused and attain adequate vaginal lubrication, or, despite adequate arousal, she may be unable to reach orgasm. Causes may include lack of estrogen, medical illness, trauma or abuse, surgery, pelvic anatomy, or psychiatric conditions.

If patient reports dryness, does she use lubricant?

Superficial pain suggests local inflammation, atrophic vaginitis, or inadequate lubrication; deeper pain may be from pelvic disorders or pressure on a normal ovary. The cause of *vaginismus* may be physical or psychological.

In addition to ascertaining the nature of a sexual problem, ask about its onset, severity (persistent or sporadic), setting, and factors, if any, that make it better or worse. What does the patient think is the cause of the problem, what has she tried to do about it, and what does she hope for? The setting of sexual dysfunction is an important but complicated topic, involving the patient's general health; medications and drugs, including use of alcohol; her partner's and her own knowledge of sexual practices and techniques; her attitudes, values, and fears; the relationship and communication between partners; and the setting in which sexual activity takes place.

More commonly, however, a sexual problem may be related to situational or psychosocial factors.

Sexually Transmitted Infections

Local symptoms or findings on physical examination may raise the possibility of *sexually transmitted infections (STIs)*. After establishing the usual attributes of any symptoms, identify sexual history. Inquire about sexual contacts and establish the number of sexual partners in the past 3 to 6 months. Ask if the patient has concerns about HIV infection, has been tested for HIV previously, desires HIV testing, or has current or past partners at risk. Also ask about oral and anal sex and, if indicated, about symptoms involving the mouth, throat, anus, and rectum. Review the past history of STIs. "Have you ever had herpes? … Any other problems such as gonorrhea? … Syphilis? … Chlamydia?… Pelvic infections?" What does the patient/partner use to prevent STIs? Continue with the more general questions suggested on pp. 81–83, The Sexual History.

PHYSICAL EXAMINATION

Important Areas of Examination

External Examination
• Mons pubis
• Labia majora and minora
• Urethral meatus, clitoris
• Vaginal introitus
• Perineum

The generalist nurse may prepare a woman for or assist with an internal pelvic examination. In addition, the nurse may inspect the external genitalia during a procedure, such as urinary catheterization; during postpartum or postabortion care; while following up on a patient complaint; or while giving a complete bed bath. Therefore, the nurse must know the normal appearance of the external genitalia.

Approach to the Pelvic Examination

Many women feel anxious or uncomfortable before and during pelvic examinations. Some women have had painful, embarrassing, or even demeaning experiences during previous examinations, whereas others may be facing a pelvic examination for the first time. Some are fearful about what the clinician may find and how findings may affect their lives. Asking the patient's permission to perform the examination shows courtesy and respect.

A woman having her first pelvic examination may not know what to expect. Using three-dimensional models, showing her the equipment and letting her handle the speculum, and explaining each step in advance and during the examination can help her learn about her body and be more comfortable. Careful and gentle technique is especially important in minimizing any pain or discomfort during the first pelvic examination.

The woman's response to the pelvic examination may reveal clues about her feelings about the examination and her sexuality. If she pulls away, adducts her thighs, or reacts negatively to the examination, you can gently comment, "I notice you are having some trouble relaxing. Is it just being here, or are you troubled by the examination? ... Is anything worrying you?" Behaviors that seem to present an obstacle may lead to a better understanding of your patient's concerns. Adverse reactions may signal prior abuse and should be explored.

Indications for a pelvic examination during adolescence include menstrual abnormalities such as amenorrhea, excessive bleeding, or dysmenorrhea; unexplained abdominal pain; vaginal discharge; the prescription of contraceptives; bacteriologic and cytologic studies in a sexually active girl; and the patient's own request for assessment.

See Chapter 23, Assessing Children: Infancy Through Adolescence, p. 899.

Tips for the Successful Pelvic Examination

The Patient	The Nurse
• Avoids intercourse, douching, or use of vaginal suppositories for 24 to 48 hours before examination • Empties bladder before examination • Lies supine, with head and shoulders elevated, arms at sides or folded across chest to enhance eye contact and reduce tightening of abdominal muscles	• Obtains permission; acts as chaperone • Explains each step of the examination in advance • Drapes patient from midabdomen to knees; folds drape between knees to provide eye contact with patient • Warms speculum with tap water • Monitors comfort of the examination by watching the patient's face

Helping the patient to relax is essential for an adequate examination. Adopting the tips above will help ensure the patient's comfort. Raising the head of the examination table and supplying a mirror for the patient to observe the examination helps her understand the process.

Note all examiners should be accompanied by an appropriate chaperone.

Rape Victims

Regardless of age, *rape* merits special evaluation, usually requiring gynecologic consultation and documentation. Often there is a special rape kit, provided in many emergency departments that must be used to ensure a chain of custody for evidence. Specimens must be labeled carefully with name, date, and time. Additional information may be needed for further legal investigation.

Equipment

Be sure the examiner has a good light, gloves, a vaginal speculum of appropriate size, water-soluble lubricant, and equipment for taking samples for Papanicolaou smears, bacteriologic cultures and DNA probes, or other diagnostic tests.

Specula are either metal or plastic and come in two basic shapes, named Pedersen and Graves. Both are available in small, medium, and large sizes. The medium Pedersen speculum is usually most comfortable for sexually active women.

Positioning the Patient

Drape the patient appropriately and then assist her into the lithotomy position. Help her to place one heel and then the other into the stirrups. She will be more comfortable with shoes or socks on than with bare feet. Then ask her to slide all the way down the examining table until her buttocks extend slightly beyond the edge. Her thighs should be flexed, abducted, and externally rotated at the hips. Make sure a pillow supports her head.

External Examination

Assess the Sexual Maturity of an Adolescent Patient

You can assess pubic hair during either the abdominal or the pelvic examination. Note its character and distribution, and rate it according to Tanner stages, described on pp. 899–900.

Delayed puberty is often familial or related to chronic illness. It may also reflect disorders of the hypothalamus, anterior pituitary gland, or ovaries.

Examine the External Genitalia

Advise the patient that you will be touching her genital area. Inspect the mons pubis, labia, and perineum. Separate the labia and inspect the:

- labia minora

- clitoris

- urethral meatus

- vaginal opening, or introitus

Note any inflammation, ulceration, discharge, swelling, lacerations, bruising, or nodules.

Excoriations or itchy, small, red maculopapules suggest *pediculosis pubis* (lice or "crabs"). Look for nits or lice at the bases of the pubic hairs.

Enlarged clitoris in masculinizing conditions.

Herpes simplex, Behçet disease, syphilitic chancre, epidermoid cyst. See Table 21-1, Chapter 21, Lesions of the Vulva, p. 780.

Lacerations and/or bruising may indicate sexual abuse.

Internal Examination

The internal pelvic examination consists of a visual examination of the vagina and cervix with a speculum that separates the walls of the vagina. The examiner can assess vaginal muscle tone as well as color, ulcerations, inflammation, discharge, or masses in the vagina or on the cervix. The Papanicolaou smear sample is obtained at this time also. The speculum holding open the vagina prevents contamination of the cervical specimen.

After the speculum is removed, the examiner will manually palpate the organs of the reproductive system. In the bimanual examination, one hand is placed on the lower abdomen and two fingers of the other hand are inserted into the vagina. The cervix and uterus can be palpated for position, size, mobility, shape, regularity, masses, and tenderness. In slender, relaxed women, the ovaries may be palpated for size, position, regularity, and tenderness. Normally the fallopian tubes cannot be felt unless infection or a tubal pregnancy exists. Some examiners may perform a rectal examination at this time.

RECORDING YOUR FINDINGS

Recording the Pelvic Examination— Female Genitalia

"No inguinal adenopathy. External genitalia without erythema, lesions, or masses."
OR
"Bilateral shotty inguinal adenopathy. External genitalia without erythema or lesions. Thin white vaginal homogeneous discharge with mild fishy odor present."

HEALTH PROMOTION AND COUNSELING

Important Topics for Health Promotion and Counseling

* Reproductive System Education
* Changes with menopause
* Cervical cancer screening: Papanicolaou (Pap) smear and human papilloma virus (HPV) infection
* Early prenatal care
* Options for family planning
* STIs including HIV

Reproductive System Education

An accurate understanding of the normal appearance and function of the reproductive system will enable the woman to take control of her reproductive health through family planning and disease prevention; to recognize pregnancy, problems, and maturational changes; and to seek appropriate care in a timely fashion. The use of three-dimensional models and charts is helpful to convey the structure and function of the system.

Changes With Menopause

Inform the patient of the psychological and physiologic changes of menopause—mood shifts and changes in self-concept, vasomotor changes ("hot flashes"), accelerated bone loss, increases in total- and low-density lipoprotein (LDL) cholesterol, and vulvovaginal atrophy leading to symptoms of vaginal drying, dysuria, and, at times, dyspareunia. Refer the woman to her midwife or gynecologist for treatment options for symptoms causing discomfort.

Cervical Cancer Screening: The Pap Smear and HPV Infection

Widespread screening with the *Pap smear* has contributed to a significant decline in cervical cancer incidence and mortality. The current estimated incidence rate is 7.8 cases per 100,000 women per year.[6] Most cases of cervical cancer occur in women who have not had appropriate screening.

The goal of cytologic screening is to sample the transformation zone of the cervix, the area where physiologic transformation from columnar endocervical epithelium to squamous (ectocervical) epithelium takes place and where dysplasia and cancer arise. HPV infection with high-risk oncogenic subtypes is found in virtually all cervical cancers.[7] Ninety percent of HPV infections are asymptomatic and resolve within 2 years. The most important risk factor for cervical cancer is *persistent infection with high-risk HPV subtypes,* especially HPV 16 or HPV 18. These two subtypes cause roughly 70% of cervical cancers worldwide. Even the 10% of women with persistent infection rarely progress to cervical cancer if they undergo regular screening, since the average estimated time for a high-grade HPV lesion to progress to cervical cancer is 10 years, allowing a long interval for detection and treatment.[6] Genital infection with low-risk subtypes, such as HPV 6 and HPV 11, is associated with genital warts.

Two notable risk factors for cervical cancer include *failure to undergo screening,* which accounts for roughly half of women diagnosed with cervical cancer, and *multiple sexual partners.* Other risk factors include smoking, immunosuppression from any cause including HIV infection, long-term use of oral contraception, coinfection with *Chlamydia,* parity, prior cervical cancer, and genetic polymorphisms affecting the entry of HPV DNA into cervical cells.[8]

Cervical Cancer Screening Guidelines, 2015

In 2012, for the first time, the U.S. Preventive Services Task Force (USPSTF), the American College of Obstetricians and Gynecologists (ACOG), and the American Cancer Society (ACS), in collaboration with the American Society for Colposcopy and Cervical Pathology and the American Society for Clinical Pathology (ASCP), released guidelines that agree on cervical cancer screening for average-risk women, summarized in the table below, which contains the important definition of average risk.[6,8–10] Note that in 2014, the American College of Physicians found no evidence supporting screening with routine pelvic examinations alone in average risk asymptomatic adult women (as distinct from cervical cancer screening or symptom-based examination).[11,12]

Current Cervical Cancer Screening Guidelines for Average-Risk Women* from the U.S. Preventive Services Task Force, American Cancer Society/American Society for Colposcopy and Cervical Pathology/American Society for Clinical Pathology, and American Congress of Obstetricians and Gynecologists

Variable	Recommendation
Age at which to begin screening	21 y
Screening method and interval	Age 21–65 y: cytology every 3 y OR Age 21–29 y: cytology every 3 y Age 30–65 y: cytology plus HPV testing (for high-risk or oncogenic HPV types) every 5 y
Age at which to end screening	>65 y, assuming 3 consecutive negative results on cytology or 2 consecutive negative results on cytology plus HPV testing within 10 y before cessation of screening, with the most recent test performed within 5 y
Screening after hysterectomy	Not recommended with removal of the cervix

HPV, human papillomavirus.
*__Definition of Average Risk:__ No history of high-grade, precancerous cervical lesion (cervical intraepithelial neoplasia grade 2 or a more severe lesion) or cervical cancer; not immunocompromised (including being HIV-infected); and no in utero exposure to diethylstilbestrol.
Source: Sawaya GF, Kulasingam S, Denberg T, et al. Cervical cancer screening in average-risk women: Best practice advice from the Clinical Guidelines Committee of the American College of Physicians. *Ann Intern Med.* 2015;162(12):851–859.

Other risk factors for cervical cancer include: early sexual activity, multiple sexual partners, a history of STIs, failure to undergo screening by Pap smear, age, nutritional status, smoking, immune status, and genetic polymorphisms affecting the entry of HPV DNA into cervical cells.

The HPV Vaccine

ROUTINE VACCINATION FOR GIRLS AND BOYS AGES 11 AND 12. The Advisory Committee on Immunization Practices (ACIP) of the Centers for Disease Control (CDC) and the American Academy of Pediatrics recommend a three-dose vaccination series over 6 months with either the quadrivalent or bivalent vaccine for *girls and boys at ages 11 or 12,* before their first sexual encounter. The series can begin as early as age 9.[13,14] The quadrivalent vaccine prevents infection from HPV subtypes 16 and 18, as well as 6 and 11, which cause 90% of genital warts. The bivalent vaccine prevents infection from subtypes 16 and 18. Vaccination with the quadrivalent HPV vaccine is also recommended for the prevention of cervical, vulvar, and vaginal cancers and precancers in females, as well as anal cancers and precancers and genital warts in both females and males.

CATCH-UP VACCINATION. Vaccination is recommended for females ages 13 through 26 and for males ages 13 through 21 who have not had prior vaccination or completed the three-dose series. Males ages 22 through 26 may also be vaccinated. If females or males reach age 27 before completing the series, the second and/or third vaccine doses can be administered after age 26 to complete the series. Prevaccination assessments to establish the need for Pap or high-risk HPV DNA testing are not recommended.

GAY AND BISEXUAL MEN; IMMUNOCOMPROMISED INDIVIDUALS. The HPV vaccine is recommended for gay and bisexual men (or any man who has sex with men) and persons with compromised immune systems, including infection with HIV, through age 26 if they have not been fully vaccinated when younger.

Starting HPV vaccination early is important. In American adolescents, the prevalence of sexual intercourse in 2013 was: 5.6% before age 13; 30% by ninth grade, and 64% by the end of high school.[15] Vaccinated women should still get cervical cancer screening since the vaccines do not prevent all HPV subtypes. Consistent use of condoms does not eliminate risk of cervical HPV infection.[16,17]

Early Prenatal Care

In 2013, the infant mortality rate was 6 deaths per 1,000 live births and the preterm (before 37 weeks of gestation) rate was 11.4% of live births.[18] Early prenatal care and preparation for pregnancy, such as stopping alcohol use and smoking, weight loss in obese women, and taking folic acid and calcium supplements, lower the perimortality rate. Women who express a desire to become pregnant or who are at risk for pregnancy should have a gynecologic examination to identify possible problems before pregnancy and be counseled on how to best prepare for pregnancy. If the history indicates the woman may be pregnant, she should be encouraged to obtain prenatal care as soon as possible.

Options for Family Planning

It is important to counsel patients, particularly adolescents, about the timing of ovulation in the menstrual cycle and how to plan or prevent pregnancy. The CDC notes that "Teen pregnancy has declined to the lowest rates in seven decades, yet still rank highest among the developed countries."[19] Significant health disparities remain: in 2013 non-Hispanic black, Hispanic and American Indian/Alaska Native teen birth rates were still one and a half to two times higher than the rate for non-Hispanic white teens. Almost half of U.S. pregnancies are unintended. Among pregnancies in teens ages 19 years and younger and under age 15, the percentage of unintended pregnancy climbs to over 80% and 98%, respectively. Nurses should be familiar with the numerous options for contraception and their effectiveness, in order to explain contraception methods to patients. Take the time to understand the patient or couple's concerns and preferences and respect these preferences whenever possible. Continued use of a preferred method is superior to a more effective method that is abandoned. For teenagers, a confidential setting eases discussion of topics that may seem private and difficult to explore.

Sexually Transmitted Infections and HIV Infection

U.S. rates of STIs are the highest in the industrialized world. *Chlamydia trachomatis* is the most commonly reported STI in the United States and the most common in women with an estimated 2.8 million cases annually.[20] Often symptoms are subtle and the infection remains undiagnosed. If untreated, 10% to 15% of women will develop pelvic inflammatory disease (PID), a polymicrobial infection with an 8% to 40% risk of tubal infertility depending on the number of episodes; a third to a half of cases are attributed to co-infection of *Chlamydia* with *Neisseria gonorrhoeae*.[21,22] Infection rates are highest in women 20 to 24 years old and second highest in women 15 to 19 years old. African-American women and American Indian/Alaska Native women have the highest infection rates.

As with other STIs, risk factors are age less than 24 and sexually active; prior infection with *Chlamydia* or other STIs; new or multiple partners; inconsistent condom use; and occupational sex work. Detection, groups most affected, and consequences of under diagnosis and treatment are similar for *gonorrhea*. Infection with *syphilis* is less common, but increasing in men.[23]

Concept Mastery Alert

Pelvic inflammatory disease (PID) is most commonly caused by sexually transmitted infections, such as Chlamydia. Vaginal infections are not a common cause because they are usually confined to the tissues of the vagina and are prevented from moving into the uterus by the cervix.

To improve detection and treatment, the CDC and the USPSTF[24] strongly recommends screening for STIs, summarized below.

CDC STI and HIV Screening Recommendations 2014

- *Chlamydia* and *gonorrhea screening* annually for *all sexually active women younger than age 25 and older women with risk factors* such as new or multiple sex partners, or a sex partner infected with an STI.
- *Chlamydia, syphilis, hepatitis B,* and *HIV screening* for *all pregnant women,* and *gonorrhea screening* for *at risk pregnant women* starting early in pregnancy, with repeat testing as needed to protect the health of mothers and their infants.
- *Chlamydia, gonorrhea,* and *syphilis screening* at least once a year for *all sexually active gay, bisexual, and other men who have sex with men (MSM).* MSM have multiple or anonymous partners should be screened more frequently for STIs (i.e., at 3- to 6-month intervals).
- *HIV testing* at least once for *all adults and adolescents from ages 13 to 64.*
- *HIV testing* at least once a year for *anyone having unsafe sex or using injection drug equipment.* Sexually active gay and bisexual men may benefit from testing every 3 to 6 months.

Source: Centers for Disease Control and Prevention. Sexually transmitted diseases. STD and HIV screening recommendations. Updated February 11, 2016. Available at http://www.cdc.gov/std/prevention/screeningreccs.htm. Accessed May 1, 2016.

HIV Infection

Over 1.2 million Americans are infected with HIV, and 1 in 7 (14%) are unaware of their infection.[25] The number of infected individuals continues to increase, although the number of new infections has remained stable. In 2013, an estimated 47,352 people were diagnosed with HIV infection and an estimated 26,688 people were diagnosed with AIDS, bringing the estimated total number of Americans diagnosed with AIDs to 1,194,039. At highest risk are gay men, bisexual men, and other MSM of all ethnicities, but especially young black/African-American MSM ages 13 to 24. In 2010, MSM represented 4% of the U.S. male population and 63% of all new infections. White MSM had the largest total number of new infections, 11,200. Blacks/African Americans and Hispanics/Latinos remain disproportionately affected.[25]

In the United States, 19% of new infections occur in women, primarily through heterosexual contact (87% in 2014) and injection drug use (13%). Women represent 25% of those living with HIV infection. Among infected women, 61% are African American, 17% are white, and 17% are Hispanic/Latina. The CDC reports that women are not accessing health care and are undertreated: "in 2013, only 55% were engaged in care, and only 30% had achieved viral suppression."[26] Heterosexual transmission is more likely in the following settings: vaginal or anal intercourse without a condom; sex exchanged for drugs; sex with multiple partners; infection with other STIs; women who have been sexually abused; sex with an infected partner with high viral load of HIV-1; cervical ectopy; sex during menstruation; and sex with a male partner without circumcision. Recurrent vulvocandidiasis, concurrent STIs, abnormal Pap smears (occurring in 40% of HIV-positive women), and HPV infection are warning indications for HIV testing. As shown in the table above, the CDC recommends *universal HIV testing for everyone in the age range of 13 to 64* due to the prevalence of infections in people without known risk factors and also of underreporting.

PATIENT COUNSELING. Nurses should assess risk factors for STIs and HIV infection by taking a careful sexual history and counseling patients about spread of disease and how to reduce high-risk practices. Key to effective clinician counseling are respect, compassion, a nonjudgmental attitude, and use of open-ended and understandable questions like "Tell me about any new sex partners" and "Have you ever had anal sex, meaning 'penis in rectum/anus sex'?"—The USPSTF review of evidence notes that successful counseling includes: "prevalence, transmission, and details on how to reduce the risk for transmission; help in identifying personal risk for STIs; training in common behavior change processes, such as problem solving, decision making, and goal-setting; training in communication surrounding condom use and safe sex; and hands-on practice with condoms."[27] The CDC recommends interactive client-centered counseling, tailored to the person's specific risk factors and situation. Training in prevention counseling improves effectiveness. The website by the CDC can provide information: https://effectiveinterventions.cdc.gov/en/home.aspx

See Chapter 4, The Health History, pp. 81–83, on eliciting the sexual history.

MALE REPRODUCTIVE SYSTEM

ANATOMY AND PHYSIOLOGY

First review the anatomy of the male genitalia.

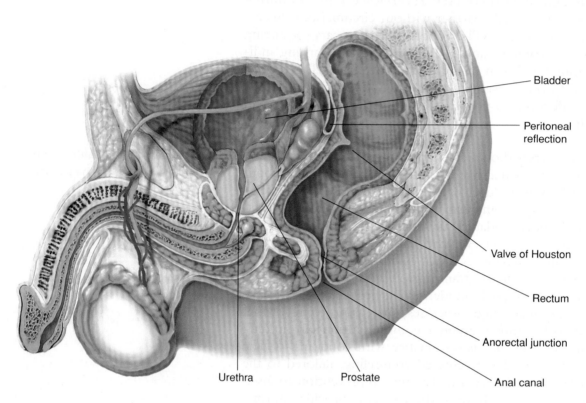

Bladder

Peritoneal reflection

Valve of Houston

Rectum

Anorectal junction

Anal canal

Urethra   Prostate

The *shaft of the penis* is formed by three columns of vascular erectile tissue: the *corpus spongiosum,* containing the urethra, and two *corpora cavernosa.* The corpus spongiosum extends from the bulb of the penis to the cone-shaped *glans* with its expanded base, or *corona.* In uncircumcised men, the glans is covered by a loose, hood-like fold of skin called the *prepuce* or *fore-skin,* where *smegma,* or secretions of the glans, may collect. The urethra is located in the ventral midline of the shaft of the penis; urethral abnormalities may sometimes be felt there. The urethra opens into the vertical, slit-like *urethral meatus,* located somewhat ventrally at the tip of the glans.

The *testes* are paired ovoid glands consisting primarily of seminiferous tubules and interstitial tissue, covered by a fibrous outer coating, the *tunica albuginea.* The testes are normally 1.5 to 2 cm in length for prepubertal boys and 4 to 5 cm postpuberty. The left testis usually lies lower than the right. The testes produce spermatozoa and testosterone. Testosterone stimulates the pubertal growth of the male genitalia, prostate, and seminal vesicles. It also stimulates the development of masculine secondary sex characteristics, including facial hair, body hair, musculoskeletal growth, and enlargement of the larynx, with its associated low-pitched voice.

Surrounding or appended to the testes are several structures. The *scrotum* is a loose, wrinkled pouch divided into two compartments, each containing a testis or testicle. Covering the testis, except posteriorly, is the serous membrane of the *tunica vaginalis*. On the posterolateral surface of each testis is the softer, comma-shaped *epididymis*, consisting of tightly coiled tubules emanating from the testis that become the *vas deferens*. The epididymis provides a reservoir for storage, maturation, and transport of sperm from the testis to the *vas deferens*.

During ejaculation, the *vas deferens*, a cord-like structure, transports sperm from the tail of the epididymis along a somewhat circular route to the urethra. The *vas* ascends from the scrotal sac into the pelvic cavity through the inguinal canal, then loops anteriorly over the ureter to the prostate behind the bladder. There it merges with the *seminal vesicle* to form the *ejaculatory duct*, which traverses the prostate and empties into the urethra. Secretions from the *vas deferens*, the seminal vesicles, and the prostate all contribute to the seminal fluid. Within the scrotum, each vas is closely associated with blood vessels, nerves, and muscle fibers. These structures make up the *spermatic cord*.

Male sexual function depends on normal levels of testosterone, arterial blood flow from the internal iliac artery to the internal pudendal artery and its penile artery and branches, and intact neural innervation from α-adrenergic and cholinergic pathways. Erection from venous engorgement of the corpora cavernosa results from two types of stimuli. Visual, auditory, or erotic cues trigger sympathetic outflow from higher brain centers to the T11 through L2 levels of the spinal cord. Tactile stimulation initiates sensory impulses from the genitalia to the S2 to S4 reflex arcs and the parasympathetic pathways through the pudendal nerve. Both sets of stimuli appear to increase levels of nitric oxide and cyclic guanosine monophosphate (GMP), resulting in local vasodilation.

Lymphatics

Lymph drainage from the *penis* passes primarily to the deep inguinal and external inguinal nodes. Lymph vessels from the *scrotum* drain into the superficial inguinal lymph nodes. When an inflammatory or possibly malignant lesion is found on these surfaces, assess the inguinal nodes for enlargement or tenderness. Lymphatic drainage from the *testes* parallels their venous drainage: the left testicular vein empties into the left renal vein, and the right testicular vein empties into the inferior vena cava. The connecting abdominal lymph nodes are clinically undetectable. See Chapter 15, p. 445 for further discussion of the inguinal nodes.

Anatomy of the Groin

Because hernias are relatively common, it is important to understand the anatomy of the groin. The basic landmarks are the anterior superior iliac spine, the pubic tubercle, and the inguinal ligament that runs between them, which are readily identified.

The *inguinal canal,* which lies medial to and approximately parallel to the inguinal ligament, forms a tunnel for the vas deferens as it passes through the abdominal muscles. The exterior opening of the tunnel—the *external inguinal ring*—is a triangular, slit-like structure palpable just above and lateral to the pubic tubercle. The internal opening of the canal—or *internal inguinal ring*—is approximately 1 cm above the midpoint of the inguinal ligament. Neither canal nor internal ring is palpable through the abdominal wall. When loops of bowel force their way through weak areas of the inguinal canal, they produce *inguinal hernias,* as illustrated in Table 21-7, Chapter 21, Course, Presentation and Differentiation of Hernias in the Groin, p. 786.

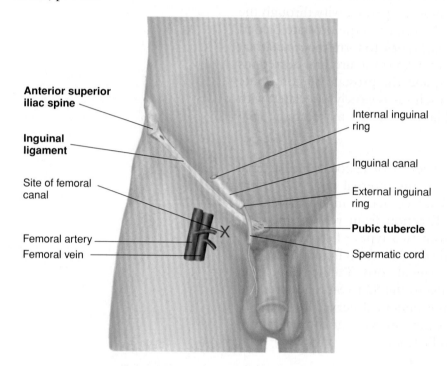

Anterior superior iliac spine

Inguinal ligament

Site of femoral canal

Femoral artery

Femoral vein

Internal inguinal ring

Inguinal canal

External inguinal ring

Pubic tubercle

Spermatic cord

Indirect inguinal hernias develop at the internal inguinal ring, where the spermatic cord exits the abdomen. *Direct inguinal hernias* arise more medially due to weakness in the floor of the inguinal canal and are associated with straining and heavy lifting.

Another potential route for a herniating mass is the *femoral canal.* This lies below the inguinal ligament. Although this canal is not visible, you can estimate its location by placing your right index finger, from below, on the right femoral artery. Your middle finger will then overlie the femoral vein; your ring finger, the femoral canal. Femoral hernias protrude at this location.

Femoral hernias are more likely to present as emergencies with bowel incarceration or strangulation.

THE HEALTH HISTORY

Common or Concerning Symptoms

- Sexual preference and gender identity
- Penile discharge or lesions
- Scrotal pain, swelling, or lesions
- Problems with urination

Sexual Preference and Gender Identity

Review the Tips for Taking the Sexual History on p. 754.

Discussing sexual orientation and gender identity touches a vital and multifaceted core of your patients' lives. Reflect on any biases you may have so they do not interfere with professional responses to your patients' disclosures and concerns. A neutral supportive approach is essential for exploring your patients' health and well-being.[5]

- Pose neutral questions about *sexual orientation* and *gender identity* such as: "Are you currently dating, sexually active, or in a relationship?" "How would you identify your sexual orientation?" The range of responses includes heterosexual or straight, lesbian, gay, women who have sex with women (WSW), men who have sex with men (MSM), bisexual, transexual, and questioning, among others.

- Continue with "How would you describe your gender identity?" Responses include male, female, transsexual, transgendered, intersex, female-to-male, male-to-female, unsure or questioning, or even "prefer not to answer."

Sexual Response

Explore the patient's sexual response.

How is sex for you?
How is your current relationship?
What about your ability to perform sexually? Are you satisfied with your relationship and your sexual activity? "Has your partner ever hurt you or forced you to have sex?"
"Are you comfortable with your partner's sexual practices?"

If the patient expresses relational or sexual concerns, explore both their psychological and physiologic dimensions.

What does this relationship mean to you?
Have you experienced any changes in desire or frequency of sexual activity?
What is your view of the cause, what responses have you tried, and what are your hopes?
Direct questions help assess each phase of the sexual response.

To assess *libido*, or desire, ask:

Have you maintained interest in sex?

Low libido may arise from depression, endocrine dysfunction, or side effects of medications.

For the *arousal phase*, ask:

Can you achieve and maintain an erection?

Explore the timing, severity, setting, and any other factors that may contribute to the issue.

Have any changes in the relationship with your partner or in your life circumstances coincided with onset of a problem?
Are there circumstances when erection is normal? On awakening in the early morning or during the night? With other partners? With masturbation?

Questions that relate to the phase of *orgasm* and *ejaculation* of semen.

If ejaculation is premature, or early and out of control, ask:

About how long does intercourse last?
Do you climax too soon?
Do you feel you have control over climaxing?
Do you think your partner would like intercourse to last longer?

For reduced or absent ejaculation:

Do you find that you cannot have reach orgasm even though you can have an erection?

Try to determine whether the problem involves the pleasurable sensation of orgasm, the ejaculation of seminal fluid, or both. Review the frequency and setting of the symptoms, medications, surgery, and neurologic causes.

Penile Discharge or Lesions

To assess the possibility of genital infection from STIs, ask:

Have you had any discharge, leaking, or dripping from your penis or staining on your underwear?

If discharge is present, ask:

When did it start?
Is it continuous or intermittent?
How much discharge is there? A teaspoon? A tablespoon?
What color is the discharge?
Is the discharge thick or thin?
Have you had any sores or growths on the penis or scrotum? Or pain or swelling in the scrotum?

Erectile dysfunction may be from psychogenic causes, especially if early morning erection is preserved; also from decreased testosterone, decreased blood flow in the hypogastric arterial system, or impaired neural innervation.[28]

Premature ejaculation is common, especially in young men. Less common is reduced or absent ejaculation affecting middle-aged or older men. Possible causes are medications, surgery, neurologic deficits, or lack of androgen. Lack of orgasm with ejaculation is usually psychogenic.

Penile discharge may accompany gonococcal (usually yellow) and nongonococcal urethritis (may be clear or white).

Have you had a fever, chills, rash, or any other symptoms?

Have you ever had these symptoms before? If yes, how were they treated?

Inquire about sores or growths on the penis.

To assess further for STIs, ask:

Have you ever been diagnosed with a sexually transmitted infection? Herpes? Gonorrhea? Syphilis?

See Table 21-3, Chapter 21, Abnormalities of the Penis and Scrotum, p. 782, Table 21-4, Chapter 21, Sexually Transmitted Infections of Male Genitalia, p. 783 and Table 21-5, Chapter 21, Abnormalities of the Testes, p. 784. In addition to STIs, many skin conditions affect the genitalia; likewise, some STIs have minimal symptoms or signs.

Because STIs may involve other parts of the body, additional questions are often indicated. An introductory explanation may be useful. "Sexually transmitted infections can involve any body opening where you have sex. It's important for you to tell me which openings you use. It's important for you to tell me if you have oral or anal sex." Ask about symptoms such as sore throat, diarrhea, rectal bleeding, anal itching, or anal pain.

Infections from oral–penile transmission include gonorrhea, chlamydia, syphilis, and herpes. Symptomatic or asymptomatic proctitis *(inflammation of the rectum and anus)* may follow anal intercourse.

Because many infected individuals do not have symptoms or risk factors, ask all patients, "Do you have any concerns about HIV infection?" and discuss the need for *universal testing for HIV.*[29–32]

Scrotal Pain or Swelling

If the patient complains of pain or swelling in his scrotum, follow the OLD CART mnemonic to gather thorough information. A sudden onset of scrotal pain may indicate torsion of the testicle, which is an emergency. A painless lump may be cancer. Ask the patient if he performs self-testicular examination and how often.

Inguinal Pain or Swelling

Inguinal pain or swelling may indicate an inguinal hernia. These hernias may be unilateral or bilateral. Ask the patient to point to the area of the pain and/or swelling and to describe it. "When did it begin? Is the pain continuous or intermittent? Achy or sharp? Does it occur with lifting heavy objects, standing, bending, or bearing down?"

Hernia pain and swelling are more likely to occur when internal abdominal pressure increases (e.g., when lifting).

Problems With Urination

The prostate gland wraps around the urethra. If the gland enlarges due to benign prostatic hyperplasia (BPH) or cancer, the patient may experience urinary symptoms. Men older than 70 years are at greatest risk. Therefore, the nurse should review the pattern of urination (see Chapter 16, The Gastrointestinal and Renal Systems). Ask the patient:

Do you have any difficulty starting or holding back the urine stream?
Is the flow weak?
How often do you urinate during the day? The night?
Is there any pain or burning as urine is passed?
Is there any blood in the urine or in your semen? Any pain with ejaculation?
Do you have any discomfort or heaviness in the prostate area at the base of the penis?

These symptoms suggest possible prostatitis.

PHYSICAL EXAMINATION

The generalist nurse does not perform prostate examinations or examine the genitalia by palpation of the male patient. However, the nurse may inspect the genitalia during a bed bath, a procedure such as urinary catheterization, or postoperative follow-up care in the genitourinary system. The nurse should be able to recognize abnormal conditions found on inspection that require referral or treatment. For younger patients, review the Tanner sexual maturity ratings in Chapter 23, Assessing Children: Infancy Through Adolescence, pp. 897–898.

Gloves should be worn. Occasionally male patients have erections during the examination or a procedure where the penis is touched. If this happens explain that this is a normal response, and finish your examination with a calm demeanor.

The Penis

Inspection

Inspect the penis, including:

- The *skin*. Inspect the skin on the ventral and dorsal surfaces and the base of the penis for excoriations or inflammation, lifting the penis when necessary.

See Table 21-3, Chapter 21, Abnormalities of the Penis and Scrotum, p. 782.

The *prepuce* (foreskin). If present, retract the prepuce or ask the patient to retract it. This step is essential for the detection of many chancres and carcinomas. Smegma, a cheesy, whitish material, may accumulate normally under the foreskin.

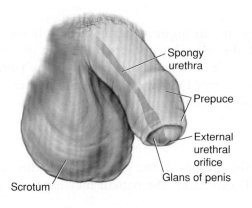

Spongy urethra

Prepuce

External urethral orifice

Glans of penis

Scrotum

Phimosis is a tight prepuce that cannot be retracted over the glans. *Paraphimosis* is a tight prepuce that, once retracted, cannot be returned. Edema ensues.

- The *glans*. Look for any ulcers, scars, nodules, or signs of inflammation.

Balanitis (inflammation of the glans); *balanoposthitis* (inflammation of the glans and prepuce)

Check the skin around the base of the penis for excoriations or inflammation. Look for nits or lice at the bases of the pubic hairs.

Note the location of the urethral meatus.

Inspect it for discharge. Normally there is none.

If you retracted the foreskin, replace it before proceeding on to examine the scrotum.

The Scrotum and Its Contents

Inspection

Inspect the scrotum, including:

* The *skin*. Lift up the scrotum so that you can inspect its posterior surface. Note any lesions or scars. Inspect the pubic hair distribution.

* The *scrotal contours*. Inspect for swelling, lumps, or veins bulging masses, or asymmetry of the left and right hemi-scrotum.

* The *inguinal areas*. Note any erythema, excoriation, or visible adenopathy.

There may be dome-shaped white or yellow papules or nodules formed by occluded follicles filled with keratin debris of desquamated follicular epithelium. Such *epidermoid cysts* are common, frequently multiple, and benign.

EPIDERMOID CYSTS

Hernias

Inspection

If the patient has complained of a bulge or pain in his lower abdomen, especially with lifting or straining, he should be examined for hernias. Standing is the preferred position, because the upright position causes gravity to accentuate the bulge. Inspect the inguinal and femoral areas for bulging and asymmetry. As you observe, ask the patient to strain and bear down (the Valsalva maneuver) to increase intra-abdominal pressure, making it easier to

---

Pubic or genital excoriations suggest the possibility of lice (crabs) or sometimes scabies.

Hypospadias is a congenital, ventral displacement of the meatus on the penis (Table 21-3, Chapter 21, Abnormalities of the Penis and Scrotum, p. 782).

Profuse yellow discharge in *gonococcal urethritis;* scanty white or clear discharge in *nongonococcal urethritis.* Definitive diagnosis requires Gram stain and culture.

See Table 21-3, Chapter 21, Abnormalities of the Penis and Scrotum, p. 782.

Rashes, epidermoid cysts, rarely skin cancer

A poorly developed scrotum on one or both sides suggests *cryptorchidism* (an undescended testicle). Common scrotal swellings include indirect *inguinal hernias, hydroceles,* and *scrotal edema.*

Erythema and mild excoriation point to fungal infection, not uncommon in this moist area.

A bulge that appears on straining suggests a *hernia.*

observe a hernia. If a bulge is present, the patient should be referred to a physician or advanced practitioner for follow-up.

Absence of a bulge during inspection does not guarantee absence of a hernia, especially in an obese patient. If suspicious history findings have been reported, the patient should be referred to an advanced practitioner for further examination.

RECORDING YOUR FINDINGS

Recording the Physical Examination—Male Genitalia and Hernias

"Circumcised. No penile discharge or lesions. No scrotal swelling or discoloration. Testes descended bilaterally. No apparent inguinal or femoral hernias."

HEALTH PROMOTION AND COUNSELING

Important Topics for Health Promotion and Counseling

- Prevention of STIs and HIV
- Testicular self-examination (TSE)
- Screening for prostate cancer

Prevention of Sexually Transmitted Infections and HIV Infection

The Institute of Medicine has called STIs a "hidden epidemic of enormous health and economic consequence in the United States."[33] Nurses play a vital role in educating patients about prevention, as well as in detecting and treating STIs. The growing burden of STIs affects the health of all segments of the population, but especially adolescents and young adults.

Facts About STIs

- The Centers for Disease Control and Prevention (CDC) recently estimated that nearly 20 million new STIs occur each year, with almost half in between the ages of 15 and 24; the associated health care costs are nearly $16 billion.[34,35]
- Of the nearly 1.8 million new STI cases reported in 2013, nearly 80% were infections from chlamydia, 18% from gonorrhea, and 3% from syphilis (all stages). In recent years, rates of gonorrhea and syphilis infections have been increasing, and chlamydia infections have been declining.

- The CDC notes that these figures underestimate the "true national burden" of STIs; many cases of gonorrhea, chlamydia, and syphilis are unreported, and mandatory reporting is not required for infections such as HPV, trichomoniasis, and genital herpes.

Screening Recommendations

The USPSTF has given a grade B recommendation for chlamydia and gonorrhea screening in sexually active women age 24 years and younger; the evidence is insufficient to make a recommendation for sexually active men.[36] However, substantial proportions of those with high-risk sexual behaviors are not being tested for STIs (or HIV).

Nurses should master the skills of eliciting the sexual history and asking frank but tactful questions about sexual practices. Key information includes the patient's sexual orientation, the number of partners in the past month, and any history of past STIs. Careful screening for alcohol and drug use, especially injection drugs, is also important. Counseling should be interactive and combine messages about general risk reduction relevant to the patient with education about specific actions for reducing the patient's risk (see also p. 765). Important topics include limiting the number of partners, using condoms or dental dams, and establishing regular medical care for treatment of STIs and HIV. Men should seek prompt attention for any genital lesions or penile discharge.

HIV and AIDS

Despite advances in detection and treatment, HIV and AIDS remain significant threats to health, particularly for younger Americans, MSM, and injection drug users.

Facts About HIV and AIDS

- The CDC estimates that over 1.2 million Americans age 13 and older are currently infected with HIV, with approximately 50,000 new infections annually.[37]
- Over 600,000 Americans have died with an AIDS diagnosis. At highest risk are men who have sex with men (78% of new infections among males), African Americans (44% of new infections), and Hispanics/Latinos (21% of new infections); injection drug users represent 8% of new HIV infections.
- In 2011, an estimated 14% of infected individuals were unaware of their infected status and only 37% were prescribed antiretroviral therapy (ART).[38]

Screening Recommendations

Identifying early HIV infection and initiating combined ART decreases the risk of progressing to AIDS. Treatment also reduces the risk of transmitting HIV to uninfected heterosexual partners and from a pregnant mother to her child.[39] Current screening recommendations are summarized below.

Summary: Screening Recommendations for HIV

- The USPSTF gives a *Grade A recommendation for HIV screening adolescents and adults from ages 15 to 65 and for screening all pregnant women*.[39]
- The CDC recommends *universal HIV testing for adolescents and adults from ages 13 to 64 in health care settings and prenatal testing of all pregnant women*.[40]
- The CDC recommends an opt-out approach to HIV testing—verbally notifying the patient that testing will be performed unless the patient declines. Separate written consent is not required.
- The American College of Physicians recommends extending the upper age for screening to 75 years.[41] The proportion of adults who have ever been tested for HIV increased from 37% in 2000 to 45% in 2010.[42]
- One-time testing for low-risk patients is reasonable, but at least *annual testing is recommended for high-risk groups* (including adolescents younger than 15 and older adults), defined as men with male sex partners, individuals with multiple sexual partners, past or present injection drug users, persons who exchange sex for money or drugs, and sex partners of persons who are HIV-infected, bisexual, or injection-drug users.[40] *The presence of any STI, or requests for STI testing, warrants testing for co-infection with HIV.*

As you counsel patients, encourage them to seek prompt attention for any genital lesions or penile discharge. Address preventive behaviors such as using condoms and dental dams, limiting the number of sexual partners, and establishing regular health care for treatment of STIs and HIV. *Correct use of male condoms* is highly effective in preventing the transmission of HIV, HPV, and other STIs.[43] Key instructions should include:

- Using a new condom with each sex act

- Applying the condom before any sexual contact occurs

- Adding only water-based lubricants

- Immediately withdrawal if the condom breaks during sexual activity, and holding the condom during withdrawal to keep it from slipping off.

HPV Vaccination

The ACIP recommends routine quadrivalent *HPV vaccination in males age 11 or 12 and through age 21 if not vaccinated previously* (age 26 if immunocompromised or having sex with other men).[44] The vaccine can prevent HPV-related diseases in males (genital warts, anal cancer, and penile cancer) and possibly reduce HPV transmission to female sex partners and lower the risk of oropharyngeal cancers.

Testicular Self-Examination

The incidence of testicular cancer is low, about 5 per 100,000 men, but it is the most common cancer of young men between the ages of 15 and 35. When detected early, testicular carcinoma has an excellent prognosis. Although the USPSTF and the American Cancer Society have not recommended routine TSE for screening, the clinician may wish to teach the TSE to enhance health awareness and self-care, especially for men at high risk. Risk factors include cryptorchidism, which confers a high risk for testicular carcinoma in the undescended testicle; a history of carcinoma in the contralateral testicle; mumps orchitis; an inguinal hernia; a hydrocele in childhood and a positive family history. Teach men, especially young men, how to perform TSEs and to seek physician evaluation for the following findings: any painless lump, swelling, or enlargement in either testicle; pain or discomfort in a testicle or the scrotum; a feeling of heaviness or a sudden fluid collection in the scrotum; or a dull ache in the lower abdomen or the groin.

Prostate Cancer

Prostate cancer is the second leading cancer diagnosed in U.S. men after skin cancer. It is the second leading cause of cancer death in American men, behind lung cancer. About one man in seven will be diagnosed with prostate cancer during his lifetime.[45] Age, ethnicity, and family history are the primary risk factors.

- *Age.* Prostate cancer occurs mainly in older men. About 6 cases in 10 are diagnosed in men aged 65 or older, and it is rare before age 40. The average age at the time of diagnosis is about 66.[45]

- *Ethnicity.* For undetermined reasons, prostate cancer occurs more often in African-American men and in Caribbean men of African ancestry than in men of other races. African-American men are more than twice as likely to die of prostate cancer as white men.[46]

- *Family history.* From 5% to 10% of prostate cancer cases are believed to be primarily caused by high-risk inherited genetic factors or prostate cancer susceptibility genes. Having a first-degree relative diagnosed with prostate cancer is a relative risk of 2.48. Having two first-degree relatives with prostate cancer approximately doubles the risk to 4.39.[47] Inheritance of certain gene variations, such as BRCA1 and BRCA2 increase a man's risk of prostate cancer.

- **_Diet._** A series of studies suggests an association between intake of dietary fat, especially saturated fats and fats from animal sources, and risk of prostate cancer. However, the evidence remains inconclusive.

The optimal approach to prostate cancer _screening_ remains controversial. The USPSTF in 2012 found insufficient evidence to recommend routine screening using _prostate-specific antigen (PSA) testing_ due to lack of evidence that the benefits of testing outweigh potential harm. The USPSTF is currently researching an update to this recommendation. The USPSTF, the American Cancer and the American Urological Association recommend an individualized patient approach to screening based on the man's age and risk factors. The greatest benefit of screening appears to be in men ages 55 to 69 years. However, men younger than 55 with high risk of prostate cancer should be individually evaluated for screening.[48,49]

For the American Urological Associations Guidelines go to: https://www.auanet.org/education/guidelines/prostate-cancer-detection.cfm

Men _with symptoms_ of prostate disorders—incomplete emptying of the bladder, urinary frequency or urgency, weak or intermittent stream or straining to initiate flow, hematuria, nocturia, or even bony pains in the pelvis—should be referred to a urologist. Men may be reluctant to report such symptoms but should be encouraged to seek evaluation and treatment early.

Patient Instructions for the Testicular Self-Examination

This examination is best performed after a warm bath or shower. This way the scrotal skin is warm and relaxed. It is best to do the test while standing.

- Standing in front of a mirror, check for any swelling on the skin of the scrotum.
- With the penis out of the way, gently feel your scrotal sac to locate a testicle. Examine each testicle separately.
- Use one hand to stabilize the testicle. Using the fingers and thumb of your other hand, firmly but gently feel or roll the testicle between your fingers. Feel the entire surface. Find

the epididymis. This is a soft, tube-like structure at the back of the testicle that collects and carries sperm, and is not an abnormal lump. Check the other testicle and epididymis the same way.

- If you find a hard lump, an absent or enlarged testicle, a painful swollen scrotum, or any other differences that do not seem normal, don't wait. See your health care provider right away.

As noted by the American Cancer Society, "It's normal for one testicle to be slightly larger than the other, and for one to hang lower than the other. You should also know that each normal testicle has a small, coiled tube (epididymis) that can feel like a small bump on the upper or middle outer side of the testicle. Normal testicles also have blood vessels, supporting tissues, and tubes that carry sperm. Some men may confuse these with abnormal lumps at first. If you have any concerns, ask your doctor."

Sources: American Cancer Society. Testicular self-exam. Updated January 21, 2015. Available at http://www.cancer.org/cancer/testicularcancer/moreinformation/doihavetesticularcancer/do-i-have-testicular-cancer-self-exam. Accessed January 6, 2016.; U.S. National Library of Medicine, National Institutes of Health. MedlinePlus—Testicular self-exam. Updated December 27, 2013. Available at http://www.nlm.nih.gov/medlineplus/ency/article/003909.htm. Accessed January 6, 2016.

LESBIAN, GAY, BISEXUAL, AND TRANSGENDER HEALTH CARE

Several recent surveys provide some of the first national data sets on the lesbian, gay, bisexual, and transgender (LGBT) population. For the first time, in 2013, the National Health Interview Survey included a measure of sexual orientation: in a sample of over 34,000 adults, 1.6% identified as gay or lesbian, 0.7% identified as bisexual, and 1.1% responded either "other" or "do not know." Most gay and lesbian respondents were between the ages of 18 and 64, with a higher percentage of bisexual respondents between 18 and 44.[50]

LGBT patients have higher rates of depression, suicide, anxiety, drug use, sexual victimization, and risk of infection with HIV and STI.[51–54] The Institute of Medicine has stated that barriers to accessing quality health care for LGBT adults are "a lack of providers who are knowledgeable about LGBT health needs as well as a fear of discrimination in health care settings."

During clinical encounters, LGBT and sexual minority patients often experience significant anxiety related to fears of being accepted. They may be uncomfortable disclosing their sexual behaviors and still fluctuating in their sexual identity. When they experience bias or discrimination, they are unlikely to reveal their sexual identity or concerns.[55–57]

TABLE
21-1

Lesions of the Vulva

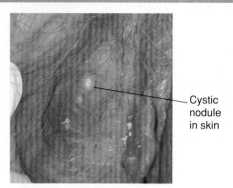

Epidermoid Cyst

A small, firm, round cystic nodule in the labia suggests an epidermoid cyst. These are yellowish in color. Look for the dark punctum marking the blocked opening of the gland.

Venereal Wart (Condyloma Acuminatum)

Warty lesions on the labia and within the vestibule are often condyloma acuminata from infection with *human papillomavirus*.

Syphilitic Chancre

This firm painless ulcer from primary syphilis forms ~21 days after exposure to *Treponema pallidum*. It may remain hidden and undetected in the vagina, and heals regardless of treatment in 3–6 weeks.

Uterine Prolapse

Uterine prolapse occurs when the uterus protrudes into the vagina.

Genital Herpes

Shallow, small, painful ulcers on red bases point to infection from genital herpes simplex virus 1 or 2. Ulcers may take 2–4 weeks to heal. Recurrent outbreaks of localized vesicles then ulcers are common.

Bartholin Gland Infection

Causes of a Bartholin gland infection include trauma, gonococci anaerobes like bacteroides and peptostreptococci, and *Chlamydia trachomatis*. Acutely, the gland appears as a tense, hot, very tender abscess. Look for pus emerging from the duct or erythema around the duct opening. Chronically, a nontender cyst is felt that may be large or small.

TABLE
21-2

Vaginal Discharge

Discharge from a vaginal infection must be distinguished from a physiologic discharge. A physiologic discharge is clear or white and may contain white clumps of epithelial cells; it is not malodorous. It is also important to distinguish vaginal from cervical discharges. The examiner will use a large cotton swab to wipe off the cervix. If no cervical discharge is present in the os, a vaginal origin is suspected and consider the causes below. Note that the diagnosis of cervicitis or vaginitis hinges on careful collection and analysis of the appropriate laboratory specimens.[58,59]

	Trichomonal Vaginitis	Candidal Vaginitis	Bacterial Vaginosis
			Lactobacilli
Cause	*Trichomonas vaginalis,* a protozoan; often but not always acquired sexually	*Candida albicans,* a yeast (normal overgrowth of vaginal flora); many factors predispose, including antibiotic therapy	Bacterial overgrowth probably from anaerobic bacteria; often transmitted sexually
Discharge	Yellowish green or gray, possibly frothy; often profuse and pooled in the vaginal fornix; may be malodorous	White and curdy; may be thin but typically thick; not as profuse as in trichomonal infection; not malodorous	Gray or white, thin, homogeneous, malodorous; coats the vaginal walls; usually not profuse, may be minimal
Other Symptoms	Pruritus (though not usually as severe as with *Candida* infection); pain on urination (from skin inflammation or possibly urethritis); dyspareunia	Pruritus; vaginal soreness; pain on urination (from skin inflammation); dyspareunia	Unpleasant fishy or musty genital odor reported to occur after intercourse
Vulva and Vaginal Mucosa	Vestibule and labia minora erythematous. The vaginal mucosa may be diffusely reddened. Vaginal mucosa may be diffusively reddened, with small red granular spots or petechiae in the posterior fornix. In mild cases, the mucosa looks normal.	The vulva and even the surrounding skin are often inflamed and sometimes swollen to a variable extent. The vaginal mucosa is often reddened, with white, often tenacious patches of discharge. The mucosa may bleed when these patches are scraped off. In mild cases, the mucosa looks normal.	The vulva and vaginal mucosa usually appear normal.
Laboratory Evaluation	Scan saline wet mount for trichomonads	Scan potassium hydroxide (KOH) preparation for the branching hyphae of *Candida.*	Scan saline wet mount for *clue cells* (epithelial cells with stippled borders); sniff for fishy odor after applying KOH ("whiff test"); test the vaginal secretions for pH >4.5

TABLE
21-3

Abnormalities of the Penis and Scrotum

Hypospadias

Congenital displacement of the urethral meatus to the inferior surface of the penis. A groove extends from the actual urethral meatus to its normal location on the tip of the glans.

Scrotal Edema

Pitting edema may make the scrotal skin taut; seen in congestive heart failure or nephrotic syndrome.

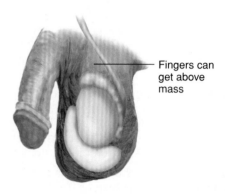

Fingers can get above mass

Epispadias

The urethral meatus is located on the top of the glans (dorsal side). This condition is a congenital defect and occurs rarely.

Hydrocele

A nontender, fluid-filled mass within the tunica vaginalis. It transilluminates, and the examining fingers can palpate above the mass within the scrotum.

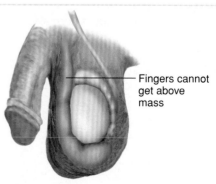

Fingers cannot get above mass

Carcinoma of the Penis

An indurated nodule or ulcer that is usually nontender. Limited almost completely to men who are not circumcised, it may be masked by the prepuce. Any persistent penile sore is suspicious.

Scrotal Hernia

Usually an *indirect inguinal hernia* that comes through the external inguinal ring, so the examining fingers cannot get above it within the scrotum.

TABLE
21-4
Sexually Transmitted Infections of Male Genitalia

Genital Warts (condylomata acuminata)

- *Appearance:* Single or multiple papules or plaques of variable shapes; may be round, acuminate (or pointed), or thin and slender. May be raised, flat, or cauliflower-like (verrucous).
- *Causative organism: Human papillomavirus (HPV),* usually from subtypes 6, 11; carcinogenic subtypes rare, approximately 5–10% of all anogenital warts. *Incubation:* weeks to months; infected contact may have no visible warts.
- Can arise on penis, scrotum, groin, thighs, anus; usually asymptomatic, occasionally cause itching and pain.
- May disappear without treatment.

Genital Herpes Simplex

1. *Appearance:* Small scattered or grouped vesicles, 1–3 mm in size, on glans or shaft of penis. Appear as erosions if vesicular membrane breaks.
2. *Causative organism:* Usually *herpes simplex virus 2* (90%), a double-stranded DNA virus. *Incubation:* 2–7 days after exposure.
3. Primary episode may be asymptomatic; recurrence usually less painful, of shorter duration.
4. Associated with fever, malaise, headache, arthralgias; local pain and edema, lymphadenopathy.
5. Need to distinguish from genital herpes zoster (usually in older patients with dermatomal distribution) and candidiasis.

Primary Syphilis

- *Appearance:* Small red papule that becomes a *chancre,* or *painless* erosion up to 2 cm in diameter. Base of chancre is clean, red, smooth, and glistening; borders are raised and indurated. Chancre heals within 3–8 weeks.
- *Causative organism: Treponema pallidum,* a spirochete. *Incubation:* 9–90 days after exposure.
- May develop inguinal lymphadenopathy within 7 days; lymph nodes are rubbery, nontender, mobile.
- Twenty to 30% of patients develop secondary syphilis while chancre still present (suggests coinfection with HIV).
- Distinguish from genital herpes simplex; chancroid; granuloma inguinale from *Klebsiella granulomatis* (rare in U.S.; four variants, so difficult to identify).

Chancroid

- *Appearance:* Red papule or pustule initially, then forms a *painful* deep ulcer with ragged nonindurated margins; contains necrotic exudate, has a friable base.
- *Causative organism: Haemophilus ducreyi,* an anaerobic bacillus. *Incubation:* 3–7 days after exposure.
- Painful inguinal adenopathy; suppurative buboes in 25% of patients.
- Need to distinguish from primary syphilis; genital herpes simplex; lymphogranuloma venereum, granuloma inguinale from *Klebsiella granulomatis* (both rare in U.S.).

TABLE
21-5

Abnormalities of the Testis

Cryptorchidism

The testis is atrophied and lies outside the scrotum in the inguinal canal, abdomen, or near the pubic tubercle; it may also be congenitally absent. As above, there is no palpable left testis or epididymis in the unfilled scrotum. Cryptorchidism, even with surgical correction, markedly raises the risk for testicular cancer.[60]

Small Testis

In adults, testicular length is usually ≤3.5 cm. Small, firm testes usually ≤2 cm suggest *Klinefelter syndrome*. Small, soft testes suggesting atrophy are seen in cirrhosis, myotonic dystrophy, use of estrogens, and hypopituitarism; may also follow orchitis.

Acute Orchitis

The testis is acutely inflamed, painful, tender, and swollen. It may be difficult to distinguish from the epididymis. The scrotum may be reddened. Seen in mumps and other viral infections; usually unilateral.

Early

Late

Tumor of the Testis

Usually appears as a painless nodule. Any nodule within the testis warrants investigation for malignancy.

As a testicular neoplasm grows and spreads, it may seem to replace the entire organ. The testicle characteristically feels heavier than normal.

TABLE
21-6
Abnormalities of the Epididymis and Spermatic Cord

Spermatocele and Cyst of the Epididymis
A painless, movable cystic mass just above the testis suggests a spermatocele or an epididymal cyst. Both transilluminate. The former contains sperm, and the latter does not, but they are clinically indistinguishable.

Varicocele of the Spermatic Cord
Varicocele refers to varicose veins of the spermatic cord, usually found on the left. It feels like a soft "bag of worms" in the spermatic cord above the testis, and if prominent, appears to distort the contours of the scrotal skin. A varicocele collapses in the supine position, so examination should be both supine and standing. If the varicocele does not collapse when the patient is supine, suspect a left spermatic vein obstruction within the abdomen.

Acute Epididymitis
An acutely inflamed epididymis is indurated, swollen and notably tender, making it difficult to distinguish from the testis. The scrotum may be reddened and the vas deferens inflamed. Causes include infection from *Neisseria gonorrhoeae* and *Chlamydia trachomatis* in younger adults, *Escherichia coli* and *Pseudomonas* in older adults, trauma, and autoimmune disease. Barring urinary symptoms, urinalysis is often negative.

Torsion of the Spermatic Cord
Torsion, or twisting, of the testicle on its spermatic cord produces an acutely painful, tender, and swollen organ that is often retracted upward in the scrotum. If the presentation is delayed, the scrotum becomes red and edematous. There is no associated urinary infection. Torsion is most common in neonates and adolescents, but can occur at any age. It is a surgical emergency because of obstructed circulation.

Internal inguinal ring

COURSE AND PRESENTATION OF FEMORAL HERNIA

Femoral artery

Femoral vein

COURSE AND PRESENTATION OF INDIRECT INGUINAL HERNIA

Inguinal canal

COURSE AND PRESENTATION OF DIRECT INGUINAL HERNIA

External inguinal ring

	Inguinal Hernias		Femoral Hernias
	Indirect	**Direct**	
Frequency, Age, and Sex	Most common, all ages, both sexes. Often in children; may occur in adults	Less common. Usually in men older than 40; rare in women	Least common. More common in women than in men
Point of Origin	Above inguinal ligament, near its midpoint (the internal inguinal ring)	Above inguinal ligament, close to the pubic tubercle (near the external inguinal ring)	Below the inguinal ligament; appears more lateral than an inguinal hernia. Can be hard to differentiate from lymph nodes
Course (Examining finger in inguinal canal during coughing or straining)	Often into the scrotum	Rarely into the scrotum	Never into the scrotum
	The hernia comes down the inguinal canal and touches the fingertip.	The hernia bulges anteriorly and pushes the side of the finger forward.	The inguinal canal is empty.

BIBLIOGRAPHY

CITATIONS

Female Reproductive System

1. Johnson CT, Hallock JL, Bienstock JL, et al., eds. Chapter 26: Anatomy of the female pelvis. *Johns Hopkins Manual of Gynecology and Obstetrics.* 5th ed. Philadelphia, PA: Wolters Kluwer – Lippincott Williams and Wilkins; 2015:338.
2. American College of Obstetricians and Gynecologists. Premenstrual syndrome. Available at http://www.acog.org/Patients/FAQs/Premenstrual-Syndrome-PMS. Accessed December 18, 2015.
3. Pachman DR, Jones JM, Loprinzi CL. Management of menopause-associated vasomotor symptoms: current treatment options, challenges and future directions. *Int J Womens Health.* 2010;2:123–135.
4. North American Menopause Society. Estrogen and progestogen use in postmenopausal women: 2010 position statement of the North American menopause society. *Menopause.* 2010;17:242–255.
5. Barbara AM, Doctor F, Gloria C. Asking the right questions 2. Talking with clients about sexual orientation and gender identity in mental health, counselling and addiction settings. Toronto, Canada: Centre for Addiction and Mental Health 2007. Available at http://www.camh.ca/en/education/about/camh_publications/Pages/Asking_Right_Questions.aspx. Accessed January 6, 2016.
6. Centers for Disease Control and Surveillance. 2013 sexually transmitted disease surveillance. Human papillomavirus. Available at http://www.cdc.gov/std/stats13/other.htm#hpv. Accessed April 30, 2016.
7. Sawaya GF, Kulasingam S, Denberg TD, et al. Cervical cancer screening in average-risk women: best practice advice from the Clinical Guidelines Committee of the American College of Physicians. *Ann Intern Med.* 2015;162(12):851–859.
8. Moyer A; U.S. Preventive Services Task Force. Screening for cervical cancer: U.S. Preventive Services Task Force recommendation statement. *Ann Intern Med.* 2012;150: 880–891.
9. Committee on Practice Bulletins—Gynecology. ACOG Practice Bulletin No. 131: screening for cervical cancer. *Obstet Gynecol.* 2012;120:1222–1238.
10. Saslow D, Solomon D, Lawson HW, et al. American Cancer Society, American Society for Colposcopy and Cervical Pathology, and American Society for Clinical Pathology screening guidelines for the prevention and early detection of cervical cancer. *CA Cancer J Clin.* 2012;62:147–172.
11. Bloomfield HE, Olson A, Greer N, et al. Screening pelvic examinations in asymptomatic, average-risk adult women: an evidence report for a clinical practice guideline from the American College of Physicians. *Ann Intern Med.* 2014; 161:46–53.
12. Qaseem A. Humphrey LL, Harris R, et al. Screening pelvic examination in adult women: a clinical practice guideline from the American College of Physicians. *Ann Intern Med.* 2014;161:67–72.
13. Advisory Committee on Immunization Practices, Centers for Disease Control and Prevention. Human papillomavirus vaccination. Recommendations of the Advisory Committee on Immunization Practices. *MMWR.* 2014;63(RR #5): 1–30.
14. Centers for Disease Control and Prevention. Human papillomavirus. HPV Vaccine Information for Clinicians—Fact Sheet. Page last reviewed July 8, 2012. Available at http://www.cdc.gov/std/hpv/STDFact-HPV-vaccine-hcp.htm. Accessed May 1, 2016.
15. Centers for Disease Control and Prevention. Youth risk behavior surveillance—United States 2013. Available at http://www.cdc.gov/healthyyouth/data/yrbs/results.htm. Accessed May 1, 2016.
16. Centers for Disease Control and Prevention. Condom effectiveness. Fact sheet for public health personnel. Page last updated March 25, 2013. Available at http://www.cdc.gov/condomeffectiveness/latex.html. Accessed May 1, 2016.
17. Pierce Campbell CM, Lin HY, Fulp W, et al. Consistent condom use reduces the genital human papillomavirus burden among high-risk men: the HPV infection in men study. *J Infect Dis.* 2012; 208:373–384.
18. National Center for Health Statistics. final natality data. Available at http://www.marchofdimes.org/peristats/Peristats.aspx. Accessed May 2, 2016.
19. Centers for Disease Control and Prevention. Reproductive health. Teen pregnancy—About teen pregnancy. Page last updated April 26, 2016. Available at http://www.cdc.gov/teenpregnancy/about/index.htm. Accessed May 1, 2016.
20. Centers for Disease Control and Prevention. 2013 Sexually transmitted disease surveillance. Chlamydia. Page last updated December 16, 2014. Available at http://www.cdc.gov/std/stats13/chlamydia.htm. Accessed May 1, 2016.
21. Centers for Disease Control and Prevention. Pelvic inflammatory disease—CDC fact sheet. Page last updated May 4, 2015. Available at http://www.cdc.gov/std/pid/stdfact-pid-detailed.htm. Accessed May 1, 2016.
22. Centers for Disease Control and Prevention. Sexually transmitted diseases. STDs and infertility. Page last updated December 16, 2014. Available at http://www.cdc.gov/std/infertility/default.htm. Accessed May 1, 2016.
23. Centers for Disease Control and Prevention. Sexually transmitted diseases. Page last updated May 15, 2015. Available at http://www.cdc.gov/std/default.htm. Accessed May 1, 2016.
24. U.S. Preventive Services Task Force. Recommendations (search "Category—Infectious diseases"). Page current as of July 2016. Available at http://www.uspreventiveservicestaskforce.org/Search. Accessed May 1, 2016.
25. Centers for Disease Control and Prevention. HIV in the United States: At a glance. Page last updated July 11, 2016. Available at http://www.cdc.gov/hiv/statistics/basics/ataglance.html. Accessed May 1, 2016.
26. Centers for Disease Control and Prevention. HIV/AIDS. HIV among women. Page last updated March 16, 2016. Available at http://www.cdc.gov/hiv/risk/gender/women/facts/index.html. Accessed May 1, 2016.

BIBLIOGRAPHY

27. U.S. Preventive Services Task Force. September 2014. Sexually transmitted infections. Behavioral counseling. Page current as of May 2016. Available at http://www.uspreventiveservicestaskforce.org/Page/Topic/recommendation-summary/sexually-transmitted-infections-behavioral-counseling1?ds=1&s=Counseling. Accessed May 1, 2016.

Male Reproductive System

28. Gareri P, Castagna A, Francomano D. Erectile dysfunction in the elderly: an old widespread issue with novel treatment perspectives. *Int J Endocrin.* 2014;2014:878670.

29. U.S. Preventive Services Task Force. USPSTF recommendations for STI screening. February 2014. Current as of March 2008. Available at http://www.uspreventiveservicestaskforce.org/Page/Name/uspstf-recommendations-for-sti-screening. Accessed May 1, 2016.

30. U.S. Preventive Services Task Force. Human immunodeficiency virus (HIV) infection: Screening. April 2013. Available at http://www.uspreventiveservicestaskforce.org/Page/Topic/recommendation-summary/human-immunodeficiency-virus-hiv-infection-screening?ds=1&s=HIV. Accessed May 1, 2016.

31. Skarbinski J, Rosenberg E, Paz-Bailey G, et al. Human Immunodeficiency virus transmission at each step of the care continuum in the United States. *JAMA Intern Med.* 2015; 175:588–596.

32. Meanley S, Gale A, Harmell C, et al. The role of provider interactions on comprehensive sexual healthcare among young men who have sex with men. *AIDS Educ Prev.* 2015;27:15–26.

33. Institute of Medicine, Eng TR, Butler WT, eds. *The Hidden Epidemic: confronting Sexually Transmitted Diseases: Summary.* Washington, DC: National Academies Press (US); 1997. Available at http://www.ncbi.nlm.nih.gov/pubmed/25165803. Accessed May 1, 2016.

34. Centers for Disease Control and Prevention. Sexually Transmitted Disease Surveillance 2013. Atlanta, GA: U.S. Department of Health and Human Services; 2014. Available at http://www.cdc.gov/std/stats13/default.htm . Accessed April 30, 2016.

35. Centers for Disease Control and Prevention. CDC Fact Sheet. Reported STDs in the United States. 2014 National Data for Chlamydia, Gonorrhea, and Syphilis, 2014. Available at http://www.cdc.gov/std/stats14/default.htm. Accessed May 2, 2016.

36. LeFevre ML, U.S. Preventive Services Task Force. Screening for Chlamydia and gonorrhea: U.S. Preventive Services Task Force recommendation statement. *Ann Intern Med.* 2014;161:902–910.

37. Centers for Disease Control and Prevention. HIV in the United States: At a glance. July 2015. Available at http://www.cdc.gov/hiv/pdf/statistics_basics_ataglance_factsheet.pdf. Accessed May, 2016.

38. Bradley H, Hall HI, Wolitski RJ, et al. Vital signs: HIV diagnosis, care, and treatment among persons living with HIV–United States, 2011. *MMWR Morb Mortal Wkly Rep.* 2014;63:1113–1117.

39. Moyer VA; U.S. Preventive Services Task Force. Screening for HIV: U.S. Preventive Services Task Force Recommendation. Statement. *Ann Intern Med.* 2013;159:51–60.

40. Branson BM, Handsfield HH, Lampe MA, et al. Revised recommendations for HIV testing of adults, adolescents, and pregnant women in health-care settings. *MMWR Recomm Rep.* 2006;55(RR-14):1–17.

41. Qaseem A, Snow V, Shekelle P, et al. Screening for HIV in health care settings: a guidance statement from the American College of Physicians and HIV Medicine Association. *Ann Intern Med.* 2009;150:125–131.

42. Centers for Disease Control and Prevention. CDC Fact Sheet. HIV Testing in the United States, 2014. Available at www.cdc.gov/nchhstp/newsroom/docs/factsheets/. Accessed May 2, 2016.

43. Centers for Disease Control and Prevention. Condom effectiveness. Condom Fact Sheet in Brief, 2013. Available at www.cdc.gov/condomeffectiveness/brief.html. Accessed May 2, 2016.

44. Markowitz LE, Dunne EF, Saraiya M, et al. Human papillomavirus vaccination: recommendations of the Advisory Committee on Immunization Practices (ACIP). *MMWR Recomm Rep.* 2014;63(RR-05):1–30.

45. American Cancer Society. What are the key statistics about prostate cancer? Available at http://www.cancer.org/cancer/prostatecancer/detailedguide/prostate-cancer-key-statistics. Accessed May 2, 2016.

46. American Cancer Society. What are the risk factors for prostate cancer? 2015. Available at http://www.cancer.org/cancer/prostatecancer/detailedguide/prostate-cancer-risk-factors. Accessed May 2, 2016.

47. NIH. National Cancer Institute. Prostate Cancer Health Professional Version. Available at http://www.cancer.gov/types/prostate/hp. Accessed May 2, 2016.

48. U.S. Preventive Services Task Force. Final recommendation statement, Prostate cancer: screening. Current as of May 2012. Available at http://www.uspreventiveservicestaskforce.org/Page/Document/RecommendationStatementFinal/prostate-cancer-screening. Accessed July 7, 2016.

49. American Urological Association. AUA Releases New Clinical Guideline On Prostate Cancer Screening, 2013. Available at https://www.auanet.org/advnews/press_releases/article.cfm?articleNo=290. Accessed July 7, 2016.

Lesbian, Gay, Bisexual, and Transgender Health Care

50. Centers for Disease Control and Prevention. Sexual orientation and health among U.S. adults. National Health Interview Survey, 2013. Available at http://www.cdc.gov/lgbthealth/. Accessed May 1, 2016.

51. Centers for Disease Control and Prevention. Lesbian and bisexual women. Available at http://www.cdc.gov/lgbthealth/women.htm. Gay and bisexual men. Updated March 25, 2014. Available at http://www.cdc.gov/lgbthealth/msm.htm. Accessed May 1, 2016.

52. Centers for Disease Prevention and Control. CDC fact sheet. HIV among gay and bisexual men. March 2015. Available at http://www.cdc.gov/msmhealth/hiv.htm. Accessed May 1, 2016.

53. Matarazzo BB, Barnes SM, Pease JL, et al. Suicide risk among lesbian, gay, bisexual, and transgender military personnel and veterans: what does the literature tell us?. *Suicide Life Threat Behav.* 2014;44:200–217.

788 BATES' NURSING GUIDE TO PHYSICAL EXAMINATION AND HISTORY TAKING

54. Haas AP, Eliason M, Mays VM, et al. Suicide and suicide risk in lesbian, gay, bisexual, and transgender populations: review and recommendations. *J Homosex.* 2011;58:10–51.

55. Durso LE, Meyer IH. Patterns and predictors of disclosure of sexual orientation to healthcare providers among lesbians, gay men, and bisexuals. *Sex Res Social Policy.* 2013;10:35–42.

56. Polek CA, Hardie TL, Crowley EM. Lesbians' disclosure of sexual orientation and satisfaction with care. *J Transcult Nurs,* 2008;19:243–249.

57. Friedman MR, Dodge B, Schick V, et al. From bias to bisexual health disparities: attitudes toward bisexual men and women in the United States. *LGBT Health.* 2014;1:309–318.

58. Wilson JF. In the clinic: vaginitis and cervicitis. *Ann Intern Med.* 2009;151:ITC3-1–ITC3-15;Quiz ITC3-16.

59. Eckhert LO. Clinical practice. Acute vulvovaginitis. *N Engl J Med.* 2006;355:1244–1252.

60. Kolon TF, Herndon CD, Baker LA, et al. American Urological Association. Evaluation and treatment of cryptorchidism: AUA guideline. *J Urol.* 2014;192:337–345.

ADDITIONAL REFERENCES

Alvarez-Blasco F, Botella-Carretero JI, San Millan JL, et al. Prevalence and characteristics of the polycystic ovary syndrome in overweight and obese women. *Arch Intern Med.* 2006;166:2081–2086.

Anderson MR, Klink K, Cohrsson A. Evaluation of vaginal complaints. *JAMA.* 2004;291(11):368–379.

Collaborative Group on Epidemiological Studies of Ovarian Cancer; Beral V, Doll R, et al. Ovarian cancer and oral contraceptives: collaborative reanalysis of data from 45 epidemiological studies including 23,257 women with ovarian cancer and 87,303 controls. *Lancet.* 2008; 371(9609):303–314.

Datta SD, Sternberg M, Johnson RE, et al. Gonorrhea and chlamydia in the United States among persons 14 to 39 years of age, 1999 to 2002. *Ann Intern Med.* 2007;147(2):89–96.

Future II Study Group. Quadrivalent vaccine against human papillomavirus to prevent high-grade cervical lesions. *N Engl J Med.* 2007;356(19):1915–1927.

Gupta R, Warren T, Wald A. Genital herpes. *Lancet.* 2007; 370(9605):2127–2137.

Hwang LY, Shafer MA, Pollack LM, et al. Sexual behaviors after universal screening of sexually transmitted infections in healthy young women. *Obstet Gynecol.* 2007;109(1):105–113.

Mayrand MH, Duarte-Franco E, Rodriques I, et al. Human papillomavirus DNA versus Papanicolaou screening tests for cervical cancer. *N Engl J Med.* 2007;357(16):1579–1588.

Nelson HD. Menopause. *Lancet.* 2008;371(9614):760–770.

Peipert JF. Genital chlamydial infections. *N Engl J Med.* 2003;349(25):2424–2430.

Reif S, Whetten K, Thielman N. Association of race and gender with use of antiretroviral therapy among HIV-infected individuals in the Southeastern United States. *South Med J.* 2007; 100(8):775–781.

Simon V, Ho DD, Abdool Karim Q. HIV/AIDS epidemiology, pathogenesis, prevention, and treatment. *Lancet.* 2006;368(9534):489–504.

Sirovich BE, Welch HG. Cervical cancer screening among women without a cervix. *JAMA.* 2004;291(24):2990–2993.

LEARNING OBJECTIVES

The student will:

1. Identify the components of the physical examination.

2. Identify the best approach for the physical examination based on individual patient needs.

3. Create an appropriate environment to ensure an accurate physical examination.

4. Demonstrate a head-to-toe physical examination.

The integration of history taking and physical examination produces the health assessment. This combination of information for each body system provides the nurse with the knowledge of the individual to develop a plan of care and specific nursing interventions. The previous system chapters are structured for nurses to first ask questions to elicit the subjective information and then use the techniques of inspection, palpation, percussion, and auscultation to identify the objective information. Learning each system in depth is important. Equally important is the integration of all systems into a complete physical examination, as well as the ability to critically evaluate the individual patient and decide which system or systems to focus on during the patient visit.

Assessments are performed with every patient contact. Generally, a complete assessment is performed on new patients or new admissions to a health care agency. The patient may be a healthy individual arriving at the clinic for a school physical or an ill patient admitted to the hospital.

A focused assessment targets specific body systems. The decision to limit the number of systems assessed is based on history findings, timing, severity of illness, pain, or limited access to the patient. The nurse caring for a patient who arrives with a chief complaint of a painful arm will focus on the following systems: musculoskeletal, cardiovascular, peripheral vascular, and neurologic. Based on the information obtained in the health history, systems may be excluded from the examination. If the pain was caused by an injury to the arm that did not impact the heart and there is no cardiac history, cardiac examination may be eliminated, but musculoskeletal, neurologic, and peripheral vascular systems would still be important to evaluate.

Initially, the complete examination may seem cumbersome and time-consuming. The student may wonder how to condense all the information and skills into an orchestrated, consistent examination. At the same time, the student wants to exude confidence and demonstrate comprehension of the examination.

This will take time but also, most importantly, practice. During laboratory sessions it is important to use the time with your partner and the guidance of your instructor to ensure proper technique and positioning for the examination. After laboratory sessions it is imperative to take additional time for repeat practice. Repetition is necessary to refine skills and coordinate the techniques into a thorough examination.

Generally, a complete assessment is performed in a head-to-toe (cephalic to caudal) sequence comparing side to side (bilaterally) for symmetry. Prior to trying the head-to-toe examination, review the systems and plot the best flow for the examination. Some systems overlap and can be interwoven during the examination. This limits the number of times patients need to change position from sitting to lying to standing, which can be difficult for patients who have pain, dyspnea, or limited range of motion. There are many correct choices when organizing the examination. Continued practice will assist you to gain proficiency and find the best flow for you and the patient. For example, some nurses cover the musculoskeletal examination, including range of motion, toward the beginning of the examination, while others prefer to wait until after assessing the core components (cardiac, pulmonary, abdomen). Determining the most efficient format for the physical examination is the initial step.

It is time to prepare for the actual examination. The equipment should be available and in working order, prior to the start of the examination. The environment should be assessed for comfort, privacy, and safety.

Equipment

- Hand sanitizer
- Examination gloves
- Alcohol wipes

- Paper and pen, or computer
- Draw sheet or drape
- Stadiometer
- Scale
- Examination light/Gooseneck lamp
- Thermometer
- Watch with a second hand
- Sphygmomanometer
- Stethoscope
- Pulse oximeter
- Doppler
- Ophthalmoscope
- Otoscope/Speculums
- Nasal speculum
- Sense of smell (e.g., mint, coffee, or alcohol swab if other scents not available)
- Snellen chart or visual acuity card to test distant vision
- Near vision card
- Opaque card
- Penlight
- Tongue depressors
- 2 × 2 gauze pads
- Cup of water
- Ruler and flexible tape measure, preferably marked in centimeters
- Goniometer
- Scoliometer
- Reflex hammer
- Tuning forks 128 Hz and 512 Hz
- Q-tips, paper clips, or other disposable objects
- Cotton
- Mini-mental status examination tool
- Your note cards, developed throughout the semester, with highlights for individual systems

During the examination, remember to consider the patient's privacy. Close the door or curtain and use a sheet to cover parts of the body not being examined at the time. While examining the patient, explain procedures and findings throughout the entire examination. Letting the patient know what you are doing and your findings, such as blood pressure results, creates teaching/learning moments and develops a rapport with your patient.

Many students find it beneficial to make note cards, which can be used as cues for each system. Do not write too much or you might be distracted. As a new practitioner, your examination of the patient should take less than 1 hour from start to finish. Below is a basic guide for conducting a physical examination while minimizing the number of position changes for the patient. Another sequence may work better for you; this is acceptable

As students become more proficient and comfortable with physical examination techniques and flow, the note cards can be re-written with less detail.

as long as the examination proceeds in a logical flow, includes all the necessary components, and limits patient position changes. However, if an assessment is missed, it may be inserted at another convenient place in the examination. The more you practice and repeat the techniques, the less likely this is to occur. Now assess your demeanor, and take a breath before entering the room.

A SAMPLE OF THE SEQUENCING FOR A HEAD-TO-TOE ASSESSMENT

Physical Examination Overview

On entering the room the nurse should: wash his or her hands, introduce self and purpose and begin the history taking component while the patient is dressed and sitting in a chair. During this conversation, the general survey and observation of the patient can be done simultaneously and throughout the examination.

Patient Seated

General Survey and Observation

- Assess the environment for:
  - a. Noise
  - b. Safety
  - c. Privacy
  - d. Lighting

- Assess the individual for:
  - a. Age—stated age versus apparent age
  - b. Emotional state—compare verbal description and nonverbal
  - c. Developmental stage—compare with behavior
  - d. Cultural background
  - e. Health requirements and learning needs

*Mental Status**
Mental status is assessed throughout the history and examination beginning with the General Survey; this includes assessment obtained when speaking to the patient. Assess for:

  a. Level of consciousness
  b. Facial expressions
  c. Speech, language, articulation, speed, tone
  d. Thought processes and perception
  e. Mood and affect
  f. Grooming and hygiene
  g. Posture, gait, and body movements
  h. Assistive devices

---

*If changes are noted, then a mini-mental status examination should be performed.

Vital Signs

a. Temperature
b. Pulse
c. Respirations
d. Blood pressure—check each arm, position at heart level
e. Pain

Body Measurements
a. Height
b. Weight
c. Body mass index and ideal body weight

Integument

At the end of the history interview, ask the patient to change into a gown. This can be done before or after vital signs are taken as long as the arm can be exposed for the blood pressure.

The **patient is sitting** on the edge of the bed or examining table. Stand in front of the patient, moving to either side as needed.

Assess the skin throughout the examination as you examine each part of the body.

a. Inspect the hands and arms for color, lesions, scars, rashes, or any changes in the skin.
b. Palpate for moisture, temperature, and texture.

   c. Palpate for skin turgor.
   d. Inspect the hair for color, distribution, and texture.
   e. Inspect and palpate the nails for size, shape, color, texture, angle, refill, and any changes.

Head
   a. Inspect the skull for size and shape.
   b. Inspect and palpate the scalp for tenderness, lesions, and bumps.

Face
   a. Inspect facial features, movements, and expressions for symmetry.

Cranial nerve VII, facial: symmetry of face—raise eyebrows, frown, close eyes, smile, puff out cheeks

   b. Palpate temporal and masseter strength.
   c. Assess temporomandibular joint for pain, crepitus, and swelling.
   d. Assess sensation to sharp and light on face—forehead, cheeks, and chin (continue assessing arms and feet for sharp and light touch).

Cranial Nerve V, trigeminal

Eyes
   a. Acuity (if a hand held eye chart is available, otherwise do in the beginning before the patient is seated or hold this part until the patient is standing for other parts of the assessment).

b. Inspect:
- Eyelids
- Eyelashes
- Eyebrows
- Lacrimal apparatus
- Conjunctiva
- Sclera
- Cornea
- Lens
- Pupils
  - Size
  - Shape
  - Direct light reaction
  - Consensual light reaction

Cranial nerve II, optic; cranial nerve III, occulomotor

Cranial nerve II, optic cranial nerve III, occulomotor; cranial nerve IV, trochlear; cranial nerve VI, abducens

c. Test visual fields by confrontation
d. Eye muscle examinations
- Test six cardinal directions of gaze
- Convergence
- Near reaction (accommodation)
- Cover–uncover test

AP e. Ophthalmoscope examination—inspect:
- Optic disc for color, size, shape
- Retina for color, abnormalities
- Arteries and veins for changes

Ears
a. Inspect pinna, lobe, and tragus for:
- position
- shape
- ulcers
- lesions
- discharge
b. Palpate pinna and tragus for:
- tenderness
- lumps
c. Palpate mastoid firmly for tenderness

d. Otoscopic examination—inspect:
- inner canal
- tympanic membrane
- cone of light

e. Hearing acuity   Cranial nerve VIII, acoustic
- Whisper test
- Weber (512 Hz on top of head)
- Rinne (512 Hz on mastoid bone and compare to air conduction)

Nose and Sinuses

a. Inspect for:
- symmetry
- alignment
- deformity

b. Palpate for tenderness and patency

c. Palpate frontal and maxillary sinuses

d. Inspect mucous membrane, septum, and turbinates for:
- inflammation
- polyps
- ulcers
- deviation

e. Sense of smell—have patient identify two different scents with eyes closed.   Cranial nerve I, olfactory

Mouth and Pharynx

   a. Inspect lips, oral mucosa, gums, roof of mouth, and floor of mouth
      for:
- color
- lesions
- moisture

   b. Inspect dentition for condition, number, and placement

   c. Tongue—inspect for:
- size
- shape
- color
- moisture
- lesions
- texture

   d. Listen for articulation of words   Cranial nerve XII, hypoglossal
- Movement—assess at-rest, raised, protruding, and
  side-to-side movements
- Taste

                                                          Cranial nerve VII, facial; cranial
                                                          nerve IX, glossopharyngeal

   e. Pharynx—inspect rise of palate and uvula.   Cranial nerve IX, glossopharyngeal;
                                                          cranial nerve X, vagus

Neck

   a. Inspect anteriorly for symmetry, masses, enlarged lymph nodes, or
      deviation.

   b. Inspect trachea position.

   c. Palpate head, neck and subclavicular lymph nodes.

   d. Test sternocleidomastoid and lower trapezius muscle strength.   Cranial nerve XI, spinal accessory

e. Test head and neck range of motion (flexion, extension, rotation, and lateral flexion).
f. Inspect thyroid.
g. Palpate thyroid (may be from front or back of patient).

The nurse will assess the following from the back of the patient:

Posterior Thorax
a. Inspect
  • shape
  • deformities
  • retractions
  • symmetry
  • skin integrity
b. Palpate for
  • tenderness
  • tactile fremitus
  • respiratory expansion

Move behind the sitting patient to feel the thyroid gland and to examine the back, posterior thorax, and lungs. Take necessary equipment with you to the posterior to limit trips around the patient (stethoscope, ruler, and pen). Have the patient open the back of the gown to expose the back to assess the skin and to percuss and auscultate the lung fields, leaving the gown on the shoulders and covering the front of the patient.

    c. Percuss lung sounds in all fields and diaphragmatic excursion on both sides.

    d. Auscultate lung sounds and identify adventitious sounds and their location.

Assess the cervical spine (inspection, palpation).

Assess for pain at the costovertebral angles (CVA tenderness).

Assess for CVA tenderness when the patient is standing or sitting.

As the nurse returns to the front of the patient, some portions of the anterior thorax, cardiac, and breast examinations can be performed sitting or lying down.

Anterior Thorax
(Can also be performed with patient lying down if preferred)

    a. Inspect for shape, deformities, retractions, symmetry, and skin integrity.

    b. Palpate for
       • tenderness
       • tactile fremitus
       • respiratory expansion

    c. Percuss sounds.

    d. Auscultate lung sounds.

Cardiac
(Patient should be sitting)

Auscultate with the bell at the apical impulse while the patient is leaning forward—listening for aortic stenosis/murmur.

Breasts

(Patient should be sitting)

    Inspect with:

- arms at side
- arms raised over head
- hands pressed into hips
- leaning forward

Axillary Nodes

Palpate axillary nodes (central, lateral, pectoral, subscapular).

Patient Lying Down

Cardiovascular

Head of bed or table should be elevated at a 30-degree angle.

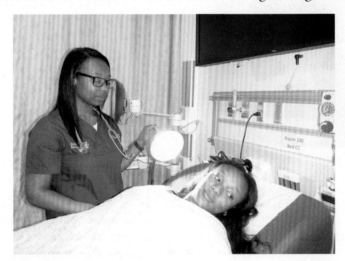

a. Inspect carotid arteries for pulsations.

b. Palpate carotid arteries.

c. Auscultate carotid for bruits with the bell while patient holds breath. Auscultate the other carotid artery with breath held.

d. Inspect external jugular vein.
e. Inspect precordium.
f. Auscultate heart with the diaphragm at the:
  • right sternal border (RSB) 2nd intercostal space (ICS)
  • left sternal border (LSB) 2nd ICS
  • left sternal border 3rd ICS
  • left sternal border 4th ICS

  • left sternal border 5th ICS
  • left midclavicular line (MCL) 5th ICS.
g. Auscultate heart with the bell at the:
  • right sternal border (RSB) 2nd intercostal space (ICS)
  • left sternal border (LSB) 2nd ICS
  • left sternal border 3rd ICS
  • left sternal border 4th ICS
  • left sternal border 5th ICS
  • left midclavicular line (MCL) 5th ICS.
h. Auscultate with the bell at the apical impulse while in the left lateral decubitus position (listening for mitral murmur, S_3, S_4).

If patient is being followed for cardiac issues, assess the heart sounds in both the supine and left lateral positions.

Breast Examination
a. Before examining the breast place the arm that is on the side of the breast being examined under the head and drape the opposite breast.
b. Examine the breast using the vertical pattern technique.

Abdomen
a. Inspect for:
  • contour
  • pulsations
  • bulges
  • skin integrity

b. Auscultate for bowel sounds and aortic pulsation.

c. Percuss abdominal sounds and liver, kidneys, and spleen.
d. Abdominal reflex—lightly stroke inward in all quadrants.
e. Lightly palpate all four quadrants noting masses, tenderness, and patient's expression.
f. Deeply palpate all four quadrants noting masses, tenderness, and patient's expression.
g. Palpate for the liver, kidneys, and spleen.

Peripheral Vascular
a. Inspect arms and legs for:
   * symmetry
   * color
   * edema
   * hair distribution
   * nail bed color
b. Palpate pulses
   * Radial
   * Brachial
     * At this time, palpate the epitrochlear lymph nodes
   * Femoral
     * At this time, palpate the remaining lymph nodes: inguinal lymph nodes (vertical then horizontal groups)
   * Popliteal
   * Posterior tibial

   * Dorsalis pedis
c. Palpate for pitting edema in feet and legs

Musculoskeletal (Lower Body)

a. Inspect for deformity, swelling, nodules, redness, and muscle bulk of:
- Hips
- Knees
- Ankles, feet and toes

b. Palpate for tenderness, crepitus, swelling, and increased warmth of:
- Hips
- Knees
- Ankles, feet and toes

c. Palpate strength and range of motion
- Hips (flexion, extension, abduction, adduction, internal and external rotation)
- Knees (flexion and extension)
- Ankles (dorsiflexion, plantar flexion, inversion, eversion)
- Toes (flexion, extension, abduction, adduction)

Patient Seated

Musculoskeletal—Upper Body

a. Inspect for deformity, swelling, nodules, redness, and muscle bulk of:
- Shoulders
- Elbows
- Wrists, hands, and fingers

b. Palpate for tenderness, crepitus, swelling, and increased warmth of:
- Shoulders
- Elbows
- Wrists, hands, and fingers

c. Palpate strength and range of motion
- Shoulders (flexion, extension, abduction, adduction, internal and external rotation)
- Forearm (pronation, supination)
- Elbow (flexion, extension)
- Wrists (extension [dorsiflexion], flexion [palmar flexion], radial and, ulnar deviation)
- Fingers (grip and flexion, extension, abduction, adduction)
- Thumb (flexion, extension, opposition, abduction, adduction)

Neurologic—Motor

    a. Inspect body position, noting tremors.

    b. Deep tendon reflexes

- Biceps
- Triceps
- Brachioradialis
- Patellar
- Achilles

Neurologic—Sensory

(If sensory assessments not incorporated previously, then complete now)

    a. Pain and light touch—if the patient is unable to feel pain and light touch, then assess for vibration and temperature

    b. Position sense

    c. Vibration

    d. Stereognosis

    e. Finger to nose

    f. Rapid alternating movements

Patient Standing

Musculoskeletal—Spine

    a. Inspect for deformity, symmetry, and skin integrity.

    b. Palpate spinous processes.

    c. Assess range of motion (flexion, extension, lateral bends, rotation).

Neurologic

a. Perform Romberg, gait, balance, and other appropriate neurologic screenings.

It is recommended that visual acuity be assessed at the beginning or at the end of the examination to alleviate the patient getting up another time.

Visual Acuity

Cranial nerve II, optic

If a hand-held Snellen is not available, then performing the visual acuity examination of the eye now is appropriate.

Continue to practice and refine your physical examination skills. The integration of the subjective and objective data guides the nurse in preparing the best nursing plan of care for the patient.

RECORDING YOUR FINDINGS

Refer to Chapter 2, Critical Thinking in Health Assessment, for documentation of a complete physical examination.

BIBLIOGRAPHY

Azer SA, Guerrero AP, Walsh A. Enhancing learning approaches: practical tips for students and teachers. *Med Teach.* 2013; 35(6):433–443.

Duvivier RJ, van Geel K, van Dalen J, et al. Learning physical examination skills outside timetabled training sessions: what happens and why?. *Adv Health Sci Educ Theory Pract.* 2012; 17(3):339–355.

Osborne S, Douglas C, Reid C, et al. The primacy of vital signs—acute care nurses' and midwives' use of physical assessment skills: a cross sectional study. *Int J Nurs Stud.* 2015;52(5):951–962.

Peitzman SJ, Cuddy MA. Performance in physical examination on the USMLE step 2 clinical skills examination. *Acad Med.* 2015;90(2):209–213.

Rush S, Firth F, Burke L, et al. Implementation and evaluation of peer assessment of clinical skills for first year student nurses. *Nurs Ed in Prac.* 2012;12(4):219–226.

Verghese A, Charlton B, Kassirer J, et al. Inadequacies of physical examination as a cause of medical errors and adverse events: a collection of vignettes. *Am J Med.* 2015;128(12): 1322–1324.

UNIT
3
Special Lifespan

Assessing Children: Infancy Through Adolescence

Adapted from the chapter originally written by Peter G. Szilagyi, MD, MPH

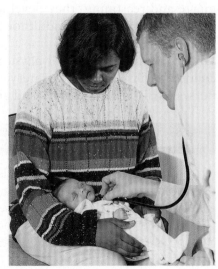

LEARNING OBJECTIVES

The student will:

1. Obtain a history on an infant, child, and adolescent.

2. Perform a developmental assessment on infants, children, and adolescents.

3. Use age-appropriate techniques to perform a physical examination on infants, children and adolescents.

4. Analyze findings against age-appropriate norms and standards.

5. Identify education topics for anticipatory guidance, health promotion and risk reduction.

6. Correctly document infant, child, and adolescent assessment findings.

This chapter begins with general principles of development and key components of health promotion. It then includes sections on infants, young and school-aged children, and adolescents, with relevant discussions of development, history taking, health promotion and counseling, and physical examination for each.

Often, students are intimidated when approaching a tiny baby or a screaming child, especially under the critical eyes of anxious parents.

When examining infants and children, the sequence should vary according to the child's age and comfort level. *Perform nondisturbing maneuvers early and potentially distressing maneuvers near the end of the examination.* For example, palpate the head and neck and auscultate the heart and lungs early, and examine the ears and mouth and palpate the abdomen near the end. If the child reports pain in one area, examine that part last.

The format of the pediatric medical record is the same as that of the adult record. Although the sequence of the physical examination may vary, convert your clinical findings into the traditional documentation format.

GENERAL PRINCIPLES OF CHILD DEVELOPMENT

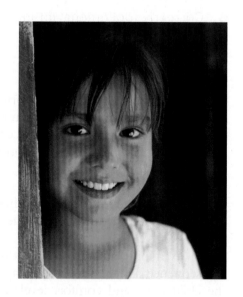

Childhood is a period of remarkable physical, cognitive, and social growth—by far the greatest in a person's lifetime. Within a few short years, children's size increases 20-fold, they acquire sophisticated language and reasoning, they develop complex social interactions, and they progress toward mature adulthood.

Understanding the normal physical, cognitive, and social development of children facilitates effective interviews and physical examinations, and helps nurses to distinguish normal and abnormal findings.

Four Principles of Child Development[1,2]

1. Child development proceeds along a predictable pathway.
2. The range of normal development is wide.
3. Various physical, social, and environmental factors, as well as diseases, can affect child development and health.
4. The child's developmental level affects how you conduct the history and physical examination.

1. *Child development proceeds along a predictable pathway* governed by the maturing brain. You can measure age-specific milestones and characterize development as normal or abnormal according to the child's achievement of them. Because the child's health visit and physical examination takes place at one point in time, determine where the child fits along a developmental trajectory. Milestones are achieved in an order than can be anticipated. Loss of milestones is always concerning.

2. The *range of normal development is wide*. Children mature at different rates. Each child's physical, cognitive, and social development should fall within a broad developmental range.

3. *Various physical, social, and environmental factors, as well as diseases, can affect child development and health.* For example, chronic illnesses, child abuse, and poverty can all cause detectable physical abnormalities and alter the rate and course of development. Additionally children with physical or cognitive disabilities may not follow the expected age-specific developmental trajectory. Tailor the physical examination to the child's developmental level.

4. *The child's developmental level affects how you conduct the history and physical examination.* For example, interviewing a 5-year-old is fundamentally different than interviewing an adolescent. Before performing a physical examination, attempt to ascertain the child's approximate developmental level and adapt your physical examination to that level. An understanding of normal child development helps you make that decision.

HEALTH PROMOTION AND COUNSELING: KEY COMPONENTS

Benjamin Franklin noted that "an ounce of prevention is worth a pound of cure." This adage is particularly true for children and adolescents because prevention and health promotion at a young age can result in improved health outcomes for decades. Pediatric clinicians dedicate substantial time to health supervision visits and health promotion activities.

Several national and international organizations have developed guidelines for health promotion for children.[3–5] Current concepts of health promotion include the detection and prevention of disease as well as active promotion of the well-being of children and their families, spanning physical, cognitive, emotional, and social health.

Every interaction with a child and family is an opportunity for health promotion. From the interview to the physical examination, think about your interactions as opportunities for two things: the traditional detection of medical problems and the promotion of health. Capitalize on your examination to offer age-appropriate guidance about the child's development. Provide suggestions about reading, conversing, playing music, and optimizing opportunities for gross and fine motor development. Advise parents about upcoming developmental stages and strategies to encourage their child's development. *Parents are the major agents of health promotion for children, and your advice is implemented through them.*

The American Academy of Pediatrics (AAP) publishes guidelines for *health supervision visits* and key age-appropriate components of these visits (see www.healthychildren.org). Remember that children and adolescents who have a chronic illness or high-risk family or environmental circumstances will probably require more frequent visits and more intensive health promotion. Key health promotion issues and strategies, tailored for specific age groups, are found throughout this chapter.

Integrate explanations of your physical findings with health promotion. For example, provide advice about expected maturational changes or how health behaviors can affect physical findings (e.g., exercise may reduce blood pressure and prevent obesity). Be sure to demonstrate the relationship between healthy lifestyles and physical health.

Childhood immunizations are a mainstay for health promotion and have been heralded as the most significant medical achievement of public health worldwide. The childhood immunization schedule changes yearly, and updates are published widely and disseminated on websites of the Centers for Disease Control and Prevention (CDC) and the AAP.[6,7] To view the most current immunization schedule, go to the CDC's website: www.cdc.gov/vaccines.

Screening procedures are performed at specific ages. For all children, these include growth parameters and developmental screening at all ages, blood pressure after age 3, BMI screening after age 2, vision and hearing screening at key ages, and behavioral and mental health screening. Increasingly, standardized screening instruments are being used to assist clinicians in identifying abnormalities. In addition, screening procedures particularly recommended for all children at certain ages or for specific high-risk patients (depending on the test) include tests for lead poisoning, tuberculosis exposure, anemia, dyslipidemia, urinary tract infections, and sexually transmitted diseases. There is variation worldwide in recommendations for screening tests; the AAP recommendations are provided at www.aap.org. *Anticipatory guidance* is a major component of the pediatric visit.[4] Key areas for health promotion cover a broad range of topics, from purely "medical" to developmental, social and emotional health. All these factors affect children's health.

Key Components of Pediatric Health Promotion

1. Age-appropriate developmental achievement of the child
   - Physical (maturation, growth, puberty)
   - Motor (gross and fine motor skills)
   - Cognitive (achievement of milestones, language, school performance)
   - Emotional (self-regulation, mood, temperament, self-efficacy, self-esteem, independence)
   - Social (social competence, self-responsibility, integration with family and community, peer interactions)
2. Health supervision visits
   - Periodic assessment of medical and oral health
   - Children with special health care needs often require more frequent health supervision visits
3. Integration of physical examination findings with healthy lifestyle recommendations
4. Immunizations
5. Screening procedures
6. Anticipatory guidance[4]
   - Healthy habits
   - Nutrition and healthy eating
   - Safety and prevention of injury or illness
   - Sexual development and sexuality
   - Self-responsibility, efficacy, and healthy self-esteem
   - Family relationships (interactions, strengths, supports)
   - Positive parenting strategies
   - Emotional and mental health
   - Oral health
   - Recognition of illness
   - Sleep
   - Prevention of risky behaviors (e.g., tobacco, alcohol and drug use, unprotected sex)
   - School and vocation
   - Peer relationships
   - Community interactions
7. Partnership among health care provider, child/adolescent, and family

ASSESSING THE INFANT

DEVELOPMENT

Physical Development[8]

Physical growth during infancy is faster than at any other age. By 1 year, the infant's birth weight should have tripled and height increased by 50% from birth.

Newborns have surprising abilities, such as fixing upon and following human faces. Neurologic development progresses centrally to peripherally.

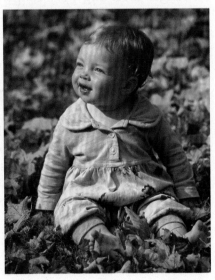

Thus, newborns learn head control before trunk control and use of arms and legs before use of hands and fingers. The graph of milestones shows the amazing developmental progression in infancy.

Activity, exploration, and environmental manipulation contribute to learning. By 3 months, normal infants lift the head and clasp the hands. By 6 months, they roll over, reach for objects, turn to voices, and possibly sit with support. With increasing peripheral coordination, infants reach for objects, transfer them from hand to hand, crawl, stand by holding on, and play with objects by banging and grabbing. A 1-year-old child may be standing and putting objects in the mouth.[9]

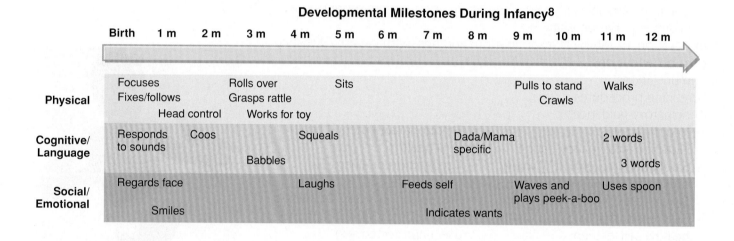

Developmental Milestones During Infancy[8]

	Birth	1 m	2 m	3 m	4 m	5 m	6 m	7 m	8 m	9 m	10 m	11 m	12 m
Physical	Focuses Fixes/follows Head control			Rolls over Grasps rattle Works for toy		Sits				Pulls to stand Crawls		Walks	
Cognitive/ Language	Responds to sounds	Coos		Babbles		Squeals			Dada/Mama specific			2 words	3 words
Social/ Emotional	Regards face		Smiles			Laughs			Feeds self Indicates wants	Waves and plays peek-a-boo		Uses spoon	

Cognitive and Language Development

Exploration fosters increased understanding of self and environment. Infants learn cause and effect (e.g., shaking a rattle produces sound), object permanence, and use of tools. By 9 months, they may recognize the examiner as a stranger deserving wary cooperation, seek comfort from parents during examinations, and actively manipulate reachable objects (e.g., equipment). Language development proceeds from cooing at 2 months, to babbling at 6 months, to saying 1 to 3 words by 1 year.[10]

Social and Emotional Development

Understanding of self and family also matures. Social tasks include bonding, attachment to caregivers, and trust that caregivers will meet their needs. Temperaments vary. Some infants are predictable, adaptable, and respond positively to new stimuli; others are less so and respond intensely or negatively. Because environment affects social development, observe the infant's interactions with caregivers.

THE HEALTH HISTORY

The health history is an important tool for assessing health, growth, and development. After a full history is obtained, subsequent visits should ask about the child's health, growth, development, and health patterns as well as other changes (e.g., family life) since the previous visit.

Birth History

At the initial appointment ask the parent about the mother's pregnancy and the infant's birth.

> Were there any problems during the pregnancy?
> Did the mother use alcohol during pregnancy? If yes, when, how often and how much?
> Did the mother use any medications/drugs or supplements during pregnancy? If yes, what medications or supplements, how much and when?
> How close was the infant's birth to the due date?
> Were there any problems during labor or birth?
> Was the child born vaginally or by C-section?

Past History

If this is the first visit of the infant to this health care practice or clinic, ask where the infant was seen before; and when and why was the infant seen.

Ask if the infant has any allergies.

> Is he on any medications, including vitamins or fluoride drops?
> Has he had any illnesses? Ask the parent to describe the illness, treatment, and outcome.

Family History

The family history may reveal hereditary disease patterns. Inquire about the age and health status of siblings, parents, grandparents, and aunts and uncles. A genogram is helpful to trace patterns emerging within a family.

Also inquire about *family structure*. Who lives in the house with the infant? What is their relationship to the infant?

Health Maintenance

- *Immunizations:* What immunizations has the infant had? Did he have any reaction to the "shots"?

- *Safety measures:* Inquire about the baby's position during sleep, blankets or toys in crib, use of car seats, and presence of smoke/carbon monoxide detectors in the house.

- *Risk factors:* The infant's environment may be affected by the parent's behaviors; therefore, inquire about:

  Tobacco: Do you smoke? In the house? In the presence of the infant? Does anyone else in your house smoke?
  Alcohol: Do you or your spouse drink alcoholic beverages? How much alcohol do you drink per sitting and per week?
  Substance abuse: Do you or your spouse use marijuana, cocaine, heroin, or other recreational drugs?
  Environmental hazards: Inquire about lead paint or other household hazards.

Conduct a Review of Systems, asking the parent about each system in turn.

Have you noted any problems with your infant's skin? Head or scalp? etc.

When the review is complete ask the parents if they have any concerns about their infant. Then move on to the infant's developmental status according to the infant's age. For example, ask the parents of a 6-month-old if he or she can sit alone. Inquire at what age the infant achieved each milestone.

Health Patterns

Complete the history by asking about the infant's health patterns.

- *Nutrition:* What does the infant drink? How many ounces at one time? Or how long does the infant nurse at each breast? How many times a day?

- Does the infant eat cereal or other foods?

- Does the infant have any problems during or after feedings?

- *Elimination:* Describe your infant's typical urination pattern and bowel pattern, including amount, consistency, and number.

- *Sleep:* Tell me about your infant's sleep pattern (including time of day the infant sleeps and hours of sleep). Do you, another family member, or a pet ever sleep with the child?

- *Activity/play:* What amuses your infant? How do you play with your infant?

Approaching the Infant

Use developmentally appropriate methods such as *distraction* and *play* to examine the infant. Because infants pay attention to one thing at a time, it is relatively easy to distract the infant's attention from the examination as it is being performed. Distract the infant with a moving object, a flashing light, a game of peek-a-boo, or any sort of noise.

If you cannot distract the infant or engage the awake infant with an object, your face, or a sound, consider a possible *visual* or *hearing deficit.*

Tips for Examining Infants

- Approach the infant gradually, using a toy or object for distraction.
- Perform as much of the examination as possible with the infant in the parent's lap.
- Speak softly to the infant or mimic the infant's sounds to attract attention.
- If the infant is cranky, make sure he or she is well fed before proceeding.
- Ask a parent about the infant's strengths to elicit useful developmental and parenting information.
- Do not expect to do a head-to-toe examination in a specific order. Work with what the infant gives you and save the mouth and ear examination for last.

General Guidelines

Start with the infant sitting or lying in the parent's lap. If the infant is tired, hungry, or ill, ask the parent to hold the baby against the parent's chest. Make sure appropriate toys, a blanket, or other familiar objects are nearby. A hungry infant may need to be fed before initiating the examination.

Close observation of an awake infant sitting on the parent's lap can reveal potential abnormalities such as *hypotonia* or *hypertonia,* conditions with abnormal skin color, jaundice or cyanosis, jitteriness, or respiratory problems.

Observe parent–infant interactions. Watch the parent's affect when talking about the infant. Note the parent's manner of holding, moving, dressing, and comforting the infant. Assess and comment on positive interactions, such as the obvious pride in the mother's face above.

Observation of the infant's communication with the parent can reveal abnormalities such as *developmental delay, language delay, hearing deficits,* or *inadequate parental attachment.* Likewise, such observations may identify maladaptive nurturing patterns that may stem from *maternal depression* or *inadequate social support.*

Infants usually do not object to having their clothing removed. To keep yourself and your surroundings dry, it is wise to leave the diaper in place throughout the examination; remove it only to examine the skin underneath, genitals, rectum, lower spine, and hips.

Testing for Developmental Milestones

Because you will want to measure the infant's best performance, checking milestones is best at the end of the interview, just before the examination. This "fun and games" interlude also enhances cooperation during the examination. Experienced nurses can weave the developmental examination into the other parts of the examination. The table on p. 814 shows some key physical or motor, cognitive or language, and social–emotional milestones during the first year. As an example, the infant in the photo on p. 817 can sit unsupported, uses a thumb-finger grasp, and is indicating wants—an 8-month level.

Many disorders cause delays in more than one milestone. For most children with developmental delay, the causes are unknown. Some known causes include *abnormality in embryonic development* (e.g., prenatal insult, chromosomal problem), *hereditary and genetic disorders* (e.g., inborn errors, genetic abnormalities), *environmental and social problems* (e.g., insufficient stimulation), *pregnancy or perinatal problems* (e.g., placental insufficiency, prematurity), and *childhood diseases* (e.g., infection, trauma, chronic illness).

The AAP recommends that health care providers use a standardized developmental screening instrument for infants as young as several months of age.[11] Several developmental screening instruments have been tested widely and validated in many nations. In general, these instruments assess *five critical domains of infant/child development: gross motor, fine motor, cognitive (or problem-solving), communication, and personal/social domains of development.* Pediatric health providers are recommended to use these standardized instruments periodically during preventive health visits because they perform better than a clinician's physical examination in identifying developmental delays which can often be subtle and challenging to determine because of the wide spectrum of normal development in children. These screening instruments are practical to use in clinical settings and have reasonable sensitivity and specificity for identifying developmental delays. Some useful developmental screening instruments include the Ages and Stages Questionnaire (ASQ), the Early Language Milestone Scale (ELM Scale-2), the Modified Checklist for Autism in Toddlers (MCHAT), and the Parents' Evaluation of Developmental Status (PEDS). Combined with your findings on interview and physical examination, results from these screening tests can help determine an appropriate management strategy.

One standard for measuring developmental milestones throughout infancy and childhood is the DENVER II Screening Test. It is designed to detect developmental delays in four domains of development from birth through 6 years: personal–social, fine motor–adaptive, language, and gross motor.

The DENVER II form is shown on the following two pages and includes instructions for recording specific observations. Each test item is represented on the form under the age by a bar, which indicates when 25%, 50%, 75%, and 90% of children attain the milestones depicted. The *DENVER II is a measure of developmental attainment only in the categories indicated. The DENVER II is not a measure of intelligence.*

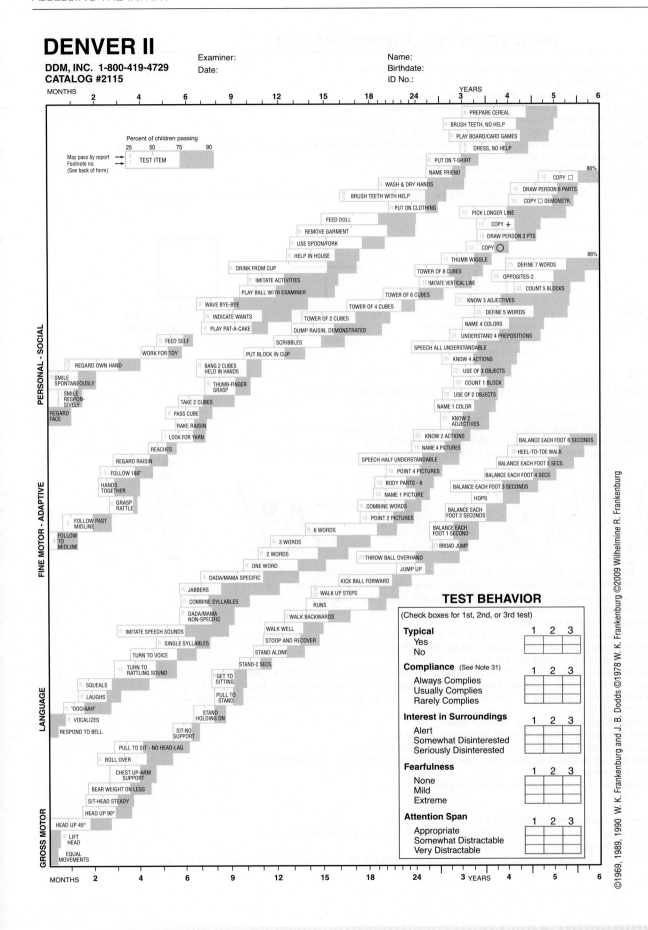

DENVER II

DDM, INC. 1-800-419-4729
CATALOG #2115

Examiner:
Date:

Name:
Birthdate:
ID No.:

DIRECTIONS FOR ADMINISTRATION

1. Try to get child to smile by smiling, talking or waving. Do not touch him/her.
2. Child must stare at hand several seconds.
3. Parent may help guide toothbrush and put toothpaste on brush.
4. Child does not have to be able to tie shoes or button/zip in the back.
5. Move yarn slowly in an arc from one side to the other, about 8" above child's face.
6. Pass if child grasps rattle when it is touched to the backs or tips of fingers.
7. Pass if child tries to see where yarn went. Yarn should be dropped quickly from sight from tester's hand without arm movement.
8. Child must transfer cube from hand to hand without help of body, mouth, or table.
9. Pass if child picks up raisin with any part of thumb and finger.
10. Line can vary only 30 degrees or less from tester's line. |/
11. Make a fist with thumb pointing upward and wiggle only the thumb. Pass if child imitates and does not move any fingers other than the thumb.

| 12. Pass any enclosed form. Fail continuous round motions. | 13. Which line is longer? (Not bigger.) Turn paper upside down and repeat. (pass 3 of 3 or 5 of 6) | 14. Pass any lines crossing near midpoint. | 15. Have child copy first. If failed, demonstrate. |

When giving items 12, 14, and 15, do not name the forms. Do not demonstrate 12 and 14.

16. When scoring, each pair (2 arms, 2 legs, etc.) counts as one part.
17. Place one cube in cup and shake gently near child's ear, but out of sight. Repeat for other ear.
18. Point to picture and have child name it. (No credit is given for sounds only.)
    If less than 4 pictures are named correctly, have child point to picture as each is named by tester.

19. Using doll, tell child: Show me the nose, eyes, ears, mouth, hands, feet, tummy, hair. Pass 6 of 8.
20. Using pictures, ask child: Which one flies?...says meow?...talks?...barks?...gallops? Pass 2 of 5, 4 of 5.
21. Ask child: What do you do when you are cold?...tired?...hungry? Pass 2 of 3, 3 of 3.
22. Ask child: What do you do with a cup? What is a chair used for? What is a pencil used for? Action words must be included in answers.
23. Pass if child correctly places <u>and</u> says how many blocks are on paper. (1,5).
24. Tell child: Put block **on** table; **under** table; **in front of** me, **behind** me. Pass 4 of 4. (Do not help child by pointing, moving head or eyes.)
25. Ask child: What is a ball?...lake?...desk?...house?...banana?...curtain?...fence?...ceiling? Pass if defined in terms of use, shape, what it is made of, or general category (such as banana is fruit, not just yellow). Pass 5 of 8, 7 of 8.
26. Ask child: If a horse is big, a mouse is ___? If fire is hot, ice is ___? If the sun shines during the day, the moon shines during the ___? Pass 2 of 3.
27. Child may use wall or rail only, not person. May not crawl.
28. Child must throw ball overhand 3 feet to within arm's reach of tester.
29. Child must perform standing broad jump over width of test sheet (8 1/2 inches).
30. Tell child to walk forward, ⚮⚮⚮⚮➜ heel within 1 inch of toe. Tester may demonstrate. Child must walk 4 consecutive steps.
31. In the second year, half of normal children are non-compliant.

OBSERVATIONS:

Denver Developmental Materials, Inc.
For permission to publish DENVER II material contact the copyright holder via:
denverdevelopmentalmaterials@gmail.com
DENVER II and associated materials can be downloaded on line, free, for the non-publishing individual user.

The DENVER II is a highly specific screening test, so that normal children will test as normal. If the child refuses to cooperate or performs below age level, ask the parent if this is typical behavior for the child.

If a cooperative infant fails items on the DENVER II or another instrument, developmental delay is possible, necessitating more precise testing and evaluation.

An infant or toddler who has developmental skills that plateau or are out of sequence may have *autism* or *cerebral palsy*.

Use the screening instruments as an adjunct to a comprehensive developmental examination. Suspected delays from the general examination or developmental screening instrument warrant further evaluation. For babies born prematurely, adjust expected developmental milestones for the gestational age up to approximately 24 months.

PHYSICAL EXAMINATION OF THE INFANT

General Survey and Vital Signs

Measure the infant's body size (length, weight, and head circumference) and vital signs (blood pressure, starting age 3, pulse, respiratory rate, and temperature). Compare vital signs or body proportions with age-specific norms, because they change dramatically as children grow. Pediatric nurses also assess pain regularly, using standardized pain scales.

Variations beyond two standard deviations for age, or above the 95th percentile or below the 5th percentile, are indications for more detailed evaluation. These deviations may be the first and only indicators of disease (see examples on thePoint).

Somatic Growth

Measurement of growth is one of the most important indicators of infant health. Deviations may provide an early indication of an underlying problem. Compare growth parameters with respect to:

- Normal values for age and sex

- Prior readings on the same child, to assess trends

Measure growth parameters carefully, using consistent technique and, optimally, the same scales to measure weight and a standardized infant length board to measure length.

A common cause of an apparent deviation in somatic growth is *measurement error,* attributed partly to the challenge of measuring a squirming infant or child. Confirm abnormalities by repeat measurement.

The most important tools for assessing somatic growth are the growth charts, which are published by the National Center for Health Statistics and the World Health Organization (go to thePoint for links to these charts).[12] All charts include length, weight, and head circumference for age, for children up to 36 months and height and weight for children 2 to 18 years. Charts plotting BMI are also available. These growth charts have percentile lines indicating the percentage of normal children above and below the child's measurement by chronologic age. Special growth charts are available for use in infants born prematurely, to correct for this result.

Although many healthy infants cross percentiles on growth charts, a sudden or significant change in growth may indicate systemic disease or inappropriate feeding.

Abnormalities that can cause deviation from normal growth patterns include *Down syndrome* or *prematurity*. Growth charts are also available for children with specific conditions such as *Down syndrome* or *Turner syndrome.*

The AAP, NIH, and CDC now recommend that clinicians use the 2006 WHO International growth charts for children 0 to 23 months of age. CDC growth charts should be used in the United States to assess growth in children 2 to 19 years of age.

Length

For children younger than 2 years, two people are needed to measure body length. Place the child supine on a length board, as shown. Direct measurement of the infant using a tape measure or drawing on the paper on an examination table is inaccurate. Velocity growth curves are helpful for older children, especially those who are suspected of having endocrine disorders.

Reduced growth velocity, shown by a drop in height percentile on a growth curve, may signify a chronic condition. Comparison with normal standards is essential, because growth velocity normally is less during the second year than during the first year.

Chronic conditions causing reduced length or height include *neurologic, renal, cardiac,* gastrointestinal and *endocrine disorders as well as cystic fibrosis.*

Weight

Weigh infants directly with an infant scale; this is more accurate than an indirect method based on weighing the parent and child together and subtracting the weight of the parent from the total weight. Infants should be clothed only in a dry diaper or weighed naked.

Failure to thrive is inadequate weight gain for age. Common scenarios are:

- Growth below 5th percentile for age
- Growth drop greater than 2 quartiles in 6 months
- Weight for height below 5th percentile

Causes include environmental or psychosocial factors and a variety of gastrointestinal, neurologic, cardiac, endocrine, renal, and other diseases.

If the infant's weight is unexpectedly and significantly different than anticipated, redo the measurement to ensure accuracy.

Head Circumference

The head circumference should always be measured during the first 2 years of life, but measurement can be useful at any age to assess growth of the head. The head circumference in infants reflects the rate of growth of the cranium and the brain. Measuring the circumference of the head, with a non-elastic tape measure just above the ears, as seen in the picture, produces the most accurate results.

A small head size may be from premature closure of the sutures or microcephaly. Microcephaly may be familial or the result of various chromosomal abnormalities, congenital infections e.g. Zika virus, maternal metabolic disorders, and neurologic insults.

An abnormally large head size (greater than 97th percentile or 2 standard deviations above the mean) is *macrocephaly,* which may be from *hydrocephalus, subdural hematoma,* or rare causes like *brain tumor or inherited syndromes. Familial megaloencephaly* (large head) is a benign familial condition with normal brain growth.

Vital Signs

Blood Pressure

Although obtaining accurate blood pressure readings in infants is challenging, this measurement is nevertheless important for some high-risk infants and should be performed routinely after age 3 years. You will need your skills in distraction or play, as shown in the photo on the next page.

Electronic blood pressure machines are commonly used today for infants. Be sure to choose the correct size cuff, apply it correctly, and control the child's movement in order to obtain a correct measurement.

The systolic blood pressure gradually increases throughout childhood. For example, normal systolic pressure in males is about 70 mm Hg at birth, 85 mm Hg at 1 month, and 90 mm Hg at 6 months.[13]

Causes of *sustained hypertension* in infants include renal artery disease (stenosis, thrombosis), congenital renal malformations, and coarctation of the aorta.

Pulse

The heart rate of infants is more sensitive to the effects of illness, exercise, and emotion than that of adults.

A pulse rate that is too rapid to count (usually greater than 180/min) may indicate *paroxysmal supraventricular tachycardia.* See Table 23-1, Abnormalities in Heart Rhythm and Blood Pressure, p. 908.

Heart Rates From Birth to 1 Year		
Age	Average Heart Rate	Range
Birth–2 months	140	90–190
0–6 months	130	80–180
6–12 months	115	75–155

You may have trouble obtaining an accurate pulse rate in a squirming infant. The best strategy is to auscultate the heart or to palpate the femoral arteries in the inguinal area or the brachial arteries in the antecubital fossa.

Bradycardia may be from drug ingestion, hypoxia, intracranial or neurologic conditions, or, rarely, cardiac dysrhythmia such as heart block.

Respiratory Rate

The respiratory rate in infants has a greater range and is more responsive to illness, exercise, and emotion *than that of adults or older children*. The rate of respirations per minute ranges between 30 and 60 in the newborn.

Extremely rapid and shallow respiratory rates are seen in newborns with *cyanotic cardiac disease* and right-to-left shunting, and metabolic acidosis.

The respiratory rate may vary considerably from moment to moment in the infant, with alternating periods of rapid and slow breathing (called "periodic breathing"). The sleeping respiratory rate is most reliable. Respiratory rates during active sleep compared with quiet sleep may be up to 10 breaths per minute faster. The respiratory pattern should be observed for at least 60 seconds. In infancy and early childhood, diaphragmatic breathing is predominant; thoracic excursion is minimal.

Fever can raise respiratory rates in infants by up to 10 respirations per minute for each degree centigrade of fever.

Commonly accepted cutoffs for defining *tachypnea* are:

- Birth to 2 months, greater than 60/min

- 2 to 12 months, greater than 50/min

Tachypnea and increased respiratory effort in an infant are signs of lower respiratory disease such as *bronchiolitis* or *pneumonia*.

Temperature

Because fever is so common in infants and children, obtain an accurate body temperature when you suspect infection. The techniques for obtaining rectal, oral, temporal artery, and tympanic membrane temperatures in adults are described on Chapter 7, Beginning the Physical Exam, pp. 135–137. Oral temperatures are not recommended for infants.

Fever (greater than 38.0°C or greater than 100.4°F) in infants less than 2 to 3 months may be a sign of *serious infection* or *disease*. These infants should be evaluated promptly.

When necessary to obtain a rectal temperature on an infant the technique differs slightly from the adult procedure. Place the infant prone, separate the buttocks with the thumb and forefinger on one hand, and with the other hand gently insert a well-lubricated digital rectal thermometer, to a depth of 1.3 to 2.5 cm (0.5 to 1 in). Keep the thermometer in place until the thermometer signals completion.

Body temperature in infants and children is less constant than in adults. The average rectal temperature is higher in infancy and early childhood, usually above 99.0°F (37.2°C) until after age 3 years. Body temperature may fluctuate as much as 3°F during a single day, approaching 101°F (38.3°C) in normal children, particularly in late afternoon and after vigorous activity.

Anxiety may elevate the body temperature of children. *Excessive bundling* of infants may elevate skin temperature but not core temperature.

Temperature instability in a newborn may result from sepsis, metabolic abnormality, or other serious conditions. Older infants rarely manifest temperature instability.

The Skin

Inspection

Carefully examine the infant's general color for cyanosis, paleness, ruddiness, or jaundice. To detect jaundice, apply pressure to blanch the skin of the normal pink or brown color. A yellowish color indicates jaundice.

Central cyanosis in a baby or child of any age should raise suspicion of *congenital heart disease*. The best area to look for central cyanosis is the tongue and oral mucosa, not the nail beds, lips, or the extremities.

 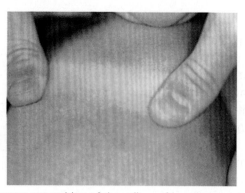

Pressing the red color from the skin allows better recognition of the yellow of jaundice. The infant on the left has no appreciable jaundice, while the infant on the right has a bilirubin level of 13 mg/dL (222 mmol/L). From Fletcher M. *Physical Diagnosis in Neonatology.* Philadelphia, PA: Lippincott-Raven; 1998.

Next examine the infant for normal and abnormal skin markings, such as birthmarks. Document their appearance and compare to the infant's last visit. See Table 23-2, Common Skin Rashes and Skin Findings in Newborns and Infants, p. 909 for examples.

Pigmented light brown lesions (less than 1 to 2 cm at birth) are *café-au-lait spots*. Isolated lesions have no significance, but multiple lesions with sharp borders suggest *neurofibromatosis*.

- A dark or bluish pigmentation over the buttocks and lower lumbar regions is common in newborns of African, Asian, and Mediterranean descent. This is congenital dermal melanocytosis, formerly called Mongolian spots, due to pigmented cells in the deep layers of the skin; they become less noticeable with age and usually disappear during childhood. Document these pigmented areas to avoid later concern about bruising or abuse.

Midline hair tufts over the lumbosacral spine region suggest a *spinal cord defect*.

- A common *vascular marking* is the "salmon patch" (also known as *nevus simplex,* telangiectatic nevus, or capillary hemangioma). These flat, irregular, light pink patches (see p. 827) are most often seen on the nape of the neck ("stork bite"), upper eyelids, forehead, or upper lip ("angel kisses"). They are not true nevi, but result from distended capillaries. They almost all disappear by 1 year of age.

Jaundice that persists beyond 2 to 3 weeks should raise suspicions of *biliary obstruction* or *liver disease*.

Palpation

Palpate the infant's skin to assess the degree of hydration, or *turgor*. Gently pinch a fold of loosely adherent skin on the abdominal wall between your thumb and forefinger to determine its consistency. The skin in well-hydrated infants returns to its normal position immediately upon release. Delay in return is a phenomenon called "tenting" and usually occurs in children with significant *dehydration*.

Dehydration is a common problem in infants. Usual causes are insufficient intake or excess loss of fluids from diarrhea.

Benign Birthmarks

Finding	Description
Eyelid patch 	This birthmark fades, usually within the first year of life.
Salmon patch 	Also called the "stork bite," this splotchy pink mark fades with age.
Café-au-lait spots 	These light brown pigmented lesions usually have borders and are uniform. They are noted in more than 10% of black infants. *If more than five café-au-lait spots exist, consider the diagnosis of neurofibromatosis.*
Congenital dermal melanocytosis (Mongolian spots) 	These are more common among dark-skinned babies. It is important to note them so that they are not mistaken for bruises or abuse.

The Head

A newborn's head accounts for one fourth of the body length and one third of the body weight; these proportions change, so that by adulthood, the head accounts for one eighth of the body length and about one tenth of the body weight.

Sutures and Fontanelles

Membranous tissue spaces called sutures separate the bones of the skull from one another. The areas where the major sutures intersect in the anterior and posterior portions of the skull are known as *fontanelles*. Examine the *sutures* and *fontanelles* carefully (see the figure below).

An enlarged posterior fontanelle may be present in *congenital hypothyroidism.*

On palpation, the sutures feel like ridges and the fontanelles like soft concavities. The *anterior fontanelle* at birth measures 4 cm to 6 cm in diameter and usually closes between 4 and 26 months of age (90% between 7 and 19 months). The *posterior fontanelle* measures 1 cm to 2 cm at birth and usually closes by 2 months.

A bulging, tense fontanelle is observed in infants with *increased intracranial pressure,* which may be caused by *central nervous system infections, neoplastic disease,* or *hydrocephalus* (obstruction of the circulation of cerebrospinal fluid within the ventricles of the brain; see Table 23-3, Abnormalities of the Head, p. 910).

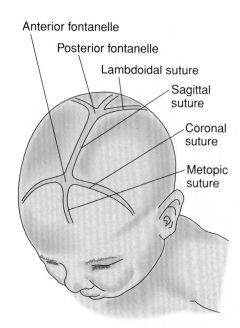

Anterior fontanelle
Posterior fontanelle
Lambdoidal suture
Sagittal suture
Coronal suture
Metopic suture

Carefully examine the fontanelle, because its fullness reflects *intracranial pressure*. Palpate the fontanelle while the baby is sitting quietly or being held upright. Experienced pediatric nurses often palpate the fontanelles at the beginning of the examination. In normal infants, the anterior fontanelle is soft and flat. Increased intracranial pressure produces a bulging, full anterior fontanelle and is seen when a baby cries, vomits, or has underlying pathology. Pulsations of the fontanelle reflect the peripheral pulse and are normal.

A depressed anterior fontanelle may be a sign of *dehydration.*

Inspect the scalp veins carefully to assess for dilatation.

Dilated scalp veins are indicative of long-standing *increased intracranial pressure.*

Skull Symmetry and Head Circumference

Assess skull symmetry. Careful inspection of the skull from the front or back of the infant helps you assess its symmetry.

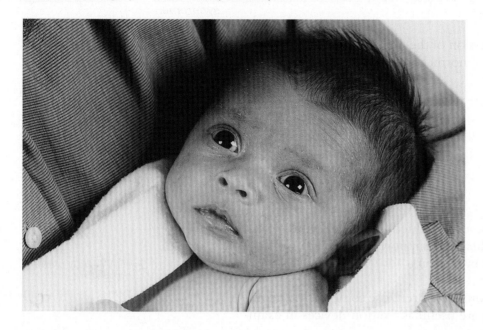

Look for asymmetric head swelling, which after the newborn period, may be due to trauma from a fall or abuse.

Asymmetry of the cranial vault (*plagiocephaly*) occurs when an infant lies mostly on one side, resulting in a flattening of the parieto-occipital region on the dependent side and a prominence of the frontal region on the opposite side. It disappears as the baby becomes more active and spends less time in one position, and symmetry is almost always restored. Interestingly, the current trend to have newborns and infants sleep on their backs to reduce the risk for sudden infant death syndrome (SIDS) has resulted in more cases of plagiocephaly. This condition can be prevented by frequent repositioning (providing "tummy time" when the infant is awake).

Plagiocephaly may also reflect pathology such as *torticollis* from injury to the sternocleidomastoid muscle at birth, or *lack of stimulation* of the infant.

Measure the head circumference (p. 829) to detect abnormally large head size (*macrocephaly*) or small head size (*microcephaly*), which may signify an underlying disorder affecting the brain. Palpate along the suture lines. A raised, bony ridge at a suture line suggests craniosynostosis.

Premature closure of cranial sutures causes *craniosynostosis* (Table 23-5, Abnormalities of the Head, p. 912), with an abnormally shaped skull. *Sagittal suture* synostosis causes a narrow head from lack of growth of the parietal bones.

Palpate the infant's skull with care. The cranial bones usually appear "soft" or pliable; they will normally become firmer with increasing age.

In *craniotabes,* the cranial bones feel springy. Craniotabes can result from increased intracranial pressure, as with *hydrocephaly,* metabolic disturbances such as *rickets,* and infection such as *congenital syphilis.*

Facial Symmetry

Check the *face* of infants for symmetry. In utero positioning may result in transient facial asymmetries. If the head is flexed on the sternum, a shortened chin (*micrognathia*) may result.

Examine the face for an overall impression of the *facies;* it is helpful to compare with the face of the parents. An abnormal-appearing facies can identify specific syndromes.[14]

Micrognathia may also be part of a syndrome, such as the *Pierre Robin syndrome.*

A child with abnormal shape or length of palpebral fissures: see Table 23-6, Diagnostic Facies in Infancy and Childhood, pp. 913–914.

Upslanting (Down syndrome)

Downslanting (Noonan syndrome)

Short (fetal alcohol effects)

The Eyes

Inspection

Bright light causes infants to blink, so use subdued lighting. If you awaken the baby gently, turn down the lights, and support the baby in a sitting position, you will often find that the eyes open.

To examine the eyes of infants and young children, use some tricks encourage cooperation. Small colorful toys are useful as fixation devices in examining the eyes.

Newborns may look at your face and follow a bright light if you catch them during an alert period. By 2 months most infants can follow an object.

Examine infants for *eye movements.* Hold the baby upright, supporting the head. Rotate yourself with the baby slowly in one direction. This usually causes the baby's eyes to open, allowing you to examine the sclerae, pupils, irises, and extraocular movements. The baby's eyes gaze in the direction you are turning. When the rotation stops, the eyes look in the opposite direction, after a few nystagmoid movements.

Nystagmus (wandering or shaking eye movements) persisting after a few days after birth or persisting after the maneuver described on the left may indicate *poor vision* or *central nervous system disease.*

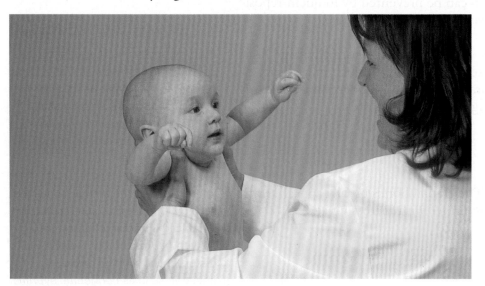

During the first few months of life, some infants have intermittent crossed eyes (*intermittent alternating convergent strabismus,* or *esotropia*) or laterally deviated eyes (*intermittent alternating divergent strabismus,* or *exotropia*).

Alternating convergent or divergent *strabismus* persisting beyond 3 months, or persistent strabismus of any type, may indicate *ocular motor weakness* or another abnormality in the visual system.

Observe pupillary reactions by response to light or by covering each eye with your hand and then uncovering it. They should be equal in size and reaction to light.

Inspect the irises carefully for abnormalities.

Brushfield spots (seen with an ophthalmoscope) are a ring of white specks in the iris. Although sometimes present in normal children, these strongly suggest *Down syndrome.* See Table 23-7, Abnormalities of the Eyes, Ears and Mouth, p. 915.

Examine the *conjunctiva* for swelling or redness.

Visual acuity of infants cannot be measured. Visual reflexes can be used to indirectly assess vision: direct and consensual pupillary constriction in response to light, blinking in response to bright light (*optic blink reflex*), and blinking in response to quick movement of an object toward the eyes. During the first year of life, visual acuity sharpens as the ability to focus improves. Infants achieve the following visual milestones:

Persistent ocular discharge and tearing since birth may be from *dacryocystitis* or *nasolacrimal duct obstruction.*

Visual Milestones of Infancy[15]	
Birth	**Blinks, May Regard Face**
1 month	Fixes on objects
1/2–2 months	Coordinated eye movements
3 months	Eyes converge, baby reaches toward a visual stimulus
12 months	Acuity around 20/80

Failure to progress along these visual developmental milestones may indicate *delayed visual maturation.*

Ophthalmoscopic Examination

For the *ophthalmoscopic examination,* with the infant awake and eyes open, examine the red retinal reflex by setting the ophthalmoscope at 0 diopters and viewing the pupil from about 10 in. Normally, a red or orange color is reflected from the fundus through the pupil.

Congenital glaucoma may cause cloudiness of the cornea. A dark light reflex can result from *cataracts, retinopathy of prematurity,* or other disorders. A white retinal reflex (*leukokoria*) is abnormal, and *cataract, retinal detachment, chorioretinitis,* or *retinoblastoma* should be suspected.

If history or examination findings indicate the need for a thorough ophthalmologic examination, refer the infant to a pediatric ophthalmologist.

The Ears

The physical examination of the ears of infants is important because many abnormalities can be detected, including structural problems, otitis media, and hearing loss. The goals are to determine the *position, shape,* and *features of the ear* and to detect abnormalities. Note ear position in relation to the eyes. An imaginary line drawn across the inner and outer canthi of the eyes should cross the auricle; if the auricle is below this line, the infant has low-set ears. Draw this imaginary line across the face of the child on p. 834; note that it crosses the auricle.

Small, deformed, or low-set auricles may indicate associated *congenital defects,* especially renal disease.

A small skin tab, cleft, or pit found just forward of the tragus represents a remnant of the *first branchial cleft* and usually has no significance.

The infant's ear canal is directed downward from outside; therefore, pull the auricle gently downward, not upward, for the best view of the eardrum. Once the tympanic membrane is visible, note that the light reflex is diffuse and does not become cone-shaped for several months.

In the absence of universal hearing screening many children with *hearing deficits* are not diagnosed until 2 years of age. Clues to hearing deficits include parental concern about hearing, delayed speech, and lack of developmental indicators of hearing.

Signs That an Infant Can Hear	
Age (months)	**Sign**
0–2	Startle response and blink to a sudden noise Calming down with soothing voice or music
2–3	Change in body movements in response to sound Change in facial expression to familiar sounds
3–4	Turning eyes and head to sound
6–7	Turning to listen to voices and conversation Appropriate language development

The Nose and Sinuses

The most important component of the examination of the nose of infants is to test for patency of the nasal passages. You can do this by gently occluding each nostril alternately while holding the infant's mouth closed. This normally will not cause stress because most infants are nasal breathers. Indeed, some infants are *obligate nasal breathers* and have difficulty breathing through their mouths. Do not occlude both nares simultaneously—this will cause considerable distress!

The nasal passages in newborns may be obstructed in *choanal atresia.*

Inspect the nose to ensure that the nasal septum is midline

The Mouth and Pharynx

Use both inspection with a tongue depressor and flashlight and palpation to inspect the mouth and pharynx. The newborn's mouth is edentulous, and the alveolar mucosa is smooth, with finely serrated borders. Occasionally, pearl-like retention cysts are seen along the alveolar ridges and are easily mistaken for teeth—they disappear within 1 or 2 months. Petechiae are commonly found on the soft palate after birth. Palpate the upper hard palate to make sure it is intact. *Epstein pearls,* tiny white or yellow, rounded mucous retention cysts, are located along the posterior midline of the hard palate. They disappear within months.

Rarely, *supernumerary teeth* are noted. These are usually dysmorphic and are shed within days but are removed to prevent aspiration.

Cysts may be noted on the tongue or mouth. Thyroglossal duct cysts may open under the tongue.

Infants produce little saliva during the first 3 months. Older infants produce lots of saliva and drool frequently.

Inspect the tongue. The frenulum varies in tightness; sometimes it extends almost to the tip and other times it is short, limiting protrusion of the tongue (ankyloglossia or tongue tie).

Although unusual, a prominent, protruding tongue may signal *congenital hypothyroidism* or *Down syndrome.*

You will often see a whitish covering on the tongue. If this coating is from milk, it can be easily removed by scraping or wiping it away. Use a tongue depressor or your gloved finger to wipe away the coating.

Oral candidiasis (thrush) is common in infants. The white plaques are difficult to wipe away and have an erythematous raw base. See Table 23-7, Abnormalities of the Eyes, Ears and Mouth, p. 915.

The pharynx of the infant is best seen while the baby is crying. You will likely have difficulty using a tongue depressor because it produces a strong gag reflex. Infants do not have prominent lymphoid tissue so you will probably not visualize the tonsils, which increase in size as children grow. Listen to the quality of the *infant's cry*. Normal infants have a lusty, strong cry. The following box lists some unusual types of infant cries.

A congenital fissure of the median line of the palate is a **cleft palate.**

Macroglossia is associated with several systemic conditions. If associated with hypoglycemia and omphalocele, the diagnosis is likely Beckwith–Wiedemann syndrome.

Abnormal Infant Cries

Type	Possible Abnormality
Shrill or high-pitched	Increased intracranial pressure. Also in newborns born to narcotic-addicted mothers
Hoarse	Hypocalcemic tetany or congenital hypothyroidism
Continuous inspiratory and expiratory stridor	Upper airway obstruction from various lesions (e.g., a polyp or hemangioma), a relatively small larynx (infantile laryngeal stridor), or a delay in the development of the cartilage in the tracheal rings (tracheomalacia)
Absence of cry	Severe illness, vocal cord paralysis, or profound brain damage

Inspiratory stridor beginning at birth suggests a congenital abnormality as described in this table. Stridor that appears following birth can be due to infections such as *croup, a foreign body, or gastroesophageal reflux.*

While there is a predictable pattern of tooth eruption there is wide variation in the age at which teeth appear. A rule of thumb is that a child will have one tooth for each month of age between 6 and 26 months, up to a maximum of 20 primary teeth.

The Neck

Palpate the *lymph nodes of the neck* and assess for any additional masses such as *congenital cysts*. Because the necks of infants are short, it is best to palpate the neck while infants are lying supine, whereas older children are best examined while sitting. Check the position of the thyroid cartilage and trachea.

Preauricular cysts and sinuses are common, pinhole-size pits, usually located anterior to the helix of the ear. They are often bilateral and may occasionally be associated with *hearing deficits* and renal disorders.

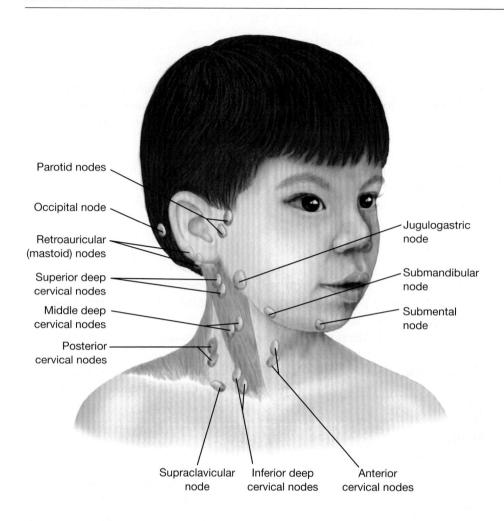

Parotid nodes

Occipital node

Retroauricular (mastoid) nodes

Superior deep cervical nodes

Middle deep cervical nodes

Posterior cervical nodes

Jugulogastric node

Submandibular node

Submental node

Supraclavicular node

Inferior deep cervical nodes

Anterior cervical nodes

Palpate the *clavicles* and look for evidence of a fracture. If present, you may feel a break in the contour of the bone, tenderness, crepitus at the fracture site, and may notice limited movement of the arm on the affected side.

The Thorax and Lungs

The infant's *thorax* is more rounded than that of older children and adults. The thin chest wall has little musculature; thus, lung and heart sounds are transmitted quite clearly. The bony and cartilaginous rib cage is soft and pliant. The tip of the xiphoid process often protrudes anteriorly, immediately beneath the skin.

Two types of chest wall abnormalities noted in childhood include *pectus excavatum,* or "funnel chest," and *pectus carinatum,* or "chicken breast deformity."

Inspection

Carefully assess respirations and breathing patterns.

Apnea is cessation of breathing for more than 20 seconds. It is often accompanied by bradycardia and may indicate *respiratory disease, central nervous system disease,* or, rarely, a *cardiopulmonary condition.* Apnea may be a high-risk factor for *SIDS.*

Do not rush to the stethoscope. Instead, observe the infant carefully. Inspection is easiest when infants are not crying; thus, work with the parents to settle the child. On observation, note general appearance, respiratory rate, color, nasal component of breathing, audible breath sounds, and work of breathing, as described below.

Because infants are obligate nasal breathers, observe their nose as they breathe. Look for *nasal flaring*. Observe breathing with the infant's mouth closed or during nursing or sucking on a bottle to assess for nasal patency. Listen to the sounds of breathing; note any *grunting, audible wheezing,* or *lack of breath sounds (obstruction)*. *Nasal flaring, grunting, retractions and wheezing are all signs of respiratory distress.*

Observe two aspects of the infant's breathing: *audible breath sounds* and *work of breathing*. These are particularly relevant in assessing both upper and lower respiratory illness.

Nasal flaring may be the result of *upper respiratory infections,* with subsequent obstruction of their small nares, but it may also be caused by pneumonia or other serious respiratory infections.

Observing Respiration—Before You Touch the Child	
Type of Assessment	**Specific Observable Pathology**
General appearance	Inability to feed or smile
	Lack of consolability
Respiratory rate	Tachypnea, apnea (see Table 13-4, p. 365, Abnormalities of Rate and Rhythm of Breathing)
Color	Pallor or cyanosis
Nasal component of breathing	Nasal flaring (enlargement of both nasal openings during inspiration)
Audible breath sounds	Grunting (repetitive, short expiratory sound) Wheezing (musical expiratory sound) Stridor (high-pitched, inspiratory noise) Obstruction (lack of breath sounds)
Work of breathing	Nasal flaring (excessive movement of nares) Grunting (expiratory noises) Retractions (chest indrawing): Supraclavicular (soft tissue above clavicles) Intercostal (indrawing of the skin between ribs) Subcostal (just below the costal margin) Paradoxical (seesaw) breathing (abdomen moves outward while chest moves inward during inspiration)

Any of the abnormalities listed on the left should raise concern about underlying respiratory pathology.

Lower respiratory infections, defined as infections below the vocal cords, are common in infants and include *bronchiolitis* and *pneumonia.*

Acute stridor is a potentially serious condition; causes include laryngotracheobronchitis (croup), epiglottitis, bacterial tracheitis, foreign body, or a vascular ring.

In infants, abnormal work of breathing plus abnormal findings on auscultation are the best findings for ruling in *pneumonia.* The best sign for ruling *out* pneumonia is the absence of tachypnea.

In healthy infants, the ribs do not move much during quiet breathing. Any outward movement is produced by descent of the diaphragm, which compresses the abdominal contents and in turn shifts the lower ribs outward.

Asymmetric chest movement may indicate a space-occupying lesion. Pulmonary disease causes increased abdominal breathing and can result in *retractions (chest indrawing),* an indicator of pulmonary disease before 2 years of age. Retractions are inward movement of the skin between the ribs during inspiration.

Obstructive respiratory disease in infants can result in the *Hoover sign,* or paradoxical (seesaw), breathing.

Suprasternal retractions
Intercostal retractions
Substernal retractions
Subcostal retractions

LOCATIONS OF RETRACTIONS

Palpation

Assess tactile fremitus by *palpation.* Place your hand on the chest when the infant cries or makes noise. Place your hand or fingertips over each side of the chest and feel for symmetry in the transmitted vibrations. Percussion is not helpful in infants except in extreme instances. The infant's chest is hyperresonant throughout, and it is difficult to detect abnormalities on percussion.

Because of the excellent transmission of sounds throughout the chest, any abnormalities of tactile fremitus or on percussion suggest severe pathology, such as a large *pneumonic consolidation.*

Auscultation

After performing these maneuvers, it is time for *auscultation.* Infant breath sounds are louder and harsher than those of adults because the stethoscope is closer to the origin of the sounds. Also, it is often difficult to distinguish transmitted upper airway sounds from sounds originating in the chest. The table that follows has some useful hints. Upper airway sounds tend to be loud, transmitted symmetrically throughout the chest, and loudest as you move your stethoscope toward the neck. They are usually coarse inspiratory sounds. Lower airway sounds are loudest over the site of pathology, are often asymmetric, and often occur during expiration.

Biphasic sounds (wheezing) imply severe obstruction from intrathoracic airway narrowing or severe obstruction from extrathoracic airway narrowing.

Expiratory sounds usually arise from an intrathoracic source, while inspiratory sounds typically arise from an extrathoracic airway such as the trachea. During expiration, the diameter of the intrathoracic airways decreases because radial forces from the surrounding lung do not "tether" the airways open as occurs during inspiration. Higher flow rates during inspiration produce turbulent flow, resulting in appreciable sounds.

Distinguishing Upper Airway From Lower Airway Sounds in Infants		
Technique	**Upper Airway**	**Lower Airway**
Compare sounds from nose/stethoscope	Same sounds	Often different sounds
Listen to harshness of sounds	Harsh and loud	Variable
Note symmetry (left/right)	Symmetric	Often asymmetric
Compare sounds at different locations (higher or lower)	Sounds louder as stethoscope is moved up chest	Often sounds louder lower in chest toward abdomen
Inspiratory vs. expiratory	Almost always inspiratory	Often has expiratory phase

Diminished breath sounds in one side of the chest suggest unilateral lesions (e.g., *congenital diaphragmatic hernia or pneumothorax*).

The characteristics of the *breath sounds,* such as vesicular and bronchovesicular, and of the adventitious lung sounds, such as crackles, wheezes, and rhonchi, are the same as those for adults, except that they may be more difficult to distinguish in infants and often occur together. Wheezes and rhonchi are common in infants. *Wheezes,* often audible without the stethoscope, occur more frequently because of the smaller size of the tracheobronchial tree. *Rhonchi* reflect obstruction of larger airways, or bronchi. *Crackles* (rales) are discontinuous sounds (Chapter 13, pp. 346–347), near the end of inspiration; they are usually caused by lung disorders and are far less likely to represent cardiac failure in infants than in adults. They tend to be harsher than in adults.

Upper respiratory infections are not serious in infants but can produce loud inspiratory sounds that are transmitted to the chest.

Wheezes in infants occur commonly from *asthma* or *bronchiolitis.*

Crackles (rales) can be heard with *pneumonia* and *bronchiolitis.*

The Heart

Inspection

Before examining the heart itself, observe the infant carefully for any cyanosis. It is important to detect *central cyanosis* because it is always abnormal and because many congenital cardiac abnormalities, as well as respiratory diseases, present with cyanosis.

Central cyanosis without acute respiratory symptoms suggests cardiac disease. See Table 23-9, Cyanosis in Children, p. 917, and Table 23-10, Congenital Heart Murmurs, pp. 918–919.

Recognizing minimal degrees of cyanosis requires care. Look at the tongue, or at the conjunctivae, in addition to assessing skin color. A true strawberry pink is normal, whereas any hint of raspberry red suggests desaturation and requires urgent evaluation.

The distribution of the cyanosis should be evaluated. An oximetry reading will confirm desaturation.

Observe the infant for *general signs of health*. The infant's nutritional status, responsiveness, happiness, and irritability and fatigue are all clues that may be useful in evaluating cardiac disease. Note that noncardiac findings can be present in infants with cardiac disease.

Tachypnea, tachycardia, and hepatomegaly in infants suggest *congestive heart failure.*

Common Noncardiac Findings in Infants With Cardiac Disease		
Poor feeding	Tachypnea	Poor overall appearance
Failure to thrive	Hepatomegaly	Weakness
Irritability	Clubbing	Fatigue

Observe the respiratory rate and pattern to help distinguish the degree of illness and cardiac versus pulmonary diseases. An increase in respiratory effort is expected from pulmonary diseases, whereas in cardiac disease there may be tachypnea without increased work of breathing (called "peaceful tachypnea") until congestive heart failure becomes significant.

A diffuse bulge outward of the left side of the chest suggests long-standing *cardiomegaly.*

Palpation

PULSES. The major branches of the aorta can be assessed by evaluation of the *peripheral pulses.* In neonates and infants, the brachial artery pulse in the antecubital fossa is easier to feel than the radial artery pulse at the wrist. Both temporal arteries should be felt just in front of the ear.

Palpate femoral pulses. They lie in the midline just below the inguinal crease, between the iliac crest and the symphysis pubis. Take your time and search for femoral pulses; they are difficult to detect in chubby, squirming infants. If the infant's thighs are flexed on the abdomen first, this may overcome the reflex flexion that occurs when you then extend the legs.

The absence or diminution of femoral pulses is indicative of *coarctation of the aorta.* If femoral pulses cannot be detected, measure blood pressures of the lower and upper extremities. Normally the blood pressure in the lower extremity is slightly higher than in the upper extremities. If they are equal or lower in the legs, coarctation is likely to be present.

Palpate the dorsalis pedis and posterior tibial pulses (see photo to the right), which may be difficult to feel unless there is an abnormality involving aortic run-off. Normal pulses should have a sharp rise and should be firm and well localized.

A weak or *thready,* difficult-to-feel pulse may reflect *myocardial dysfunction* and *congestive heart failure,* particularly if associated with an unusual degree of tachycardia.

As discussed on pp. 823–824, carefully measure the *blood pressure* of infants and children as part of the cardiac examination.

APICAL IMPULSE. The apical impulse is not always palpable in infants and is affected by respiratory patterns, a full stomach, and the infant's positioning. It is usually an interspace higher than in adults during the first few years of life because the heart lies more horizontally within the chest.

A *"rolling" heave* at the left sternal border suggests an *increase in right ventricular work,* whereas the same kind of motion closer to the apex suggests the same thing for the left ventricle.

CHEST WALL. *Palpation* of the chest wall will allow you to assess volume changes within the heart. For example, a hyperdynamic precordium reflects a big volume change.

THRILLS. *Thrills* are palpable when turbulence within the heart or great vessels is transmitted to the surface. Knowledge of the structures of the precordium helps pinpoint the origin of the thrill. Thrills are easiest to feel with your palm or the base of your fingers rather than your fingertips. Thrills have a somewhat rough, vibrating quality. The figure below shows locations of thrills from various cardiac abnormalities that occur in infants and children.

Visible and palpable chest pulsations suggest a hyperdynamic state from either increased metabolic rate or inefficient pumping as a result of an underlying cardiac effect.

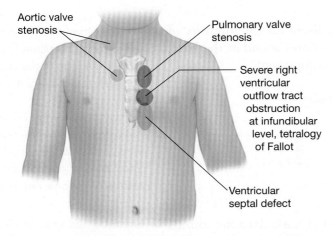

LOCATION OF THRILLS IN INFANTS AND CHILDREN

Auscultation

The *heart rhythm can be evaluated* more easily in infants by listening to the heart than by feeling the peripheral pulses; in older children it can be done either way. Infants and children commonly have a normal sinus arrhythmia, with the heart rate increasing on inspiration and decreasing on expiration, sometimes quite abruptly. This normal finding can be identified by its repetitive nature and its correlation with respiration.

The most common dysrhythmia in infants is *paroxysmal supraventricular tachycardia (PSVT)*, or *paroxysmal atrial tachycardia (PAT)*. It can occur at any age, including in utero. It is remarkably well tolerated by some infants and children and is found on examination. The child may look perfectly healthy or may be mildly pale or with tachypnea. The heart rate is sustained and regular at around 240 beats per minute or more. Some children, particularly neonates, may appear very ill. In older children, this dysrhythmia is more likely to be truly paroxysmal, with episodes of varying duration and frequency.

See Table 23-1, Abnormalities in Heart Rhythm and Blood Pressure, p. 908.

Many infants and some older children have premature atrial or ventricular beats that are often appreciated as "skipped" beats.

HEART SOUNDS. Heart sounds are challenging to assess in infants because they are rapid and often obscured by respiratory or other sounds. Nevertheless, evaluate the S_1 and S_2 heart sounds carefully and systematically. They are normally crisp. You can usually hear the second sounds (S_2) at the base separately, but they should fuse into a single sound in deep expiration. In the neonate, you should be able to detect a split S_2 if you examine the infant when the infant is completely quiet or asleep. Detecting this split eliminates many, but not all, of the more serious congenital cardiac defects.

Distant heart tones suggest *pericardial effusion;* mushy, less distinct heart sounds suggest *myocardial dysfunction.*

In addition to trying to detect splitting of the S_2, listen for the intensity of A_2 and P_2. The aortic, or first component of the second sound at the base, is normally louder than the pulmonic, or second component.

A louder-than-normal pulmonic component, particularly when louder than the aortic sound, suggests *pulmonary hypertension.*

Persistent splitting of S_2 may indicate a right ventricular volume load such as *atrial septal defect, anomalies of pulmonary venous return,* or *chronic anemia.*

A *third heart sound may be detected*. It is low-pitched, early diastolic sounds best heard at the lower left sternal border, or apex. These are frequently heard in children and are normal. They reflect rapid ventricular filling.

The third heart sound (S_3) should be differentiated from the higher-intensity third heart sound gallop, which is a sign of underlying pathology.

Fourth heart sounds (S4), which are not often heard in children, are low-frequency, late diastolic sounds, occurring just before the first heart sound.

Fourth heart sounds represent decreased ventricular compliance, suggesting *congestive heart failure.*

Heart Murmurs

One of the most challenging aspects of cardiac examination in children is the evaluation of *heart murmurs*. A major challenge is distinguishing common benign murmurs from unusual or pathologic ones. Characterize heart murmurs in infants and children by noting their specific location (e.g., left upper sternal border, not just left sternal border), timing, intensity, and quality.

An important rule of thumb is that, by definition, *benign murmurs in children have no associated abnormal findings.* Many (but not all) children with serious cardiac malformations have signs and symptoms other than a heart murmur obtainable on careful history or examination. Many have other noncardiac signs and symptoms, including evidence of genetic defects that may offer helpful diagnostic clues.

Most children will have one or more *functional, or benign, heart murmurs* before reaching adulthood.[16–18] It is important to identify functional murmurs by their specific qualities rather than by their intensity.

See Table 23-10, Congenital Heart Murmurs, pp. 918–919.

Any of the *noncardiac findings* that frequently accompany cardiac disease in children markedly raises the possibility that a murmur is pathologic.

A newborn with a heart murmur and central cyanosis likely has congenital heart disease and requires urgent cardiac evaluation.

Physiologic Basis for Some Pathologic Heart Murmurs

Change in Pulmonary Vascular Resistance
Heart murmurs that are dependent on a postnatal drop in pulmonary vascular resistance, allowing turbulent flow from the high-pressure systemic circuit to the lower-pressure pulmonary circuit, are not audible until such a drop has occurred. Therefore, except in premature infants, murmurs of a *ventricular septal defect* or *patent ductus arteriosus* are not heard in the first few days of life and usually become audible after a week to 10 days.

Obstructive Lesions
Obstructive lesions, such as *pulmonic and aortic stenosis,* are caused by normal blood flow through two small valves. They are not dependent on a drop in pulmonary vascular resistance. They are audible at birth.

Pressure Gradient Differences
Murmurs of *atrioventricular valve regurgitation* are audible at birth because of the high-pressure gradient between the ventricle and its atrium.

Changes Associated With Growth of Children
Some murmurs do not follow the rules above, but become audible because of alterations in normal blood flow that occurs with growth. For example, even though it is an obstructive defect, *aortic stenosis* may not be audible until considerable growth has occurred and, indeed, is frequently not heard until adulthood, although a congenitally abnormal valve is responsible. Similarly, the pulmonary flow murmur of an *atrial septal defect* may not be heard for a year or more because right ventricular compliance gradually increases and the shunt becomes larger, eventually producing a murmur caused by too much blood flow across a normal pulmonic valve.

When any murmur in a child is detected, note all of the qualities described in Chapter 14 to help you distinguish *pathologic murmurs* from the benign murmurs.

The Breasts

The breasts of the infant should be undeveloped and flush with the chest wall. Residual enlargement from maternal estrogen effect may last for several months after birth. The breasts may also be engorged with a white liquid, sometimes colloquially called "witch's milk," which may last 1 or 2 weeks.

In *premature thelarche,* breast development occurs, most often between 6 months and 2 years. Other signs of puberty or hormonal abnormalities are not present.

The Abdomen

Inspection

Inspect the abdomen with the infant lying supine (and, optimally, asleep). The infant's abdomen is protuberant as a result of poorly developed abdominal musculature. Abdominal wall blood vessels and intestinal peristalsis are easily noticed.

Inspect the area around the umbilicus for redness or swelling. *Umbilical hernias* are detectable by a few weeks of age. Most disappear by 1 year, nearly all by 5 years.

Umbilical hernias in infants are caused by a defect in the abdominal wall and can be up to 6 cm in diameter and quite protuberant with intra-abdominal pressure.

In some normal infants, a *diastasis recti may be noticed.* This involves separation of the two rectus abdominis muscles, causing a midline ridge, most apparent when the infant contracts the abdominal muscles. A benign condition in most cases, it resolves during early childhood.

Auscultation

Auscultation of a quiet infant's abdomen is easy. Do not be surprised if you hear an orchestra of musical tinkling bowel sounds upon placement of your stethoscope on the infant's abdomen.

An increase in pitch or frequency of bowel sounds is heard with *gastroenteritis* or, rarely, with *intestinal obstruction.*

Percussion and Palpation

The infant's abdomen can be percussed as an adult's, but be prepared to note greater tympanitic sounds because of the infant's propensity to swallow air. Percussion is useful for determining the size of organs and abdominal masses.

A silent, tympanic, distended and tender abdomen suggests *peritonitis.*

It is easy to *palpate* an infant's abdomen because infants like being touched. A useful technique to relax the infant, shown here, is to hold the legs flexed at the knees and hips with one hand and palpate the abdomen with the other. A pacifier may be used to quiet the infant in this position.

Start gently palpating the liver of infants low in the abdomen, moving upward with your fingers. This technique helps you avoid missing an extremely enlarged liver that extends down into the pelvis. With a careful examination, you can feel the liver edge in most infants, 1 to 2 cm below the right costal margin.

One technique for assessing liver size in infants is simultaneous percussion and auscultation.[19] Percuss and simultaneously auscultate, noting a change in sound as you percuss over the liver or beyond it. A scratch test (described on p. 879 for older children) can be attempted in infants.

The *spleen*, like the liver, is felt easily in most infants. It too is soft with a sharp edge, and it projects downward like a tongue from under the left costal margin. The spleen is moveable and rarely extends more than 1 to 2 cm below the left costal margin.

Palpate the *other abdominal structures*. You will commonly note pulsations in the epigastrium caused by the aorta. This is felt on deep palpation to the left of the midline.

The kidneys of infants may be palpated by carefully placing the fingers of one hand in front of and those of the other behind each kidney. The descending colon is a sausage-like mass in the left lower quadrant.

Once the normal structures in the infant's abdomen have been identified, use palpation to identify abnormal masses.

An enlarged, tender liver may be due to *congestive heart failure* or to *storage diseases.* Among newborns, causes of hepatomegaly include *hepatitis, storage diseases, vascular congestion,* and *biliary obstruction.*

Several diseases can cause splenomegaly, including *infections, hemolytic anemias, infiltrative disorders, inflammatory* or *autoimmune diseases,* and *portal hypertension.*

Abnormal abdominal masses in infants can be associated with the kidney (e.g., *hydronephrosis*), bladder (e.g., *urethral obstruction*), bowel (e.g., *Hirschsprung disease* or *intussusception*), and tumors.

In *pyloric stenosis,* deep palpation in the right upper quadrant or midline can reveal an "olive," or a 2-cm firm pyloric mass. While feeding, some infants with this condition will have visible peristaltic waves pass across their abdomen, followed by projectile vomiting. Infants with this condition tend to present at about 4 to 6 weeks of age.

Male Genitalia

Inspect the male genitalia with the infant supine, noting the appearance of the penis, testes, and scrotum. The *foreskin completely covers the glans penis.* It is nonretractable at birth, though you may be able to retract it enough to visualize the external urethral meatus. The foreskin gradually loosens over months to years and becomes retractable. The rate of circumcision has declined recently in North America and varies worldwide, depending on cultural practices, but is now recommended by the AAP and by experts in many parts of the world (often due to reduced rates of HIV and other infection among circumcised males).

Hypospadias refers to an abnormal location of the urethral orifice at some point along the ventral surface of the glans or shaft of the penis (see Table 23-12, p. 921). The foreskin is incompletely formed ventrally.

Inspect the *shaft of the penis*, noting any abnormalities on the ventral surface. Make sure the penis appears straight.

A fixed, downward bowing of the penis is a *chordee;* this may accompany a hypospadias.

Inspect the *scrotum*, noting rugae, which should be present by 40 weeks of gestation. Palpate the testes in the scrotal sacs, proceeding downward from the external inguinal ring to the scrotum. If you feel a testis up in the inguinal canal, gently milk it downward into the scrotum. The newborn's testes should be about 10 mm in width and 15 mm in length and should lie in the scrotal sacs most of the time. If infant's testicle has not descended by 6 months, he should be referred to a specialist.

In newborns with an *undescended testicle (cryptorchidism)*, the scrotum often appears underdeveloped and tight, and palpation reveals an absence of scrotal contents (see Table 23-12, p. 921).

Examine the testes for swelling within the scrotal sac and over the inguinal ring. If you detect swelling in the scrotal sac, try to differentiate it from the testis. Note whether the size changes when the infant increases abdominal pressure by crying. Two common scrotal masses in newborns are *hydroceles* and *inguinal hernias;* frequently both coexist, and both are more common on the right side. See Table 21-3, Abnormalities of the Penis and Scrotum, p. 910.

TRANSILLUMINATION OF A HYDROCELE.

From Fletcher M. *Physical Diagnosis in Neonatology.* Philadelphia, PA: Lippincott-Raven; 1998.

Hydroceles overlie the testes and the spermatic cord, are not reducible, and can be transilluminated (see photo). During transillumination of the scrotum, the light will pass through the clear fluid of the hydrocele causing the scrotum to appear red. Most hydroceles resolve by 18 months. Hernias are separate from the testes, are usually reducible, and often do not transilluminate. They do not resolve.

Female Genitalia

In the infant female, the labia majora and minora have a dull pink color in light-skinned infants and may be hyperpigmented in dark-skinned infants.

Ambiguous genitalia, involving masculinization of the female external genitalia, is a rare condition caused by endocrine disorders such as *congenital adrenal hyperplasia.*

Examine the female genitalia with the infant supine.

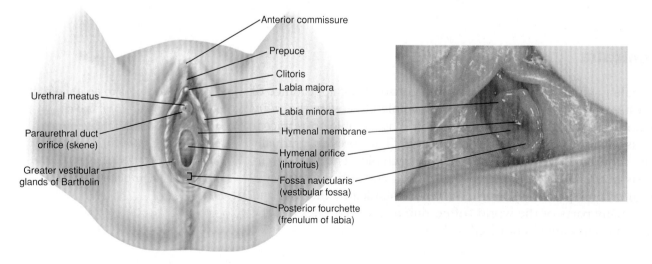

Anterior commissure
Prepuce
Clitoris
Labia majora
Urethral meatus
Labia minora
Hymenal membrane
Paraurethral duct orifice (skene)
Hymenal orifice (introitus)
Greater vestibular glands of Bartholin
Fossa navicularis (vestibular fossa)
Posterior fourchette (frenulum of labia)

Examine the different structures systematically, including the size of the clitoris, the color and size of the labia majora, and any rashes, bruises, or external lesions. Next, separate the labia majora at their midpoint with the thumb of each hand for young infants. Infants will not mind the examination because they are used to having their diapers changed and their bodies washed.

Labial adhesions occur not infrequently, tend to be paper thin, and often disappear without treatment.

Inspect the urethral orifice and the labia minora. Inspect the hymen, which in infants is a thickened, avascular structure with a central orifice, covering the vaginal opening. You should note a vaginal opening, although the hymen is thickened. Note any discharge.

An imperforate hymen may be noted at birth.

Rectal Examination

The rectal examination generally is not performed for infants or children, unless there is question of patency of the anus or an abdominal mass. Refer the patient to the pediatrician or pediatric nurse practitioner, if an imperforate anus is found.

The Musculoskeletal System

Enormous changes in the musculoskeletal system occur during infancy. Much of the examination of the infant focuses on detection of congenital abnormalities, particularly in the hands, spine, hips, legs, and feet. With a little practice, you will be able to combine the musculoskeletal examination with the neurologic and developmental examination.

Careful inspection can reveal gross deformities such as dwarfism, congenital abnormalities of the extremities or digits, and annular bands that constrict an extremity.

Palpate along the *clavicle*, noting any lumps, tenderness, or crepitus; these may indicate a fracture.

Inspect the *spine* carefully. Subtle abnormalities such as pigmented spots, hairy patches, or deep pits within 1 cm or so of the midline may overlie external openings of sinus tracts that extend to the spinal canal. Palpate the spine in the lumbosacral region, noting any deformities of the vertebrae.

Spina bifida occulta (a defect of the vertebral bodies) may be associated with defects of the spinal cord, which can cause severe neurologic dysfunction.

Examine the infant's *hips* carefully at each examination for signs of dislocation.[20,21] Positive Ortolani and Barlow tests, limited abduction, and leg-length discrepancy are signs of a dislocated hip. Positive findings need to be referred for further evaluation and possible treatment. The Ortolani maneuver moves a dislocated hip back into the acetabulum, while the Barlow maneuver will dislocate the femoral head in an unstable hip joint.

A soft audible "click" heard with these maneuvers does not prove a dislocated hip, but should prompt a careful examination.

Make sure the baby is relaxed. For the *Ortolani test,* place the baby supine with the legs pointing toward you. Flex the legs to form right angles at the hips and knees, placing your index fingers over the greater trochanter of each femur and your thumbs over the lesser trochanters. Abduct both hips until the lateral aspect of each knee touches the examining table.

ORTOLANI TEST

Signs of *developmental dysplasia of the hip are* any limitation of abduction in either or both hips and feeling a "clunk" as the femoral head, which lies posterior to the acetabulum, enters the acetabulum. A palpable movement of the femoral head back into place constitutes a *positive Ortolani sign.*

For the *Barlow test,* position the infant as you did with the Ortolani test, supine with legs flexed 90 degrees at the hips and knees with your fingers along the femur. Adduct the thighs and apply gentle downward pressure and feel for a "clunk" as the femoral head slips over the rim of the acetabulum.

BARLOW TEST

Dislocation of the femur head during the Barlow test is a sign of developmental dysplasia of the hip.

Developmental dysplasia is important to detect as early appropriate treatment has excellent outcomes.

Femoral shortening may also be seen with hip dysplasia. *The Galeazzi or Allis test will show femoral shortening.* With the child lying supine on a firm flat table or surface, flex the hips and knees and place the feet flat on the table near the buttocks. With the knees together, check the height of the knees, which should be even. If the knee height is uneven, the shorter knee will indicate the leg with hip dysplasia.

In addition to examining the hips, it is important to examine an infant's *legs and feet* to detect developmental abnormalities. Assess symmetry, bowing, and torsion of the legs. There should be no discrepancy in leg length. It is common for normal infants to have asymmetric thigh skin folds, but if you do detect asymmetry, make sure you perform the instability tests because dislocated hips are commonly associated with this finding.

Most infants are *bowlegged*, reflecting their curled-up intrauterine position.

Severe bowing of the knees can be normal, but it can also be due to **rickets** or **Blount disease.** The most common cause of bowing is tibial torsion.

Some normal infants exhibit twisting or *torsion of the tibia* inwardly or outwardly on its longitudinal axis. Parents may be concerned about a toeing in or toeing out of the foot and an awkward gait, all of which are usually normal. Tibial torsion corrects itself during the second year of life after months of weight bearing.

Pathologic tibial torsion occurs only in association with *deformities of the feet or hips.*

Now examine the feet. At birth, the feet may appear deformed from retaining their intrauterine positioning, often turned inward as shown below. You should be able to correct the feet to the neutral and even to an overcorrected position. You can also scratch or stroke along the outer edge to see if the foot assumes a normal position.

True *deformities of the feet* do not return to the neutral position even with manipulation.

The infant's foot appears flat because of a plantar fat pad. There is often inversion of the foot, elevating the outer margin. Other babies will have adduction of the forefoot without inversion, called *metatarsus adductus,* which requires close follow-up. Still others will have adduction of the entire foot. Finally, most toddlers have some pronation during early stages of weight bearing, with eversion of the foot. In all of these normal variants, the abnormal position can be easily overcorrected past midline. They all tend to resolve within 1 or 2 years.

See Table 23-13, Common Musculoskelital Findings in Young Children, p. 921. The most common severe congenital foot deformity is talipes equinovarus (talipes calcaneovalgus), or *clubfoot.*

The Nervous System

The examination of the nervous system in infants includes techniques that are highly specific to this particular age. Further, unlike many neurologic abnormalities in adults that produce asymmetric localized findings, neurologic abnormalities in infants often present as developmental abnormalities such as failure to do age-appropriate tasks. Therefore, the neurologic and developmental examinations need to proceed hand in hand. Finding a developmental abnormality should prompt you to pay particular attention to the neurologic examination.

Signs of severe neurologic disease in infants include *extreme irritability, persistent asymmetry of posture, persistent extension of extremities, constant turning of the head to one side, marked extension of the head, neck, and extremities (opisthotonus), severe flaccidity, limited response to pain,* and sometimes *seizures.*

The neurologic screening examination of all infants should include assessment of mental status, gross and fine motor function, tone, cry, deep tendon reflexes, and primitive reflexes. More detailed examination of cranial nerve function and sensory function, are indicated if you suspect any abnormalities from the history or screening.[22]

The neurologic examination can reveal extensive disease but will not pinpoint specific functional deficits or minute lesions.

Subtle neonatal behaviors such as fine tremors, irritability, and poor self-regulation may indicate *withdrawal from nicotine,* if the mother smoked during pregnancy.

Mental Status

Infants should appear alert when awake, regard faces, and attend to their parents' voices. The infant should display mental activity appropriate for his or her age.

Persistent irritability in the newborn may be a sign of *neurologic insult* or may reflect a variety of *metabolic, infectious,* or other *constitutional abnormalities,* or environmental conditions such as *drug withdrawal.*

Motor Function and Tone

Assess the *motor tone* of infants, first by carefully watching their position at rest and testing their resistance to passive movement.

Further assess *tone* as you move each major joint through its range of motion, noting any spasticity or flaccidity. Hold the baby in your hands, as shown in the photo, to determine whether the tone is normal, increased, or decreased. Either increased or decreased tone may indicate intracranial disease, although such disease is usually accompanied by a number of other signs.

Infants with *hypotonia* often lie in a frog-leg position, with arms flexed and hands near the ears. Hypotonia can be caused by a variety of *central nervous system abnormalities* and *disorders of the motor unit.*

Sensory Function

The *sensory function* of the infant can be tested in only a limited way. Test for pain sensation by flicking the infant's palm or sole with your finger. Observe for withdrawal, arousal, and change in facial expression. Do not use a pin to test for pain.

If changes in facial expression or cry follow a painful stimulus but no withdrawal occurs, weakness or *paralysis* may be present.

Cranial Nerves

The *cranial nerves* of the infant can be tested, but requires methods that differ from those used for the older child or adult. The following table provides useful strategies.

Strategies to Assess Cranial Nerves in Newborns and Infants		
Cranial Nerve		**Strategy**
I	Olfactory	Difficult to test
II	Visual acuity	Have baby regard your face and look for facial response and tracking.
II, III	Response to light	Darken room; raise baby to sitting position to open eyes. Use light and test for *optic blink reflex* (blinking in response to light). Use the otoscope light (without speculum) to assess papillary responses.
III, IV, VI	Extraocular movements	Observe how well the baby tracks your smiling face (or a bright light) and whether the eyes move together.
V	Motor	Test rooting reflex. Test sucking reflex (watch baby suck breast, bottle, or pacifier) and strength of suck.
VII	Facial	Observe baby crying and smiling; note symmetry of face and forehead.
VIII	Acoustic	Test acoustic blink reflex of both eyes in response to loud noise (blinking) Observe tracking in response to sound.

(continued)

Abnormalities in the cranial nerves suggest an intracranial lesion such as hemorrhage or a congenital malformation.

Congenital facial nerve palsy can result from birth trauma or developmental defects.

Dysphagia, or difficulty in swallowing, can occasionally be due to injury to CN IX, X, and XII.

IX, X	Swallow Gag	Observe coordination during swallowing. Test for gag reflex.
XI	Spinal accessory	Observe symmetry of shoulders.
XII	Hypoglossal	Observe coordination of sucking, swallowing, and tongue thrusting. Pinch nostrils; observe reflex opening of mouth with tip of tongue to midline.

Deep Tendon Reflexes

The *deep tendon reflexes* are variable in infants because the corticospinal pathways are not fully developed. Thus, their exaggerated presence or their absence has little diagnostic significance, unless this response is different from results of previous testing or extreme responses are observed or they are very asymmetric.

A progressive increase in deep tendon reflexes during the first year of life may indicate central nervous system disease such as *cerebral palsy,* especially if it is coupled with increased tone.

Use the same techniques to elicit deep tendon reflexes as you would for an adult. You can substitute your index or middle finger for the reflex hammer, as shown below.

As in adults, asymmetric reflexes suggest a lesion of the peripheral nerves or spinal segment.

The triceps, brachioradialis, and abdominal reflexes are difficult to elicit before 6 months of age. The *anal reflex* is present at birth and important to elicit if a spinal cord lesion is suspected.

An absent anal reflex suggests loss of innervation of the external sphincter muscle caused by a spinal cord abnormality such as a congenital anomaly (e.g., *spina bifida*), *tumor,* or *injury.*

In newborns, a *Babinski response* to plantar stimulation (dorsiflexion of big toe and fanning of other toes) can be elicited and may persist for several months. In order to best elicit the ankle reflex of an infant, grasp the infant's malleoli with one hand and quickly dorsiflex the ankle. Do not be surprised if you note rapid, rhythmic plantar flexion of the newborn's foot (*ankle clonus*) in response to this maneuver. Up to 10 beats are normal in newborns and young infants; this is *unsustained ankle clonus.*

When the contractions are continuous (*sustained ankle clonus*), *central nervous system disease* should be suspected.

Primitive Reflexes

Evaluate the infant's developing central nervous system by assessing *infantile automatisms,* called *primitive reflexes.* These develop during gestation, are generally demonstrable at birth, and disappear at defined ages. Abnormalities in these primitive reflexes suggest neurologic disease and merit more intensive investigation.[23] The most important primitive reflexes are illustrated on the next page.

A *neurologic* or *developmental abnormality* is suspected if primitive reflexes are
- Absent at appropriate age
- Present longer than normal
- Asymmetric
- Associated with posturing or twitching

Development

Refer to the developmental milestones on p. 814, or use a validated developmental assessment tool, such as the DENVER II on pages 818–820 to learn which age-specific developmental tasks to evaluate. By observation and play with the infant, you can do both a developmental screening examination and an assessment for gross and fine motor achievement. Specifically, look for *weakness* by observing sitting, standing, and transitions. Note *station,* or the posture of sitting or standing. Carefully observe the *gait* of the toddler, including balance and fluidity of movements. Fine motor development can be assessed in a similar way, combining the neurologic and developmental examination. Key milestones include the development of the pincer grasp, ability to manipulate objects with the hands, and more precise tasks, such as building a tower of cubes or scribbling. Fine and gross motor development progresses in a proximal to distal direction.

Assess the infant's cognitive and social–emotional development as you proceed with the comprehensive neurologic and developmental examination. Some neurologic abnormalities produce deficits or slowing in cognitive and social development. As stated, infants who have developmental delay may have abnormalities on the neurologic examination because much of the examination is based on age-specific norms.

Developmental delay across more than one domain (e.g., motor plus cognitive) suggests more severe disease.

Primitive Reflex

Primitive Reflex		Maneuver	Ages	
Palmar Grasp Reflex		Place your fingers into the baby's hands and press against the palmar surfaces. The baby will flex all fingers to grasp your fingers.	Birth to 3–4 months	Persistence of palmar grasp reflex beyond 4 months suggests pyramidal tract dysfunction. Persistence of clenched hand beyond 2 months suggests central nervous system damage, especially if fingers overlap thumb.
Plantar Grasp Reflex		Touch the sole at the base of the toes. The toes will curl.	Birth to 6–8 months	Persistence of palmar grasp reflex beyond 8 months suggests pyramidal tract dysfunction.
Moro Reflex (Startle Reflex)		Hold the baby supine, supporting the head, back, and legs. Abruptly lower the entire body about 2 ft. The arms will abduct and extend, hands will open, and legs flex. Baby may cry.	Birth to 4 months	Persistence beyond 4 months suggests neurologic disease (e.g., cerebral palsy); beyond 6 months strongly suggests it. Asymmetric response suggests fracture of clavicle or humerus or brachial plexus injury.
Asymmetric Tonic Neck Reflex		With baby supine, turn head to one side, holding jaw over shoulder. The arms/legs on side to which head is turned will extend while the opposite arm/leg will flex. Repeat on other side.	Birth to 2 months	Persistence beyond 2 months suggests asymmetric central nervous system development and sometimes predicts the development of cerebral palsy.

Positive Support Reflex		Hold the baby around the trunk and lower until the feet touch a flat surface. The hips, knees, and ankles extend; the baby stands up, partially bearing weight, and sagging after 20–30 seconds.	Birth or 2 months until 6 months	Lack of reflex suggests hypotonia or flaccidity. Fixed extension and adduction of legs (scissoring) suggests spasticity from neurologic disease, such as cerebral palsy.
Rooting Reflex		Stroke the perioral skin at the corners of the mouth. The mouth will open and baby will turn the head toward the stimulated side and suck.	Birth to 3–4 months	Absence of rooting indicates severe generalized or central nervous system disease.
Trunk Incurvation (Galant) Reflex		Support the baby prone with one hand, and stroke one side of the back 1 cm from midline, from shoulder to buttocks. The spine will curve toward the stimulated side.	Birth to 2 months	Absence suggests a transverse spinal cord lesion or injury. Persistence may indicate delayed development.
Stepping Reflex		Hold baby upright from behind as in positive support reflex. Have one sole touch the tabletop. The hip and knee of that foot will flex and the other foot will step forward. Alternate stepping will occur.	Birth (best after 4 days). Variable age to disappear	Absence of stepping may indicate paralysis. Babies born by breech delivery may not have stepping reflex.
Landau Reflex		Suspend the baby prone with one hand. The head will lift up, and the spine will straighten.	Birth to 6 months	Persistence may indicate delayed development.
Parachute Reflex		Suspend the baby prone and slowly lower the head toward a surface. The arms and legs will extend in a protective fashion.	4–6 months and does not disappear	Delay in appearance may predict future delays in voluntary motor development.

HEALTH PROMOTION AND COUNSELING

The AAP and an expert group, Bright Futures, recommend health supervision visits for infants and their parents when infants are the following ages: birth, at 3 to 5 days, by 1 month, and at 2, 4, 6, 9, and 12 months. This is called the *Infant Periodicity Schedule*. Health supervision visits provide opportunities to answer questions for parents, assess the infant's growth and development, perform a comprehensive physical examination, and provide anticipatory guidance. Age-appropriate anticipatory guidance includes healthy habits and behaviors, social competence of caregivers, parenting techniques, family relationships, and community interactions.

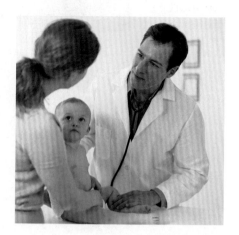

Regular visits provide an opportunity to plot a course for health and successful development. That infants generally are well during these visits, which enhances the quality of the experience. Parents are usually receptive to suggestions about health promotion which can have major, long-term influences on the child and family. Strong interviewing skills are necessary as you discuss strategies to optimize the health and well-being of their infants.

As an exercise review the critical components of a health supervision visit for a 6-month-old. Adjust the content to the appropriate developmental level of the infant.

Components of a Health Supervision Visit for a 6-Month-Old

Discussions With Parents
* Address parents' concerns/questions
* Provide advice
* Obtain social history
* Assess development, nutrition, sleep, elimination, safety, oral health, family relationships, stressors, parenting beliefs, community factors

Developmental Assessment
* Use a standardized developmental instrument to measure milestones, for example, the Denver II or the Ages and Stages Questionnaires (ASQ-3)
* Assess milestones by history
* Measure milestones by examination

Physical Examination
* Perform a careful examination, including growth parameters with percentiles for age

Screening Tests
* Vision and hearing (by examination), possibly hematocrit and lead (if high risk), screen for social risk factors

Immunizations
* See CDC schedule at http://www.cdc.gov/vaccines/schedules/index.html

Anticipatory Guidance

Healthy Habits and Behaviors
- Injury and illness prevention
  - Use infant car seat, watch for rolling, poisons, tobacco exposure, "back to sleep" position
- Nutrition
  - Breast-feeding or bottle, solids, no juice, prevent choking, overfeeding
- Oral health
  - No bottle in bed, fluoride, brushing teeth

Parent–Infant Interaction
- Promoting development (play, reading, music, talking)

Family Relationships
- Time for self; babysitters, support system

Community Interaction
- Child care, resources

The AAP recommends against the use of baby walkers, due to the many injuries sustained by children in walkers, even when the child is under adult supervision.[24]

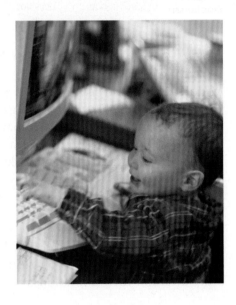

ASSESSING YOUNG AND SCHOOL-AGED CHILDREN

DEVELOPMENT

Early Childhood: 1 to 4 Years

Physical Development

After infancy, the rate of physical growth slows by approximately half. After 2 years, toddlers gain about 2 to 3 kg (4.5 to 6.5 lb) and grow 5 cm (2 in) per year. Physical changes are impressive. Chubby, clumsy toddlers transform into leaner, more muscular preschoolers.

Gross motor skills also develop quickly. Almost all children walk by 15 months, run well by 2 years, and pedal a tricycle and jump by 4 years. Fine motor skills develop through neurologic maturation and environmental manipulation. The 18-month-old who scribbles becomes a 2-year-old who draws lines and then a 4-year-old who makes circles.

Cognitive and Language Development

Toddlers move from sensorimotor learning (through touching and looking) to symbolic thinking, solving simple problems, remembering songs, and engaging in imitative play. Language develops with extraordinary speed. An 18-month-old with 10 to 20 words becomes a 2-year-old with three-word sentences, and then a 3-year-old who converses well. By 4 years, preschoolers form complex sentences. They remain preoperational, however, without sustained logical thought processes.

Social and Emotional Development

New intellectual pursuits are surpassed only by an emerging drive for independence. Because toddlers are impulsive, temper tantrums are common. Self-regulation is an important developmental task with wide range of normal.

Developmental Milestones During Early Childhood

	1 yr	2 yr	3 yr	4 yr	5 yr
Physical/ Motor	Walks	Throws	Jumps in place Balances on 1 foot	Hops Pedals tricycle	Skips Balances well
Cognitive/ Language	2-3 words	2-3 word phrases	Sentences	Speech all understandable	Copies figures Defines words
Social/ Emotional	Plays games (peek-a-boo)	Imitates activities	Feeds self	Imaginative Sings	Dresses self Plays games

Middle Childhood: 5 to 10 Years

Middle childhood is an active period of growth and development. Goal-directed exploration, increased physical and cognitive abilities, and achievements by trial and error mark this stage. The physical examination is more straightforward during at this age period, but always consider the developmental stages and tasks that school-aged children are facing.

Physical Development

Children grow steadily but more slowly. Nevertheless, strength and coordination improve dramatically, with more participation in activities. This is also when children with physical disabilities or chronic illnesses become more aware of their limitations.

Cognitive and Language Development

Children become "concrete operational"—capable of limited logic and more complex learning. They remain rooted in the present, with little ability to understand consequences or abstractions. School, family, and environment greatly influence learning. A major developmental task is self-efficacy, or the ability to thrive in different situations. Language becomes increasingly complex.

Social and Emotional Development

Children become progressively more independent, initiating activities and enjoying accomplishments. Achievements are critical for self-esteem and developing a "fit" within major social structures—family, school, and peer activity groups. Guilt and poor self-esteem also may emerge. Family and environment contribute enormously to the child's self-image. Moral development remains simple and concrete, with a clear sense of "right and wrong."

Developmental Tasks During Middle Childhood		
Task	**Characteristic**	**Health Care Needs**
Physical	Enhanced strength and coordination Competence in various tasks and activities	Screening for strengths, assessing problems Involving parents Support for disabilities Anticipatory guidance: safety, exercise, nutrition, sleep
Cognitive	"Concrete operational": focus on the present Achievement of knowledge and skills, self-efficacy	Emphasis on short-term consequences Support; screening for skills and school performance
Social	Achieving good "fit" with family, friends, school Sustained self-esteem Evolving self-identity	Assessment, support, advice about interactions Support, emphasis on strengths Understanding, advice, support

THE HEALTH HISTORY

An important and unique aspect of examining children is that parents are usually watching and taking part in the interaction, providing you the opportunity to observe the parent–child interaction. Note whether the child displays age-appropriate behaviors. Assess the "goodness of fit" between parents and child. Although some abnormal interactions may result from the unnatural setting of the examination room, others may be a consequence of interactional problems. Careful *observation* of the child's interactions with parents and the child's unstructured play in the examination room can reveal *abnormalities in physical, cognitive, and social development or issues with parent–child relationship.*

The health history of the child is similar to the infant health history on pp. 815–816, updated for the child's developmental level. A complete history and prior health care information would be obtained if the child is a new patient. Otherwise, the history is continuously updated at each visit.

Normal toddlers are occasionally terrified or angry at the examiner. Often, they are completely uncooperative. Most eventually warm up to you. If this behavior continues or is not developmentally appropriate, there may be an *underlying behavioral or developmental abnormality.* Older, school-aged children have more self-control and prior experience with nurses and are generally cooperative with the examination. You can detect a surprising amount by using observation.

Abnormalities Detected While Observing Play

Behavioral Problems*
Poor parent–child interactions
Sibling rivalry
Inappropriate parental discipline
"Difficult temperament"

Developmental Delay
Gross motor delay
Fine motor delay
Language delay (expressive, receptive)
Delay in social or emotional tasks (may use Denver II)

Social or Environmental Problems
Parental problem (e.g., stress, depression)
Risk for abuse or neglect

Neurologic Problems
Weakness
Abnormal posture
Spasticity
Clumsiness
Attentional problems and hyperactivity
Autistic features
Musculoskeletal abnormalities

---

*Note: The child's behavior during the visit may not represent typical behavior, but your observations may serve as a springboard for discussion with parents.

Assessing Younger Children

One challenge in examining children in this age group is avoiding a physical struggle, a crying child, or a distraught parent.

The child should remain dressed during the interview to minimize the child's apprehension. It also allows you to interact more naturally and observe the child playing, interacting with the parents, and undressing and dressing.

Toddlers who are 9 to 15 months may have *stranger anxiety,* a fear of strangers that is developmentally normal. It signals the toddler's growing awareness that the stranger is "new." You should not approach these toddlers quickly. Play can help the child warm up to you. Make sure they remain solidly in their parent's lap throughout much of the examination and that the parent remains close when the child is on the examination table.

The following are useful tips in examining young children.

Some Tips for Examining Young Children (1–4-Year-Olds)	
Useful Strategies for Examination	**Useful Toys and Aids**
Examine a child sitting on parent's lap. Try to be at the child's eye level.	"Blow out" the otoscope light.
First examine the child's toy or teddy bear, then the child.	"Beep" the stethoscope on your nose.
Let the child do some of the examination (e.g., move the stethoscope). Then go back and "get the places we missed."	Make tongue-depressor puppets.
Ask the toddler who keeps pushing you away to "hold your hand." Then have the toddler "help you" with the examination.	Use the child's own toys for play.
Some toddlers believe that if they cannot see you, then you are not there. Perform the examination while the child stands on the parent's lap, facing the parent.	Jingle your keys to test for hearing.
If 2-year-olds are holding something in each hand (such as tongue depressors), it is more difficult for them to fight or resist.	Shine the otoscope through the tip of your finger (or the child's finger) to show it doesn't hurt, "lighting it up," and then examine the child's ears with it.
	Use age-appropriate toys and books.

Engage children in age-appropriate conversation. Ask simple questions about their illness or toys. Compliment their appearance or behavior, tell a story, or play a simple game to "break the ice." If a child is shy, turn your attention to the parent to allow the child to warm up gradually.

With certain exceptions, physical examination does not require use of the examining table—it can be done on the floor or with the child in a parent's lap. The key is to engage the child's cooperation. For young children who resist undressing, expose only the body part being examined. When examining siblings, begin with the oldest child, who is more likely to cooperate and set a good example. Approach the child pleasantly. Explain each step as you perform it. Continue conversing with the family to provide distraction.

Plan the examination to start with the least distressing procedures and end with the most distressing (usually involving the throat and ears). Begin with parts that can be done with the child sitting, such as examining the eyes or palpating the neck. Lying down may make a child feel vulnerable, so change positions with care. Once a child is supine, start with the abdomen, saving the throat and ears or genitalia for last. A parent's help may be needed to hold the child for examination of the ears or throat; however, use of formal restraints is inappropriate. Patience, distraction, play, flexibility in the order of the examination, and a caring but firm and gentle approach are all key to successfully examining the young child.

More Tips for Examining the Young Child

- Use a reassuring voice throughout the examination.
- Let the child see and touch the examination tools you will be using.
- Avoid asking permission to examine a body part because you will do the examination anyway. Instead, ask the child which ear or which part of the body he or she would like you to examine "first."
- Examine the child in the parent's lap. Let the parent undress the child.
- If unable to console the child, give the child a short break.
- Make a game out of the examination! For example, "Let's see how big your tongue is!" or, for lung examination, "Blow out the light" using a penlight.

Reassure parents that resistance to examination is developmentally appropriate. Some embarrassed parents scold the child, compounding the problem. Involve parents in the examination. Learn which techniques and approaches work best and are most comfortable for you.

Assessing Older Children

Many children at this age are modest. Providing gowns and leaving underwear in place as long as possible are wise approaches. Suggest that children disrobe behind a curtain. Consider leaving the room while they change with their parents' help. Some children may prefer opposite-sex siblings to leave, but most prefer a parent of either sex to remain in the room. Parents of children younger than 11 years should stay with them.

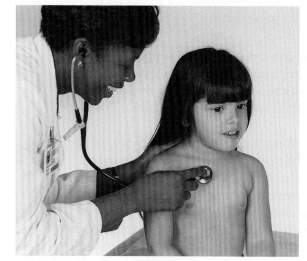

Children usually are accompanied by a parent or caregiver. Even when alone, they are often seeking health care at the request of their parents—indeed, the parent is usually sitting in the waiting room. When interviewing a child, you need to consider the needs and perspectives of both the child and the caregivers.

Establishing Rapport

Begin the interview by greeting and establishing rapport with each person present. Refer to the child by name rather than by "him" or "her." Clarify the role or relationship of all of the adults and children. "Now, are you Jimmy's grandmother?" "Please help me by telling me Jimmy's relationship to everyone here." Address the parents as "Mr. Smith" and "Ms. Smith" rather than by their first names or "Mom" or "Dad." When the family structure is not immediately clear, you may avoid embarrassment by asking directly about other members. "Who else lives in the home?" "Who is Jimmy's father?" "Do you live together?" Do not assume that just because parents are separated, only one parent is actively involved in the child's life. Families come in many varieties—these include traditional families, single parents, separated/divorced parents, blended, same-sex parents, kinship families, foster families, adoptive families.

Use your personal experiences with children to guide how you interact in a health care setting. To establish rapport, meet children on their own level. Eye contact on their level, participating in playful engagement, and talking about what interests them are always good strategies. Ask children about their clothes, one of their toys, what book or TV show they like, or their adult companion in an enthusiastic but gentle style. Spending time at the beginning of the interview to calm down and connect with an anxious child can put both the child and the caregiver at ease.

Working With Families

One challenge when several people are present is deciding to whom to direct your questions. While eventually you need to get information from both the child and the parent, it is useful to start with the child. Asking simple open-ended questions like "Are you sick? ... Tell me about it," followed by more specific questions, often provides much of the clinical data. The parents can then verify the information, add details that give you the larger context, and identify other issues you need to address. Sometimes children are embarrassed to begin, but once the parent has started the conversation, direct questions back to the child: Characterize symptom attributes the same way you do with adults.

> Your mom tells me that you get stomachaches. Tell me about them. Show me where you get the pain. What does it feel like?

Is it sharp like a pin prick, or does it ache?
Does it stay in the same spot, or does it move around?
What helps make it go away? What makes it worse?
What do you think causes it?

The presence of family members allows you to observe how they interact with the child. A child may be able to sit still or may get restless and start fidgeting. Watch how the parents set limits or fail to set limits when needed.

PHYSICAL EXAMINATION OF YOUNG AND SCHOOL-AGED CHILDREN

The order of the examination now begins to follow that used for adults. Examine painful areas last, and forewarn children about areas you are going to examine. If a child resists part of the examination, you can return to it at the end.

General Survey and Vital Signs

Somatic Growth

Height

After 2 years of age, children can be measured standing up provided they can stand up straight and remain still. Prior to measurement; shoes, hats, and hair ornaments are removed. A measuring device, such as a stadiometer, which is mounted on the wall is used. The child stands with the back of the head, shoulders, buttocks and heels, with feet together, against the wall. The patient is looking straight ahead and the head plate is at a right angle. Stand-up weight scales with a height attachment are not accurate.

Short stature, defined as height less than the 5th percentile, can be a normal variant or caused by endocrine or other diseases. Normal variants include *familial short stature* and *constitutional delay.* Chronic diseases include *growth hormone deficiency,* other endocrine diseases, *gastrointestinal disease, renal* or *metabolic disease,* and *genetic syndromes.*

Rule of thumb on height: After age 2 years, children should grow at least 5 cm (2 in) per year. *During puberty growth velocity increases.*

Weight

Young children who can stand and school-aged children should be weighed in a gown (or in clothing without shoes) on a stand-up scale. Although initially nervous, most young children can be coaxed onto such scales. Use the same scale if possible for each visit.

Young children can have inadequate weight and height gain if caloric intake is insufficient. Etiologies of failure to thrive include *psychosocial, interactional, gastrointestinal,* and *endocrine disorders.*

Head Circumference

In general, head circumference is measured until the child reaches 24 months. Afterward, head circumference measurement may be helpful if you suspect a genetic or central nervous system disorder.

Body Mass Index for Age

Age- and sex-specific charts are now available to assess BMI in children (see the following table for interpreting a child's BMI). BMI in children is associated with body fat, related to subsequent health risks for obesity. BMI measurements are helpful for early detection of obesity in children older than 2 years. Obesity is now a major childhood epidemic, and it often begins before 6 to 8 years. Consequences of childhood obesity include hypertension, diabetes, metabolic syndrome, and poor self-esteem. Childhood obesity often leads to adult obesity and shortened lifespan. It is helpful to give parents their child's BMI results together with information about the impact of healthy eating and physical activity.

Most children with exogenous obesity are also tall for their age. Children with endocrine causes of obesity tend to be short.

Childhood obesity is a major epidemic: 32% of U.S. children have a BMI greater than 85th percentile, and 17% have a BMI greater than or equal to 95th percentile.[25] Long-term morbidity from childhood obesity spans many organ systems, including cardiovascular, endocrine, renal, musculoskeletal, gastrointestinal, and psychological. Prevention, early detection, and aggressive management are needed.

Interpreting BMI in Children	
Group	**BMI for Age**
Underweight	<5th percentile
Healthy Weight	5th–85th percentile
At risk of overweight	≥85th percentile
Overweight	≥95th percentile

Vital Signs

Blood Pressure

Hypertension during childhood is more common than previously thought, and it is important to recognize, confirm, and appropriately manage it. Children have elevated blood pressure during exercise, crying, and anxiety. Although young children may be anxious at first, when the procedure is explained and demonstrated beforehand, most children are cooperative. If the blood pressure is initially elevated, you can perform blood pressure readings again at the end of the examination; one trick is to leave the cuff on the arm (deflated) and repeat the reading later. Elevated readings must always be confirmed by subsequent measurements.

A very common cause of apparent hypertension is anxiety or "white-coat hypertension." The most frequent "cause" of an elevated blood pressure in children is an *improperly performed examination*, often due to an incorrect cuff size.

A proper cuff size is essential for accurate determinations of blood pressure in children.

Select the blood pressure cuff as you would for adults. It should be wide enough to cover two thirds of the upper arm or leg. A cuff that is too narrow falsely elevates the blood pressure reading, whereas a wider cuff lowers it and may interfere with proper placement of the stethoscope diaphragm over the artery.

In children, as in adults, systolic blood pressure readings from the thigh are approximately 10 mm Hg higher than those from the upper arm. If they are the same or lower, *coarctation of the aorta* should be suspected.

With children, as with adults, *the first Korotkoff sound indicates systolic pressure and* the point at which the Korotkoff sounds disappear constitutes the diastolic pressure. If the sounds continue to be heard to 0, record three numbers, the first Korotkoff sound, fourth sound (where the sound softens and 0, e.g., 98/62/0). At times, especially among chubby young children, the Korotkoff sounds are not easily heard. In such instances, use palpation to determine the systolic blood pressure, remembering that the systolic pressure is approximately 10 mm Hg lower by palpation than by auscultation.

An electronic sphygmomanometer can be used if the Korotkoff sounds are inaudible. The child's limb must be still during the measurement. Gentle restraint may be necessary to prevent movement.

Transient hypertension in children can be caused by some common childhood medications, including those to treat asthma (e.g., prednisone) and attention deficit hyperactivity disorder (ADHD; e.g., Ritalin).

In 2004, the National Heart, Lung, and Blood Institute's National High Blood Pressure Working Group on Hypertension Control in Children and Adolescents defined normal, high-normal, and high blood pressure as follows, with measurements on at least three separate occasions.[26]

Causes of *sustained hypertension*[27] in childhood include renal parenchymal or artery disease, coarctation of the aorta, and primary hypertension. Obesity is highly associated with hypertension in childhood.

See Table 23-1, Abnormalities in Heart Rhythm and Blood Pressure, p. 908.

Blood Pressure	
Blood Pressure Category	**Average Systolic and/or Diastolic Blood Pressure for Age, Sex, and Height**
Normal	<90th percentile
Prehypertensive	90th–95th percentile
Hypertensive Stage 1 Stage 2	≥95th percentile 95th percentile to 5 mm Hg above 99th percentile ≥99th percentile plus 5 mm Hg*

*Refer to standard blood pressure tables based on age.

The epidemic of childhood obesity has also resulted in a rising prevalence of childhood hypertension.[28]

Children who have hypertension should be evaluated extensively to determine the cause. For infants and young children, a specific cause can usually be found. An increasing proportion of older children and adolescents, however, have essential or primary hypertension. In all cases, it is important to repeat measurements to reduce the possibility that the elevation reflects anxiety. Sometimes repeating measurements in school is a way to obtain readings in a more relaxed environment. Hypertension and obesity often coexist in children.

It is important not to *falsely label* a child or adolescent as having hypertension, because of the stigma of labeling, potential limitations to activities, and possible side effects of treatment.

Pulse

Average heart rates and normal ranges are shown in the table below. Measure the heart rate over a 60-second interval.

Average Heart Rate of Children at Rest		
Age (years)	Average Rate	Range (Two Standard Deviations)
1–2	110	70–150
2–6	103	68–138
6–10	95	65–125

Sinus bradycardia is a heart rate less than 100 beats per minute in infants and toddlers, and less than 60 beats per minute in children 3 to 9 years.

Respiratory Rate

The rate of respirations per minute ranges from 20 to 40 during early childhood, and 15 to 25 during late childhood, reaching adult levels at around 15 years of age.[29]

Children with respiratory diseases such as *bronchiolitis* or *pneumonia* have rapid respirations (up to 80 to 90/min) but *also* increased work of breathing such as grunting, nasal flaring, or use of accessory muscles.

For young children, observe the movements of the chest wall for two 30-second intervals or over 1 minute, preferably before stimulating them. Direct auscultation of the chest or placing the stethoscope in front of the mouth is also useful for counting respirations, but the measurement may be falsely elevated if the child becomes agitated. For older children, use the same technique as that used for adults.

The commonly accepted cutoff for tachypnea in children older than 1 year is a respiratory rate greater than 40 breaths per minute.

The best single physical finding for ruling out *pneumonia* is an absence of tachypnea.

Temperature

In children, auditory canal or temporal artery temperature recordings are preferable because they can be obtained quickly with essentially no discomfort.

Young children with infections can have extremely high fevers (up to 104°F or 40°C). Children younger than 3 years, who appear very ill with a fever, should be evaluated for possible sepsis, urinary tract infection, pneumonia, or other infectious etiology.

The Skin

After a child's first year of life, the techniques of examination are the same as those for the adult (see Chapter 9).

See Table 23-3, Warts, Lesions That Resemble Warts and Other Raised Lesions, p. 910, and Table 23-4, Common Skin Lesions During Childhood, p. 911.

The Head

In examining the head and neck, tailor your examination to the child's stage of growth and development.

Even before touching the child, carefully observe the shape of the head, its symmetry, and the presence of abnormal facies. Abnormal facies may not be apparent until later in childhood; therefore, carefully examine the face as well as the head of all children.

See Table 23-6, Diagnostic Facies in infancy and Childhood, pp. 913–914.

The Eyes

The two most important components of the eye examination for young children are to determine whether the gaze is conjugate or symmetric and to test visual acuity in each eye.

Strabismus in children requires treatment by an ophthalmologist.

Conjugate Gaze

Use the methods described in Chapter 11 for adults to assess *conjugate gaze,* or the *position and alignment of the eyes,* and the function of the extraocular muscles. The corneal light reflex test and the cover–uncover test are particularly useful in young children.

Perform the cover–uncover test as a game by having the young child watch your nose or tell you if you are smiling or not while you cover one of the child's eyes. When you uncover the eye, watch for any deviation of that eye. Repeat for the other eye. Latent strabismus is indicated by movement of either eye when uncovered.

Both *ocular strabismus* and *anisometropia* (eyes with significantly different refractive errors) can result in *amblyopia,* or reduced vision in an otherwise normal eye. *Amblyopia* can lead to a "lazy eye," with permanently reduced visual acuity if not corrected early (generally by 6 years).

Visual Acuity

It may not be possible to measure the visual acuity of children younger than 3 years who cannot identify pictures on an eye chart. For these children, the simplest examination is to assess for fixation preference by alternately covering one eye; the child with normal vision will not object, but a child with poor vision in one eye will object to having the good eye covered. In all tests of visual acuity, it is important that both eyes show the same result. If you or the parent have any doubts about visual acuity, it is wise to refer to an optometrist or ophthalmologist because this aspect of the physical examination is insensitive.

Reduced visual acuity is more likely among children who were born prematurely, and among those with other neurologic or developmental disorders.

Visual Acuity	
Age	**Acuity**
3 months	Eyes converge, baby reaches for object
12 months	~20/200
Younger than 4 years	20/40
4 years and older	20/30

Visual acuity in children 4 years and older can usually be formally tested using an eye chart with one of a variety of optotypes (characters or symbols).[30] A child who does not know letters or numbers reliably can be tested using pictures, symbols, or the "E" chart. Using the "E" chart, most children will cooperate by telling you in which direction the "E" is pointing.

Any difference in visual acuity between the eyes (e.g., 20/20 on the left and 20/30 on the right) is abnormal by age 5 years, and the patient should be referred to an ophthalmologist.

The most common visual disorder of childhood is *myopia* (abnormalities in near vision), which can be easily detected using this examination technique. Myopia can lead to reading difficulties, headaches, and school problems, as well as double vision.

Visual Fields

The *visual fields* can be examined in infants and young children with the child sitting on the parent's lap. One eye should be tested at a time with the other eye covered. Hold the child's head in the midline while bringing an object such as a toy into the field of vision from behind the child. The overall method is the same as that for adults, except that you will have to make this into a game for your patient.

The Ears

Examining the *ear canal and drum* can be difficult in young children who are sensitive and fearful because they cannot observe the procedure. If the child is not too fearful, examine the ears with the child sitting on a parent's lap. Make a game out of the otoscopic examination, or talk playfully to allay fears during the examination. It may help to place the otoscopic speculum gently into the external auditory canal of one ear and then withdraw it so the child gets used to the procedure, before the actual examination. Unfortunately, many young children need to be briefly restrained during this examination, which is why you may want to leave it for the end.

Ask the parent for a preference regarding the positioning of the child for the examination. There are two common positions—the child lying down and restrained, and the child sitting in the parent's lap. If the child is held supine, have the parent hold the arms either extended or close to the sides to limit motions. Hold the head and retract the tragus with one hand while you hold the otoscope with your other hand. If the child is on the parent's lap, the child's legs should be between the parent's legs. The parent could help by placing one arm around the child's body and using the second arm to steady the head (with the parent's hand on the child's forehead).

Tympanic Membranes

Until approximately 3 years the external auditory canal is directed downward similar to infants and the auricle must be pulled downward and backward to afford the best view. After about 3 years the ear canal assumes an adult like slope and the auricle is pulled upward and backward. Steady the child's head with one hand (your left hand if you are right-handed), and with that same hand pull on the auricle. With your other hand, position the otoscope.

Tips for Conducting the Otoscopic Examination

Use the best angle of the otoscope.
Use the largest possible speculum.
   A larger speculum allows you to better visualize the tympanic membrane and is less painful since it is not inserted as far as a smaller speculum.
Do not apply too much pressure, which will cause the child to cry.
Insert the speculum ¼ to ½ inch into the canal.
First find the landmarks.
   Be careful, as sometimes the ear canal resembles the tympanic membrane.
Note whether the tympanic membrane is abnormal.

There are two ways to hold the otoscope, as illustrated by the following photos:

- The first is with the otoscope handle pointing upward or laterally while you pull on the auricle. Hold the lateral aspect of your hand that has the otoscope against the child's head to provide a buffer against sudden movements by the patient.

- The second technique may be used because of the different angle of the auditory canal in children. Hold the otoscope with the handle pointing down toward the child's feet while you pull on the auricle. Hold the head and pull up on the auricle with one hand while you hold the otoscope with the other hand.

Acute otitis media is a common condition of childhood. A symptomatic child typically has a red, bulging tympanic membrane, with a dull or absent light reflex. Purulent material may also be seen behind the tympanic membrane. See Table 23-7, Abnormalities of the Eyes, Ears and Mouth, p. 915. The most useful symptom in making the diagnosis is ear pain, if combined with the above signs.[31,32]

Gently move and pull on the *auricle* before or during your otoscopic examination. Carefully inspect the area behind the auricle, over the mastoid bone.

With *otitis externa* (but not otitis media), movement of the auricle elicits pain.

With acute *mastoiditis,* the auricle may protrude forward and outward, and the area over the mastoid bone is red, swollen, and tender.

Formal Hearing Testing

Although formal hearing testing is necessary for accurate detection of hearing deficits in young children, you can grossly test for hearing by using the whispered voice test. To do this, stand behind the child (so that the child cannot read your lips), cover one of the child's ear canals, and rub the tragus, using a circular motion. Whisper letters, numbers, or a word and have the child repeat it; then test the other ear. This technique has relatively high sensitivity and specificity compared with formal testing.[33]

The AAP recommends that *all children older than 4 years have a full-scale acoustic screening test using standardized equipment.*[4] Even though a normal hearing screen at birth is reassuring, some hearing loss is acquired as

Younger children who fail these screening maneuvers or who have speech delay should have audiometric testing. These children may have *hearing deficits* or central auditory processing disorders.

children age and hearing loss can dramatically affect a child's language and development.

Up to 15% of school-aged children have at least mild hearing loss, emphasizing the importance of screening for hearing prior to school age.[31]

The Nose and Sinuses

Inspect the anterior portion of the nose by using a large speculum on your otoscope. Inspect the nasal mucous membranes, noting their color and condition. Look for nasal septal deviation and the presence of polyps.

Pale, boggy nasal mucous membranes are found in children with *chronic (perennial) allergic rhinitis.*

Purulent rhinitis is common in viral infections but may also be a symptom of *sinusitis.*

Foul-smelling, purulent, unilateral discharge from the nose may be due to a *foreign body* in the nose. This is particularly common among young preschool children, who tend to stick objects into any body orifice.

Nasal polyps are flesh-colored growths inside the nares. They are generally isolated findings but in some cases are present as part of a syndrome.

Maxillary sinuses are noted on x-rays by age 4 years, sphenoid sinuses by age 6, and frontal sinuses by ages 6 to 7. The sinuses of older children can be palpated as in adults, looking for tenderness.[34]

Children with purulent rhinorrhea (generally unilateral) for more than 10 days and also headache, sore throat, and tenderness over the sinuses may have *sinusitis.*

The Mouth and Pharynx

For anxious or young children, it is wise to leave this part of the examination until the end, because it may require parental assistance. The young, cooperative child may be more comfortable sitting in the parent's lap.

The accompanying figure demonstrates some tricks to getting children to open their mouths. The child who can say "ahhh" will usually offer a sufficient (albeit brief) view of the posterior pharynx so that a tongue blade is unnecessary. Healthy children are more likely to cooperate with this examination than sick children, especially if the sick child sees the tongue blade or has had previous experience with throat cultures.

If you need to use the tongue depressor, push down and pull slightly forward toward yourself while the child says "ahhh," being careful not to place the blade too far posteriorly, eliciting a gag reflex.

Examine the *teeth* for the timing and sequence of eruption, number, character, condition, and position. Abnormalities of the enamel may reflect local or general disease.

How to Get Children to Open Their Mouths (aka, "Would You Please Say 'Ahhh'?")

- Turn it into a game.
  - "Now let's see what's in your mouth."
  - "Can you stick out your *whole tongue*?"
  - "I bet you can't open your mouth *really wide*!"
  - "Let me see the inside of your teeth."
- Don't show a tongue depressor unless really necessary.
- Demonstrate first on an older sibling (or even the parent).
- Offer enthusiastic praise for opening their mouths a little, and encourage them to open even wider.

Dental caries are the most common health problem in children. They are particularly prevalent in impoverished populations and can cause both short-term and long-term problems.[35] Caries are highly treatable, but require a dental visit.

Carefully inspect the upper teeth. This is a common location for *nursing-bottle caries*. The technique, called "lift the lip," can facilitate visualization of dental caries. Gently raise the child's upper lip with your gloved thumb to visualize the outside of the upper teeth. Visualize the inside of the upper teeth by having the child look up at the ceiling with the mouth wide open.

Dental caries are caused by bacterial activity. Caries are more likely among young children who are put to bed nursing from a bottle, allowing formula to pool around the teeth ("nursing-bottle caries"). See Table 23-8, Abnormalities of the Teeth, Pharynx and Neck, p. 916.

The table below displays the common pattern of tooth eruption. In general, lower teeth erupt a bit earlier than upper teeth.

Tooth Types and Age of Eruption[36]		
	Approximate Age of Eruption	
Tooth Type	Primary (months)	Permanent (years)
Central incisor	5–8	6–8
Lateral incisor	5–11	7–9
Cuspids	24–30	11–12
First bicuspids	—	10–12
Second bicuspids	—	10–12
First molars	16–20	6–7
Second molars	24–30	11–13
Third molars	—	17–22

Staining of the teeth may be intrinsic or extrinsic. Intrinsic stains may be from tetracycline use before 8 years (yellow, gray, or brown stain). Iron preparation (black stain) is an example of extrinsic stain. Extrinsic stains can be polished off; intrinsic stains cannot. See Table 23-8, Abnormalities of the Teeth, Pharynx and Neck, p. 916.

Look for abnormalities of the position of the teeth. These include malocclusion, maxillary protrusion (*overbite*), and mandibular protrusion (*underbite*). You can demonstrate the latter two by asking the child to bite down hard while either you or the child parts the lips. Observe the true bite. In normal children, the lower teeth are contained within the arch formed by the upper teeth.

Malocclusion and misalignment of teeth can be from thumb sucking, a hereditary condition or from premature loss of primary teeth.

Carefully inspect the *tongue,* including the underside. Most children will happily stick their tongue out at you, move it from side to side, and demonstrate its color.

Common abnormalities include *coated tongue* in viral infections, and *strawberry tongue,* found in scarlet fever.

Some young children have a tight frenulum. Children who are severely "tongue-tied" might have a speech impediment. Have the child touch the tongue to the roof of the mouth to diagnose this condition, which often does not require treatment unless it interferes with eating or speech.

Note the size, position, symmetry, and appearance of the *tonsils*. The peak growth of tonsillar tissue is between 8 and 16 years (see figure in Table 23-8, p. 916). The size of the tonsils varies considerably in children and is often categorized on a scale of 1+ to 4+, with 1+ being easy visibility of the gap between the tonsils, and 4+ being tonsils that touch in the midline with the mouth wide open. The tonsils in children often appear more obstructive than they really are.

Streptococcal pharyngitis typically produces a strawberry tongue, white or yellow exudates on the tonsils or posterior pharynx, a beefy-red uvula, and palatal petechiae. See Table 23-8, Abnormalities of the Teeth, Pharynx and Neck, p. 916. Together with these signs, the most helpful historical information is exposure to strep throat infection within 2 weeks.[37]

Tonsils in children usually have deep crypts on their surfaces, which often have white concretions or food particles protruding from their depths. This does not indicate disease.

A *peritonsillar abscess* is suggested by erythema and asymmetric enlargement of one the tonsils and lateral displacement of the uvula.

Look for clues of a submucosal cleft palate, such as notching of the posterior margin of the hard palate or a bifid *uvula*. Because the mucosa is intact, the underlying defect is easily missed, but needs referral to otolaryngology.

Rarely, you may encounter a child who has a sore throat and has difficulty swallowing saliva, and who is sitting up stiffly in a "tripod" position because of throat obstruction. Do not open this child's mouth because he or she may have acute epiglottitis.

Acute epiglottitis is now rare in the United States because of immunization against *Haemophilus influenzae* type B. *Suspected epiglottitis is* contraindication to examination of the throat because of potential gagging and laryngeal obstruction.

Note the quality of the child's voice. Certain abnormalities can change the pitch and quality of the voice.

> *Bacterial tracheitis* can cause airway obstruction.
> *Tonsillitis* can be caused by bacteria, such as *Streptococcus*, or viruses. The "rocks in the mouth" voice is accompanied by enlarged tonsils with exudates.
> The epidemic of childhood obesity has resulted in many children who snore and have *sleep apnea*.
> You may note an abnormal breath odor, which may help lead to a specific diagnosis.

Halitosis in a child can be caused by upper respiratory, pharyngeal, or mouth infection; foreign body in the nose; dental disease; sinusitis and gastroesophageal reflux (among other causes).

The Neck

Beyond infancy, the techniques for examining the neck are the same as for adults. Lymphadenopathy is unusual during infancy but very common during childhood. The child's lymphatic system reaches its zenith of growth at 12 years, and cervical or tonsillar lymph nodes reach their peak size between 8 and 16 years.

Lymphadenopathy is usually from viral or bacterial infections. See Table 23-8, Abnormalities of the Teeth, Pharynx and Neck, p. 916.

The vast majority of enlarged lymph nodes in children are due to infections (mostly viral but also bacterial) and not to malignant disease, even though the latter is a concern for many parents. It is important to differentiate normal lymph nodes from abnormal ones or from congenital cysts of the neck.

Malignancy is more likely if the node is greater than 2 cm, is hard, is fixed to the skin or underlying tissues (i.e., not mobile), or is accompanied by serious systemic signs such as weight loss.

The figure on p. 834 demonstrates the typical anatomic locations of lymph nodes.

Check for *neck mobility.* It is important to ensure that the neck of all children is supple and easily mobile in all directions. This is particularly important when the patient is holding the head in an asymmetric manner, and when central nervous system disease such as meningitis is suspected.

In young children with small necks, it may be difficult to differentiate low posterior cervical lymph nodes from *supraclavicular lymph nodes* (which are always abnormal and raise suspicion for malignancy).

In children, the presence of nuchal rigidity is a more reliable indicator of meningeal irritation than the *Brudzinski sign* or *Kernig sign.* To detect nuchal rigidity in older children, ask the child to sit with legs extended on the examining table. Normally, children should be able to sit upright and touch their chins to their chests. Younger children can be persuaded to flex their necks by having them follow a small toy or light beam. You also can test for nuchal rigidity with the child lying on the examining table, as shown. Nearly all children with nuchal rigidity will be extremely sick, irritable, and difficult to examine.

Nuchal rigidity is marked resistance to movement of the head in any direction. It suggests meningeal irritation due to *meningitis, bleeding, tumor,* or *other causes.* These children are extremely irritable and difficult to console and may have "paradoxical irritability"—increased irritability when being held.

When meningeal irritation is present, the child assumes the *tripod position* and is unable to assume a full upright position to perform the chin-to-chest maneuver.

The Thorax and Lungs

As children age, lung examination becomes similar to that for adults. Cooperation is critical. Auscultation is usually easiest when a child barely notices (as when in a parent's lap). Let a toddler who seems fearful of the stethoscope play with it before touching the child's chest.

Assess the relative proportion of time spent on inspiration versus expiration. The normal ratio is about 1:1. Prolonged inspirations or expirations are a clue to disease location. Degree of prolongation and effort, or "work of breathing," are related to disease severity.

Young children asked to "take deep breaths" often hold their breath, further complicating auscultation. It is easier to let preschoolers breathe normally. Demonstrate to older children how to take nice, quiet, deep breaths. Make it a game. To accomplish a forced expiratory maneuver, ask the child to blow out candles on an imaginary birthday cake.

Older children will be cooperative for the respiratory examination and can even go through the maneuvers of assessing fremitus or listening to "E to A" changes (egophony) (see p. 348). As children grow, the evaluation by observation discussed on the previous page, such as assessing the work of breathing, nasal flaring, and grunting, becomes less helpful in assessing for respiratory pathology. Palpation, percussion, and auscultation achieve greater importance in a careful examination of the thorax and lungs.

With upper airway obstruction such as croup, inspiration is prolonged and accompanied by other signs such as stridor, cough, or rhonchi. With lower airway obstruction such as asthma, expiration is prolonged and often accompanied by wheezing.

Pneumonia in young children generally is manifested by fever, tachypnea, dyspnea, and increased work of breathing.

While *upper respiratory infections* due to viruses can cause young infants to appear quite ill, in children they present with the same signs as in adults, and children can appear well, without lower respiratory signs.

Childhood asthma is an extremely common condition throughout the world. Children with acute asthma present with varying severity and often have increased work of breathing. Expiratory wheezing and a prolonged expiratory phase, caused by reversible bronchospasm, may be heard without the stethoscope and are apparent on auscultation. Wheezes, often accompanied by inspiratory rhonchi, are most commonly caused by upper respiratory infections; these can also trigger asthma attacks.[38]

Children in respiratory distress may assume a *"tripod position"* in which they lean forward to optimize airway patency. This same position can also be caused by pharyngeal obstruction.

The Heart

The examination of the heart and vascular systems in infants and children is similar to that in adults; however, a child's fearfulness or inability to cooperate may make the examination difficult while their desire to play will make the examination easier and more productive. Use your knowledge of the developmental stage of each child. A 2-year-old may be easiest to examine while standing or sitting on the mother's lap, facing her shoulder, or being held, as shown.

Give young children something to hold in each hand. They cannot figure out how to drop one object and therefore have no hand free to push you away. Endless chatter to small children will hold their attention and they will forget you are examining them. Let older children move the stethoscope themselves, going back to listen properly. Use your imagination to make the examination work.

Benign Murmurs

Preschool and school-aged children often have benign murmurs (see figure on next page). The most common (*Still's murmur*) is a grade I–II/VI, musical, vibratory, early and midsystolic murmur with multiple overtones, located over the mid- or lower left sternal border, it may also be heard over the carotid arteries. Carotid artery compression will usually cause the precordial murmur to disappear. This murmur may be extremely variable and may be accentuated when cardiac output is increased, as occurs with fever or exercise.

In preschool or school-aged children, you may detect a *venous hum*. This is a soft, hollow, continuous sound, louder in diastole, heard just below the right clavicle. It can be completely eliminated by maneuvers that affect venous return, such as lying supine, changing head position, or jugular venous compression. It has the same quality as breath sounds and therefore is frequently overlooked.

Among young children, murmurs without the recognizable features of the two common benign sounds below may signify underlying heart disease and should be evaluated thoroughly by a pediatric cardiologist.

Pathologic murmurs that signify cardiac disease can first appear after infancy and during childhood. Examples include aortic stenosis and mitral valve disease. See Table 23-10, Congenital Heart Murmurs, pp. 918–919.

Location and Characteristics of Benign Heart Murmurs in Children

Typical Age	Name	Characteristics	Description and Location
Preschool or early school age	*Still's murmur*	I ⟋⌵⌵⌵ II	Grade I–II/VI, musical, vibratory Multiple overtones Early and midsystolic Mid-/lower left sternal border Frequently also a carotid bruit
Preschool or early school age	*Venous hum*	I ⟋⌣⌢ II II	Soft, hollow, continuous Louder in diastole Under clavicle Can be eliminated by maneuvers
Preschool and later	*Carotid bruit*	I ⢀⣀⣀ II	Early and midsystolic Usually louder on left Eliminated by carotid compression
Preschool and school age	*Pulmonary flow murmur*		Grade II–III systolic ejection Loudest at pulmonary auscultation area Harsh, nonvibratory Intensity increases when in the supine position

The Abdomen

Toddlers and young children commonly have protuberant abdomens, most apparent when they are upright. The examination can follow the same order as for adults, except the child may need to be distracted during the examination.

An exaggerated "pot-belly appearance" may indicate malabsorption from *celiac disease, cystic fibrosis,* or *constipation* or *aerophagia.*

Most children are ticklish when a hand is first placed on their abdomens for *palpation*. This reaction tends to disappear, particularly if the child is distracted with conversation and the whole hand is placed flush on the abdominal surface for a few moments without probing. For children who are particularly sensitive and who tighten their abdominal muscles, start by placing the child's hand under yours. Eventually the child's hand can be removed and the abdomen freely palpated.

Also try flexing the knees and hips to relax the child's abdominal wall, as shown. Palpate lightly in all areas, then deeply, leaving the site of potential pathology to the end.

A common condition of childhood that can occasionally cause a protuberant abdomen is constipation. The abdomen is often tympanic on percussion, and stool is often felt on palpation.

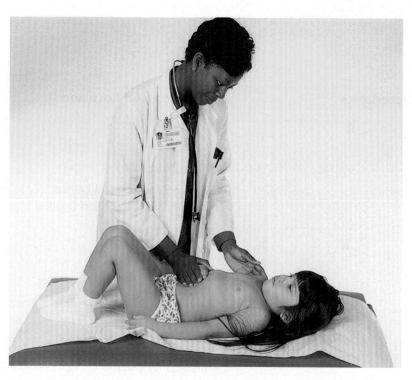

Many children present with abdominal pain from *acute gastroenteritis*. Despite pain, their physical examination is relatively normal except for increased bowel sounds on auscultation and mild tenderness on palpation.

Expected Liver Span of Children by Percussion		
	Mean Estimated Liver Span (cm)	
Age in Years	**Males**	**Females**
2	3.5	3.6
3	4.0	4.0
4	4.4	4.3
5	4.8	4.5
6	5.1	4.8
8	5.6	5.1
10	6.1	5.4

One method to determine the lower border of the liver involves the *scratch test*, shown below. Place the diaphragm of your stethoscope just above the right costal margin at the midclavicular line. With your fingernail, lightly scratch the skin of the abdomen along the midclavicular line, moving from below the umbilicus toward the costal margin. When your scratching finger reaches the liver's edge, you will hear a change in the scratching sound as it passes through the liver to your stethoscope.[39]

Hepatomegaly in young children is unusual. It can be caused by cystic fibrosis, protein malabsorption, parasites, fatty liver, and tumors.

Various diseases can cause splenomegaly, including *infections, hematologic disorders* such as *hemolytic anemias, infiltrative disorders,* and *inflammatory or autoimmune diseases,* as well as congestion from *portal hypertension.*

The *spleen,* like the liver, is felt easily in most children. It too is soft with a sharp edge, and it projects downward like a tongue from under the left costal margin. The spleen is moveable and rarely extends more than 1 cm to 2 cm below the costal margin.

Palpate the *other abdominal structures.* You will commonly note pulsations in the epigastrium caused by the aorta. This is felt most easily to the left of the midline, on deep palpation.

Palpating for abdominal tenderness in an older child is the same as for the adult; localization of tenderness may help you pinpoint the abdominal structures most likely to be causing the abdominal pain.

In a child with an acute abdomen, as in *acute appendicitis,* special techniques are helpful, such as checking for involuntary rigidity, rebound tenderness, a Rovsing sign, or a positive psoas or obturator sign (see Chapter 16, Assessing Possible Appendicitis, pp, 507–508).[40] *Gastroenteritis, constipation,* and *gastrointestinal obstruction* are other possible etiologies of acute abdominal pain.

Male Genitalia

Inspect the penis. The size in prepubertal children has little significance unless it is abnormally large. In obese boys, the fat pad over the symphysis pubis may obscure the penis.

In *precocious puberty,* the penis and testes are enlarged, with signs of pubertal changes. This is caused by a variety of conditions associated with excess androgens, including *adrenal or pituitary tumors.* Other pubertal changes also occur.

There is an art to *palpation* of the young boy's scrotum and testes because many have an extremely active cremasteric reflex that may cause the testis to retract upward into the inguinal canal and thereby appear to be undescended. Examine the child when he is relaxed because anxiety stimulates the cremasteric reflex. With warm hands, palpate the lower abdomen, working your way downward toward the scrotum along the inguinal canal. This will minimize retraction of the testes into the canal.

A useful technique is to have the boy sit cross-legged on the examining table, as shown here. You can also give him a balloon to inflate or an object to lift to increase intra-abdominal pressure. If you can detect the testis in the scrotum, it is descended even if it spends much time in the inguinal canal.

The cremasteric reflex can be tested by scratching the medial aspect of the thigh. The testis on the side being scratched will move upward.

Cryptorchidism may be noted at this age. It requires surgical correction. It should be differentiated from a retractable testis. See Table 23-12, The Male Genitourinary System, p. 921.

A painful testicle requires rapid treatment; common causes include infection such as *epididymitis* or *orchitis, torsion of the testicle,* or *torsion of the appendix testis.*

Inguinal hernias in older boys present as they do in adult men with swelling in the inguinal canal, particularly following a Valsalva maneuver.

Female Genitalia

The genital examination can be anxiety provoking for the older child and adolescent (especially if you are of the opposite sex), for parents, and for you; however, if not performed, a significant finding may be missed. Depending on the child's developmental stage, explain what parts of the body you will check, and that this is part of the routine examination.

After infancy, the labia majora and minora flatten out, and the hymenal membrane becomes thin, translucent, and vascular, with the edges easily identified.

The appearance of pubic hair before 7 years should be considered *precocious puberty* and requires evaluation to determine the cause.

The genital examination is the same for all ages of children, from late infancy until adolescence. Use a calm, gentle approach, including a developmentally appropriate explanation as you do the examination. A bright light source is essential. Most children can be examined in the supine, frog-leg position.

Rashes on the external genitals can be from various causes such as physical irritation, sweating, and candidal or bacterial infections.

If the child seems reluctant, it may be helpful to have the parent sit on the examination table with the child; alternatively, the examination may be performed while the child sits in the parent's lap. Do not use stirrups, as these may frighten the child. The following diagram demonstrates a 5-year-old child sitting on her parent's lap with the parent holding her knees outstretched.

Examine the genitalia in an efficient and systematic manner. Inspect the external genitalia for pubic hair, the size of the clitoris, the color and size of the labia majora, and the presence of rashes, bruises, or other lesions.

Next, visualize the structures by separating the labia with your fingers as shown below. *Labial adhesions*, or fusion of the labia minora, may be noted in prepubertal children and can obscure the vaginal and urethral orifices. They may be a normal variant.

A *vaginal discharge* in early childhood can be from *perineal irritation* (e.g., bubble baths or soaps), *foreign body, vaginitis,* or a *sexually transmitted disease* from sexual abuse.

Vaginal bleeding is always concerning. Etiologies include *vaginal irritation, accidental trauma, sexual abuse, foreign body,* and *tumors. Precocious puberty* from many causes can induce menses in a young girl.

Purulent, profuse, malodorous, and blood-tinged discharge should be evaluated for the presence of *infiltration, foreign body,* or *trauma.*

Sexual abuse is unfortunately far too common throughout the world. Up to 25% of women report some history of sexual abuse; while many of these do not involve severe physical trauma, some do.[41–43] See Table 23-11, Physical Signs of Sexual Abuse, p. 920.

Avoid touching the hymenal edges because the hymen is exquisitely tender without the protective effects of hormones. Examine for discharge, labial adhesions, lesions, and hygiene. A thin, white discharge (leukorrhea) is often present. A speculum examination of the vagina and cervix is not necessary in a prepubertal child unless there is suspicion of severe trauma or foreign body. An experienced gynecologist or advanced practice nurse should perform the speculum examination.

Abrasions or signs of trauma of the external genitalia can be from benign causes such as masturbation, irritants, or accidental trauma, but should also raise the possibility of *sexual abuse.*

The physical examination may reveal signs that suggest *sexual abuse,* and the examination is particularly important if there are suspicious clues in the history. Bear in mind that, even with known abuse, the great majority of examinations will be unremarkable; thus, a normal genital examination does not rule out sexual abuse.

The Rectal Examination

The rectal examination is not routine. If intra-abdominal, pelvic, or perirectal disease is suspected, the child should be referred to an advanced care provider.

The Musculoskeletal System

In older children, abnormalities of the upper extremities are rare in the absence of injury.

Toddlers may acquire *nursemaid's elbow* or subluxation of the radial head from a tugging injury. They will hold their arms slightly flexed at the elbows but will resist using their arm.

The normal young child has increased lumbar concavity and decreased thoracic convexity compared with the adult, and often has a protuberant abdomen.

Observe the child standing and walking barefoot. You can also ask the child to touch the toes, rise from sitting, run a short distance, and pick up objects. You will detect most abnormalities by watching carefully from both front and behind. To indirectly assess the child's gait pattern, you can also look at the soles of the shoes to see whether one side of the soles is worn down.

The cause of *acute limp* in childhood is usually trauma or injury although infection of the bone, joint, or muscle should be considered. In an obese child, consider *slipped capital femoral epiphysis.*

During early infancy, there is a common and normal progression from bow-leggedness (see top of next page, on the left), which begins to disappear at about 18 months of age, often followed by transition toward knock-knees. The *knock-knee pattern* (see top of next page, on the right) is usually maximal by age 3 to 4 years and gradually corrects by age 9 or 10 years.

Severe bowing of the legs (*genu varum*) may still be physiologic bowing that will spontaneously resolve. Extreme bowing or unilateral bowing may be from pathologic causes such as *rickets* or *tibia vara (Blount disease).*

The most common lower extremity pathology in childhood is injury from accidents. Joint injuries, fractures, sprains, strains, and serious ligament injuries such as anterior cruciate ligament (ACL) tears of the knee are all too common in children.

Children may *toe in* when they begin to walk. This may increase up to 4 years of age and then gradually disappear by about 10 years of age.

Inspect any child who can stand for *scoliosis,* using techniques described under "Adolescents."

Also, have the child stand straight and place your hands horizontally over the iliac crests from behind. Small discrepancies can be appreciated. If such a discrepancy is noted and you suspect leg-length discrepancy, with one iliac crest higher than the other, a clever trick is to place a book under the shorter leg; this should eliminate the discrepancy.

Test for severe hip disease, with its associated weakness of the gluteus medius muscle. Observe from behind as the child shifts weight from one leg to the other. A pelvis that remains level when weight is shifted from one foot to the other is normal or a *negative Trendelenburg sign.*[44] An abnormal positive sign is seen in *severe hip disease,* that is, the pelvis tilts toward the unaffected hip during weight bearing on the affected side (positive Trendelenburg sign).

Normal hip abductors

Weak hip abductors

NEGATIVE TRENDELENBURG SIGN

POSITIVE TRENDELENBURG SIGN

The Nervous System

Beyond infancy, the neurologic examination includes the components evaluated in adults. Again, you should combine the neurologic and developmental assessment and will need to turn this into a game with the child to assess optimal development and neurologic performance.

Perform the DENVER II, up to 6 years, as shown on pp. 818–820, or another validated developmental screening examination. Children usually enjoy this component, and you can too. Remember that the DENVER II is better at detecting delays in motor skills than in language or cognitive milestones.

Children with *spastic diplegias* will often have hypotonia as infants and then excessive tone with spasticity, scissoring, and perhaps clenched fists as toddlers and young children.

Problems with social interaction, verbal and nonverbal communication, restricted interests, and repetitive behaviors could be signs of *autism*.

Sensation

The sensory examination can be performed by using a cotton ball or cotton swab. This is best performed with the child's eyes closed. Do not use pin pricks, which may scare the child.

Gait, Strength, and Coordination

Observe the child's gait while the child is walking and, optimally, running. Note any asymmetries, weakness, undue tripping, or clumsiness. You can follow the developmental milestones to test for appropriate maneuvers such as heel-to-toe walking (photo below), hopping, and jumping. Use a toy to test for coordination and strength of the upper extremities.

In children with uncoordinated gait, be sure to distinguish *orthopedic causes* such as positional deformities of the hip, knee, or foot from *neurologic abnormalities* such as *cerebral palsy, ataxia,* or *neuromuscular conditions.*

If you are concerned about the child's strength, have the child lie on the floor and then stand up, and closely observe the stages. Most normal children will first sit up, then flex the knees and extend the arms to the side to push off from the floor and stand up.

Hand preference is demonstrated in most children by age 2. If a younger child has clear hand preference, check for weakness in the nonpreferred upper extremity.

In certain forms of *muscular dystrophy* with weakness of the pelvic girdle muscles, children will rise to standing by rolling over prone and pushing off the floor with the arms while the legs remain extended (*Gower sign*).

Deep Tendon Reflexes

Deep tendon reflexes can be tested as in adults. First demonstrate the use of the reflex hammer on the child's hand to assure the child that it will not hurt. Children love to feel their legs bounce when their patellar reflexes are tested. The child must cooperate and keep the eyes closed during some of this examination because tensing will disrupt the results. One trick is to ask the child to pretend the arms or legs "are asleep."

Children with mild cerebral palsy may have both slightly increased tone and hyperreflexia.

Development

You can ask children older than 3 years to draw a picture, copy objects as seen in the DENVER II, and then discuss their pictures to test simultaneously for fine motor coordination, cognition, and language.

Among school-aged children, the best test for development is their school performance. You can obtain school records or psychological testing results, obviating the need for the clinician to formally test an older child's development.

Cerebellar Function

The cerebellar examination can be tested using finger-to-nose and rapid alternating movements of the hands or fingers. The younger child may be slower than an adult when performing the rapid alternating movements. Children enjoy this game. Children older than 5 years should be able to tell right from left, so you can assign them right–left discrimination tasks, as is done in the adult patient.

Distinguish between isolated delays in one aspect of development (e.g., coordination or language) and more generalized delays that occur in several components. The latter is more likely to reflect global neurologic disorders such as *cognitive disabilities* that can be caused by many etiologies.

Some children with *ADHD* will have great difficulty cooperating with your neurologic and developmental examination because of problems focusing. These children often have high-energy levels, cannot stay still for extended periods, and have a history of difficulty in school or structured situations. However, other conditions may have similar symptoms so a complete history and physical examination is warranted.

Cranial Nerves

The cranial nerves can be assessed quite well using developmentally appropriate strategies, as shown in the following table:

Strategies to Assess Cranial Nerves in Young Children		
Cranial Nerve		**Strategy**
I	Olfactory	Testable in older children.
II	Visual acuity	Use Snellen chart after age 3 years.
		Test visual fields as for an adult. A parent may need to hold the child's head.

(continued)

Localizing neurologic signs are rare in children but can be caused by trauma, brain tumor, intracranial bleed, or infection.

Children with meningitis, encephalitis, or cerebral abscess can have abnormalities of cranial nerves although they also have altered consciousness and other signs.

III, IV, VI	Extraocular movements	Have the child track a light or an object (a toy is preferable). A parent may need to hold the child's head steady.
V	Motor	Play a game with a soft cotton ball to test sensation. Have the child clench the teeth and chew or swallow some food.
VII	Facial	Have the child "make faces" or imitate you as you make faces (including moving your eyebrows), and observe symmetry and facial movements.
VII	Acoustic	Perform auditory testing after age 4 years. Whisper a word or command behind the child's back and have the child repeat it.
IX, X	Swallow and gag	Have the child stick the "whole tongue out" or "say 'ah'." Observe movement of the uvula and soft palate. Test the gag reflex.
XI	Spinal accessory	Have the child push your hand away with his or her head. Have the child shrug his or her shoulders while you push down with your hands to "see how strong you are."
XII	Hypoglossal	Ask the child to "stick out your tongue all the way."

HEALTH PROMOTION AND COUNSELING

Children 1 to 4 Years

The AAP and Bright Futures periodicity schedules for children include health supervision visits at 12, 15, 18, and 24 months, followed by annual visits when the child is 3 and 4 years old.[45] An additional visit at 30 months is also recommended to assess the child's development.

During these health supervision visits, nurses address concerns and questions from parents, evaluate the child's growth and development, perform a comprehensive physical examination, and provide anticipatory guidance about healthy habits and behaviors, social competence of caregivers, family relationships, and community interactions.

This is a critical age for preventing childhood obesity: many children begin their trajectory toward obesity between ages 3 and 4. It is also important to adequately assess the child's development. Standardized developmental screening instruments are increasingly being recommended to measure the different dimensions of a child's development. Similarly, it is important to differentiate normal (but potentially challenging) childhood behavior from abnormal behavioral or mental health problems.[46]

The following box demonstrates the major components of a health supervision visit for a 3-year-old, stressing health promotion. You do not have to wait for a health supervision visit to address many of these health promotion issues—they can be addressed during other types of visits, even when the child is mildly ill.

Components of a Health Supervision Visit for a 3-Year-Old[4]

Discussions With Parents
- Address parent concerns
- Provide advice
- Assess childcare, school, social environments
- Assess major topic areas: development, nutrition, safety, oral health, family relationships, community

Developmental Assessment
- Assess milestones: gross and fine motor, personal-social, language, cognitive; use a validated developmental screening tool.

Physical Examination
- Perform a careful examination, including growth parameters with percentiles for age.

Screening Tests
Vision and hearing (formal testing at age 4), hematocrit and lead (if high risk or at ages 1–3), screen for social risk factors

See Table 23-14, The Power of Prevention: Vaccine Preventable Diseases, p. 922.

Immunizations

See schedule on the CDC website: http://www.cdc.gov/vaccines/schedules/hcp/child-adolescent.html

Anticipatory Guidance

Healthy Habits and Behaviors

- Injury and illness prevention
  Car seat, poisons, tobacco exposure, supervision of activities
- Nutrition
  Obesity assessment; healthy meals and snacks
- Oral health
  Brushing teeth; dentist visits

Parent–Infant Interaction

- Reading and fun times, child directed play, limiting screen time

Family Relationships

- Activities, babysitters

Community Interaction

- Childcare, family resources

Children 5 to 10 Years

The AAP and Bright Futures periodicity schedules for children recommend annual health supervision visits during this period.[45] As for earlier ages, these visits present wonderful opportunities to assess the child's physical, mental, and developmental health and the parent–child relationship and the child's relationships with peers and school performance. Once again, health promotion should be incorporated into all interactions with children and families—take advantage of any opportunity to promote optimal health and development and to enhance the child's involvement in normalizing activities.

In addition to discussing issues of health, safety, development, and anticipatory guidance with parents, include the child in these conversations, using age-appropriate language and concepts. For example, the child's major environment beyond the family involves school. Discuss the child's experience and perceptions of school, interactions with peers, as well as other cognitive and social activities. During these discussions, focus on healthy habits such as good nutrition, exercise, reading, stimulating activities, health sleep hygiene, screen time, and safety.

School-aged children often begin participating in organized sports. Anticipatory guidance should include the appropriate safety equipment for sports the child plays. Parent should learn the signs and symptoms for concussions, if the child plays a sport with increased risk of head injuries.

It is estimated that 20% of children in the United States are affected by at least one chronic physical disease, although the burden of chronic conditions is greater for minority populations of children.[47] In addition, 13% to 20% of children living in the United States experience a mental disorder in a given year.[48]

These children should be seen more frequently for monitoring, disease management, and preventive care. Some behaviors that become established at this age can lead to or exacerbate chronic conditions such as obesity or eating disorders. Therefore, health promotion is critical to optimize healthy habits and minimize unhealthy ones. Helping families and children with chronic diseases deal most effectively with these disorders is a key part of health promotion. For all children, the well-being of the family is critical to the child's health; thus, health promotion involves assessing and promoting the family's overall health.

The specific components of the health supervision visit for older children are the same as the components for younger children, shown in the box on pp. 887–888. "Components of a Health Supervision Visit for a 3-Year-Old." Emphasize school performance and experiences, as well as appropriate and safe sports and activities and healthy peer relationships.

ASSESSING ADOLESCENTS

DEVELOPMENT: 11 TO 20 YEARS

Adolescence can be divided into three stages: early, middle, and late. Your interview and examination techniques will vary widely depending on the adolescent's physical, cognitive, and social–emotional levels of development.

Physical Development

Adolescence is the period of transition from childhood to adulthood. The physical transformation generally occurs over a period of years, beginning at an average age of 10 in girls and 11 in boys. On average, girls end pubertal development with a growth spurt by age 14 and boys by age 16. The age of onset and duration of puberty vary widely, although the stages follow the same sequence in all adolescents. Early adolescents are preoccupied with these physical changes.

Cognitive Development

Although less obvious, cognitive changes during adolescence are as dramatic as changes in physique. Most adolescents progress from concrete to formal operational thinking, acquiring an ability to reason logically and abstractly and to consider future implications of current actions. Although the interview and examination resemble those of adults, keep in mind the wide variability in cognitive development of adolescents and their often erratic and still limited ability to see beyond simple solutions. Moral thinking becomes sophisticated, with lots of time spent debating issues. Recent evidence shows brain development (especially in the right prefrontal cortex) probably continues well into the twenties.

Social and Emotional Development

Adolescence is a tumultuous time, marked by the transition from family-dominated influences to increasing autonomy and peer influence. The struggle for identity, independence, and eventually intimacy leads to much stress, many health-related problems, and, often, high-risk behaviors. This struggle also provides you with an important opportunity for health promotion.

Developmental Tasks of Adolescence		
Task	**Characteristic**	**Health Care Approaches**
Early Adolescence (10–14-year-olds)		
Physical	Puberty (F: 10–14; M: 11–16) variable	Confidentiality; privacy
Cognitive	"Concrete operational"	Emphasis on short term
Social Identity	Am I normal? Peers increasingly important	Reassurance and positive attitude
Independence	Ambivalence (family, self, peers)	Support for growing autonomy

Middle Adolescence (15–16-year-olds)

Physical	Females more comforta-ble, males awkward	Support if patient varies from "normal"
Cognitive	Transition; many ideas, often highly emotional thinker	Problem solving; decision making, increased responsibility
Social Identity	Who am I? Much intro-spection; global issues	Nonjudgmental acceptance
Independence	Limit testing; "experimen-tal" behaviors; dating	Consistency; limit setting

Late Adolescence (17–20-year-olds)

Physical	Adult appearance	Minimal unless chronic illness present
Cognitive	"Formal operational" (for many but not all 17–20-year-olds)	Approach as an adult
Social Identity	Role with respect to others; sexuality; future	Encouragement of identity to allow growth, safety, and healthy decision making
Independence	Separation from family; toward real independence	Support, anticipatory guidance

THE HEALTH HISTORY

A complete history and prior health care information would be obtained if the adolescent is a new patient. Otherwise, the history is continuously updated at each visit as with the child's history. The key to successfully examining adolescents is a comfortable, confidential environment. This makes the examination more relaxed and informative. Consider the teen's cognitive and social development when deciding issues of privacy, parental involvement, and confidentiality.

Like most people, adolescents usually respond positively to anyone demonstrating a genuine interest in them. Show such interest early and then sustain the connection for effective communication.

Adolescents are more likely to open up when the interview focuses on them rather than on their problems. In contrast to most other interviews, *start with specific questions* to build trust and rapport and get the conversation going. The nurse has to do more talking than usual, at the beginning. A good way to start is to chat informally about friends, school, hobbies, and family. Using silence in an attempt to get adolescents to talk or asking about feelings directly is usually not a good idea.

It is particularly important to use summarization and transitional statements and to explain what will happen during the physical examination. The physical examination can also be an opportunity to engage young persons. Once rapport is established, return to more open-ended questions. At that point, make sure to ask what concerns or questions the adolescent may have. Because adolescents are often reluctant to ask their most important questions (which are sometimes about sensitive topics), ask if the adolescent has anything else to discuss. A useful phrase to use is "tell me what other questions you have." Another option is to use the phrase: "other kids your age often have questions about …"

Adolescents' behavior is related to their developmental stage, and not necessarily to chronologic age or physical maturation. Their age and appearance may fool you into assuming that they are functioning on a more future-oriented and realistic level. This is particularly true regarding "early bloomers," who look older than their age. The reverse can also be true, especially in teens with delayed puberty or chronic illness.

Issues of *confidentiality* are important in adolescence. Explain to both parents and adolescents that the best health care allows adolescents some degree of independence and confidentiality. It helps if the nurse starts asking the parent to leave the room for part of the interview when the child is age 10 or 11 years. This prepares both parents and teens for future visits when the patient spends time alone with the nurse.

Before the parent leaves, obtain relevant medical history, such as certain elements of past history, and clarify the parent's agenda for the visit. Also discuss the need for confidentiality. Explain that the purpose of confidentiality is to improve health care, not to keep secrets. Adolescents need to know that you will hold in confidence what they discuss. However, never make confidentiality unlimited. Always state explicitly that you will act on information if concerned about safety: "I will not tell your parents what we talk about unless you give me permission or I am concerned about your safety. For example, if you were to talk to me about hurting yourself or someone else or you are being hurt or bullied, I would discuss it with others."

The goal is to help adolescents bring their concerns or questions to their parents. Encourage adolescents to discuss sensitive issues with their parents and offer to be present or help. Although young people may believe that their parents would "kill them if they only knew," you may be able to promote more open dialogue. Occasionally you will encounter a parent who is very rigid and punitive. It is important to carefully assess the parents' perspective prior to further discussion, and to obtain the explicit consent of the young person.

As in middle childhood, modesty is important. The patient should remain dressed until the examination begins, and should have privacy while putting on a gown. Not all adolescents are willing to don a gown so partially uncovering as the examination proceeds to preserve the patient's modesty is important. Most adolescents older than 13 years prefer to be examined without a parent in the room, but this depends on the patient's developmental level, familiarity with the examiner, relationship with the parent, and cultural and medical issues. For younger adolescents, ask the adolescent and parent their preferences. It is advisable to have a chaperone in the room when examining a female patient's breasts or genitalia of both sexes.

The sequence and content of the physical examination of the adolescent are similar to those in the adult. Keep in mind, however, particular issues unique to adolescents, such as puberty, growth, development, family and peer relationships, sexuality, healthy decision making, and high-risk behaviors.

PHYSICAL EXAMINATION OF THE ADOLESCENT

General Survey and Vital Signs

Somatic Growth

Adolescents should wear gowns to be weighed, or have them remove their shoes and heavy clothing. This is particularly important for adolescent girls being evaluated for underweight problems. Ideally, serial weights (and heights) should use the same scale.

Both obesity and eating disorders (anorexia and bulimia) among adolescents are major public health problems, requiring frequent assessments of weight, monitoring for complications, and promoting healthy choices and self-concept.

Vital Signs

Ongoing evaluations of blood pressure are important for adolescents. The average heart rate from age 10 to 14 years is 85 beats per minute, with a range of 55 to 115 beats per minute considered normal. Average heart rate for those 15 years and older is 60 to 100 beats per minute.

Causes of sustained hypertension for this age group include *primary hypertension, renal parenchymal disease,* and *drug use.*

The Skin

Examine the adolescent's skin carefully. Many teens will have concerns about various skin lesions, such as acne, dimples, blemishes, and moles. Stretch marks have come to the forefront as an issue with the epidemic of obesity.

Adolescent acne, a very common skin condition, tends to resolve eventually but often benefits from proper treatment. It tends to begin during middle to late puberty.

Many adolescents spend considerable time in the sun and at tanning salons. You may detect this during a comprehensive health history or by noticing signs of tanning during the physical examination. This is a good opportunity to counsel adolescents about the dangers of excessive ultraviolet exposure, the need for sunscreen, and the risks of tanning salons.

Counsel older adolescents to begin performing a regular self-examination of the skin, as shown on pp. 189–191 of Chapter 9.

Moles or benign nevi may appear during adolescence. Their characteristics differentiate them from atypical nevi, discussed in Chapter 9, The Integumentary System.

Head, Ears, Eyes, Throat, and Neck

The examination of these body parts is generally the same as for adults.

The methods used to examine the eye, including testing for visual acuity, are the same as those for adults. Refractive errors become common and it is important to test visual acuity of each eye separately during the annual health supervision visit.

An adolescent with persistent fever, tonsillar pharyngitis, and cervical lymphadenopathy may have infectious mononucleosis.

The ease and techniques of examining the ears and testing the hearing approach the methods used for adults. There are no ear abnormalities or variations of normal unique to this age group.

The Heart

The technique and sequence of examination are the same as those for adults. Murmurs are a continued cardiovascular issue for evaluation.

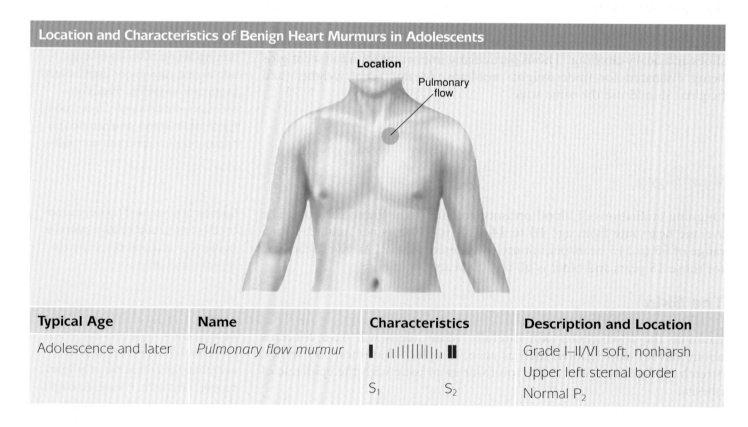

Location and Characteristics of Benign Heart Murmurs in Adolescents

Typical Age	Name	Characteristics	Description and Location
Adolescence and later	*Pulmonary flow murmur*	S_1 ‖ ⫫⫫⫫⫫ ‖ S_2	Grade I–II/VI soft, nonharsh Upper left sternal border Normal P_2

The *benign pulmonary flow murmur* is a grade I–II/VI soft, nonharsh murmur, beginning after the first sound and ending before the second sound. An adolescent with a benign pulmonary ejection murmur will have normal intensity and normally split second heart sounds.

A pulmonary flow murmur accompanied by a fixed split-second heart sound suggests right-heart volume load such as an *atrial septal defect*. See Table 23-10, Congenital Heart Murmurs, pp. 918–919.

The Breasts

Physical changes in a young girl's breasts are one of the first signs of puberty. As in most developmental changes, there is a systematic progression. Generally, over a 4-year period, the breasts progress through five stages, called Tanner stages or Tanner sex maturity rating (SMR) stages, as shown on p. 896. Breast buds in the preadolescent enlarge, changing the contour of the breasts and areola (the areola also darkens in color). These stages are accompanied by the development of pubic hair and other secondary sexual characteristics, as shown on pp. 899–900. Menarche usually occurs when a girl is in breast stage 3 or 4, and by then she has passed her peak growth spurt (see the figure on p. 900).

For years, the normal range for onset of breast development and pubic hair was 8 to 13 years (average, 11 years), with earlier onset considered abnormal.[50,52,53] Some studies suggest that the *lower age cutoff should be 7 years for white girls and 6 years for African-American and Hispanic girls.* Breast development varies by age, race, and ethnicity.[52,53] Breasts develop at different rates in approximately 10% of girls, with resultant asymmetry of size or Tanner stage. Reassurance that this generally resolves is helpful to the patient.

Masses or nodules in the breasts of adolescent girls should be examined carefully. They are usually *benign fibroadenomas* or *cysts;* less likely etiologies include *abscesses* or *lipomas.* Breast carcinoma is extremely rare in adolescence and nearly always occurs in families with a strong history of the disease.[49]

Breast asymmetry is common in adolescents, particularly when adolescents are between Tanner stages 2 and 4. This is nearly always a benign condition.

Older adolescent girls around 18 years should undergo a comprehensive breast examination with instructions for self-examination, if they would like to learn (see pp. 552–553). A second person (parent or health care provider) should be present during the examination.

Breasts in boys consist of a small nipple and areola. During puberty about one third of boys develop a breast bud 2 cm or more in diameter, usually in one breast. Obese boys may develop substantial breast tissue.

Many adolescent boys develop *gynecomastia* (enlarged breasts) on one or both sides. Although usually slight, it can be embarrassing. It generally resolves in a few years.

Sex Maturity Ratings in Girls: Breasts

Stage 1	Preadolescent. Elevation of nipple only	
Stage 2	Breast bud stage. Elevation of breast and nipple as a small mound; enlargement of areolar diameter	
Stage 3	Further enlargement of elevation of breast and areola, with no separation of their contours	
Stage 4	Projection of areola and nipple to form a secondary mound above the level of breast	
Stage 5	Mature stage; projection of nipple only. Areola has receded to general contour of the breast (although in some normal individuals, the areola continues to form a secondary mound).	

Tanner JM. *Growth at Adolescence*. 2nd ed. Oxford: Blackwell Scientific Publications; 1962. Photos from the American Academy of Pediatrics, *Assessment of Sexual Maturity Stages in Girls*, 1995.

The Abdomen

Techniques of abdominal examination are the same as for adults. The size of the liver approaches the adult size as the teen progresses through puberty, and is related to the adolescent's overall height.

Hepatomegaly in teens may be from *infections* such as hepatitis or infectious mononucleosis, inflammatory bowel disease, or tumors.

Male Genitalia

The genital examination of the adolescent boy proceeds like the examination of the adult male. Be aware of the embarrassment many boys experience during this examination.

Important anatomic changes in the male genitalia accompany puberty and help to define its progress. The first reliable sign of puberty, starting between ages 9 and 13.5 years, is an increase in the size of the testes. Next, pubic hair appears, along with progressive enlargement of the penis. The complete change from preadolescent to adult anatomy requires about 3 years, with a range of 1.8 to 5 years.[51]

Delayed puberty is suspected in boys who have no signs of pubertal development by 14 years of age.

When examining the adolescent male, assign a sexual maturity rating. The five stages of sexual development, first described by Tanner, are outlined and illustrated below. These involve changes in the penis, testes, and scrotum. In addition, in about 80% of men, pubic hair spreads farther up the abdomen in a triangular pattern pointing toward the umbilicus; this phase is not completed until the 20s.

The most common cause of delayed puberty in males is *constitutional delay,* frequently a familial condition involving delayed bone and physical maturation but normal hormonal levels.

Sex Maturity Ratings in Boys

In assigning SMRs in boys, observe each of the three characteristics separately because they may develop at different rates. Record two separate ratings: pubic hair and genital. If the penis and testes differ in their stages, average the two into a single figure for the genital rating.

	Pubic Hair	Penis	Testes and Scrotum	
Stage 1	Preadolescent—no pubic hair except for the fine body hair (vellus hair) similar to that on the abdomen	Preadolescent—same size and proportions as in childhood	Preadolescent—same size and proportions as in childhood	
Stage 2	Sparse growth of long, slightly pigmented, downy hair, straight or only slightly curled, chiefly at the base of the penis	Slight or no enlargement	Testes larger; scrotum larger, somewhat reddened, and altered in texture	
Stage 3	Darker, coarser, curlier hair spreading sparsely over the pubic symphysis	Larger, especially in length	Further enlarged	

(continued)

| Stage 4 | Coarse and curly hair, as in the adult; area covered greater than in stage 3 but not as great as in the adult and not yet including the thighs | Further enlarged in length and breadth, with development of the glans | Further enlarged; scrotal skin darkened | |
| Stage 5 | Hair adult in quantity and quality, spread to the medial surfaces of the thighs but not up over the abdomen | Adult in size and shape | Adult in size and shape | |

Tanner JM. *Growth at Adolescence*. 2nd ed. Oxford: Blackwell Scientific Publications; 1962. Photos from Wales & Wit, *Pediatric Endocrinology and Growth*. 2nd ed. Elsevier; 2003.

An important developmental principle is that physical pubertal changes progress along a well-established sequence (below). Although age ranges for start and completion are wide, the sequence for each boy is nevertheless the same. This is helpful in counseling anxious adolescents about current and future maturation and the wide range of normal for puberty. It is also helpful for detecting abnormal physical changes.

Although nocturnal or daytime ejaculation tends to begin around sexual maturity rating 3, a finding on either history or physical examination of penile discharge may indicate a *sexually transmitted disease*.

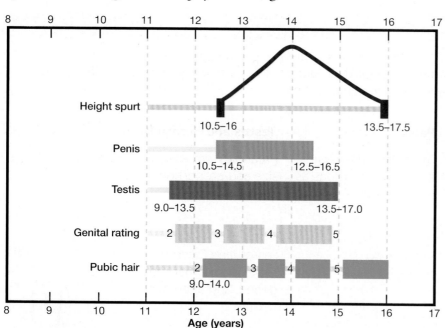

Male adolescents: *Numbers below the bars indicate the ranges in age within which certain changes occur.* (*Redrawn from* Marshall WA, Tanner JM. Variations in the patterns of pubertal changes in boys. *Arch Dis Child.* 1970;45:22.)

Observe the penis for sores and discharge as you would in an adult male.

In uncircumcised males, the foreskin should be easily retractable by adolescence. This is also an opportunity to discuss normal hygiene. Discuss testicular examination in older boys by age 18.

Female Genitalia

The external examination of adolescent female genitalia proceeds in the same manner as for school-age children. An adolescent's first pelvic examination should be performed by an experienced health care provider. If it is necessary to complete a full pelvic examination on an adolescent, the actual technique is the same as that used for an adult, including the rectal examination. A full explanation of the steps of the examination, demonstration of the instruments, and a gentle, reassuring approach are necessary because the adolescent is usually quite anxious. A parent or another health care provider must be present.

A girl's initial signs of puberty are hymenal thickening and redundancy secondary to estrogen, widening of the hips, and beginning of a height spurt, although these changes are difficult to detect. The first easily detectable sign of puberty is usually the appearance of breast buds, although pubic hair sometimes appears earlier. The average age of the appearance of pubic hair has decreased in recent years, and current consensus is that the appearance of pubic hair as early as 7 years can be normal, particularly in dark-skinned girls who develop secondary sexual characteristics at an earlier age.

Assign a sexual maturity rating to every female, irrespective of chronologic age. The assessment of sexual maturity in girls is based on both growth of pubic hair and the development of breasts. Counsel girls about this sequence and their current stage. The assessment (Tanner staging) of pubic hair growth is shown in the figure below. See p. 896 for breast development assessment.

Vaginal discharge in a young adolescent should be treated as in the adult. Causes include *physiologic leukorrhea, sexually transmitted diseases* from consensual sexual activity or *sexual abuse, bacterial vaginosis, foreign body,* and *external irritants.*

Pubertal development prior to the normal age ranges may signify *precocious puberty,* which has a variety of endocrine and central nervous system causes.

Sex Maturity Ratings in Girls: Pubic Hair	
Stage 1	Preadolescent—no pubic hair except for the fine body hair (vellus hair) similar to that on the abdomen

Stage 2	**Stage 3**
Sparse growth of long, slightly pigmented, downy hair, straight or only slightly curled, chiefly along the labia	Darker, coarser, curlier hair, spreading sparsely over the pubic symphysis

(continued)

Stage 4

Coarse and curly hair as in adults; area covered greater than in stage 3 but not as great as in the adult and not yet including the thighs

Stage 5

Hair adult in quantity and quality, spread on the medial surfaces of the thighs but not up over the abdomen

Tanner JM. *Growth at Adolescence*. 2nd ed. Oxford: Blackwell Scientific Publications; 1962.

Although there is a wide variation in the age of onset and completion of puberty, remember that the stages occur in a predictable sequence, as shown below.

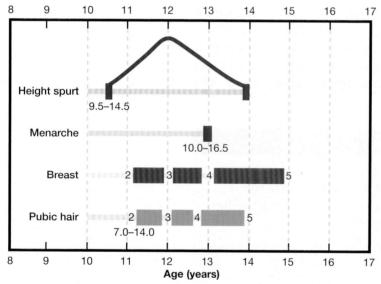

Female adolescents: *Numbers below the bars indicate the ranges in age within which certain changes occur.* (*Redrawn from* Marshall WA, Tanner JM. Variations in the pattern of pubertal changes in girls. *Arch Dis Child.* 1970;45:22.)

Delayed puberty (no breasts or pubic hair development by age 12) is usually caused by inadequate gonadotropin secretion from the anterior pituitary due to defective hypothalamic GnRH production. A common cause is anorexia nervosa.

Delayed puberty in an adolescent female below the 3rd percentile in height may be from Turner syndrome or chronic disease. The two most common causes of delayed sexual development in an extremely thin adolescent girl are anorexia nervosa and chronic disease.

Obesity in females can be associated with early onset of puberty.

Amenorrhea in adolescence can be primary (no menarche by age 16) or secondary (cessation of menses in an adolescent who had previously menstruated). While primary amenorrhea is usually due to anatomic or genetic causes, secondary amenorrhea can be due to a variety of etiologies such as *stress, excessive exercise, eating disorders, and pregnancy.*

The Musculoskeletal System

Evaluations for scoliosis and screening for participation in sports remain common components of examination in adolescents. Other segments of the musculoskeletal examination are the same as for adults.

Assessing for Scoliosis

First, examine the patient standing assessing symmetry of shoulders, scapula, and hips. Then have the child/adolescent bends forward with the knees straight and head hanging straight down between extended arms (Adams forward bend test). Next evaluate any asymmetry in positioning. Scoliosis in a young child is unusual and abnormal; mild scoliosis in an older child is not uncommon. Scoliosis appears as an asymmetrical rise in the thoracic region (as shown in the photo) or lumbar region, or both.

If scoliosis is detected, use a scoliometer to test for the degree of scoliosis. Have the teen bend forward again as described above. Place the scoliometer over the spine at a point of maximum prominence, making sure that the spine is parallel to the floor at that point, as shown above. If needed, move the scoliometer up and down the spine to find the point of maximal prominence. An angle greater than 7 degrees on the scoliometer is a reason for concern and often used as a threshold for referral to a specialist. Of note, the sensitivity and specificity of both the Adams forward bend test and scoliometer vary greatly according to the skill and experience of the examiner.

Several types of *scoliosis* may present during childhood. Idiopathic scoliosis (75% of cases), seen mostly in girls, is usually detected in early adolescence. As seen in the girl in the photo, the right hemithorax is generally prominent. Scoliosis is more common among children and adolescents with neurologic or musculoskeletal abnormalities.

A *plumb line*, a string with a weight attached, can also be used to assess symmetry of the back. Place the top of the plumb line at C-7 and have the child stand straight. The plumb line should extend to the gluteal crease (not seen here).

Apparent scoliosis, including an abnormal plumb line test, can be caused by a *leg-length discrepancy*.

The remainder of the musculoskeletal examination is similar to that for adults, except for the sports preparticipation screening examination described on p. 902.

The Sports Preparticipation Screening Evaluation

More than 25 million children and adolescents in the United States and several other countries participate in organized sports and often require "medical clearance." Start the evaluation with a thorough medical history, focusing on cardiovascular risk factors, prior surgeries, prior injuries, including concussions, other medical problems, and a family history. The complete history is the most sensitive and specific part of the evaluation for detection of risk factors or abnormalities that would preclude participation in sports. The preparticipation physical evaluation is often the only time a healthy adolescent will see a medical professional, so it is important to include some screening questions and anticipatory guidance (see the discussion in Health Promotion and Counseling). Finally, perform a general physical, with special attention to the heart and lungs and a vision and hearing screening. Include a focused, thorough musculoskeletal examination, looking for weakness, limited range of motion, and evidence of previous injury.

Important risk factors for sudden cardiovascular death during sports include episodes of *dizziness or palpitations, prior syncope* (particularly if associated with exercise), or family history of *sudden death* or cardiomyopathy in young or middle-aged relatives.

During the preparticipation sports physical, assess carefully for *cardiac murmurs* and *wheezing* in the lungs. Also, if the adolescent has had head injuries or a concussion[54] perform a careful, focused neurologic examination.[55,56] A child or adolescent should not participate in sports until all signs and symptoms of a concussion have subsided.

The Nervous System

The neurologic examination of the adolescent and the adult is the same. Still, assess the adolescent's developmental achievement according to age-specific milestones, as described on pp. 890–891.

HEALTH PROMOTION AND COUNSELING

The AAP recommends annual health supervision visits for adolescents.[45] Because adolescents tend to be seen less frequently than do younger children for any health care visit, be sure to include health promotion during all health encounters with youth. In addition, adolescents with chronic problems or high-risk behaviors may require additional visits for health promotion and anticipatory guidance.

Most chronic diseases of adults have their antecedents in childhood or adolescence. For example, obesity, cardiovascular disease, addiction (to drugs, tobacco, or alcohol), and depression are all influenced by childhood and teen experiences and by behaviors established during adolescence. More specifically, most obese adults were obese as adolescents or had abnormal indicators such as elevated BMI scores. Almost all adults who are addicted to tobacco began their tobacco habits before 18 years. Therefore, a major component of health promotion for adolescents includes discussions about health behaviors or habits. Effective health promotion can help patients develop healthy habits and lifestyles and avoid several chronic health problems.

Because some health promotion topics involve confidential issues such as mental health, addiction, sexual behavior, and eating disorders, speak to adolescents (particularly older youth) privately during part of a visit that involves health supervision.

Components of a Health Supervision Visit for Adolescents 11–18 Years

Discussions With Parents
- Address parent concerns
- Provide advice about supervision, encouraging progressively responsible decision making
- Discuss school, activities, social interactions
- Discuss youth's behaviors and habits, mental health

Discussions With Adolescent
- *Social and Emotional Development:* mental health, friends, family
- *Physical Development:* puberty, self-concept
- *Behaviors and Habits:* nutrition, exercise, TV, video games or computer screen time, drug/alcohol, sleep
- *Relationships and Sexuality:* dating, sexual activity, forced sex
- *Family Functioning:* relations with parents and siblings
- *School Performance:* activities, strengths, goals

Physical Examination
- Perform a careful examination; note growth parameters, sexual maturity ratings

Screening Tests
- Vision and hearing, blood pressure; consider hematocrit (especially in females); assess emotional health and risk factors

Immunizations
- See schedule on the CDC website http://www.cdc.gov/vaccines/schedules/index.html

Anticipatory Guidance—Teen
Promote Healthy Habits and Behaviors:
- Injury and illness prevention Seat belts, drunk driving, helmets, sun, weapons
- Nutrition Healthy meals/snacks, healthy weight
- Oral health: dentist, brushing and flossing
- Physical activity and screen time

Sexuality:
- Confidentiality, sexual behaviors, safer sex, contraception if needed

High-Risk Behaviors:
- Prevention strategies; parent–teen interaction, peer interactions
- Communication, rules

Social Achievement:
- Activities, school, future

Community Interaction:
- Resources, involvement

Anticipatory Guidance—Parent
Positive interactions, support, safety, limit setting, family values, modeling behaviors, increased responsibility

RECORDING YOUR FINDINGS

Note the modifications necessary to accommodate reports from the small child's parent, rather than from the child.

Recording the Examination: The Pediatric Patient

3/11/xx
Brian is an active, 26-month-old boy accompanied by his mother who is concerned about his development and behavior.

Referral. None.

Source and Reliability. Mother (Mom), reliable.

Chief Complaint. Slow development and difficult behavior.

Present Illness. Brian appears to be developing more slowly than his older sister did. He uses only single words and simple phrases, rarely combines words, and appears frustrated with not being able to communicate. People understand approximately 25% of his speech. Physical development seems appropriate for his age; he can throw a ball, kick, scribble, and dress himself well. He has had no head trauma, chronic illnesses, seizures, or regression in his milestones.

Mom also is concerned about his behavior. Brian is extremely stubborn, frequently has tantrums, gets angry easily (especially with his older sister), throws objects, bites, and physically strikes others when he doesn't get his way. His behavior seems worse around Mom, who reports that he is "fine" at his childcare center. He moves from one activity to another with an inability to sit still to read or play a game. Of note, he is sometimes affectionate and cuddly. He does make eye contact and plays normally with toys. He has no unusual movements.

Brian is an extremely picky eater who eats a large quantity of junk food and little else. He will not eat fruits or vegetables and drinks enormous quantities of juice and soda. His mother has tried everything to get him to eat healthy food, to no avail.

The family has been under substantial stress during the past year because Brian's father has been unemployed. Although Brian now has Medicaid insurance, the parents are uninsured.

Brian's sleep pattern appears normal for his age.

Medications. One multivitamin daily.

Past History

Pregnancy. Uneventful. Mom reduced tobacco intake to a half-pack a day and drank a glass of wine once a month. She denies use of other drugs or any infections.

Newborn Period. Born vaginally at 40 weeks; left the hospital in 2 days. Birth weight 2.5 kg (5 lb, 8 oz). Mom does not know why Brian was small at birth.

Illnesses. Only minor illnesses; no hospitalizations.

Accidents. Required sutures last year for a facial laceration secondary to a fall on the road. He did not lose consciousness and had no sequelae.

Preventive Care. Regular preventive check-ups. Six months ago, his regular physician said that Brian was a bit behind on some developmental milestones and suggested a childcare center and increased parental attention to reading, speaking, playing, and stimulation. Immunizations up-to-date. Lead level was elevated mildly last year, and Mom reports he had "low blood." Physician recommended iron supplements and foods high in iron, but Brian won't eat these foods.

Family History

Family history of: diabetes (maternal grandmother and paternal grandfather, both diagnosed after 60 years of age), hypertension (paternal grandfather). No family history of childhood developmental, psychiatric, or chronic illnesses.

Developmental History. Sat up at 6 months, crawled at 9 months, and walked at 13 months. First words ("mama" and "car") said at approximately 1 year.

Personal and Social History. Parents are married and live with the two children in a rented single family house. Dad has not had a steady job for 1 year but has worked intermittently in construction. Mom works as a waitress part-time while Brian is in childcare.

Mom had depression during Brian's first year and attended some counseling sessions, but stopped because she could not pay for them or medications. She gets support from her mother who lives 30 minutes away, and many friends, some of whom babysit occasionally.

Despite substantial family stress, Mom describes a loving and intact family. They try to eat dinner together daily, limit television, read to both children (although Brian won't sit still), and go to the nearby park regularly to play.

Environmental Exposures. Both parents smoke, although generally outside the house.

Safety. Mom reports this as a major concern: she can barely leave Brian out of her sight without him getting into something. She fears he will run in front of a car; the family is thinking of fencing in their small yard. Brian sits in his car seat most of the time; smoke detectors work in the home. Guns are locked; medications are in a cabinet in the parents' bedroom; childproof cabinet locks on cabinets with cleaning supplies.

Review of Systems

General. Denies major illnesses.

Skin. Dry and itchy. Last year hydrocortisone prescribed, which relieved the itching.

Head, Eyes, Ears, Nose, and Throat (HEENT). *Head:* Denies trauma. *Eyes:* Vision "fine." *Ears:* Multiple infections in the past year. Frequently ignores parents' requests; they can't tell if this is purposeful or if he can't hear well. *Nose:* Often runny; Mom wonders about allergies. *Mouth:* No dentist visit yet. Brushes teeth sometimes (a frequent source of dispute).

Neck. Denies lumps but glands in neck seem "large."

Respiratory. Frequent cough and whistle in chest. Mom cannot identify trigger; it tends to go away. He can run around all day without seeming to get tired.

Cardiovascular. No known heart disease. Murmur when younger, but it "went away."

Gastrointestinal. Appetite and eating habits described above. Daily bowel movements. In the process of toilet training and wears pull-ups at night and underwear during day.

Urinary. Good stream. Denies prior urinary tract infections.

Genital. Appropriate for age.

Musculoskeletal. He is "all boy" and never gets tired. Minor bumps and bruises occasionally; denies fractures and pain.

Neurologic. Walks and runs well; seems coordinated for age. Denies stiffness, seizures, or fainting. Mom says his memory seems great, but his attention span is "poor."

Psychiatric. Generally seems happy. Cries easily; bounces back and forth from trying to be independent to needing cuddling and comforting.

Physical Examination

Active and energetic toddler. Plays with reflex hammer, pretending it is a truck. Appears closely bonded with his mother, looking at her occasionally for comfort. She seems concerned that Brian will break something. His face and clothes are clean.

Vital Signs. Ht 90 cm (90th percentile). Wt 16 kg (greater than 95th percentile). BMI 19.8 (greater than 95th percentile). Head circumference 50 cm (75th percentile). Blood pressure 108/58. Heart rate 90 and regular. Respiratory rate 30; varies with activity. Temperature (temporal artery) 37.5°C. No obvious pain.

Skin. Olive, visible bruises on anterior legs; patchy, dry skin over external surface of elbows; elastic, turgor less than 2 seconds.

HEENT. *Head:* Normocephalic; no lesions. *Eyes:* Difficult to examine due to movement. Symmetric with equal extraocular movements bilaterally. Pupils 4 to 5 mm and symmetrically reactive to light. Discs difficult to visualize; no hemorrhages noted. *Ears:* Auricle, no external lesions. External canals and tympanic membranes (TMs) without exudate, cerumen, or foreign objects bilaterally. *Nose:* Nares equal; septum midline. *Mouth:* Several darkened teeth (inside surface of upper incisors). One cavity on upper right incisor. Tongue pink, midline, full range of motion. Cobblestoning of posterior pharynx; no exudates. Tonsils +3/4, pink. No allergic shiners.

When the posterior pharynx is *bumpy,* like a cobblestone street, it may be described as being cobblestoned.

Neck. Supple, midline trachea, thyroid not palpable.

Lymph Nodes. 0.5-cm tonsillar lymph nodes bilaterally. 0.5-cm inguinal nodes bilaterally. Palpable lymph nodes round, mobile, and nontender.

Lungs. Equal expansion. No tachypnea or dyspnea. Congestion audible, but seems to be upper airway (louder near mouth, symmetric). No rhonchi, rales, or wheezes. Clear to auscultation.

Cardiovascular. Apical impulse in 4th intercostal space medial to the MCL. Positive S_1 and S_2, regular rhythm. No murmurs or abnormal heart sounds. Femoral pulses and dorsalis pedis pulses 2+ bilaterally.

Breasts. Minimal fat bilaterally.

Abdomen. Protuberant, soft; no masses or tenderness. Liver span 2 cm below right costal margin (RCM) and not tender. Spleen and kidneys not palpable.

Genitalia. Tanner I circumcised penis; no pubic hair, lesions, or discharge. Testes descended, difficult to palpate because of active cremasteric reflex. Scrotum equal bilaterally.

Musculoskeletal. FROM of upper and lower extremities and all joints BL. Spine straight. Gait coordinated, wide based.

Neurologic. *Mental Status:* Happy, cooperative, active child. *Developmental (DENVER II):* Gross motor—Jumps and throws objects. Fine motor—Imitates vertical line. Language—Does not combine words; single words only, three to four noted during examination. Personal-social—Washes face, brushes teeth, and puts on shirt. Overall—At level, except for language, which appears delayed. *Cranial Nerves:* Intact, although several difficult to elicit. *Cerebellar:* Gait age appropriate with steady balance and opposite arm swing. *Deep tendon reflexes (DTRs):* 2+ and symmetric throughout with plantar response BL. *Sensory:* Deferred.

TABLE
23-1

Abnormalities in Heart Rhythm and Blood Pressure

Supraventricular Tachycardia

Paroxysmal supraventricular tachycardia (SVT) is the most common dysrhythmia in children. Some infants with SVT look well or may be somewhat pale with tachypnea, but have a heart rate of 240 beats per minute or greater. Others are ill and in cardiovascular collapse.

SVT in infants is usually sustained, requiring medical therapy for conversion to a normal rate and rhythm. In older children, it is more likely to be truly paroxysmal, with episodes of varying duration and frequency.

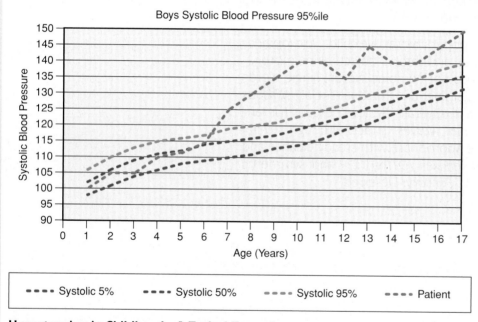

Hypertension in Childhood—A Typical Example

Hypertension can start in childhood.[26] While elevated blood pressure in young children is more likely to have a renal, cardiac, or endocrine cause, adolescents with hypertension are most likely to have primary or essential hypertension.

This child developed hypertension and it "tracked" into adulthood. Children tend to remain in the same percentile for blood pressure as they grow. This tracking of blood pressure continues into adulthood, supporting the concept that adult essential hypertension often begins during childhood.

The consequences of untreated hypertension can be severe and include cardiac, renal, and visual sequelae.

TABLE
23-2

Common Skin Rashes and Skin Findings in Newborns and Infants

Erythema Toxicum
These common yellow or white pustules are surrounded by a red base.

Neonatal Acne
Red pustules and papules are most prominent over the cheeks and nose of some normal newborns.

Seborrhea
The salmon red, scaly eruption often involves the face, neck, axilla, diaper area, and behind the ears.

Body and Extremities

Atopic Dermatitis (Eczema)
Erythema, scaling, dry skin, and intense itching characterize this condition.

Neurofibromatosis
Characteristic features include more than 5 café-au-lait spots. Later findings include axillary freckling, neurofibromas and Lish nodules (not shown).

Diaper Region

Candidal Diaper Dermatitis
This bright red rash involves the intertriginous folds, with small "satellite lesions" along the edges.

Contact Diaper Dermatitis
This irritant rash is secondary to diarrhea or irritation and is noted along contact areas (here, the area touching the diaper).

Impetigo
This infection is due to bacteria and can appear bullous or crusty and yellowed with some pus.

TABLE
23-3

Warts, Lesions That Resemble Warts, and Other Raised Lesions

Verruca Vulgaris
Dry, rough warts on hands

Verruca Plana
Small, flat warts

Plantar Warts
Tender warts on feet

Molluscum Contagiosum
Dome-shaped, fleshy lesions

Adolescent Acne
Acne in adolescents involves open comedones (blackheads) and closed comedones (whiteheads) shown at the left, and inflamed pustules (right).

TABLE
23-4

Common Skin Lesions During Childhood

Insect Bites
Intensely pruritic, red, distinct papules characterize these lesions.

Urticaria (Hives)
This pruritic, allergic sensitivity reaction changes shape quickly.

Tinea Capitis
Scaling, crusting, and hair loss are seen in the scalp, along with a painful plaque (kerion) and occipital lymph node (*arrow*).

Tinea Corporis
This annular lesion has central clearing and papules along the border.

Scabies
Intensely itchy papules and vesicles, sometimes burrows, most often on extremities

Pityriasis rosea
Oval lesions on trunk, in older children, often in a pine tree pattern, sometimes a herald patch (a large patch that appears first)

Source of bites, tinea capitis, and tinea corporis—Goodheart H. *A Photoguide of Common Skin Disorders*. Baltimore: Williams & Wilkins, 1999.

TABLE
23-5

Abnormalities of the Head

Hydrocephalus

In hydrocephaly, the anterior fontanelle is bulging, and the eyes may be deviated downward, revealing the upper scleras and creating the *setting sun* sign, as shown here. The setting sun sign is also seen briefly in some normal newborns. (From Zitelli BJ, Davis HW. *Atlas of Pediatric Physical Diagnosis.* 3rd ed. St. Louis, Mosby–Year Book; 1997. Courtesy of Dr. Albert Briglan, Children's Hospital of Pittsburgh.)

Anterior

Normal

Posterior

Craniosynostosis

Craniosynostosis is a condition of premature closure of one or more sutures of the skull. This results in an abnormal growth and shape of the skull because growth will occur across sutures that are not affected but not across sutures that are affected. The figures demonstrate different skull shapes associated with the various NAMEs of craniosynostosis. The prematurely closed suture line is noted by the absence of a suture line in each figure. Scaphocephaly and frontal plagiocephaly are the most common forms of craniosynostosis. The *blue shading* shows areas of maximal flattening. The *red arrows* show the direction of continued growth across the sutures, which is normal.

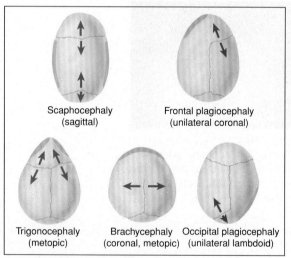

Scaphocephaly
(sagittal)

Frontal plagiocephaly
(unilateral coronal)

Trigonocephaly
(metopic)

Brachycephaly
(coronal, metopic)

Occipital plagiocephaly
(unilateral lambdoid)

Diagnostic Facies in Infancy and Childhood

Fetal Alcohol Syndrome

Babies born to women with chronic alcoholism are at increased risk for growth deficiency, microcephaly, and intellectual disability. Facial characteristics include short palpebral fissures, a wide and flattened philtrum (the vertical groove in the midline of the upper lip), and thin lips.

Congenital Hypothyroidism

The child with congenital hypothyroidism (*cretinism*) has coarse facial features, a low-set hair line, sparse eyebrows, and an enlarged tongue. Associated features include a hoarse cry, umbilical hernia, dry and cold extremities, myxedema, mottled skin, and intellectual disability. Most infants with congenital hypothyroidism have no physical stigmata; this has led to screening of all newborns in the United States and most other developed countries for congenital hypothyroidism.

Congenital Syphilis

In utero infection by *Treponema pallidum* usually occurs after the 16th week of gestation and affects virtually all fetal organs. If it is not treated, 25% of infected babies die before birth and another 30% shortly thereafter. Signs of illness appear in survivors within the first month of life. Facial stigmata often include bulging of the frontal bones and nasal bridge depression (*saddle nose*), both from periostitis; rhinitis from weeping nasal mucosal lesions (*snuffles*); and a circumoral rash. Mucocutaneous inflammation and fissuring of the mouth and lips (*rhagades*), not shown here, may also occur as stigmata of congenital syphilis, as may craniotabes tibial periostitis (*saber shins*) and dental dysplasia (*Hutchinson teeth*—see Table 12-7, p. 321).

Facial Nerve Palsy

Peripheral (lower motor neuron) paralysis of the facial nerve may be from (1) an injury to the nerve from pressure during labor and birth, (2) inflammation of the middle ear branch of the nerve during episodes of acute or chronic otitis media, or (3) unknown causes (Bell palsy). The nasolabial fold on the affected left side is flattened, and the eye does not close. This is accentuated during crying, as shown here. Full recovery occurs in ≥90% of those affected.

(table continues on page 914)

TABLE
23-6

Diagnostic Facies in Infancy and Childhood (continued)

Down Syndrome

The child with Down syndrome (trisomy 21) usually has a small, rounded head, a flattened nasal bridge, oblique palpebral fissures, prominent epicanthal folds, small, low-set, shell-like ears, and a relatively large tongue. Associated features include generalized hypotonia, transverse palmar creases (*simian lines*), shortening and incurving of the 5th fingers (*clinodactyly*), Brushfield spots (see p. 915), mild to moderate cognitive impairment.

Battered Child Syndrome

The child who has been physically abused (battered) may have old *and* fresh bruises on the head and face and may either look sad and forlorn or be actively seeking to please. Other stigmata include bruises in areas (axilla and groin) not usually subject to injury rather than the bony prominences; x-ray evidence of fractures of the skull, ribs, and long bones in various stages of healing; and skin lesions that are morphologically similar to implements used to inflict trauma (hand, belt buckle, strap, rope, coat hanger, or lighted cigarette). Of note, it is more common among abused children to note bruises on protected areas and not on bony prominences.

Perennial Allergic Rhinitis

The child suffering from perennial allergic rhinitis has an open mouth (cannot breathe through the nose) and edema and discoloration of the lower orbitopalpebral grooves ("allergic shiners"). Such a child is often seen to push the nose upward and backward with a hand ("allergic salute") and to grimace (wrinkle the nose and mouth) to relieve nasal itching and obstruction. (Photograph reproduced with permission from Marks MB. Allergic shiners: dark circles under the eyes in children. *Clin Pediatr.* 1966:5:656.)

Hyperthyroidism

Thyrotoxicosis (*Graves disease*) occurs in approximately 2 per 1,000 children younger than 10 years. Affected children exhibit hypermetabolism tachycardia, and accelerated linear growth. Facial characteristics shown in this 6-year-old girl are "staring" eyes (not true exophthalmos, which is rare in children) and an enlarged thyroid gland (*goiter*). See Table 10-4, p. 233.

TABLE
23-7
Abnormalities of the Eyes, Ears, and Mouth

Eye Abnormalities

Brushfield Spots
These abnormal speckling spots on the iris suggest Down syndrome.

Strabismus
Strabismus, or misalignment of the eyes, can lead to visual impairment. Esotropia, shown here, is an inward deviation.

Ear Abnormalities

A

B

C

Otitis Media
Otitis media is one of the most common conditions in young children. The spectrum of otitis media is shown here. **(A)** Typical acute otitis media with a red, distorted, bulging tympanic membrane in a highly symptomatic child. **(B)** Acute otitis media with bullae formation and fluid visible behind the tympanic membrane. **(C)** Otitis media with effusion, showing a yellowish fluid behind a retracted and thickened tympanic membrane. Often you can no longer visualize the normal landmarks such as the light reflex and handle of the malleus.

Mouth Abnormalities

Oral Candidiasis ("thrush")
This infection is common in infants. The white plaques do not rub off.

Herpetic Stomatitis
Tender ulcerations on the oral mucosa are surrounded by erythema.

Source of photos: *Otitis Media*—Courtesy of Alejandro Hoberman, Children's Hospital of Pittsburgh, University of Pittsburgh.

TABLE
23-8

Abnormalities of the Teeth, Pharynx, and Neck

Dental Abnormalities

Dental Caries
Dental caries is a major global health and pediatric problem. The photographs below show different characteristics of caries. White spots on the teeth (left photo) often reflect early caries.

Nursing-bottle caries

Erosion of teeth

Severe erosion

Staining of the Teeth
Various causes can lead to staining of the teeth of children, including intrinsic stains such as tetracycline (right) or extrinsic stains such as poor oral hygiene (not shown). Extrinsic stains can be removed.

Streptococcal Pharyngitis ("strep throat")
This common childhood infection has a classic presentation of erythema of the posterior pharynx and palatal petechiae (*left*). A foul-smelling exudate (*right*) is also commonly noted.

Lymphadenopathy
Enlarged and tender cervical lymph nodes are common in children. The most likely causes are viral and bacterial infections. Lymph node enlargement can be bilateral, as shown above.

Sources of photos: *Dental Caries* and *Staining of the Teeth*—Courtesy of American Academy of Pediatrics; *Streptococcal Pharyngitis* and *Lymphadenopathy*—Fleisher G, Ludwig S. *Textbook of Pediatric Emergency Medicine.* 4th ed. Philadelphia, PA: Lippincott Williams & Wilkins; 2000.

TABLE
23-9
917

Cyanosis in Children

It is important to recognize cyanosis. The best location to examine is the mucous membranes. Cyanosis is a "raspberry" color, whereas normal mucous membranes should have a "strawberry" color. Try to identify the cyanosis in these photographs before reading the captions.

Generalized Cyanosis
This baby has total anomalous pulmonary venous return and an oxygen saturation level of 80%.

Perioral Cyanosis
This baby has mild cyanosis above the lips, but the mucous membranes remain pink.

Bluish Lips, Giving Appearance of Cyanosis
Normal pigment deposition in the vermilion border of the lips gives them a bluish hue, but the mucous membranes are pink.

Acrocyanosis
This commonly appears on the feet and hands of babies shortly after birth. This infant is a 32-week newborn.

Source of photos: Fletcher M. *Physical Diagnosis in Neonatology*. Philadelphia, PA: Lippincott-Raven; 1998.

TABLE 23-10 — Congenital Heart Murmurs

Some heart murmurs reflect underlying heart disease. If you understand their physiologic causes, you will more readily be able to identify and distinguish them from innocent heart murmurs. Obstructive lesions result when blood flows through under-sized valves. Because this problem does not depend on the drop in pulmonary vascular resistance following birth, these murmurs are audible at birth. Defects with left-to-right shunts, on the other hand, depend on the drop in pulmonary vascular resistance that occurs shortly after birth. High-pressured shunts such as ventricular septal defect, patent ductus arteriosus, and persistent truncus arteriosus are not heard until 1 week or more after birth. Low-pressured left-to-right shunts, such as atrial septal defects, may not be heard until 1 year or more. Many children with congenital cardiac defects have combinations of defects or variations of abnormalities, so findings on cardiac examination may not follow these classic patterns. This table shows a limited selection of the more common murmurs, starting with murmurs that appear in the newborn period.

Congenital Defect and Mechanism	Characteristics of the Murmur	Associated Findings
Pulmonary Valve Stenosis Usually a normal valve annulus with fusion of some or most of the valve leaflets, restricting flow across the valve *Mild* *Severe* 	*Location.* Upper left sternal border *Radiation.* In mild degrees of stenosis, the murmur may be heard over the course of the pulmonary arteries in the lung fields. *Intensity.* Increases in intensity and duration as the degree of obstruction increases *Quality.* Ejection, peaking later in systole as the obstruction increases	Usually a prominent ejection click in early systole Pulmonary component of the second sounds at the base (P_2) becomes delayed and softer, disappearing as obstruction increases. Inspiration may increase murmur; expiration may increase click. Growth is usually normal. Newborns with severe stenosis may be cyanotic from right-to-left atrial shunting and rapidly develop heart failure as the ductus arteriosus closes.
Aortic Valve Stenosis Usually a bicuspid valve with progressive obstruction, but may occur as a result of a dysplastic valve or damage from rheumatic fever or degenerative disease 	*Location.* Midsternum, upper right sternal border *Radiation.* To the carotid arteries and suprasternal notch; may also be a thrill *Intensity.* Varies, louder with increasingly severe obstruction *Quality.* An ejection, often harsh, systolic murmur	May be an associated ejection click The aortic closure sound may be increased in intensity. There may be a diastolic murmur of aortic valve regurgitation (not shown in the diagram). Newborns with severe stenosis may have weak or absent pulses and severe congestive heart failure. May not be audible until adulthood even though the valve is congenitally abnormal
Tetralogy of Fallot Complex defect with ventricular septal defect, infundibular and usually valvular right ventricular outflow obstruction, malrotation of the aorta, and right-to-left shunting at ventricular septal level *With Pulmonic Stenosis* *With Pulmonic Atresia* 	*General.* Variable cyanosis, increasing with activity *Location.* Mid-to-upper left sternal border. If pulmonary atresia, there is the continuous murmur of ductus arteriosus flow at upper left sternal border or in the back. *Radiation.* Little, to upper left sternal border, occasionally to lung fields *Intensity.* Usually grade III–IV *Quality.* Mid-peaking, systolic ejection murmur	Normal pulses The pulmonary closure sound is usually not heard. May have abrupt hypercyanotic spells with sudden increase in cyanosis, air hunger, altered level of awareness Failure to gain weight with persistent and increasingly severe cyanosis Long-term persistence of cyanosis accompanied by clubbing of fingers and toes Persistent hypoxemia leads to polycythemia, which will accentuate the cyanosis.

Transposition of the Great Arteries

A severe defect with failure of rotation of the great vessels, leaving the aorta to arise from the right ventricle and the pulmonary artery from the left ventricle

General. Intense generalized cyanosis

Location. No characteristic murmur. If present, it may reflect an associated defect such as VSD.

Radiation and Quality. Depends on associated abnormalities

Single loud second sound of the anterior aortic valve

Frequent rapid development of congestive heart failure

Frequent associated defects as described at the left

Ventricular Septal Defect

Blood going from a high-pressured left ventricle through a defect in the septum to the lower-pressured right ventricle creates turbulence, usually throughout systole.

Small to Moderate

Location. Lower left sternal border

Radiation. Little

Intensity. Variable, only partially determined by the size of the shunt. Small shunts with a high-pressure gradient may have very loud murmurs. Large defects with elevated pulmonary vascular resistance may have no murmur. Grade II–IV/VI with a thrill if grade IV/VI or higher.

Quality. Pansystolic, usually harsh, may obscure S_1 and S_2 if loud enough

With large shunts, there may be a low-pitched middiastolic murmur of relative mitral stenosis at the apex.

As pulmonary artery pressure increases, the pulmonic component of the second sounds at the base increases in intensity. When pulmonary artery pressure equals aortic pressure, there may be no murmur, and P_2 will be very loud.

In low-volume shunts, growth is normal.

In larger shunts, heart failure may occur by 6–8 weeks; poor weight gain, poor feeding.

Associated defects are frequent.

Patent Ductus Arteriosus

Continuous flow from aorta to pulmonary artery throughout the cardiac cycle when ductus arteriosus does not close after birth

Small to Moderate

Location. Upper left sternal border and to left

Radiation. Sometimes to the back

Intensity. Varies depending on size of the shunt, usually grade II–III/VI.

Quality. A rather hollow, sometimes machinery-like murmur that is continuous throughout the cardiac cycle, although occasionally almost inaudible in late diastole, uninterrupted by the heart sounds, louder in systole

Full to bounding pulses

Noticed at birth in the premature infant who may have bounding pulses, a hyperdynamic precordium, and an atypical murmur

Noticed later in the full-term infant as pulmonary vascular resistance falls.

May develop heart failure at 4–6 weeks if large shunt

Poor weight gain related to size of shunt

Pulmonary hypertension affects murmur as above.

Atrial Septal Defect

Left-to-right shunt through an opening in the atrial septum, possible at various levels

Location. Upper left sternal border

Radiation. To the back

Intensity. Variable, usually grade II–III/VI

Quality. Ejection but without the harsh quality

Widely split second sounds throughout all phases of respiration, normal intensity

Usually not heard until after age of 1 year

Gradual decrease in weight gain as shunt increases

Decreased exercise tolerance, subtle, not dramatic

Heart failure is rare.

TABLE

23-11

Physical Signs of Sexual Abuse

Possible Indications

1. Marked and immediate dilatation of the anus in knee–chest position, with no constipation, stool in the vault, or neurologic disorders
2. Hymenal notch or cleft that extends greater than 50% of the inferior hymenal rim (confirmed in knee–chest position)
3. Condyloma acuminata in a child older than 3 years
4. Bruising, abrasions, lacerations, or bite marks of labia or perihymenal tissue
5. Herpes of the anogenital area beyond the neonatal period
6. Purulent or malodorous vaginal discharge in a young girl (culture and view all discharges under a microscope for evidence of a sexually transmitted disease)

Strong Indications

1. Lacerations, ecchymoses, and newly healed scars of the hymen or the posterior fourchette
2. No hymenal tissue from 3 to 9 o'clock (confirmed in various positions)
3. Healed hymenal transections, especially between 3 and 9 o'clock (complete cleft)
4. Perianal lacerations extending to external sphincter

A child with concerning physical signs must be evaluated by a sexual abuse expert for a complete history and sexual abuse examination.

Any physical sign must be evaluated in light of the entire history, other parts of the physical examination, and laboratory data.

Key to Photos

A. Acute hemorrhage and ecchymoses of tissues (10-month-old)

B. Erythema and superficial abrasions to the labia minora (5-year-old)

C. Healed interruption of hymenal membrane at 9 o'clock (4-year-old)

D. Narrowed posterior ring continuous with floor of vagina (12-year-old)

E. Copious vaginal discharge and erythema (9-year-old)

F. Extensive condylomata around the anus (2-year-old)

Source: Reece R, Ludwig S, eds. *Child Abuse Medical Diagnosis and Management*. 2nd ed. Philadelphia, PA: Lippincott Williams & Wilkins; 2001.

TABLE
23-12

The Male Genitourinary System

Hypospadias

Hypospadias is the most common congenital penile abnormality. The urethral meatus opens abnormally on the ventral surface of the penis. One form is shown above; more severe forms involve openings on the lower shaft or scrotum.

Undescended Testicle

You should distinguish between undescended testes, shown above (with testes in the inguinal canals), from highly retractile testes from an active cremasteric reflex.

Sources of photos: *Hypospadias*—Courtesy of Warren Snodgrass, MD, UT–Southwestern Medical Center at Dallas; *Undescended Testicle*—Fletcher M. *Physical Diagnosis in Neonatology*. Philadelphia: Lippincott-Raven, 1998.

TABLE
23-13

Common Musculoskeletal Findings in Young Children

Flat feet or *pes planus* from laxity of the soft-tissue structures of the foot

Inversion of the foot (*pes varus*)

Metatarsus adductus in a child. The convex ("C") shape of the child's right foot suggests metatarsus adductus.

A   **B**

Pronation in a toddler. (**A**) When viewed from behind, the hindfoot is everted. (**B**) When viewed from the front, the forefoot is everted and abducted.

TABLE
23-14

The Power of Prevention: Vaccine-Preventable Diseases

This table shows photographs of children with vaccine-preventable diseases. Childhood vaccines have been named the single most important medical intervention in the world in terms of influence on public health. Because of vaccinations, we hope you will never see many of these conditions, but you should be able to identify them. Try to identify the diseases before reading the captions.

Polio

The deformed leg of this child is from polio.

Measles

Characteristic rash of measles, in the presence of a child who also has coryza, conjunctivitis, fever, and this diffuse rash.

Rubella

Rubella rash on a child's back

Tetanus

Rigid newborn with neonatal tetanus

Haemophilus influenzae Type b

Periorbital cellulitis from this invasive bacterial disease

Meningitis

Nuchal Rigidity

Varicella

An infant with a severe form of varicella.

Pertussis

Paroxysmal cough with a "whoop" at the end.

Cervical Cancer

Largely prevented through vaccination with human papillomavirus vaccine.

Sources of photos: *Polio*—Courtesy of World Health Organization; *Haemophilus influenzae*—Courtesy of American Academy of Pediatrics; *Varicella*—Courtesy of Barbara Watson, MD, Albert Einstein Medical Center and Division of Disease Control, Philadelphia, Department of Health; all others courtesy of Centers for Disease Control and Prevention.

BIBLIOGRAPHY

CITATIONS

1. Carey WB. *Developmental-Behavioral Pediatrics.* 4th ed. Philadelphia, PA: Saunders/Elsevier; 2009.
2. Levine MD, Carey WB, Crocker AC. *Developmental-Behavioral Pediatrics.* 3rd ed. Philadelphia, PA: Saunders; 1999.
3. Clark EM. *Well-Child Care : A Bright Futures Pocket Guide for Pediatric Providers.* 1st ed. Washington, DC: Georgetown University; 2008.
4. American Academy of Pediatrics. Bright Futures. Available at https://brightfutures.aap.org/Pages/default.aspx. Accessed January 15, 2016.
5. United States Department of Health and Human Services. U.S. Preventive Services Task Force (USPSTF). Available at http://www.ahrq.gov/professionals/clinicians-providers/guidelines-recommendations/guide/. Accessed January 15, 2016.
6. Centers for Disease Control and Prevention. Immunization Schedules. Available at http://www.cdc.gov/vaccines/schedules/index.html. Accessed January 15, 2016.
7. American. Academy of Pediatrics. Immunization. Available at http://www2.aap.org/immunization/izschedule.html. Accessed January 15, 2016.
8. Johnson CP, Blasco PA. Infant growth and development. *Pediatr Rev.* 1997;18(7):224–242.
9. Colson ER, Dworkin PH. Toddler development. *Pediatr Rev.* 1997;18(8):255–259.
10. Copelan J. Normal speech and development. *Pediatr Rev.* 1995;18:91–100.
11. American Academy of Pediatrics. Developmental surveillance and screening of infants and young children. *Pediatrics.* 2001;108(1):192–196.
12. Grummer-Strawn LM, Reinold C, Krebs NF; Centers for Disease Control and Prevention (CDC). Use of World Health Organization and CDC growth charts for children aged 0–59 months in the United States. *MMWR Recomm Rep.* 2010;59:1.
13. NIH. National Heart, Lung and Blood Institute. Blood Pressure Tables for Children and Adolescents. Available at: http://www.nhlbi.nih.gov/health-pro/guidelines/current/hypertension-pediatric-jnc-4/blood-pressure-tables. Accessed January 15, 2016.
14. Fong CT. Clinical diagnosis of genetic diseases. *Pediatr Ann.* 1993;22(5):277–281.
15. Hyvarinen L. Assessment of visually impaired infants. *Ophthalmol Clin North Am.* 1994;7:219.
16. Gessner IH. What makes a heart murmur innocent? *Pediatr Ann.* 1997;26(2):82–91.
17. Frank JE, Jacobe KM. Evaluation and management of heart murmurs in children. *Am Fam Phys.* 2011;84:793–800.
18. Wierwille L. Pediatric heart murmurs: evaluation and management in primary care. *Nurse Pract.* 2011;36:22–28; quiz 8–9.
19. Callahan CW Jr, Alpert B. Simultaneous percussion auscultation technique for the determination of liver span. *Arch Pediatr Adolesc Med.* 1994;148(8):873–875.
20. Burger BJ, Burger JD, Bos CF, et al. Neonatal screening and staggered early treatment for congenital dislocation or dysplasia of the hip. *Lancet.* 1990;336(8730):1549–1553.
21. American Academy of Pediatrics. Clinical practice guideline: early detection of developmental dysplasia of the hip. Committee on Quality Improvement, Subcommittee on Developmental Dysplasia of the Hip. *Pediatrics.* 2000;105:896.
22. Zafeiriou DI. Primitive reflexes and postural reactions in the neurodevelopmental examination. *Pediatr Neurol.* 2004;31(1):1–8.
23. Schott JM, Rossor MN. The grasp and other primitive reflexes. *J Neurol Neurosurg Psychiatry.* 2003;74(5):558–560.
24. American Academy of Pediatrics. Baby Walkers: A Dangerous Choice. 2015. Available at https://www.healthychildren.org/English/safety-prevention/at-home/Pages/Baby-Walkers-A-Dangerous-Choice.aspx. Accessed January 18, 2016.
25. Ogden CL, Carroll MD, Kit BK, et al. Prevalence of obesity and trends in body mass index among US children and adolescents, 1999–2010. *JAMA.* 2012;307:483–490.
26. National High Blood Pressure Education Program Working Group on High Blood Pressure in Children and Adolescents. The Fourth Report on the Diagnosis, Evaluation, and Treatment of High Blood Pressure in Children and Adolescents. *Pediatrics.* 2004;114:555–576.
27. Ingelfinger JR. The child or adolescent with elevated blood pressure. *N Engl J Med.* 2014;370:2316–2325.
28. Falkner B. Is there a bend in the upward trend of high blood pressure in childhood?: A commentary on prevalence of and trends in dyslipidemia and blood pressure among US children and adolescents, 1999–2012. *J Am Soc Hypertens.* 2015;9(9):668–669.
29. Fleming S, Thompson M, Stevens R, et al. Normal ranges of heart rate and respiratory rate in children from birth to 18 years of age: a systematic review of observational studies. *Lancet.* 2011;377:1011.
30. Shamis DI. Collecting the "facts": vision assessment techniques: perils and pitfalls. *Am Orthop J.* 1996;46:7.
31. Rothman R, Owens T, Simel DL. Does this child have acute otitis media? *JAMA.* 2003;290:1633–1640.
32. Blomgren K, Pitkaranta A. Current challenges in diagnosis of acute otitis media. *Intl J Ped Otorhinolaryngol.* 2005;69(3):295–299.
33. Pirozzo S, Papinczak T, Glasziou P. Whispered voice test for screening for hearing impairment in adults and children: systematic review. *BMJ.* 2003;327(7421):967.
34. Wolf G, Anderhuber W, Kuhn F. Development of the paranasal sinuses in children: implications for paranasal sinus surgery. *Ann Otol Rhinol Laryngol.* 1993;102(9):705–711.
35. Tinanoff N, Reisine S. Update on early childhood caries since the Surgeon General's Report. *Acad Pediatr.* 2009;9:396–403.
36. Lunt RC, Law DB. A review of the chronology of eruption of deciduous teeth. *J Am Dent Assoc.* 1974;89:872.
37. Ebell MH, Smith MA, Barry HC, et al. Does this patient have strep throat? *JAMA.* 2000;284:2912–2918.
38. Moorman JE, Zahran H, Truman BI, et al.; Centers for Disease C, Prevention. Current asthma prevalence—United States, 2006–2008. Morbidity and mortality weekly report Surveillance summaries. 2011;60 Suppl:84–86.

39. Tucker WN, Saab S, Leland SR, et al. The scratch test is unreliable for determining the liver edge. *J Clin Gastroenterol.* 1997;25:410–414.

40. Ashcraft KW. Consultation with the specialist: acute abdominal pain. *Pediatr Rev.* 2000;21:363–367.

41. Hymel KP, Jenny C. Child sexual abuse. *Pediatr Rev.* 1996; 17(7):236–249; quiz, 249–250.

42. Maniglio R. The impact of child sexual abuse on the course of bipolar disorder: a systematic review. *Bipolar Disord.* 2013; 15:341–358.

43. Stoltenborgh M, van Ijzendoorn MH, Euser EM, et al. A global perspective on child sexual abuse: meta-analysis of prevalence around the world. *Child Maltreat.* 2011;16:79–101.

44. Bruce RW. Torsional and angular deformities. *Pediatr Clin North Am.* 1996;43:867–881.

45. AAP. 2016 Recommendations for Preventive Pediatric Health Care. *Pediatrics.* 2016;137(1):25–27.

46. Sheldrick RC, Merchant S, Perrin EC. Identification of developmental-behavioral problems in primary care: a systematic review. *Pediatrics.* 2011;128:356.

47. Kitsantas P, Kornides ML, Cantiello J, et al. Chronic physical health conditions among children of different racial/ethnic backgrounds. *Public Health.* 2013;127(6):546–553.

48. Perou R, Bitsko RH, Blumberg SJ, et al. Mental Health Surveillance Among Children—United States, 2005–2011. *MMWR Suppl.* 2013;62(02):1–35.

49. ACOG Committee on Adolescent Health Care. ACOG Committee. Opinion no. 350, November 2006: Breast concerns in the adolescent. *Obstet Gynecol.* 2006;108(5):1329–1336.

50. Herman-Giddens ME, Slora EJ, Wasserman RC, et al. Secondary sexual characteristics and menses in young girls seen in office practice: a study from the Pediatric Research in Office Settings Network. *Pediatrics.* 1997;99(4):505–512.

51. Herman-Giddens ME, Steffes J, Harris D, et al. Secondary sexual characteristics in boys: data from the Pediatric Research in Office Settings Network. *Pediatrics.* 2012; 130:e1058.

52. Biro FM, Galvez MP, Greenspan LC, et al. Pubertal assessment method and baseline characteristics in a mixed longitudinal study of girls. *Pediatrics* . 2010;126(3):e583–590.

53. Biro FM, Greenspan LC, Galvez MP, et al. Onset of breast development in a longitudinal cohort. *Pediatrics.* 2013;132:1019.

54. McCrory P, Meeuwisse WH, Aubry M, et al. Consensus statement on concussion in sport: the 4th International Conference on Concussion in Sport held in Zurich, November 2012. *Br J Sports Med.* 2013;47:250–258.

55. Metzl JD. Preparticipation examination of the adolescent athlete: part 1. *Pediatr Rev.* 2001;22(6):119–204.

56. Metzl JD. Preparticipation examination of the adolescent athlete: part 2. *Pediatr Rev.* 2001;22(7):227–239.

ADDITIONAL REFERENCES

Frankenburg WK, Dodds J, et al. DENVER II Training Manual. Denver Developmental Materials, Inc., Denver, CO. 1996:18–21

Hockenberry MJ, Wilson D. *Wong's Nursing Care of Infants and Children.* 10th Ed. St. Louis, MO: Mosby; 2015.

Kyle T, Carman S. *Essentials of Pediatric Nursing.* 3rd ed. Philadelphia, PA: Lippincott Williams Wilkins; 2016.

Shahshahani S, Vameghi R, Azari N, et al. Validity and Reliability Determination of Denver Developmental Screening Test-II in 0–6 Year-Olds in Tehran. *Iran J Pediatr.* 2010;(20):3.

Sharon R. Developmental Screening and Assessment Instruments with an Emphasis on Social and Emotional Development for Young Children Ages Birth through Five. The National Early Childhood Technical Assistance Center. 2008. Available at http://www.nectac.org/~pdfs/pubs/screening.pdf. Accessed: January 16, 2016.

Assessing Older Adults

LEARNING OBJECTIVES

The student will:

1. Use the techniques that best facilitate the health history and physical examination of the older adult.

2. Identify focus areas during the health history specific to the older adult.

3. Recognize normal physiologic changes in the older adult.

4. Use screening tools in the assessment of older adults.

5. Perform a health history on an older adult.

6. Perform a physical examination on an older adult.

7. Document the older adult assessment findings.

8. Address areas of health promotion and counseling specific to the older adult.

Older Americans now number more than 43 million, and that number is expected to reach 80 million by 2040, constituting more than 20% of the population.[1,2] Americans are living longer than previous generations: life span at birth is currently 81 years for women and 76 years for men. The population over age 85 years is projected to more than double from 6 million to over 14 million in 2040.[3] Hence, the "*demographic imperative*" to societies worldwide is to maximize not only life span but also "health span," so that older adults maintain full function as long as possible, enjoying rich and active lives in their homes and communities.

Although statistics group aging by decades, aging is hardly chronologic, measured by time in years, but rather encompasses a wealth of wisdom and lived experience in addition to the complex interplay of health and illness. The aging population is highly heterogeneous—in disposition, social networks, level of physical activity, and biology. Frailty is one of society's common myths about aging; more than 95% of Americans older than 65 years live in the community, and only 5% reside in institutional facilities.[4] For those over age 85 years, only 10% live in institutional facilities.

Self-reported health status and functional status supersede disability as measures of healthy aging. Health was rated as good to excellent in 76% of older adults, and there has been a decline in the percentage of older adults reporting functional limitations, from 49% in 1990 to 41% in 2010, even though up to 56% report at least one chronic condition.[5] However, recent trends suggest that obesity may increase future levels of disability, especially in African American and Hispanic adults ages 60 to 69 years. Now 38% of adults of age 65 years and over are obese, compared to 22% in 1988–1994. Studies show that successful aging is not strictly medical, but rests on variables such as positive cognition and mental health, physical activity, and social networks.[6] Terminology about aging is in flux. This chapter uses the term "older adult"; however, evidence about these designations is lacking, so take the time to find out which term your patient prefers.

Assessing the older adult presents special opportunities and challenges. This chapter highlights only key points, as assessment of older adults encompasses much more than a single chapter can impart. Many of these challenges are quite different from those of the disease-oriented approach of history taking and physical examination for younger patients: the focus is on healthy or "successful" aging; the need to understand and mobilize family, social, and community supports; the importance of functional assessment skills; and the opportunities for promoting the older adult's long-term health and safety. It is important to distinguish between normal aging changes and abnormalities commonly found in an elderly person.

Promoting healthy aging leads to interactive goals in clinical care—"an informed active patient interacting with a prepared proactive team, resulting in high quality satisfying encounters and improved outcomes" and a distinct set of clinical attitudes and skills.[7-9] Experts recommend "goal-oriented patient care" that is patient-centered, defined as "respectful of and responsive to individual patient preferences, needs, and values, and ensuring that patient values guide all clinical decisions."[10] For older adults, this means focusing on the patient's "individual health goals within or across a variety of dimensions (e.g., symptoms; physical functional status, including mobility; and social and role functions) and to determine how these goals are being met."[11] This approach individualizes decision-making and allows patients to express preferences about which "health states are important to them and their relative priority," for example, choosing better symptom control over a longer life span. Goal-oriented care moves beyond "preventive and disease-specific care processes… and condition-specific indicators" such as targets for glucose or blood pressure.

New paradigms also highlight the importance of shifting assessment to *geriatric syndromes* that fall outside traditional disease models but are strongly linked to activities of daily living (ADLs). These syndromes are present in almost 50% of older adults.[12] Managing these conditions, such as cognitive impairment, falls, incontinence, low body mass index (BMI), dizziness, and impaired vision and hearing, presents both opportunities and challenges. The focus is on healthy or "successful" aging, including the need to understand and mobilize family, social, and community supports; the importance of skills directed to functional assessment, which is considered "the sixth vital sign"; and the opportunities for promoting the older adult's long-term health and safety.

See Minimum Geriatric Competencies, pp. 927–929.

Minimum Geriatric Competencies

Medication Management

1. Explain impact of age-related changes on drug selection and dose based on knowledge of age-related changes in renal and hepatic function, body composition, and central nervous system sensitivity.
2. Identify medications, including anticholinergic, psychoactive, anticoagulant, analgesic, hypoglycemic, and cardiovascular drugs that should be avoided or used with caution in older adults and explain the potential problems associated with each.
3. Document a patient's complete medication list, including prescribed, herbal, and over-the-counter medications, and for each medication provide the dose, frequency, indication, benefit, side effects, and an assessment of adherence.

Cognitive and Behavioral Disorders

4. Define and distinguish the clinical presentations of delirium, dementia, and depression.
5. Formulate a differential diagnosis and implement initial evaluation in a patient who exhibits cognitive impairment.
6. Urgently initiate a diagnostic workup to determine the root cause (etiology) of delirium in an older patient.
7. Perform and interpret a cognitive assessment in older patients for whom there are concerns regarding memory or function.
8. Develop an evaluation and nonpharmacologic management plan for agitated, demented, or delirious patients.

Use assessment tools for geriatrics and geriatric syndromes, including falls, delirium/cognitive impairment, and functional dependence in every patient. The Hartford Institute for Geriatric Nursing has a clinical website, "Consult Geri," which provides access to many assessment tools: http://consultgeri.org/tools/try-this-series

Identify frail elderly patients, as they are most vulnerable to adverse outcomes and most benefit from a holistic geriatric approach.

Self-Care Capacity

9. Assess and describe baseline and current functional abilities (instrumental activities of daily living, activities of daily living, and special senses) in an older patient by collecting historical data from multiple sources and performing a confirmatory physical examination.

10. Develop a preliminary management plan for patients presenting with functional deficits, including adaptive interventions and involvement of interdisciplinary team members, such as social work, nursing, rehabilitation, nutrition, and pharmacy.

11. Identify and assess safety risks in the home environment, and make recommendations to mitigate these.

Falls, Balance, Gait Disorders

12. Ask all patients older than 65 years of age, or their caregivers, about falls in the last year; watch the patient rise from a chair and walk (or transfer); and then record and interpret the findings.

13. For a patient who has fallen, construct a differential diagnosis and evaluation plan that addresses the multiple etiologies identified by history, physical examination, and functional assessment.

Health Care Planning and Promotion

14. Define and differentiate among types of code status, health care proxies, and advanced directives in the site where one is training.

15. Accurately identify clinical situations where life expectancy, functional status, patient preference, or goals of care should override standard recommendations for screening tests in older adults.

16. Accurately identify clinical situations where life expectancy, functional status, patient preference, or goals of care should override standard recommendations for treatment in older adults.

Atypical Presentation of Disease

17. Identify at least three physiologic changes of aging for each organ system and their impact on the patient, including their contribution to homeostenosis (the age-related narrowing or homeostatic reserve mechanisms).

As people age their organs have less functional reserve to cope with biological stresses such as increasing their heart rate to cope with increased oxygen demand of heavy physical activity.

18. Generate a differential diagnosis based on recognition of the unique presentations of common conditions in older adults, including acute coronary syndrome, dehydration, urinary tract infection, acute abdomen, and pneumonia.

Palliative Care

19. Assess and provide initial management of pain and key nonpain symptoms based on the patient's goals of care.

20. Identify the psychological, social, and spiritual needs of patients with advanced illness as well as their family members, and link these identified needs with the appropriate interdisciplinary team members.

21. Present palliative care (including hospice) as a positive, active treatment option for a patient with advanced disease.

Hospital Care for Elders

22. Identify potential hazards of hospitalization for all older adult patients (including immobility, delirium, medication side effects, malnutrition, pressure ulcers, procedures, peri- and postoperative periods, and hospital-acquired infections) and identify potential prevention strategies.
23. Explain the risks, indications, alternatives, and contraindications for indwelling (Foley) catheter use in the older adult patient.
24. Explain the risks, indications, alternatives, and contraindications for physical and pharmacologic restraint use.
25. Communicate the key components of a safe discharge plan (e.g., accurate medication list, plan for follow-up), including comparing/contrasting potential sites for discharge.
26. Conduct a surveillance examination of areas of the skin at high risk for pressure ulcers and describe existing ulcers.

Source: Association of American Medical Colleges/John A. Hartford Foundation, Inc. July 2007 Consensus Conference on Competencies in Geriatrics Education Academic Medicine. 84(5):604–10, May 2009.

ANATOMY AND PHYSIOLOGY

Primary aging reflects changes in physiologic reserves over time that are independent of changes from disease. These changes are likely to appear during periods of stress, such as exposure to fluctuating temperatures, dehydration, or even shock. In aging, decreased cutaneous vasoconstriction and sweat production can impair responses to heat; declines in thirst may delay recovery from dehydration; and the physiologic drops in maximum cardiac output, left ventricular filling, and maximum heart rate (HR) present with aging may impair the response to shock.

At the same time, the aging population displays marked heterogeneity. Researchers have identified vast differences in how people age and have distinguished "usual" aging, with its complexity of diseases and impairments, from "optimal" aging. Optimal aging occurs in those people who escape debilitating disease entirely and maintain healthy lives late into their 80s and 90s. Studies of centenarians show that genes account for approximately 20% to 30% probability of living to 100. Importantly, healthy lifestyles also account for 20% to 30%.[13,14] These findings provide evidence to promote modifiable lifestyle choices like optimal nutrition, strength training, and exercise and to promote optimal function for older adults to delay the depletion of physiologic reserves and the onset of frailty.

Vital Signs

Blood Pressure

In Western societies, systolic blood pressure (SBP) tends to rise with aging. The aorta and large arteries stiffen and become atherosclerotic. As the aorta becomes less distensible, a given stroke volume causes a greater rise in SBP; *systolic hypertension* with a *widened pulse pressure* (PP) often ensues. Diastolic blood pressure (DBP) stops rising at approximately the sixth decade. At the other extreme, some older adults develop a tendency toward *postural (orthostatic) hypotension* which is a sudden drop in blood pressure upon rising to standing position.

Heart Rate and Rhythm

In older adults, resting heart rate (HR) remains unchanged, but pacemaker cells decline in the sinoatrial node and the maximal heart rate, which affect the response to exercise and physiologic stress.[15] Older adults are more likely to have abnormal heart rhythms such as atrial or ventricular ectopy. Asymptomatic rhythm changes are generally benign. However, some rhythm changes cause *syncope,* which is a temporary loss of consciousness.

Respiratory Rate and Temperature

Respiratory rate (RR) and temperature are unchanged, but changes in temperature regulation lead to a susceptibility to *hypothermia*.

Skin, Nails, and Hair

With age, the skin wrinkles, becomes lax, and loses turgor. The vascularity of the dermis decreases, causing lighter skin to look paler and more opaque. Skin on the backs of the hands and forearms appears thin, fragile, loose, and transparent. There may be purple patches or macules, termed actinic purpura, that fade over time. These spots and patches come from blood that has leaked through poorly supported capillaries and spread within the dermis.

Nails lose luster with age and may yellow and thicken, especially on the toes.

Hair undergoes a series of changes. Scalp hair loses its pigment, changing hair color to gray. Hair loss on the scalp is genetically determined. As early as 20 years, a man's hairline may start to recede at the temples and then at the vertex. In women, hair loss follows a similar but less severe pattern. In both sexes, the number of scalp hairs decreases in a generalized pattern, and the diameter of each hair gets smaller. Less familiar, but probably more important clinically, is normal hair loss elsewhere on the body: the trunk, pubic areas, axillae, and limbs. As women reach age 55 years, coarse facial hairs may appear on the chin and upper lip but do not increase further.

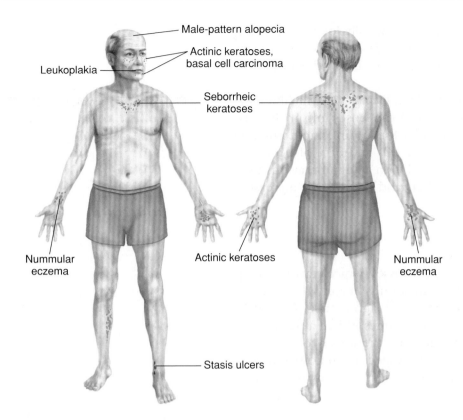

Many of the changes described here pertain to lighter-skinned people and do not necessarily apply to those with darker skin tones. For example, Native American men have relatively little facial and body hair compared with lighter-skinned men and should be evaluated according to their own norms.

Head and Neck

Eyes and Visual Acuity

The eyes, ears, and mouth show more visible changes of aging. The fat that surrounds and cushions the eye within the bony orbit may atrophy, allowing the eyeball to recede. The skin of the eyelids becomes wrinkled and may hang in looser folds. Fat may push the fascia of the eyelids forward, creating soft bulges, especially in the lower lids and the inner third of the upper lids. Because their eyes produce fewer lacrimal secretions, older patients may complain of dry eyes. The corneas lose some of their luster.

The pupils become smaller, which makes it more difficult to examine the ocular fundi. The pupils may also become slightly irregular but should continue to respond to light and show the near reaction.

Visual acuity remains fairly constant between 20 and 50 years. It diminishes gradually until approximately 70 years and then more rapidly. Nevertheless, most older adults retain good to adequate vision (20/20 to 20/70 as measured by standard charts). Near vision, however, begins to blur noticeably for virtually everyone. From childhood on, the lens gradually loses its elasticity, and the eye grows progressively less able to accommodate and focus on nearby objects. Ensuing *presbyopia* usually becomes noticeable during the 40s.

Aging affects the lenses and increases risk for *cataracts, glaucoma,* and *macular degeneration.* Thickening and yellowing of the lenses impair the passage of light to the retinas, requiring more light for reading and doing fine work. Cataracts affect 10% of patients in their 60s and 30% of people in their 80s. Because the lens continues to expand with aging, it may push the iris forward, narrowing the angle between iris and cornea and increasing the risk of *narrow-angle glaucoma.*

See Chapter 11, The Eyes, pp. 266–267.

Hearing

Hearing acuity usually declines with age. Early losses, which start in young adulthood, involve primarily the high-pitched sounds beyond the range of human speech and have relatively little functional significance. Gradually, loss extends to sounds in the middle and lower ranges. When a person fails to hear the higher tones of words but still hears the lower tones, words sound distorted and are difficult to understand, especially in noisy environments. Hearing loss associated with aging, known as *presbycusis,* becomes increasingly evident, usually after 50 years.

Mouth, Teeth, and Lymph Nodes

Diminished salivary secretions and a decreased sense of taste accompany aging. Medications and various diseases may intensify these changes. Decreased olfaction and increased sensitivity to bitterness and saltiness also affect taste. Teeth may wear down, become abraded, or be lost to dental caries or periodontal disease. In patients without teeth, the lower portion of the face looks small and sunken, with accentuated "purse-string" wrinkles radiating from the mouth. Over closure of the mouth may lead to maceration of the skin at the corners, a condition known as *angular cheilitis.* The bony ridges of the jaws that once surrounded the tooth sockets are gradually resorbed, especially in the lower jaw.

See Chapter 12, Ear, Nose, Mouth and Throat, pp. 290–292.

With aging, the cervical lymph nodes become less palpable. In contrast, the submandibular glands become easier to feel.

Thorax and Lungs

As people age, they lose lung capacity during exercise.[16] The chest wall becomes stiffer and harder to move, respiratory muscles may weaken, and the lungs lose some of their elastic recoil. Lung mass and the surface area for gas exchange decline, and residual volume increases as the alveoli enlarge. An increase in closing volumes of small airways predisposes to atelectasis and risk of pneumonia. Diaphragmatic strength declines. The speed of breathing out with maximal effort gradually diminishes, and the cough becomes less effective. There is a decrease in arterial pO_2, but the O_2 saturation normally remains above 90%.

Skeletal changes associated with aging may accentuate the dorsal curve of the thoracic spine. Osteoporotic vertebral collapse produces *kyphosis,* which increases the anteroposterior diameter of the chest. The resulting "barrel chest," however, has little effect on function.

Cardiovascular System

Cardiovascular findings vary significantly with age. Aging also affects vascular sounds in the neck and adds to the significance of extra heart sounds like S_3 and S_4 and of murmurs.

Neck Vessels

Lengthening and tortuosity of the aorta and its branches occasionally result in kinking or buckling of the carotid artery low in the neck, especially on the right. The resulting pulsatile mass, occurring chiefly in women with hypertension, may be mistaken for a carotid aneurysm—which is a true dilation of the artery. A tortuous aorta occasionally raises the pressure in the jugular veins on the left side of the neck by impairing their drainage within the thorax.

In older adults, systolic bruits heard in the middle or upper portions of the carotid arteries indicate stenosis from atherosclerotic plaque. Cervical or carotid bruits in younger people are usually innocent.

Cardiac Output

Myocardial contraction is less responsive to stimulation from β-adrenergic catecholamines. There is a modest drop in resting heart rate, but a significant drop in the maximum HR during exercise. Though HR drops stroke volume increases, so cardiac output is maintained. Diastolic dysfunction arises from decreased early diastolic filling and greater dependence on atrial contraction. There is increased myocardial stiffness, notably in the left ventricle, which also hypertrophies.

Risk of heart failure increases with loss of atrial contraction and onset of atrial fibrillation due to decreased ventricular filling.

Extra Heart Sounds—S_3 and S_4

A physiologic *third heart sound,* commonly heard in children and young adults, may persist as late as age 40, especially in women. After age 40, however, an S_3 strongly suggests heart failure from volume overload of the left ventricle in conditions such as heart failure and valvular heart disease (e.g., mitral regurgitation). In contrast, a *fourth heart sound* is seldom heard in young adults other than well-conditioned athletes. An S_4 can be heard in otherwise healthy older people, but often suggests decreased ventricular compliance and impaired ventricular filling.

See Table 14-7, Extra Heart Sounds in Diastole, p. 430.

Cardiac Murmurs

Middle-aged and older adults commonly have a *systolic aortic murmur*. This murmur is detected in approximately one third of people at age 60 years, and in more than half of those reaching 85 years. With aging, fibrotic changes thicken the bases of the aortic cusps. Calcification follows, resulting in audible vibrations. Turbulence produced by blood flow into a dilated aorta may further augment this murmur. In most older adults, the process of fibrosis and calcification, known as *aortic sclerosis*, does not impede blood flow. In some, the aortic valve leaflets become calcified and immobile, resulting in *aortic stenosis* and outflow obstruction. A brisk carotid upstroke can help distinguish aortic sclerosis from aortic stenosis, which has a delayed carotid upstroke, but clinically distinguishing these conditions is difficult. Both carry increased risk for cardiovascular morbidity and mortality.

Similar changes alter the mitral valve, approximately one decade later than the aortic valve. Calcification of the mitral valve annulus, or valve ring, impedes normal valve closure during systole, causing the systolic murmur of *mitral regurgitation*. This change in the configuration of the valve may become pathologic as volume overload increases in the left ventricle.

Peripheral Vascular System

The peripheral arteries tend to lengthen, become tortuous, and feel harder and less resilient. There is increased arterial stiffness and decreased endothelial function.[16] The trophic changes in skin, nails, and hair discussed earlier occur independently, although they may not accompany arterial disease. Although arterial and venous disorders, especially atherosclerosis, are more common in older adults, these are not normal changes of aging. Loss of arterial pulsations is not typical, however, and demands careful evaluation. Abdominal or back pain in older adults raises the important concern of possible abdominal aortic aneurysm, especially in male smokers over age 65 years. Rarely, after age 50 years, but especially after age 70 years, the temporal arteries may develop giant cell, or temporal arteritis, leading to loss of vision in 15% of patients and headache and jaw claudication.

Breasts and Axillae

The normal adult female breast is soft, and may be granular, nodular, or lumpy. This uneven texture represents physiologic nodularity palpable throughout or only in parts of the breast. With aging, the female breasts tend to become smaller, more flaccid, and more pendulous as glandular tissue atrophies and is replaced by fatty tissue. The ducts surrounding the nipple may become more palpable as firm, stringy strands. Axillary hair diminishes. Males may develop gynecomastia or increased breast fullness due to obesity and hormonal changes.

Abdomen

During the middle and later years, the abdominal muscles tend to weaken, there is decreased activity of lipoprotein lipase, and fat may accumulate in the lower abdomen and near the hips even when the weight is stable. These changes often produce a softer, more protruding abdomen, which patients may interpret as fluid or evidence of disease. The change in abdominal fat distribution increases the risk of cardiovascular disease.

Aging can blunt the manifestations of acute abdominal disease. Pain may be less severe, fever is often less pronounced, and signs of peritoneal inflammation, such as muscular guarding and rebound tenderness, may be diminished or even absent.

See Chapter 16, The Peripheral Vascular and Lymphatic System.

Female and Male Genitalia

In women, ovarian function usually starts to diminish during the fifth decade; on average, menstrual periods cease between 48 and 55 years. As estrogen stimulation falls, many women experience hot flashes, sometimes for up to 5 years. Symptoms range from flushing, sweating, and palpitations to chills and anxiety. Sleep disruption and mood changes are common. Women may report vaginal dryness, urge incontinence, or dyspareunia. Several vulvovaginal changes occur: pubic hair becomes sparse as well as gray, the labia and clitoris become smaller, the vagina narrows and shortens, and the vaginal mucosa becomes thin, pale, and dry, with loss of lubrication. The uterus and ovaries diminish in size. Within 10 years after menopause, the ovaries are usually no longer palpable. The suspensory ligaments of the adnexa, uterus, and bladder may also relax. Sexuality and sexual interest are often unchanged, particularly when women are untroubled by partner issues, partner loss, or unusual work or life stress.[17]

As men age, sexual interest appears to remain intact, although frequency of intercourse declines. Several physiologic changes accompany decreasing testosterone levels.[16] Erections become more dependent on tactile stimulation and less responsive to erotic cues. The penis decreases in size, and the testicles drop lower in the scrotum. Protracted illnesses, more than aging, lead to decreased testicular size. Pubic hair may decrease and become gray. Erectile dysfunction, or the inability to have an erection, affects approximately 50% of older men. Vascular causes are the most common, from both atherosclerotic arterial occlusive disease and corpora cavernosa venous leak. Chronic diseases such as diabetes, hypertension, dyslipidemia, and smoking, as well as medication side effects, all contribute to the prevalence of erectile dysfunction.

The prevalence of *urinary incontinence* increases with age in both women and men. Incontinence may be related to decreased innervation and contractility of the detrusor muscle, loss of bladder capacity, changes in urinary flow rate, and the ability to inhibit voiding.

In women, injury to or weakening of the supporting muscles of the pelvic floor could exacerbate incontinence. This potentially could occur because of past vaginal childbirth(s) or a surgery related to the reproductive system. Decreased production of estrogen after menopause can also exacerbate incontinence.

In men, there is androgen-dependent proliferation of prostate epithelial and stromal tissue, termed *benign prostatic hyperplasia (BPH),* that begins in the third decade, continues to the seventh decade, then appears to plateau. Only half of men will have clinically significant enlargement, and of those, only half will report symptoms such as urinary hesitancy, dribbling, and incomplete emptying.

For both, men and women, the symptoms can often be traced to other causes like coexisting disease, use of medications, and lower urinary tract abnormalities.[18]

Musculoskeletal System

Both men and women lose cortical and trabecular bone mass throughout adulthood, men more slowly, and women more rapidly after menopause, which leads to increased risk of fracture. Calcium resorption from bone rather than diet increases with aging as parathyroid hormone levels rise. Subtle losses in height begin soon after maturity; significant shortening is obvious by old age. Most loss of height occurs in the trunk and reflects thinning of the intervertebral discs and shortening or even collapse of the vertebral bodies from osteoporosis, leading to kyphosis and an increase in the anteroposterior diameter of the chest. Added flexion at the knees and hips also contributes to shortened stature. These changes cause the limbs of an elderly person tend to look long in proportion to the trunk. With aging, there is a 30% to 50% decline in muscle mass in relation to body weight in both men and women, and ligaments lose some of their tensile strength. Range of motion diminishes, partly because of osteoarthritis. *Sarcopenia* is the loss of lean body mass and strength with aging.[19] The causes of muscle loss are multifactorial, including inflammatory and endocrine changes as well as sedentary lifestyle. There is substantial evidence that strength training in older adults can slow or reverse this process.

Mental Status Assessment and Nervous System

Aging affects all aspects of the nervous system, from mental status to motor and sensory function and reflexes. Brain volume, cortical brain cells, and intrinsic regional connecting networks decrease, and both microanatomical and biochemical changes have been identified.[20] Nevertheless, most older adults maintain their self-esteem and adapt well to their changing capacities and circumstances.

Mental Status

Although older adults generally perform well on mental status examinations, they may display selected impairments, especially at advanced ages. Many older people complain about memory issues. This is usually from "benign forgetfulness," which can occur at any age. This term refers to difficulty recalling the names of people or objects or details of specific events. Identifying this common phenomenon can decrease fears of Alzheimer disease (AD). Older adults also retrieve and process data more slowly, and take more time to learn new information. Their motor responses may slow and their ability to perform complex tasks may diminish.

Frequently, the nurse distinguishes these age-related changes in the nervous system from manifestations of mental disorders that are prevalent in older adults, such as *depression* and *dementia*. Sorting out these ailments may be difficult, because both mood disturbances and cognitive changes can alter the patient's ability to recognize or report symptoms. Older patients are also more susceptible to *delirium*, a temporary state of confusion that may be the first clue to infection, problems with medications, or changes in the environment such as hospitalization. It is important to recognize these conditions promptly and to delay functional decline. Recall that sensory and motor findings in older patients that are physiologic, such as the changes in hearing, vision, extraocular movements, and pupillary size, shape, and reactivity, are abnormal in younger adults.

Review Chapter 19, Mental Status, and Table 24-1, Delirium and Dementia, p. 975.

Emotional Concerns

Older adults experience the death of loved ones and friends, retirement from valued employment, diminution in income, and often growing social isolation in addition to physiologic changes and decreased physical capacity. Including the impact of these significant life events in the assessment of mood and affect and addressing these issues may improve the patient's quality of life.

Motor System

Changes in the motor system are common. Older adults move and react with less speed and agility, and skeletal muscles decrease in bulk. The hands of an older patient often look thin and bony as a result of atrophy of the interosseous muscles that leaves concavities or grooves. Muscle wasting tends to appear between the thumb and the hand (the first and second metacarpals) then affect the other metacarpals. It may also flatten the thenar and hypothenar eminences of the palms. Arm and leg muscles can also show signs of atrophy, exaggerating the apparent size of adjacent joints. Muscle strength, though diminished, is relatively well maintained.

Occasionally, older adults develop a benign essential tremor in the head, jaw, lips, or hands that may be confused with Parkinsonism. Unlike Parkinsonian tremors, however, benign tremors are slightly faster and disappear at rest, and there is no associated muscle rigidity.

See Chapter 20, The Nervous System, Table 20-4, Abnormalities of Gait and Posture, p. 732.

Vibratory and Position Sense, Reflexes

Aging can also affect vibratory and position sense and reflexes. Older adults frequently lose some or all vibration sense in the feet and ankles (but not in the fingers or over the shins). Less commonly, position sense may diminish or disappear. The gag reflex may be diminished or absent. Abdominal reflexes may diminish or disappear. Ankle reflexes may be symmetrically decreased or absent, even when reinforced. Less commonly, knee reflexes are similarly affected. Partly because of musculoskeletal changes in the feet, the plantar responses become less obvious and more difficult to interpret. If there are associated neurologic findings, or if atrophy and reflex changes are asymmetric, search for an explanation other than aging.

THE HEALTH HISTORY

Approach to the Older Adult Patient

Modify your usual approach when obtaining the Health History and interviewing older adults. As with all patients, the nurse's demeanor should convey respect, patience, and cultural awareness. Inquire about issues regarding privacy such as: would you like a friend or family member present during the interview or may I share information about your examination with your family or friend? Be sure to address patients by an appropriate title and their last name (e.g., Mr. Jones or Mrs./Ms. Thomas).

- Adjust the environment
- Shape the content and pace of the visit
- Address the cultural dimensions of aging
- Elicit symptoms

Adjust the Environment

First, take the time to adjust the environment of the office, hospital, or nursing home to put your patient at ease. Recall the physiologic changes in temperature regulation, and make sure the office is neither too cool nor too warm. Brighter lighting helps compensate for changes in the lens and allows the older patient to see your facial expressions and gestures more clearly. Ensure the patient is not facing a window, as the glare may also impair the ability to see well. The nurse should face the patient directly and sit at eye level. Focusing on personal electronic devices or turning away from the patient to search the electronic medical record should also be avoided.

More than 50% of older adults have hearing deficits, especially for higher frequency tones, so choose a quiet room that is free of distractions or noise. Turn off the radio or television before you start the conversation. If appropriate, consider using a "pocket talker," a small, portable microphone that amplifies your voice and connects to an earpiece inserted by the patient. Speak in low tones, and make sure the patient is using glasses, hearing aids, and dentures when needed to assist with communication. Patients with quadriceps weakness benefit from chairs with higher seating and a wide stool with a handrail leading up to the examining table.

Shape the Content and Pace of the Visit

With older adults, rethink the traditional format of the visit. Older patients often measure their lives in terms of years left rather than years lived. They may reminisce about the past and reflect on previous experiences. By listening to these life reviews you gain important insights and an understanding of the individual which enables you to support patients as they work through painful feelings or recapture joys and accomplishments.

At the same time, it is important to balance the need to assess complex problems with the patient's endurance and possible fatigue. To expand time for listening to the patient but prevent exhaustion, make ample use of brief screening tools,[21,22] information from home visits and the medical record, and reports from family members, caregivers, and allied health disciplines. Consider dividing the initial assessment into two visits. Two or more shorter visits may be less fatiguing and more productive to allow more time to respond to questions, since explanations may be slow and lengthy.

See brief screening tools, p. 945.

Address Cultural Dimensions of Aging

Knowledge and skills about the cultural dimensions of aging are the cornerstone to improving health care for the rapidly growing number of older adults of diverse ethnic backgrounds. In fact, the demographic imperative for older adults can be called the *ethnogeriatric imperative,* "because by mid-century more than one in three older Americans is projected to be from one of the four populations designated as 'minority,'"[23] as shown in the graph.

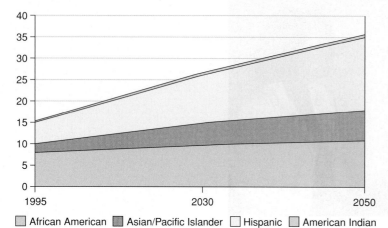

☐ African American ■ Asian/Pacific Islander ☐ Hispanic ☐ American Indian

Source: Yeo, F. How will the U.S. healthcare system meet the challenge of the ethnogeriatric imperative? *J Am Geriatr Soc.* 2009;57:1278.

Geriatric Diversity: Now and in 2050

- *Hispanic Americans* over the age of 65 years will increase in number from 2.7 million in 2010, or 6.9% of the older adult population, to 17.5 million in 2050, or 19.8% of the older adult population.[5]
- *African-American* older adults will increase in number from 3.4 million (8.5%), to 10.5 million in 2050 (11.9%).
- *Asian Americans* and other ethnic groups, although smaller in number currently, will increase in number from 1.4 million to 7.5 million, or from 3.4% to 8.5% of the older adult population.
- *Non-Hispanic whites* will increase in number from 32.2 million to 58.5 million in 2050, but will drop in percentage of the older population from 80% to 58.5%.

Source: Federal Interagency Forum on Aging Related Statistics. Older Americans 2012, Key Indicators of Well Being. Indicator 2, Racial and Ethnic Composition, p. 86. Federal Interagency Forum on Aging-Related Statistics. Washington, DC: U.S. Government Printing Office. June 2012. Available at http://agingstats.gov/agingstatsdotnet/Main_Site/Data/2012_Documents/Docs/EntireChartbook.pdf. Accessed January 20, 2016.

The changing demographics of aging only hint at how older adults of different ethnicities experience suffering, illness, and decisions about their health care. Cultural and socioeconomic attributes affect the epidemiology of illness and mental health, the process of acculturation in families, individual concerns about aging, choices about healers and when to pursue symptoms, the potential for misdiagnosis, and disparities in health outcomes.[24] Culture, including spiritual beliefs, shapes views about the entire spectrum of aging: work and retirement, perceptions of health and illness, the utility of medications, use of health care proxies, and preferences about dying, to name just a few.

The CDC Health Disparities and Inequalities Report—United States, 2013 "highlights health disparities and inequalities across a wide range of diseases, behavioral risk factors, environmental exposures, social determinants, and health care access by sex, race and ethnicity, income, education, health literacy, disability status, and other social characteristics."[25,26] Aging racial/ethnic minority populations have poorer health outcomes in cardiovascular disease, diabetes, cancer, asthma, and human immunodeficiency virus/acquired immunodeficiency syndrome as well as shorter life spans.[27] Despite advances in *ethnogeriatrics*,[28–30] information on racial and ethnic disparities in later life regarding chronic disease, ADLs, and self-rated health status remains "limited and inconsistent," and guidelines for providing individualized culturally appropriate care are sparse.[26]

Improving competence in care for diverse older populations is a critical step in improving health outcomes. The *ETHNIC(S)* mnemonic helps clinicians escape the pitfalls of group-labeling by expanding individual history taking to include *Explanation, Treatment, Healers, Negotiate, Intervention, Collaborate, and Spirituality*.[31] Nonetheless, this model may miss important information about cultural identity, social supports, health literacy, and views about health care.[32] Experts recommend letting patients establish their cultural identity by exploring four key areas during the interview: the individual's cultural identity; cultural explanations of the individual's illness; cultural factors related to the psychosocial environment and levels of function; and cultural elements in the clinician–patient relationship. Test your "ethnogeriatric IQ" at the Stanford Geriatrics Education Center website and explore the Stanford curriculum in ethnogeriatrics.[33,34] Learn to convey respect to older adults through culturally specific nonverbal communication. Direct eye contact or handshaking, for example, may not be culturally appropriate. Identify critical life experiences from the country of origin or migration history that affect the patient's outlook and psyche. Ask about family decision making, spiritual advisors, and traditional healers and practices.

The Office of Minority Health in the Department of Health and Human Services has developed *Think Cultural Health*, a resource center to improve quality of care through cultural and linguistic competencies and continuing education programs.[29]

Cultural values particularly affect decisions about the end of life. Elders, family, and even an extended community group may make these decisions with or for the older patient. Such group decision making is quite different from the focus on individual autonomy and informed consent featured in contemporary health care settings. Eliciting the stresses of migration and acculturation, using translators effectively, enlisting "patient navigators" from the family and community, and accessing culturally validated assessment tools like the Geriatric Depression Scale will help you provide empathic care of older adults.

See Chapter 3, Interviewing and Communication, on working with translators, pp. 60–61.

Elicit Symptoms From the Older Adult

Eliciting the history calls for an astute nurse: patients may accidentally or purposefully underreport symptoms; the presentation of acute illnesses may be different; common symptoms may mask a geriatric syndrome; or patients may have cognitive impairment.

Underreporting Symptoms

Older patients tend to give more positive ratings to their overall health than do younger adults, even when affected by disease and disability. It is best to start the visit with open-ended questions like "How can I help you today?" Older patients may be reluctant to report their symptoms. Some are afraid or embarrassed; others try to avoid medical expenses or the discomforts of diagnosis and treatment. Still others overlook their symptoms (e.g., pain), thinking them to be merely part of aging, or they may simply forget about them. To reduce the risk for late recognition and delayed intervention, you may need to adopt more direct questions, use well-validated geriatric screening tools, and consult with family members and caregivers.

Acute illnesses present differently in older adults. Older patients with infections are less likely to have a fever. Older patients having a myocardial infarction are less likely to report chest pain and symptoms have an atypical presentation, such as shortness of breath, palpitations, syncope, and confusion.[35] Older patients with hyperthyroidism and hypothyroidism have fewer symptoms and signs. One third of older adults with hyperthyroidism present with fatigue, weight loss, and tachycardia in lieu of the classic features of heat intolerance, sweating, and hyperreflexia.[36] Up to 35% present with atrial fibrillation. Hyperthyroidism increases the risk of osteoporosis, and, in affected women, risk of hip and vertebral fractures increases threefold. In older adults, hypothyroidism is most commonly caused by autoimmune thyroiditis (Hashimoto thyroiditis); fatigue, weakness, constipation, dry skin, and cold intolerance are often attributed to other conditions, medication side effects, or aging.

In older adults the prevalence of hyperthyroidism is 0.5% to 4% and of hypothyroidism, approximately 10% in men and 16% in women.[36]

Tips for Communicating Effectively With Older Adults

- Provide a well-lit, moderately warm setting with minimal background noise, a safe chair, and access to the examining table.
- Face the patient and speak in low tones; make sure the patient is using glasses, hearing devices, and dentures if needed.
- Adjust the pace and content of the interview to the stamina of the patient; consider two visits for initial evaluations.
- Allow time for open-ended questions and reminiscing; include family and caregivers when needed, especially if the patient has a cognitive impairment.

- Make use of brief screening instruments, the medical record, and reports from allied disciplines.
- Carefully assess symptoms, especially fatigue, loss of appetite, weight loss, incontinence, skin integrity, dizziness, falls, and pain, for clues to underlying disorders and geriatric disorders.
- Make sure written instructions are in large print and easy to read.

Geriatric Syndromes

Managing an increasing number of interrelated conditions calls for recognizing the symptom clusters typical of different *geriatric syndromes*. A geriatric syndrome represents serious issues for older adults and is often related to functional decline. Geriatric syndromes impact quality of life, and nurses need to be aware of these syndromes. One symptom may relate to several others. It is especially important to be vigilant and recognize these syndromes because symptoms may cluster in patterns unfamiliar to the patient.[37] It is important for nurses to obtain an accurate assessment using both subjective and objective information.

These syndromes have been found in more than half of adults over age 65 years, in contrast to the conventional search in younger patients for a "single unifying diagnosis."[38]

SPICES is a mnemonic which focuses on frequent geriatric syndromes of the older adult.

Sleep Disorders
Problems with Eating or Feeding
Incontinence
Confusion
Evidence of Falls
Skin Breakdown

Although not a comprehensive compilation, SPICES clearly directs attention to key areas for the nurse to begin assessing and planning for appropriate interventions.[39–41]

The Hartford Institute of Geriatric Nursing has a comprehensive website with general assessment tools designed for nurses caring for older adults. The entire assessment series site can be accessed at http://consultgeri.org/tools/try-this-series. SPICES is the first issue in the series.[42]

Cognitive Impairment

A number of parameters affect assessment of health status; however, evidence suggests that self-report continues to be reliable in older adults, especially for prevalence of chronic conditions.[43–47] When compared with healthy peers, older adults with mild cognitive impairment provide sufficient history to reveal concurrent disorders. Use simple sentences with prompts to elicit necessary information. For patients with more severe impairments, confirm key symptoms with family members or caregivers in the patient's presence and with his or her consent. To avoid invalid assumptions, explore how older patients view themselves and their situations. Listen for their priorities and coping skills. These insights strengthen your partnerships with both patients and families as you evolve plans for care and treatment. Learn to recognize and avoid stereotypes that distort your appreciation of each patient as unique, with a treasure of life experiences.

Special Areas of Concern When Assessing Common or Concerning Symptoms

Common Concerns

- Functional assessment
- Activities of daily living
- Instrumental activities of daily living
- Medications
- Nutrition
- Pain (acute and persistent)
- Sexuality
- Urinary incontinence
- Smoking and alcohol

Symptoms in the older adult can have many meanings and interconnections, as seen with the geriatric syndromes. Explore the meaning of these symptoms as you would with all patients, and for the older adults, place these symptoms in the context of the overall functional assessment of the Activities of daily living (ADLs). Several topics warrant special attention as you gather the health history. Approach these areas with extra thoroughness and sensitivity, always with the goal of helping the older adult to maintain optimal level of function and well-being.

Functional Assessment

The 10-Minute Geriatric Screener evaluates for age-related changes that help older adults maintain optimal function. It covers the three important domains of geriatric assessment: physical, cognitive, and psychosocial function. Note that it addresses vision and hearing, key sensory modalities that can be followed with additional objective testing such as using an eye chart for vision, asking the patient about hearing, followed by the whisper test and more formal testing if indicated. It also includes questions about mobility, urinary incontinence (an often unreported problem), nutrition, memory, depression, and physical disabilities. All these components can affect social interaction and self-esteem in the elderly.

10-Minute Geriatric Screener[48]

Problem	Screening Measure	Positive Screen
Vision	Two Parts: Ask: "Do you have difficulty driving, or watching television, or reading, or doing any of your daily activities because of your eyesight?" If yes, then: Test each eye with the Snellen chart while the patient wears corrective lenses (if applicable).	Yes to question and inability to read greater than 20/40 on Snellen chart
Hearing	Use audioscope set at 40 dB. Test hearing using 1,000 and 2,000 Hz	Inability to hear 1,000 or 2,000 Hz in both ears or either of these frequencies in one ear
Leg mobility	Time the patient after asking: "Rise from the chair. Walk 20 feet briskly, turn, walk back to the chair, and sit down."	Unable to complete task in 15 seconds
Urinary incontinence	Two Parts: Ask: "In the last year, have you ever lost your urine and gotten wet?" If yes, then ask: "Have you lost urine on at least 6 separate dates?"	Yes to both questions
Nutrition/weight loss	Two Parts: Ask: "Have you lost 10 lb over the past 6 months without trying to do so?" Weigh the patient.	Yes to the question or weight <100 lb
Memory	Three-item recall	Unable to remember all three items after 1 minute
Depression	Ask: "Do you often feel sad or depressed?"	Yes to the question
Physical disability	Six questions: "Are you unable to…: "Do strenuous activities like fast walking or bicycling?" "Do heavy work around the house like washing windows, walls, or floors?" "Go shopping for groceries or clothes?" "Get to places out of walking distance?" "Bathe, either a sponge bath, tub bath, or shower?" "Dress, like putting on a shirt, buttoning and zipping, or putting on shoes?"	Yes to any of the questions

Activities of Daily Living

The daily activities of older adults, especially those with chronic illness, provide an important baseline for the future. First, ask about the capacity to perform the *ADLs*, which consist of six basic self-care abilities. Then move on to higher-level functions, the *instrumental activities of daily living (IADLs)*. Can the patient perform these activities independently, does the patient need some help, or is the patient entirely dependent on others?

Start with an open-ended request such as: "Tell me about your typical day" or "Tell me about your day yesterday." Then move to a greater level of detail ... "You got up at 8 AM?" "How is it getting out of bed?" ... "What did you do next?" Ask if activity levels have changed, who is available for help, and what helpers or caregivers actually do. Remember that assessing the patient's safety is a clinical priority.

Activities of Daily Living and Instrumental Activities of Daily Living	
Physical Activities of Daily Living (ADLs)	**Instrumental Activities of Daily Living (IADLs)**
Bathing	Using the telephone
Dressing	Shopping
Toileting	Preparing food
Transferring	Housekeeping
Continence	Doing laundry
Feeding	Transportation, including driving
	Taking medicine
	Managing money

Medications

The magnitude of adverse drug events leading to hospitalization and poor patient outcomes underscores the importance of a thorough medication history. Adults over the age of 65 years receive approximately 30% of all prescriptions. Approximately 85% of adults over the age of 65 years have at least one of six chronic conditions—arthritis, current asthma, cancer, cardiovascular disease, chronic obstructive pulmonary disease (COPD), or diabetes—and 50% take at least one prescription drug each day.[49,50] Almost 40% take five or more prescription drugs daily. Older adults have more than 50% of all reported adverse drug reactions causing hospital admission, reflecting pharmacodynamic changes in the distribution, metabolism, and elimination of drugs that place them at increased risk.

- A thorough *medication history* includes name, dose, frequency, and the *patient's view* of the reason for taking each drug.

- Ask the patient to bring in all medication bottles and over-the-counter products to develop an accurate medication list.

- Explore all components of polypharmacy, a major cause of morbidity, including suboptimal prescribing, concurrent use of multiple drugs, underuse, inappropriate use, and nonadherence.

- Ask specifically about over-the-counter products; vitamin and nutritional supplements; and mood-altering drugs such as narcotics, benzodiazepines, and recreational substances.[51]

- Assess medications for drug interactions.

- Be particularly careful when treating *insomnia*, estimated to occur in 40% of older adults. A *sleep history* provides information essential for diagnosis; a *sleep diary* may be especially helpful in uncovering the origins of a poor sleep pattern.[52] Increased exercise may be the best remedy. Turn to expert guidelines on types of sleep disorders and recommended management.[53]

Medications are the single most common modifiable risk factor associated with falls. Review strategies for avoiding polypharmacy.[54,55] Keep the number of drugs prescribed to a minimum and "start low, go slow" with respect to dosing. Learn about drug–drug interactions and consult the *Beers criteria* (http://www.americangeriatrics.org/files/documents/beers/BeersCriteriaPublicTranslation.pdf), updated in 2012 by the American Geriatrics Society and widely used by health care providers, educators, and policymakers. These criteria include listing hazardous drugs for older adults.[56,57] Risk factors for adverse drug reactions in hospitalized older patients are listed below.

Hospitalized Older Adults: Risk Factors for Adverse Drug Reactions[58]

- More than four comorbid conditions
- Heart failure, renal failure, or liver disease
- Age 80 years or older
- Number of drugs, especially if eight or more
- Use of warfarin, insulins, oral antiplatelet agents, or oral hypoglycemic agents
- Previous adverse drug reaction
- Hyperlipidemia
- Raised white cell count
- Use of antidiabetic agents
- Length of stay 12 days or longer

Source: Onder G, Petrovic M, Balamurugan T, et al. Less is more. Development and validation of a score to assess risk of adverse drug reactions among the in-hospital patients 65 years or older. *Arch Intern Med*. 2010;170:1142.

Nutrition

Taking a diet history and using nutritional screening tools often reveal nutritional deficits. The prevalence of undernutrition increases with age, affecting up to 10% of nursing home residents and up to 50% of older patients at hospital discharge.[59] Recent data suggest that only 30% to 40% meet recommended guidelines for daily intake of fruit and vegetables.[60] Older adults with chronic diseases are particularly vulnerable, especially those with poor dentition, oral or gastrointestinal disorders, depression or other psychiatric illness, and drug regimens that affect appetite and oral secretions. For underweight elders, the serum albumin is an independent risk factor for all-cause mortality.

Mini Nutritional Assessment
MNA®

Last name:			First name:	
Sex:	Age:	Weight, kg:	Height, cm:	Date:

Complete the screen by filling in the boxes with the appropriate numbers. Total the numbers for the final screening score.

Screening

A Has food intake declined over the past 3 months due to loss of appetite, digestive problems, chewing or swallowing difficulties?
0 = severe decrease in food intake
1 = moderate decrease in food intake

▣

B Weight loss during the last 3 months
0 = weight loss greater than 3 kg (6.6 lbs)
1 = does not know
2 = weight loss between 1 and 3 kg (2.2 and 6.6 lbs)

▣

C Mobility
0 = bed or chair bound
1 = able to get out of bed / chair but does not go out
2 = goes out

▣

D Has suffered psychological stress or acute disease in the past 3 months?

▣

E Neuropsychological problems
0 = severe dementia or depression
1 = mild dementia

▣

F1 Body Mass Index (BMI) (weight in kg) / (height in m²)
0 = BMI less than 19
1 = BMI 19 to less than 21
2 = BMI 21 to less than 23

▣

IF BMI IS NOT AVAILABLE, REPLACE QUESTION F1 WITH QUESTION F2.
DO NOT ANSWER QUESTION F2 IF QUESTION F1 IS ALREADY COMPLETED.

F2 Calf circumference (CC) in cm
0 = CC less than 31

▣

▣ ▣

(max. 14 points)

12-14 points:	Normal nutritional status
8-11 points:	At risk of malnutrition
0-7 points:	Malnourished

Ref. Vellas B, Villars H, Abellan G, et al. *Overview of the MNA® - Its History and Challenges.* J Nutr Health Aging 2006;10:456-465.

Rubenstein LZ, Harker JO, Salva A, Guigoz Y, Vellas B. *Screening for Undernutrition in Geriatric Practice: Developing the Short-Form Mini Nutritional Assessment (MNA-SF).* J. Geront 2001;56A: M366-377.

Guigoz Y. *The Mini-Nutritional Assessment (MNA®) Review of the Literature - What does it tell us?* J Nutr Health Aging 2006; 10:466-487.

Kaiser MJ, Bauer JM, Ramsch C, et al. *Validation of the Mini Nutritional Assessment Short-Form (MNA®-SF): A practical tool for identification of nutritional status.* J Nutr Health Aging 2009; 13:782-788.

® Société des Produits Nestlé, S.A., Vevey, Switzerland, Trademark Owners

© Nestlé, 1994, Revision 2009. N67200 12/99 10M

For more information: www.mna-elderly.com

Acute and Persistent Pain

Pain and associated complaints account for 80% of clinician visits. Prevalence of pain may reach 25% to 50% in community-dwelling adults and 40% to 80% in nursing home residents. Pain usually arises from musculoskeletal complaints like back and joint pain.[61] Headache, neuralgias from diabetes and herpes zoster, nighttime leg pain, and cancer pain are also common. Older patients are less likely to report pain, leading to undue suffering, depression, social isolation, physical disability, and loss of function. The American Geriatrics Society favors the term *persistent pain*, because chronic pain is associated with negative stereotypes.[62]

Characteristics of Acute and Persistent Pain[59]	
Acute Pain	**Persistent Pain**
Distinct onset	Lasts more than 3 months
Obvious pathology	Often associated with psychological or functional impairment
Short duration	Can fluctuate in character and intensity over time
Common causes: postsurgical, trauma, headache	Common causes: arthritis, cancer, claudication, leg cramps, neuropathy, radiculopathy

Accurate assessment is the basis of effective treatment.[63,64] Inquire about pain *each time* you meet with an older patient. Assessing pain in older adults is challenging. Patients may be reluctant to report symptoms due to fears of additional testing, cost of care and medication, denial of disease, cognitive or verbal impairments, or barriers of trust, language, or cultural understanding. Patients may report multiple conditions that complicate assessment. Nonetheless, evidence shows when patients do report pain, even those with mild to moderate cognitive impairment, the self-report is reliable. Ask specifically, "Are you having any pain right now? How about during the past week?" Be alert for signs of untreated pain, such as use of the terms "burning," "discomfort," or "soreness"; depressed affect; and nonverbal change in posture or gait. Many multidimensional and unidimensional pain scales are available. Unidimensional scales such as the Visual Analog Scale, graphic pictures, and the Verbal 0–10 Scale have all been validated and are easiest to use.[63,65] Interview caregivers or family members for relevant history in patients with severe cognitive deficits.

Refer to the pain scale in Chapter 7, Beginning the Physical Examination: General Survey, Vital Signs, and Pain, p. 139.

It is important to distinguish acute pain from persistent pain and thoroughly investigate its cause. In older adults, confusion, restlessness, fatigue, or irritability often accompany conditions causing pain. Assessing pain includes evaluation of these related conditions as well as the effect of pain on quality of life, social interactions, and functional level. Consider multidisciplinary assessment is complex cases if the cause cannot be identified and risks of disability and comorbidity are high.

Be familiar with the many modalities of pain relief, ranging from analgesics to numerous nonpharmacologic therapies, especially those that actively engage patients in their treatment plan and build self-reliance. Patient education alone has been shown effective.[61] Relaxation techniques, tai chi, acupuncture, massage, and biofeedback can avert adding more medications.

See the 10-Minute Geriatric Screener for functional assessment on pp. 944–945.

Sexuality

Sex continues throughout the lifespan, and issues should be addressed as patients may have valid concerns requiring attention. The physical assessment section will address changes that occur with aging, including pain or medical conditions that may deter sexual responses such as diabetes or heart conditions. Suggestions to alleviate pain might be changes in positions, use of lubrication, heat application, and warm baths.

The PLISS IT Model has been used to initiate the discussion of sex.[66,67]

PLISS IT Model
P Obtaining **P**ermission from the client to initiate sexual discussion
LI Providing the **L**imited **I**nformation needed to function sexually
SS Giving **S**pecific **S**uggestions for the individual to proceed with sexual relations
IT Providing Intensive **T**herapy surrounding the issues of sexuality for that client

Urinary Incontinence[68,69]

Urinary incontinence is often not mentioned by patients as they may be embarrassed or may believe it is a normal part of aging.[70] During the health history, questions should address:

Onset: When did the incontinence/leaking begin? Has it occurred before? How often does it occur? Does it occur when something else happens (sneezing, laughing, jumping)?
Location: Where are you when this occurs?
Duration: Does it last all day? Occasionally? Is there a pattern?
Characteristic Symptoms: Describe the urine (color, odor, amount, and times per day).
Associated Manifestations: What else is occurring? (Use the mnemonic DIAPPERS on the next page.) How is this affecting the quality of life?
Relieving Factors: Does changing the amount, type, or timing of fluid intake influence the incontinence?
Treatment: Have you seen anyone for this? What have you done? Bladder training? Kegel exercises?

The "**DIAPPERS**" mnemonic helps students assess incontinence:

Delirium
Infection-urinary
Atrophic urethritis/vaginitis
Pharmaceuticals
Psychological disorders, especially depression
Excess urine output, for example, hyperglycemia or heart failure
Restricted mobility
Stool impaction

Smoking and Alcohol

Smoking is harmful at all ages. At each visit, advise smokers, approximately 9.5% of older adults, to quit.[71] The commitment to stop smoking may take time, but quitting is crucial for reducing risk of heart disease, pulmonary disease, malignancy, and loss of daily function.

Recommended limits for consumption of *alcohol* are lower for adults older than 65 years due to physiologic changes that alter alcohol metabolism, frequent comorbid illness, and risk of drug interactions. Older adults should have *no more than three drinks on any one day or seven drinks a week.*[72]

More than 40% of adults over age 65 years drink alcohol, about 4.5% are binge-drinkers, and 2% to 4% may have abuse or dependence.[73,74] More than 14% of older adults exceed the recommended limits.[75] When health status is taken into account, more than 53% have harmful or hazardous alcohol consumption. From 10% to 15% of older patients in primary care practices and up to 38% of hospitalized older adults are reported to have problematic alcohol consumption.[76]

Despite the high prevalence of alcohol-related problems, rates of detection and treatment are low. Screening all older adults for harmful alcohol use is especially important due to adverse interactions with most medications and exacerbation of comorbid illnesses, including cirrhosis, gastrointestinal bleeding or reflux disease, gout, hypertension, diabetes, insomnia, gait disorders, and depression in up to 30% of older patients.[74] Watch for clues of excess alcohol consumption, listed below, especially in patients with recent bereavement or losses, pain, disability or depression, or a family history of alcohol disorders.

Detecting Alcohol Use Disorders in Older Adults: Clinical Clues

- Memory loss, cognitive impairment
- Depression, anxiety
- Neglect in hygiene, appearance
- Poor appetite, nutritional deficits

- Sleep disruption
- Hypertension refractory to therapy
- Blood glucose control issues
- Seizures refractory to therapy
- Impaired balance and gait, falls
- Recurrent gastritis or esophagitis
- Difficulty managing warfarin dosing
- Use of other addictive substances such as sedatives or narcotic analgesics, illicit drugs, nicotine

The AUDIT-C is used to determine risky drinking and has been shown to perform as well as the full AUDIT and notably better than self-reporting or the CAGE questionnaire.[77,78] Although symptoms and signs are more subtle in older adults, making early detection more difficult, the AUDIT-C is sensitive and specific in this age group. Below is the AUDIT-C test

See Chapter 4, The Health History, pp. 74–75.

AUDIT-C

Q1: How often did you have a drink containing alcohol in the past year?

Answer	Points
Never	0
Monthly or less	1
Two to four times a month	2
Two to three times a week	3
Four or more times a week	4

Q2: How many drinks did you have on a typical day when you were drinking in the past year?

Answer	Points
None, I do not drink	0
1 or 2	0
3 or 4	1
5 or 6	2
7 to 9	3
10 or more	4

Q3: How often did you have six or more drinks on one occasion in the past year?	
Answer	**Points**
Never	0
Less than monthly	1
Monthly	2
Weekly	3
Daily or almost daily	4

The AUDIT-C is scored on a scale of 0–12 (scores of 0 reflect no alcohol use). In men, a score of 4 or more is considered positive; in women, a score of 3 or more is considered positive. Generally, the higher the AUDIT-C score, the more likely it is that the patient's drinking is affecting his/her health and safety.

The Alcohol Use Disorders Identification Test is a publication of the World Health Organization, @ 1990

PHYSICAL EXAMINATION OF THE OLDER ADULT

General Survey

As the patient enters the room, how does the patient walk to the chair? Move onto the examining table? Are there changes in posture or involuntary movements? Note the patient's hygiene and dress. Assess the patient's apparent state of health, degree of vitality, and mood and affect. As you talk with the patient, decide if screening for cognitive changes is needed.

Undernutrition, slowed motor performance, loss of muscle mass, or weakness suggests frailty.

Kyphosis or abnormal gait can impair balance and increase risk of falls.

Flat or impoverished affect is seen in *depression, Parkinson disease,* or Alzheimers disease.

See Screening for Dementia: The Mini-Cog, pp. 960–961, for a brief and well-validated screening tool for dementia.[79,80]

Vital Signs

Measure blood pressure using recommended techniques, checking for increased SBP and widened PP, defined as SBP minus DBP. With aging, SBP and peripheral vascular resistance increase, whereas DBP decreases. For adults ages 60 years and older, the Eighth Joint National Committee (JNC8) recommends blood pressure targets of 150/90 or lower but notes that if treatment results in SBP lower than 140 and is "well tolerated and without adverse effects to health or quality of live, treatment does not need to be adjusted."[81] However, in the "oldest old," those ages 80 years and older, other experts cite studies showing that blood pressure targets of 140

Isolated systolic hypertension (SBP ≥140) after age 50 years and PP of 60 or greater increases the risk of stroke, renal failure, and heart disease.[82]

to less than 150/70 to 80 appear optimal for notable reductions in stroke, cardiovascular events, and all-cause mortality.[83–86]

Assess the patient for orthostatic hypotension, defined as a drop in SBP of 20 mm Hg or more or DBP of 10 mm Hg or more within 3 minutes of standing. Measure blood pressure and HR in two positions: supine after the patient rests for up to 10 minutes, then within 3 minutes after standing up.

Orthostatic hypotension occurs in 20% of older adults and in up to 50% of frail nursing home residents, especially when they first get up. Symptoms include lightheadedness, weakness, unsteadiness, visual blurring, and, in 20% to 30% of patients, syncope. Causes include medications, autonomic disorders, diabetes, prolonged bed rest, volume depletion, amyloidosis, postprandial state, and cardiovascular disorders.[87–90]

Measure heart rate, respiratory rate, and temperature. The apical HR often yields better detection of about arrhythmias in older patients than does the radial pulse. Use thermometers accurate for lower temperatures. Obtain oxygen saturation using a pulse oximeter.

RR of 25 breaths per minute or greater indicates lower respiratory infection, heart failure, and COPD exacerbation.

Hypothermia is more common in elderly patients.

Weight and height are especially important in the elderly and needed for calculation of the BMI. Weight is also a key clinical measure for patients with heart failure and chronic kidney disease. Weight should be measured at every visit, preferably with footwear removed.

Low weight is a key indicator of poor nutrition, seen in depression, alcoholism, cognitive impairment, malignancy, chronic organ failure (cardiac, renal, pulmonary), medication use, social isolation, poor dentition, and poverty. Rapidly increasing daily weights occur in fluid overload.

Skin

Note physiologic changes of aging, such as thinning, loss of elastic tissue and turgor, and wrinkling. Skin may be dry, flaky, rough, and often itchy (*asteatosis*), with a latticework of shallow fissures that creates a mosaic of small polygons, especially on the legs.

Observe any patchy changes in color. Check the extensor surface of the hands and forearms for white depigmented patches, or *pseudoscars,* and for well-demarcated vividly purple macules or patches, *actinic purpura,* that may fade after several weeks.

ACTINIC PURPURA—FOREARM

Look for changes from sun exposure. Areas of skin may appear weather beaten, thickened, yellowed, and deeply furrowed; there may be *solar or actinic lentigines,* or "liver spots," and *actinic keratoses,* superficial flattened papules covered by a dry scale.

Distinguish such lesions from a *basal cell carcinoma,* a translucent nodule that spreads and leaves a depressed center with a firm elevated border, and from a *squamous cell carcinoma,* a firm reddish-appearing lesion often emerging in a sun-exposed area. A dark-raised asymmetric lesion with irregular borders may be a *melanoma.* See Table 9-9, Skin Tumors, p. 203, and Table 9-10, Benign and Malignant Nevi, p. 204.

Inspect for the benign lesions of aging, namely, *comedones,* or blackheads, on the cheeks or around the eyes; *cherry angiomas,* which often appear early in adulthood; and *seborrheic keratoses,* raised yellowish lesions that feel greasy and velvety or warty.

Vesicular lesions occurring in a dermatomal distribution are suspicious for *herpes zoster* from reactivation of latent varicella-zoster virus in the dorsal root ganglia. Risk increases with age and impaired cell-mediated immunity.[91,92]

In older bed-bound patients, especially when emaciated or neurologically impaired, inspect the skin thoroughly for damage or ulceration on the sacral and perianal areas, the lower back, heels, and elbows where pressure ulcers commonly occur.

Pressure ulcers may develop from obliteration of arteriolar and capillary blood flow to the skin or from shear forces during movement across sheets or when lifted upright incorrectly. See Table 9-12, Pressure Ulcers, p. 206.

Head and Neck

Perform a thorough evaluation of the head and neck.

See Chapter 10, The Head and Neck.

Inspect the eyelids, the bony orbit, and the eye. The eye may appear recessed from atrophy of fat in the surrounding tissues. Observe any *senile ptosis* arising from weakening of the levator palpebrae, relaxation of the skin, and increased weight of the upper eyelid. Check the lower lids for ectropion or *entropion.* Note yellowing of the sclera, and *arcus senilis,* a benign whitish ring around the limbus.

See Table 11-3, Variations and Abnormalties of the Eyelids, p. 266 and Table 11-4, Lumps and Swelling in and Around the Eyes, p. 267.

Test visual acuity with correction in each eye, using a pocket Snellen chart or wall-mounted chart. Note any *presbyopia,* the loss of near vision arising from decreased elasticity of the lens related to aging.

One in three adults suffers some form of visual loss by age 65.[93]

Test pupillary constriction to light, both the direct and consensual response and during the near response. Then swing the light beam several times between the right and left eyes. Test the six directions of gaze. Except for possible impairment in upward gaze, extraocular movements should remain intact.

If the pupil dilates as the light swings over, a relative afferent pupillary defect is present, which is suspicious for optic nerve disease. Refer to an ophthalmologist.

Using your ophthalmoscope, carefully examine the lenses and fundi.

The prevalence of cataracts, glaucoma, and macular degeneration all increase with aging.

Using the ophthalmoscope beam, check at 1 to 2 ft for a red reflex. With the ophthalmoscope lens at +10 diopters, inspect each lens close to the eye for opacities. Do not depend on the flashlight alone because the lens may look clear superficially.

A red reflex is not seen with *cataracts*. At +10 diopters, a cataract appears white.[94] Cataracts are the world's leading cause of blindness. Risk factors include cigarette smoking, exposure to UV-B light, high alcohol intake, diabetes, medications (including steroids), and trauma. See Table 11-5, Opacities of the Cornea and Lens, p. 268.

In older adults, the fundi lose their youthful shine and light reflections, and the arteries look narrowed, paler, straighter, and less brilliant. Assess the cup-to-disc ratio, usually 1:2 or less.

Retinal microvascular disease is linked to cerebral microvascular changes and cognitive impairment.[95,96]

An increased cup-to-disc ratio suggests *primary open-angle glaucoma (POAG),* caused by irreversible optic neuropathy and leading to loss of peripheral and central vision and blindness. Prevalence of POAG is four to five times higher in African Americans and Hispanics, although older, non-Hispanic white women, are highest in number affected.[97,98]

Inspect the fundi for colloid bodies causing alterations in pigmentation, called *drusen*.

Macular degeneration causes poor central vision and blindness.[99] Types include *dry atrophic* (more common but less severe) and *wet exudative,* or neovascular. Drusen may be hard and sharply defined, or soft and confluent with altered pigmentation.

Test hearing by occluding one ear and using the whispered voice technique or an audioscope. Be sure to inspect the ear canals for cerumen, because removal can quickly improve hearing.

See techniques for testing hearing, pp. 298–299. Ask if hearing loss is present in an effective screening method. Proceed to audiometry for those saying yes; check acuity to whispered voice for saying no.

Examine the oral cavity for odor, appearance of the gingival mucosa, any caries, mobility of the teeth, and quantity of saliva. Inspect closely for lesions on any of the mucosal surfaces. Ask the patient to remove the dentures to check the gums for sores.

Continue with your usual examination of the thyroid gland and lymph nodes.

In older adults common causes of hyperthyroidism are *Graves disease* and *toxic multinodular goiter*. Causes of hypothyroidism include autoimmune thyroiditis, followed by drugs, neck radiotherapy, thyroidectomy, or radio-iodine ablation.[38]

Malodor may occur with poor oral hygiene, periodontitis or caries. *Gingivitis* accompanies periodontal disease. Dental plaque and cavitation may cause caries. For increased tooth mobility from abscesses or advanced caries, consider removal to prevent aspiration. Decreased salivation results from medications, radiation, Sjögren syndrome, or dehydration. Oral tumors can cause lesions, usually on the lateral margins of the tongue and floor of the mouth.[100,101]

Thorax and Lungs

Complete the usual examination, observing for subtle signs of changes in pulmonary function.

Increased anteroposterior diameter, purse-lipped breathing, and dyspnea with talking or minimal exertion suggest *COPD.* There is considerable overlap of asthma and COPD in older adults, heralded by nonspecific symptoms like dyspnea, cough, wheezing, and nocturnal onset.

Proceed to objective testing with spirometry, which most tolerate well.[102]

Cardiovascular System

Review the findings from blood pressure and heart rate measurements.

Isolated systolic hypertension and a widened pulse pressure are cardiac risk factors, prompting a search for *left ventricular hypertrophy* (LVH).

Begin by inspecting the jugular venous pressure (JVP). Palpate the carotid upstrokes and auscultate for carotid bruits.

A *tortuous atherosclerotic aorta* can raise pressure in the left jugular veins by impairing emptying into the right atrium. It may also cause kinking of the carotid artery low in the neck on the right, chiefly in women with hypertension, which can be mistaken for a carotid aneurysm.

Carotid bruits can occur in *aortic stenosis.* The presence of bruits from *carotid stenosis* increases risk of ipsilateral stroke.

Assess the point of maximum impulse (PMI) or apical impulse and auscultate for S_1 and S_2. Listen also for the extra sounds of S_3 and S_4.

A sustained PMI is present in LVH; a diffuse PMI and an S_3 signal left ventricular dilatation from heart failure or cardiomyopathy and an S_3 signal left ventricular dilatation from heart failure or cardiomyopathy. An S_4 often accompanies hypertension.[103]

Beginning in the second right interspace, listen for cardiac murmurs in all areas of auscultation (see pp. 408–412 of Chapter 14, The Cardiovascular System). Describe the timing, shape, location of maximal intensity, radiation, intensity, pitch, and quality of each murmur you detect.

A systolic crescendo–decrescendo murmur in the second right interspace suggests *aortic sclerosis or aortic stenosis.* Both are associated with an increased risk of cardiovascular disease and death.[104,105]

A harsh holosystolic murmur at the apex radiating to the axilla suggests *mitral regurgitation,* the most common murmur in older adults.

Breasts and Axillae

Palpate the breasts carefully for lumps or masses. Include palpation of the tail of Spence that extends into the axilla. Examine the axillae for lymphadenopathy. Note any scaly, vesicular ulcerated lesions on or near the nipple.

Any lumps or masses in older women, and more rarely, in older men, mandate further investigation for possible breast cancer.

Paget disease with eczematoid scaling of the nipple is uncommon, but peaks between the ages of 50 and 60 years.[106]

Abdomen

Inspect the abdomen for masses or visible pulsations. Auscultate for bruits over the aorta, and the renal and femoral arteries. Palpate to the right and left of the midline for aortic pulsations. Try to assess the width of the aorta by pressing more deeply with one hand on each of its lateral margins (see Chapter 16, The Gastrointestinal and Renal Systems, p. 504–505).

Abdominal bruits are suspicious for atherosclerotic vascular disease.

A widened aorta of 3 cm or greater and pulsatile mass are found in *abdominal aortic aneurysm,* especially in older male smokers.

Peripheral Vascular System

Carefully palpate the brachial, radial, femoral, popliteal, and pedal pulses.

Diminished or absent pulses are present in *peripheral arterial disease (PAD).* Confirm your findings with an office ankle–brachial index (ABI); if less than 0.9, the ABI has a sensitivity of 70% and specificity of 90%. In patients with PAD, 30% to 60% report no leg symptoms.[107]

See Chapter 15, The Peripheral Vascular System and Lymphatic System, pp. 460–462.

Female Genitalia[108]

Inspect for changes related to menopause such as thinning of the skin or loss of pubic hair. Note redness, discharge, lesions, prolapsed uterus, or mutilation.

Erythema with satellite lesions results from *Candida* infection; erythema with ulceration or a necrotic center is suspicious for *vulvar carcinoma*. Multifocal reddened lesions with white scaling plaques occur in extramammary *Paget disease,* a form of intraepithelial adenocarcinoma.

Male Genitalia

Examine the penis, retracting the foreskin if present. Examine the scrotum, testes, and epididymis. Note redness, lesions, discharge, or lumps.

Findings include smegma, penile cancer, and scrotal hydroceles.

Musculoskeletal System

The evaluation of this system began with leg mobility testing during the *10-Minute Geriatric Screener* (p. 945) at the onset of the visit. Leg mobility is routinely tested by the *"Timed Get Up and Go,"* or *TUG, test* for gait and balance, an excellent screen for risk of falling. Ask the patient to get up from a chair, walk 10 feet, turn, and return to the chair. Older adults should complete this test in 10 seconds.

If the patient has joint deformities, deficits in mobility, pain with movement, or a delayed "get up and go" perform a more thorough examination of individual joints and a more comprehensive neurologic examination.

Assess for degenerative joint changes in *osteoarthritis* and joint inflammation from *rheumatoid* or *gouty arthritis.*

See Chapter 18, The Musculoskeletal System, Tables 18-1 to 18-8, pp. 636–644.

Timed Get Up and Go Test[109,110]

Performed with patient wearing regular footwear, using usual walking aid if needed, and sitting back in a chair with armrest.

On the word, "Go," the patient is asked to do the following:
1. Stand up from the arm chair
2. Walk 3 meters (in a line)
3. Turn
4. Walk back to chair
5. Sit down

Time the second effort.

Observe patient for postural stability, steppage, stride length, and sway.

Scoring:
- **Normal:** completes task in less than 10 seconds
- **Abnormal:** completes task in more than 20 seconds

Low scores correlate with good functional independence; high scores correlate with poor functional independence and higher risk of falls.

Reproduced from Get-up and Go Test. In: Mathias S, Nayak USL, Isaacs B. "Balance in elderly patient" The "Get Up and Go" Test. *Arch Phys Med Rehabil.* 1986;67:387; Podsiadlo D, Richardson S. The Timed "Up and Go": A test of basic functional mobility for frail elderly persons. *J Am Geriatr Soc.* 1991;39:142.

Nervous System and Mental Status

As with the musculoskeletal examination, begin your evaluation of the nervous system with the *10-Minute Geriatric Screener* (p. 945). Carefully assess memory and affect.

Learn to distinguish delirium from depression and dementia (see Table 24-1, p. 975). Search carefully for underlying causes. Mini-Cog Screening for Cognitive Impairment in Older Adults is available at: http:www.mini-cog.com and The Montreal Cognitive Assessment (MoCA).

Instructions for Administration & Scoring

ID: _____ Date: _____

Step 1: Three Word Registration

Look directly at person and say, "Please listen carefully. I am going to say three words that I want you to repeat back to me now and try to remember. The words are [select a list of words from the versions below]. Please say them for me now." If the person is unable to repeat the words after three attempts, move on to Step 2 (clock drawing).

The following and other word lists have been used in one or more clinical studies.[1-3] For repeated administrations, use of an alternative word list is recommended.

Version 1	Version 2	Version 3	Version 4	Version 5	Version 6
Banana	Leader	Village	River	Captain	Daughter
Sunrise	Season	Kitchen	Nation	Garden	Heaven
Chair	Table	Baby	Finger	Picture	Mountain

Step 2: Clock Drawing

Say: "Next, I want you to draw a clock for me. First, put in all of the numbers where they go." When that is completed, say: "Now, set the hands to 10 past 11."

Use preprinted circle (see next page) for this exercise. Repeat instructions as needed as this is not a memory test. Move to Step 3 if the clock is not complete within three minutes.

Step 3: Three Word Recall

Ask the person to recall the three words you stated in Step 1. Say: "What were the three words I asked you to remember?" Record the word list version number and the person's answers below.

Word List Version: _____   Person's Answers: _____   _____   _____

Scoring

Word Recall: _____ (0-3 points)	1 point for each word spontaneously recalled without cueing.
Clock Draw: _____ (0 or 2 points)	Normal clock = 2 points. A normal clock has all numbers placed in the correct sequence and approximately correct position (e.g., 12, 3, 6 and 9 are in anchor positions) with no missing or duplicate numbers. Hands are pointing to the 11 and 2 (11:10). Hand length is not scored. Inability or refusal to draw a clock (abnormal) = 0 points.
Total Score: _____ (0-5 points)	Total score = Word Recall score + Clock Draw score. A cut point of <3 on the Mini-Cog™ has been validated for dementia screening, but many individuals with clinically meaningful cognitive impairment will score higher. When greater sensitivity is desired, a cut point of <4 is recommended as it may indicate a need for further evaluation of cognitive status.

Clock Drawing

ID: _____ Date: _____

MONTREAL COGNITIVE ASSESSMENT (MOCA)
Version 7.1 Original Version

NAME :
Education :
Sex :

Date of birth :
DATE :

VISUOSPATIAL / EXECUTIVE		POINTS

Ⓔ End
Ⓐ
⑤
①Begin
Ⓑ
②
Ⓓ
④
③
Ⓒ

Copy cube

[ ]

Draw CLOCK (Ten past eleven)
(3 points)

[ ]

[ ]
Contour

[ ]
Numbers

[ ]
Hands

__/5

NAMING

[ ]   [ ]   [ ]   __/3

MEMORY	Read list of words, subject must repeat them. Do 2 trials, even if 1st trial is successful. Do a recall after 5 minutes.		FACE	VELVET	CHURCH	DAISY	RED	No points
		1st trial						
		2nd trial						

ATTENTION	Read list of digits (1 digit/ sec.).	Subject has to repeat them in the forward order	[ ] 2 1 8 5 4	__/2
		Subject has to repeat them in the backward order	[ ] 7 4 2	

Read list of letters. The subject must tap with his hand at each letter A. No points if ≥ 2 errors

[ ]   F B A C M N A A J K L B A F A K D E A A A J A M O F A A B   __/1

Serial 7 subtraction starting at 100   [ ] 93   [ ] 86   [ ] 79   [ ] 72   [ ] 65

4 or 5 correct subtractions: **3 pts**, 2 or 3 correct: **2 pts**, 1 correct: **1 pt**, 0 correct: **0 pt**   __/3

LANGUAGE	Repeat : I only know that John is the one to help today. [ ]	__/2
	The cat always hid under the couch when dogs were in the room. [ ]	

Fluency / Name maximum number of words in one minute that begin with the letter F   [ ] _____ (N ≥ 11 words)   __/1

ABSTRACTION	Similarity between e.g. banana - orange = fruit [ ] train – bicycle [ ] watch - ruler	__/2

DELAYED RECALL	Has to recall words WITH NO CUE	FACE [ ]	VELVET [ ]	CHURCH [ ]	DAISY [ ]	RED [ ]	Points for UNCUED recall only	__/5
Optional	Category cue							
	Multiple choice cue							

ORIENTATION	[ ] Date [ ] Month [ ] Year [ ] Day [ ] Place [ ] City	__/6

© Z.Nasreddine MD   www.mocatest.org   Normal ≥ 26 / 30

TOTAL   __/30

Administered by: _____

Add 1 point if ≤ 12 yr edu

Pay close attention to gait and balance, particularly standing balance; timed 10-foot walk; stride characteristics including width, pace, and length of stride; and careful turning. A recent study of neurologic versus nonneurologic (primarily hip and knee orthopedic) gait disorders showed that neurologic disorders like Parkinsonian, sensory ataxic, spastic, higher-level gait, and, particularly, multiple neurologic gait disorders tripled the risk for recurrent falls.[118] Investigators are looking at the neurobiology of gait disorders as markers of preclinical dementia and other neurologic conditions that may lead to earlier diagnosis and new preventive strategies.[119]

When gait abnormalities are detected, pursue a more detailed neurologic examination.[122,123] Distinguishing neurologic changes of aging from abnormal findings is challenging, as neurologic abnormalities without identifiable disease are common in the older population and increase with age, occurring in up to 50% of older adults.[124] Examples of age-related abnormalities include unequal pupil size, decreased arm swing and spontaneous movements, increased leg rigidity and abnormal gait, presence of the snout and grasp reflexes, and decreased toe vibratory sense.

Examine for evidence of **T**remor, **R**igidity, **A**kinesia, and **P**ostural instability, or **TRAP,** which are several of the most common features of Parkinson disease.[125] Also look for bradykinesia, the most characteristic clinical sign, and micrographia, shuffling "freezing" gait, and difficulty rising from a chair.

In summary, the assessment of the older adult does not follow the traditional format of the history and physical examination. It calls for enhanced techniques of interviewing, special emphasis on daily function and key topics related to elder health, and a focus on functional assessment during the physical examination.

RECORDING YOUR FINDINGS

As you read through this physical examination, you will notice some atypical findings. Try to test yourself. See if you can interpret these findings in the context of all you have learned about the examination of the older adult.

Abnormalities of gait and balance, especially widening of the base, slowing and lengthening of stride, and difficulty turning, are correlated with risk for falls.[120,121]

These findings are seen in *Parkinson disease,* found in approximately 60,000 new cases a year and affecting about 1 million people in the United States.[126] Tremor is of slow frequency and occurs at rest, with a "pill-rolling" quality. It is aggravated by stress and inhibited during sleep or movement. Prodromal nonmotor symptoms including depression, rapid eye movement behavior disorder, and daytime sleepiness are now being identified.[125]

Essential tremor is bilateral and symmetric, with a positive family history and commonly diminished by alcohol.

Persistent blinking after tap on forehead and difficulty walking heel-to-toe in *Parkinson disease* are also more common.

Recording the Physical Examination—The Older Adult

Mr. J, 82-year-old man appears healthy but overweight, with positive muscle bulk and tone. He is alert and interactive, with recall of his life history. Accompanied by his son.

Vital Signs
Ht (without shoes) 5'10" (178 cm). Wt (dressed) 195 lb. BMI 28. BP 145/88 right arm, supine; 154/94 left arm, supine. Orthostatic BP without changes. HR 98 and regular. RR 18, regular. Temperature (oral) 98.6°F.

10-Minute Geriatric Screener
(See p. 945) *Vision.* Patient reports difficulty reading. Visual acuity 20/60 (R eye), 20/40 (L eye) on Snellen chart with glasses.

Needs further evaluation for glasses.

Hearing. Whisper test R with difficulty, L with increased difficulty, third attempt. Cannot hear 1,000 or 2,000 Hz with audioscope in either ear.

Needs further evaluation for hearing.

Leg Mobility. Can walk 10 ft briskly, turn, walk back to chair, and sit down in 9 seconds.

Urinary Incontinence. Has lost urine and gotten wet on 20 separate days in the past 2 months.

Needs further evaluation for incontinence, including "DIAPPERS" assessment (see p. 951), referral for prostate examination, bladder scan and post-void residual, which is normally ≤50 mL (requires bladder catheterization)

Nutrition. Has lost 15 lb over the past 6 months without trying.

Needs nutritional screen, p. 948

Memory. Can remember three items after 1 minute.

Depression. Does not often feel sad or depressed.

Physical Disability. Can walk fast but cannot ride a bicycle (never learned). Can do moderate but not heavy work around the house. Can go shopping for groceries or clothes. Can go to places out of walking distance (son drives). Can bathe each day without difficulty. Can dress independently, including buttoning, zippering, and tying shoes.

Consider exercise regimen with strength and balance.

Physical Examination
Skin, Hair, Nails. Tan, warm and moist. 1.5 cm solar lentigo above R eyebrow. Gray hair thinning at crown, dry with moderate amount of flakes, gray hairs evenly distributed over body. Nails without clubbing or cyanosis, slightly yellow and thick.

Head, Eyes, Ears, Nose, Throat (HEENT). Scalp without lesions. Skull NC/AT (normocephalic/atraumatic).

Eyes—symmetrical, lids—close BL, no ptosis or edema, conjunctiva pink, sclera muddy, iris brown. Lacrimal apparatus moist without additional drainage PERRLA (pupils equal, round, reactive to light and accommodation), 2 mm constricting to 1 mm BL. EOMs (extraocular movements) intact.

Disc margins sharp, without hemorrhages or exudates. Mild arteriolar narrowing. Snellen with corrective glasses on 20/60 (R eye), 20/40 (L eye).

Ears—pinna without lumps, lesions or tenderness, TMs (tympanic membranes) with cone of light, minimal tan, sticky cerumen BL. Weber midline, AC ≥ BC, whisper test R with difficulty, L, third attempt.

Nose—patent BL, mucosa and turbinates pink. No odor, frontal or maxillary sinus tenderness, exudates, polyps or bleeding. Septum midline.

Lips—pink, moist, without lesions or ulcerations. Oral mucosa pink, moist, without lesions or bleeding. Dentition fair, some loose teeth. Caries present. Tongue midline, slight beefy redness, no lesions. Uvula midline. Pharynx without exudates.

Neck. Supple. Trachea midline. Thyroid lobes slightly enlarged, no nodules.

Lymph Nodes. No preauricular, postauricular, occipital, tonsillar, submandibular, submental, superficial, posterior cervical, deep cervical chain, supraclavicular, cervical, axillary, epitrochlear, or inguinal lymph nodes.

Thorax and Lungs. A&P (anterior and posterior) thorax symmetric without retraction. Mild kyphosis. No tenderness, crepitus or lesions. Positive tactile fremitus. Lungs resonant throughout. Equal expansion. Diaphragmatic excursion descends 4 cm BL (bilateral). Vesicular breath sounds in all fields. No adventitious sounds.

Cardiovascular. R JVP 2 cm at 30 degrees. Carotid upstrokes brisk, without bruits. PMI 2 cm in diameter, tapping, in the fifth ICS L MCL (intercostal space, left, midclavicular line). II/VI harsh holosystolic murmur at the apex, radiating to the axilla. No S_3, S_4, or other murmurs.

Abdomen. Protuberant, symmetric without lesions, peristalsis, pulsations or increased vasculature. Active bowel sounds, no aortic, renal or iliac bruits. Soft, nontender. No masses or hepatosplenomegaly. Liver span 7 cm in R MCL; edge smooth and palpable. No CVAT (costal vertebral angle tenderness).

Genitourinary. Circumcised male. No penile lesions. Testes descended BL, smooth without masses or tenderness.

Extremities. Upper and lower—warm, without edema, bruising, pain, or increased vascularity.

Peripheral Vascular. BL radial, brachial, femoral, popliteal, dorsalis pedis, and posterior tibial pulses 2+ and symmetric.

Musculoskeletal. Mild degenerative changes in spine and at the knees, with quadriceps wasting. FROM in all joints. Motor: Decreased quadriceps bulk. Tone intact. Strength 4/5 throughout.

Neurologic. O×4 (person, place, time, situation), dressed appropriately for the weather, good spirits. Mini-Mental Status examination: score 29. Cranial Nerves II–XII intact. BL RAMs, finger-to-nose sequence intact. Gait with widened base. Sensation intact to pinprick, light touch, position, and vibration (upper/lower extremities intact). Romberg negative. BL biceps, triceps, brachioradialis, knee, and ankle reflexes 2+ and symmetric, with plantar response.

HEALTH PROMOTION AND COUNSELING

> **Important Topics for Health Promotion and Counseling in the Older Adult**
>
> - When to screen
> - Vision and Hearing
> - Exercise
> - Safety, including fall assessment
> - Immunizations
> - Cancer screening
> - Depression
> - Dementia, mild cognitive impairment, and cognitive decline
> - Elder mistreatment and abuse
> - Advanced directives and palliative care

When to Screen

As more adults live into their 80s and beyond, decisions about screening become more complex, and the evidence base for screening decisions becomes more limited.[127,128] The aging population is physiologically heterogeneous, many with numerous chronic diseases but also many with delayed or absent disability. Moreover, level of function in "successful aging" does not always parallel the number of chronic ailments, and there are substantial regional gaps in availability and use of preventive services.[129] Although there is relative consensus about immunization recommendations and falls prevention, screening for specific disease states remains more controversial. In general, individual screening decisions should be based on each older adult's health and functional status, including presence of comorbidity, rather than age alone.[130,131]

The American Geriatrics Society recommends a five-step approach to screening decisions[132]:

1. Assess patient preferences

2. Interpret the available evidence

3. Estimate prognosis

4. Consider treatment feasibility

5. Optimize therapies and care plans.

If life expectancy is short, give priority to treatment that benefits the patient in the time that remains. Consider deferring screening if it overburdens the older adults who have multiple medical problems, shortened life expectancy, or dementia. Tests that help with prognosis and planning may still be warranted even if the patient does not want to pursue treatment.

Vision and Hearing

Screening for age-related changes in *vision* and *hearing* is important in helping older adults maintain optimal function as they are vital sensory modalities for daily living. They are key items in the 10-Minute Geriatric Screener.

- Test *vision* objectively using an eye chart.

See 10-Minute Geriatric Screener, p. 945.

- Ask the patient about any *hearing* loss is effective for screening, then proceed to the whisper test and more formal testing if indicated. Among adults ages 65 to 69 years, 1% have visual impairment, increasing to 17% of those over age 80 years. About a third of adults over age 65 years have hearing loss, increasing to 80% in those over age 80 years.

See Chapter 12, Ear, Nose, Mouth and Throat, techniques for assessing hearing, pp. 298–299.

Exercise

Exercise is one of the most effective ways to promote healthy aging. Abundant literature documents the many benefits of physical activity in older adults, even in those who are frail.[133–136] These include a "decrease in all-cause mortality; reduced risk of functional limitation and role limitation, falls, hypertension, diabetes, colorectal cancer, and breast cancer; and improvement in cognitive function, physical function, quality of life, gait speed, balance, and performance of activities of daily living" as well as preservation of cognition.[137]

Recommendations emphasize combining aerobic exercise with graded resistance training in major muscle groups to increase strength. Guidelines from the Centers for Disease Control and Prevention (CDC) are listed below. The CDC website provides information on higher targets for exercise and explanations of aerobic and muscle-strength training. For help with exercise plans, turn to the Exercise in Medicine program of the American College of Sports Medicine.[138,139] The many benefits of individualized, supervised exercise plans usually outweigh the risks of joint pain, falls, and cardiac events.

CDC Exercise Recommendations for Older Adults[140]

Adults need at least:
- 2 hours and 30 minutes (150 minutes) of moderate-intensity aerobic activity (i.e., brisk walking) every week **and**
- muscle-strengthening activities on 2 or more days a week that work all major muscle groups (legs, hips, back, abdomen, chest, shoulders, and arms).

OR
- 1 hour and 15 minutes (75 minutes) of vigorous-intensity aerobic activity (i.e., jogging or running) every week **and**
- muscle-strengthening activities on 2 or more days a week that work all major muscle groups (legs, hips, back, abdomen, chest, shoulders, and arms).

OR

- an equivalent mix of moderate- and vigorous-intensity aerobic activity **and**
- muscle-strengthening activities on 2 or more days a week that work all major muscle groups (legs, hips, back, abdomen, chest, shoulders, and arms).

Source: Centers for Disease Control and Prevention. How much physical activity do older adults need? Physical activity is essential to healthy aging. Updated June 4, 2015. Available at http://www.cdc.gov/physicalactivity/basics/older_adults/index.htm. Accessed January 17, 2016.

Safety, Including Fall Assessment

The CDC reported that 2.5 million nonfatal falls among older adults were treated in emergency departments, and more than 734,000 of these patients were hospitalized at a direct medical cost of $34 billion.[139] Many have hip fractures and traumatic brain injuries that impact daily function and independence. Emergency room visits and deaths are most likely to involve yard and garden equipment, ladders and stepstools, personal use items like hair dryers and flammable clothing, and bathroom and sports injuries. Encourage older adults to adopt corrective measures for poor lighting, chairs at awkward heights, slippery or irregular surfaces, and environmental hazards.

See also Fall Assessment, p. 969.

Home Safety Tips for Older Adults[139]

- Install bright lighting and lightweight curtains or shades.
- Install handrails and lights on all staircases. Pathways and walkways should be well-lit.
- Remove items that cause tripping like papers, books, clothes, and shoes from stairs and walkways.
- Remove or secure small throw rugs and other rugs with double-sided tape.
- Wear shoes both inside and outside the house. Avoid bare feet and wearing slippers.
- Store medications safely.
- Keep commonly used items in cabinets that are easy to reach without using a step stool.
- Install grab bars and nonslip mats or safety strips in baths and showers.
- Repair faulty plugs and electrical cords.
- Install carbon monoxide and smoke alarms and have a plan for escaping fire.
- Secure all firearms.
- Have a medical alert device/system for emergency contacts or easy access to 911.

Fall Assessment

A veritable avalanche of evidence links falls to morbidity and mortality in our older population. Each year approximately 35% to 40% of healthy community-dwelling older adults experience falls. Incidence rates in nursing homes and hospitals are almost three times higher, with related injuries in approximately 25%. Loss of confidence from fear of falling and postfall anxiety further impair full recovery.[25,26]

Fall-related assessments should include details about the how the fall occurred, especially from witnesses, and identification of risk factors, medical comorbidities, functional status, and environmental risks—coupled with interventions for prevention.[131] Gait velocity is also emerging as a significant predictor of falls and related adverse events.[132] The Hendrich II Fall Risk Model tool is able to screen for those at risk of falling. Effective single

Hendrich II Fall Risk Model ™		
RISK FACTOR	**RISK POINTS**	**SCORE**
Confusion/Disorientation/Impulsivity	4	
Symptomatic Depression	2	
Altered Elimination	1	
Dizziness/Vertigo	1	
Gender (Male)	1	
Any Administered Antiepileptics (anticonvulsants): (Carbamazepine, Divalproex Sodium, Ethotoin, Ethosuximide, Felbamate, Fosphenytoin, Gabapentin, Lamotrigine, Mephenytoin, Methsuximide, Phenobarbital, Phenytoin, Primidone, Topiramate, Trimethadione, Valproic Acid)[1]	2	
Any Administered Benzodiazepines:[2] (Alprazolam, Chloridiazepoxide, Clonazepam, Clorazepate Dipotassium, Diazepam, Flurazepam, Halazepam[3], Lorazepam, Midazolam, Oxazepam, Temazepam, Triazolam)	1	
Get-Up-and-Go Test: "Rising from a Chair" If unable to assess, monitor for change in activity level, assess other risk factors, document both on patient chart with date and time.		
Ability to rise in single movement - No loss of balance with steps	0	
Pushes up, successful in one attempt	1	
Multiple attempts but successful	3	
Unable to rise without assistance during test If unable to assess, document this on the patient chart with the date and time.	4	
(A score of 5 or greater = High Risk)	**TOTAL SCORE**	
© 2013 AHI of Indiana, Inc. All rights reserved. United States Patent No. 7,282,031 and U.S. Patent No. 7,682,308.		
Reproduction of copyright and patented materials without authorization is a violation of federal law.		

On-going Medication Review Updates:

Levetiracetam (Keppra) was not assessed during the original research conducted to create the Hendrich Fall Risk Model. As an antiepileptic, levetiracetam does have a side effect of somnolence and dizziness which contributes to its fall risk and should be scored (effective June 2010).

The study did not include the effect of benzodiazepine-like drugs since they were not on the market at the time. However, due to their similarity in drug structure, mechanism of action and drug effects, they should also be scored (effective January 2010).

Halazepam was included in the study but is no longer available in the United States (effective June 2010).

V2012.1

interventions include gait and balance training and exercise to strengthen muscles, reduction of home hazards, discontinuation of psychotropic medication, and multifactorial assessment with targeted interventions. Additional useful strategies include addressing change in postural blood pressure, attention to concurrent acute illness, reduction in medications to fewer than four, detection of sensory neuropathy and impairment of proprioception, investigation of any episodes of syncope, patient and family education, treatment of osteoporosis, and possible use of hip protectors.[141]

Immunizations

Recommend vaccination for influenza; pneumonia, both PPSV23 and PCV13; herpes zoster (shingles); and tetanus/diphtheria and pertussis (Tdap and Td). The immunization schedule is updated annually. For the most up-to-date recommendations, consult the latest guidelines and contraindications provided by the CDC at http://www.cdc.gov/vaccines/schedules/hcp/adult.html.[2,142,143] Note that vaccination rates still lag behind for Hispanics and African Americans.

See also Chapter 13, The Respiratory System, pp. 357–359.

Cancer Screening

Cancer screening recommendations for older adults remain controversial. The American Geriatrics Society recommends no screening for, "breast, colorectal, prostate, or lung cancer without considering life expectancy and the risks of testing, overdiagnosis and overtreatment."[144] Advocates for older adults are suggesting individualized decision making based on the principles outlined in "When to Screen" discussed earlier, since "guidelines become less robust and evidenced-based as individuals age and/or develop declining health status and disabilities."[73] Recent more complex published frameworks include "weighing quantitative information, such as risk of cancer death and likelihood of beneficial and adverse screening outcomes, as well as qualitative factors, such as individual patients' values and preferences."[135] The recommendations of the USPSTF as of 2015, which target straightforward age cutoffs, are summarized below.[96]

Screening Recommendations for Older Adults: U.S. Preventive Services Task Force

- **Breast cancer** (2009): Recommends mammography every 2 years for women ages 50 to 74 and cites insufficient evidence for screening women ages ≥75 years.
- **Cervical cancer** (2012): Recommends against routine screening for women over age 65 if they have had adequate recent screening with normal Pap smears and are not otherwise at high risk for cervical cancer, based on fair evidence.
- **Colorectal cancer** (2008): Recommends screening with colonoscopy every 10 years, sigmoidoscopy every 5 years with high-sensitivity fecal occult blood tests (FOBTs) every 3 years, or FOBTs every year begin-

ning age 50 years through age 75 years. Recommends against routine screening for adults ages 76 to 85 years, due to moderate certainty that the net benefit is small.

- **Prostate cancer** (2012): Recommends against routine prostate-specific antigen–based screening for prostate cancer in men of all ages due to evidence that expected harms are greater than expected benefits.
- **Lung cancer** (2013): For adults ages 55 to 80 years with a 30-pack/year smoking history, and those who currently smoke or have quit within the past 15 years, recommends annual screening with low-dose computed tomography. Screening should be discontinued once a person has not smoked for 15 years or develops a health problem that substantially limits life expectancy or the ability or willingness to have curative lung surgery.
- **Skin cancer** (2009; updated in 2015): States that evidence is insufficient to balance the benefits and harms of whole-body skin examination.

Depression

Depression affects 5% to 7% of community-dwelling older adults and approximately 10% of older men and 18% of older women, but is often undiagnosed, untreated, or undertreated.[135,145] Prevalence rises in those with multiple comorbidities and hospitalizations. Screening for the general adult population, with services in place for diagnosis, treatment, and follow-up, is now recommended by the USPSTF (2015)[146] and requires only one or two questions. The single screening question, "Do you often feel sad or depressed?" has a sensitivity of 69% and specificity of 90%. The two screening questions below are 100% sensitive and 77% specific.

See Chapter 19, Mental Status, p. 664–665.

- "Over the past 2 weeks have you felt down, depressed, or hopeless?" (screens for depressed mood)

- "Over the past 2 weeks have you felt little interest or pleasure in doing things?" (screens for anhedonia)

Positive responses should prompt further investigation with scales such as the Geriatric Depression Scale or the 9-item Patient Health Questionnaire (PHQ-9).[145,147] Depressed men over age 65 years are at increased risk for suicide and require particularly careful evaluation. Effective treatment for older adults both reduces morbidity and extends life, and includes exercise, supportive and group therapy, and medication.[148]

Dementia, Mild Cognitive Impairment, and Cognitive Decline

Dementia is "an acquired condition that is characterized by a decline in at least two cognitive domains (e.g., loss of memory, attention, language, or visuospatial or executive functioning) that is severe enough to affect social or occupational functioning." Affected patients may also exhibit behavioral and psychological symptoms. In the *Diagnostic and Statistical Manual of Mental Disorders 5* (DSM-5), dementia is classified as a "major neurocognitive disorder."[149] The major dementia syndromes include Alzheimer's Disease (AD), vascular dementia, frontotemporal dementia, dementia with Lewy bodies, Parkinson disease with dementia, and dementia of mixed etiology. AD, the predominant form, affects 11% of Americans over the age of 65 years, or roughly 5.1 million people; more than two thirds are women.[150] By 2050, the prevalence is estimated to increase to 13.8 million cases. Risk factors include advancing age, family history, and the gene mutation apolipoprotein (APOE) ε4. Risk of AD more than doubles in first-degree relatives. Risk doubles in the presence of one APOE ε4 allele and increases fivefold or more in the presence of two alleles, although only 2% of the population carries these genes.[151]

The diagnosis of AD is challenging because the mechanisms of disease are still under intense investigation; the absence of a consistent and uniformly applied definition of disease hampers investigation of risk factors; between 60% and 90% of Alzheimer patients have coexisting ischemic disease; and distinguishing *age-related cognitive decline* from *mild cognitive impairment* and AD can be subtle. In addition, delirium and depression can further complicate a diagnosis.[152,153] Some distinguishing clinical features are highlighted below.

See Table 24-1, Delirium and Dementia, p. 975

Once you identify cognitive changes, a number of steps are helpful for planning patient care.

Caring for Patients With Altered Cognition

- Obtain collateral information from family members and caretakers.
- Consider formal neuropsychological testing.
- Investigate contributing factors such as medications; metabolic abnormalities; depression; delirium; and other medical and psychiatric conditions, including vascular risk from diabetes and hypertension.
- Counsel families about the challenges for caregivers. The NIH Senior Health website *http://nihseniorhealth.gov/alzheimerscare/afterthediagnosis/01.html* is about "Alzheimer Caregiving" and is especially helpful. Review household safety measures.
- Learn the laws about reporting *drivers with dementia* in your state. Consult the American Academy of Neurology evidence-based practice parameters for drivers with dementia, updated in 2010, and guidelines from numerous professional organizations, including the American Medical Association. Note, however, that underlying quantitative evidence linking assessment to road safety is limited.[154] A 2013 Cochrane review details the pitfalls of disqualifying impaired drivers, which can lead to depression and social withdrawal if disqualification is premature.[155,156] The review concludes that for drivers with dementia, there

---

is no good evidence that neuropsychological or on-road assessment will maintain mobility and improve safety. The authors call for more research to develop assessment tools "that can reliably identify unsafe drivers with dementia in an office setting" and determine what changes in function provide a threshold for disqualification, as no single validated test is available.

- Encourage patient and family discussion of appointing a health care proxy and arranging for power of attorney, health care power of attorney, and advance directives while the patient can still contribute to active decision making.

Elder Mistreatment and Abuse

Screen vulnerable older adults for possible *elder mistreatment,* which includes abuse, neglect, exploitation, and abandonment. Prevalence ranges from 5% to 10%, depending on the population studied, and is even higher among older adults with depression and dementia.[157–159] Many cases are undetected due to the patient's fear of reprisal, physical or cognitive inability to report, and unwillingness to expose the abuser, of whom 80% to 90% are family members. Self-neglect, or "the behavior of an elderly person that threatens his/her own health and safety," is also a growing national concern and represents more than 50% of adult protective service referrals. Although several screening instruments are available, no valid reliable screening tools to identify abuse of elderly or vulnerable adults in the primary care setting and therefore cited insufficient evidence for recommending screening.[131] Consequently, a careful history and high index of suspicion are important. Assess for physical signs, such as bruising, black eyes, fractures, bleeding, lacerations, or burns, and other signs such as a change in behavior, odor, the caregiver refusing to allow assessment of older adult alone, or use of restraints.

Advance Directives and Palliative Care

Many older patients are interested in discussing end-of-life decisions and would like providers to initiate these discussions *before* the onset of serious illness.[160] *Advance care planning* involves several tasks: providing information, clarifying the patient's preferences, and identifying the surrogate decision maker. You can begin this discussion by linking these decisions to a current illness or experiences with relatives or friends. Ask the patient about "Do Not Resuscitate" orders specifying life support measures "if the heart or lungs were to stop or give out." Also encourage the patient to designate in writing a health care proxy or durable power of attorney for health care, "someone who can make decisions reflecting your wishes in case of confusion or emergency."

Roughly half of hospitalized older adults require surrogate decision making within 48 hours of admission. Common topics include life-sustaining care, surgeries and procedures, and discharge planning.[161] Conversations about life care choices help patients and their families prepare openly and in advance for a peaceful death. Pursue these discussions during office visits rather than in the stressful environment of the emergency department or intensive care unit.

Experts note that *advance care directives* can be more flexible, depending on the situation. These directives "may range from general statements of values to such specific orders as [Do Not Resuscitate], do not intubate, do not hospitalize, do not provide artificial hydration or nutrition, or do not administer antibiotics. Different situations, including different stages of health and illness, demand different types of advanced care directives and thus require both different conversations and different training in leading such discussions."[70] Moreover, always consult competent patients about current options because their decisions supersede prior written instructions.

For patients with advanced or terminal illnesses, include the review of advanced directives in an overall plan for *palliative care*. Palliative care encompasses the alleviation of pain and suffering and the promotion of optimal quality of life across all phases of treatment, including curative interventions and rehabilitation. Its goals are "to consider the physical, mental, spiritual, and social well-being of patients and their families in order to maintain hope while ensuring patient dignity and respecting autonomy" both for patients with serious illnesses and for patients considering hospice care at the end of life.[71] To ease patient and family distress, use good communication skills: make good eye contact; ask open-ended questions; respond to anxiety, depression, or changes in the patient's affect; show empathy; and be sure to consult caregivers.

See also Chapter 3, Death and the Dying Patient, pp. 58–60.

TABLE 24-1 Delirium and Dementia

Delirium and dementia are common. They each affect multiple aspects of mental status and have many possible causes. Some clinical features and their effects on mental status are compared below. Note: A delirium may be superimposed on dementia.

	Delirium	Dementia
Clinical Features		
Onset	Acute	Insidious
Course	Fluctuating, with lucid intervals; worse at night	Slowly progressive
Duration	Hours to weeks	Months to years
Sleep/Wake Cycle	Always disrupted	Sleep fragmented
General Medical Illness or Drug Toxicity	Either or both present	Often absent, especially in Alzheimer disease
Mental Status		
Level of Consciousness	Disturbed. Person less clearly aware of the environment and less able to focus, sustain, or shift attention	Usually normal until late in the course of the illness
Behavior	Activity often abnormally decreased (somnolence) or increased (agitation, hypervigilance)	Normal to slow; may become inappropriate
Speech	May be hesitant, slow or rapid, incoherent	Difficulty in finding words, aphasia
Mood	Fluctuating, labile, from fearful or irritable to normal or depressed	Often flat, depressed
Thought Process	Disorganized, may be incoherent	Impoverished. Speech gives little information.
Thought Content	Delusions common, often transient	Delusions may occur.
Perceptions	Illusions, hallucinations, most often visual	Hallucinations may occur.
Judgment	Impaired, often to a varying degree	Increasingly impaired over the course of the illness
Orientation	Usually disoriented, especially for time. A known place may seem unfamiliar.	Fairly well maintained, but becomes impaired in the later stages of illness
Attention	Fluctuates, with inattention. Person easily distracted, unable to concentrate on selected tasks	Usually unaffected until late in the illness
Memory	Immediate and recent memory impaired	Recent memory and new learning especially impaired
Examples of Cause	Delirium tremens (due to withdrawal from alcohol) Infection Uremia Acute hepatic failure Acute cerebral vasculitis Atropine poisoning	*Reversible:* Vitamin B$_{12}$ deficiency, thyroid disorders *Irreversible:* Alzheimer disease, vascular dementia (from multiple infarcts), dementia due to head trauma

BIBLIOGRAPHY

CITATIONS

1. Administration on Aging. Census data and population estimates, 2013. Available at http://www.aoa.acl.gov/aging_statistics/Census_Population/Index.aspx. Accessed January 20, 2016.

2. Administration on Aging. A profile of older Americans: 2013. Available at http://www.aoa.acl.gov/Aging_Statistics/Profile/2013/index.aspx. Accessed January 20, 2016.

3. Centers for Disease Control and Prevention, U.S. Department of Health and Human Services. Health, United States, 2013. DHHS Publication No. 2014–1232. Available at http://www.cdc.gov/nchs/data/hus/hus13.pdf#018. Accessed January 20, 2016.

4. Ortman JM, Veloff V, Hogan H. An Aging Nation: The Older Population in the United States Population Estimates and Projections Current Population Reports. Available at https://www.census.gov/prod/2014pubs/p25–1140.pdf. Accessed January 20, 2016.

5. Federal Interagency Forum on Aging Related Statistics. *Older Americans 2012, Key Indicators of Well Being. See Indicators 16, Chronic Health Conditions (p. 27); 18, Respondent Assessed Health Statistics (p. 29); 20, Functional Limitations (p. 32); and 45, Obesity (p. 41). Federal Interagency Forum on Aging-Related Statistics.* Washington, DC: U.S. Government Printing Office. 2012. Available at http://agingstats.gov/agingstatsdotnet/Main_Site/Data/2012_Documents/Docs/EntireChartbook.pdf. Accessed January 20, 2016.

6. Sabia S, Singh-Manoux A, Hagger-Johnson G, et al. Influence of individual and combined healthy behaviours on successful aging. *CMAJ.* 2012;184:1985.

7. Davy C, Bleasel J, Liu H, et al. Effectiveness of chronic care models: opportunities for improving healthcare practice and health outcomes: a systematic review. *BMC Health Serv Res.* 2015;15:194.

8. Partnership for Health in Aging Workgroup on Interdisciplinary Team Training in Geriatrics. Position statement on interdisciplinary team training in geriatrics: an essential component of quality health care for older adults. *J Am Geriatr Soc.* 2014;62:961.

9. Bodenheimer T, Wagner EH, Brumbach K. Improving primary care for patients with chronic illness. *JAMA.* 2002;288:1775.

10. Institute of Medicine. Crossing the quality chasm: a new health system for the 21st century. Washington, DC: National Academy Press; 2011.

11. Reuben DB, Tinetti ME. Goal-oriented patient care—an alternative health outcome paradigm. *N Engl J Med.* 2012;366:777.

12. Carlson C, Merel SE, Yukawa M. Geriatric syndromes and geriatric assessment for the generalist. *Med Clin N Am.* 2015;99:263.

13. Sebastiani P, Bae H, Sun FX, et al. Meta analysis of genetic variants associated with human exceptional longevity. *Aging.* 2014;5:653.

14. Sebastiani P, Sun FX, Andersen SL, et al. Families enriched for exceptional longevity also have increased health-span: findings from the Long Life Family Study. *Front Public Health.* 2013;1:38.

15. Kane EL, Ouslander JG, Abrass IB, et al. Chapter 3, Evaluating the geriatric patient. *In Essentials of Clinical Geriatrics,* 7th ed. New York, NY: McGraw Hill Medical; 2013.

16. Morley JE, Tolsen DT. Chapter 3: The physiology of aging. In: *Pathy's Principles and Practice of Geriatric Medicine.* 5th ed. Vellas BJ, Pathy MS, Sinclair A, et al., eds. Oxford: John Wiley & Sons, Inc.; 2012:33.

17. Morley JE, Tolsen DT. Chapter 9: Sexuality and aging. In: *Pathy's Principles and Practice of Geriatric Medicine.* 5th ed. Vellas BJ, Pathy MS, Sinclair A, et al., eds. Oxford: John Wiley & Sons, Inc.; 2012:93.

18. Hollingsworth JM, Wilt TJ. Lower urinary tract symptoms in men. *BMJ.* 2014;14(349):g4474. doi: 10.1136/bmj.g4474.

19. Evans WJ. Sarcopenia should reflect the contribution of age-associated changes in skeletal muscle to risk of morbidity and mortality in elderly people. *J Am Med Dir Assoc.* 2015;16:5464.

20. Demonet J-F, Celsis P. Chapter 5: Aging of the brain. In: Vellas BJ, ed. *Pathy's Principles and Practice of Geriatric Medicine.* 5th ed. John Wiley & Sons, Inc.; 2012:49.

21. Iowa Geriatric Education Center, University of Iowa. Geriatric Assessment Tools. Available at https://www.healthcare.uiowa.edu/igec/tools./. Accessed January 20, 2016.

22. Rosen SL, Reuben DB. Geriatric assessment tools. *Mt Sinai J Med.* 2011;78:489.

23. Yeo G. How will the U.S. Healthcare system meet the challenge of the ethnogeriatric imperative? *J Am Geriatr Soc.* 2009;57:1278.

24. Jackson CS, Gracia JN. Addressing health and health-care disparities: the role of a diverse workforce and the social determinants of health. *Pub Health Rep.* 2014;129:57.

25. Centers for Disease Control and Prevention. Health Disparities and Inequalities Report 2013. Available at http://www.cdc.gov/minorityhealth/CHDIReport.html. Accessed January 20, 2016.

26. August KJ, Sorkin DH. Racial and ethnic disparities in indicators of physical health status: do they still exist throughout late life? *J Am Geriatr Soc.* 2010;58:2009.

27. Ng JH, Bierman AS, Elliott MN, et al. Beyond black and white: race/ethnicity and health status among older adults. *Am J Manag Care.* 2014;20:239.

28. Stanford School of Medicine. Ethnogeriatrics. Available at http://geriatrics.stanford.edu/. Accessed January 2016.

29. Office of Minority Health, Department of Health and Human Services. Think Cultural Health. Available at https://www.thinkculturalhealth.hhs.gov/index.asp. Accessed January 20, 2016.

30. Aggarwal NK, Glass A, Tirado A, et al. The development of the DSM-5 Cultural Formulation Interview-Fidelity Instrument (CFI-FI): a pilot study. *J Health Care Poor Underserved.* 2014;25:1397.

31. Kobylarz FA, Heath JM, Lide RC. The ETHNIC(S) mnemonic: a clinical tool for ethnogeriatric education. *J Am Geriatr Soc.* 2002;50:1852.

32. Aggarwal NK. Reassessing cultural evaluations in geriatrics: insights from cultural psychiatry. *J Am Geriatr Soc.* 2010;58:2191.

33. Stanford Geriatrics Education Center. "Test your Ethnogeriatric IQ." Available at http://sgec.stanford.edu/resources/training/iq.html. Accessed January 20, 2016.

34. Stanford Geriatric Education Center. Modules—EthnoGeriatrics Overview. Available at https://geriatrics.stanford.edu/culturemed.html. Accessed January 20, 2016.

35. Bhatia LC, Naik RH. Clinical profile of acute myocardial infarction in elderly patients. *Cardiovasc Dis Res.* 2013;4:107.

36. Papaleontiou M, Haymart MR. Approach to and treatment of thyroid disorders in the elderly. *Med Clin North Am.* 2012;96:297.

37. Koroukian SM, Warner DF, Owusu C, et al. Multimorbidity redefined: prospective health outcomes and the cumulative effect of co-occurring conditions. *Prev Chronic Dis.* 2015;12:E55.

38. Strandberg TE, Pitkälä KH, Tilvis RS, et al. Geriatric syndromes—vascular disorders? *Ann Med.* 2013;45:265.

39. Fulmer T. How to try this: Fulmer SPICES. *AJN.* 2007; 107(10):40–48.

40. Kagan SH. Geriatric syndromes in practice: Delirium is not the only thing. *Geriatr Nurs.* 2010;31(4):299–304.

41. Nurses Improving Care for Healthsystem Elders (NICHE). Program at the Hartford Institute for Geriatric Nursing. http://www.nicheprogram.org./ Accessed January 17, 2016.

42. Fulmer T, Wallace M. Fulmer SPICES: An Overall Assessment Tool for Older Adults Hartford Institute of Geriatric Nursing Assessment Series. Available at https://consultgeri.org/try-this/general-assessment/issue-1. Accessed July 6, 2016.

43. Montlahuc C, Soumaré A, Dufouil C, et al. Self-rated health and risk of incident dementia: A community-based elderly cohort, the 3C Study. *Neurology.* 2011;77:1457.

44. Mendonça MD, Alves L, Bugalho P. From subjective cognitive complaints to dementia: who is at risk?: A systematic review. *Am J Alzheimers Dis Other Demen.* 2015;pii: 1533317515592331.

45. Fernández-Ruiz M, Guerra-Vales JM, Trincado R, et al. The ability of self-rated health to predict mortality among community-dwelling elderly individuals differs according to the specific cause of death: data from the NEDICES cohort. *Gerontology.* 2013;59:368.

46. Vogelsang EM. Self-rated health changes and oldest-old mortality. *J Gerontol B Psychol Sci Soc Sci.* 2014;69:612.

47. Iecovich E, Biderman A. Concordance between self-reported and physician-reported chronic co-morbidity among disabled older adults. *Can J Aging.* 2013;32:287.

48. Moore AA, Siu AL. Screening for common problems in ambulatory elderly: clinical confirmation of a screening instrument. *Am J Med.* 1996;100:438–440.

49. Centers for Disease Control and Prevention, U.S. Department of Health and Human Services. Percent of U.S. adults 55 and over with chronic conditions (2009). Available at http://www.cdc.gov/nchs/health_policy/adult_chronic_conditions.htm. Accessed January 21, 2015.

50. Centers for Disease Control and Prevention, U.S. Department of Health and Human Services. Special feature on prescription drugs, p. 20; see Figure 20, Prescription drug use in the past 30 days, p. 21, in Health, United States, 2013. 2013:DHHS Publication No. 2014–1232. Available at http://www.cdc.gov/nchs/data/hus/hus13.pdf#018. Accessed August 12, 2015.

51. Wang YP, Andrade LH. Epidemiology of alcohol and drug use in the elderly. *Curr Opin Psychiatry.* 2013;26:343.

52. Rodriguez JC, Dzierzewski JM, Alessi CA. Sleep problems in the elderly. *Med Clin North Am.* 2015;99:431.

53. Bloom HG, Ahmed I, Alessi CA, et al. Evidence-based recommendations for the assessment and management of sleep disorders in older persons. *J Am Geriatr Soc.* 2009;57:761.

54. Wooten JM. Rules for improving pharmacotherapy in older adult patients: part 1 (rules 1–5). *South Med J.* 2015;108:97.

55. Wooten JM. Rules for improving pharmacotherapy in older adult patients: part 2 (rules 6–10). *South Med J.* 2015;108:145.

56. American Geriatrics Society 2012 Beers Criteria Update Expert Panel. American Geriatrics Society updated Beers criteria for potentially inappropriate medication use in older adults. *J Am Geriatr Soc.* 2012;60:616.

57. Reuben DB, Herr KA, Pacala JT, et al. *Geriatrics at Your Fingertips.* 16th ed. New York, NY: American Geriatrics Society; 2014.

58. Onder G, Petrovic M, Balamurugan T, et al. Less is more. Development and validation of a score to assess risk of adverse drug reactions among the in-hospital patients 65 years or older. *Arch Intern Med.* 2010;170:1142.

59. Morley JE. Undernutrition in older adults. *Fam Pract.* 2012;29(Suppl 1):89.

60. National Center for Chronic Disease Prevention and Health Promotion. Centers for Disease Control and Prevention. Table 1, The national report card on healthy aging. How healthy are older adults in the United States, p. 15. Atlanta: Centers for Disease Control and Prevention, U.S. Department of Health and Human Services; 2013. Available at http://www.cdc.gov/aging/pdf/state-aging-health-in-america-2013.pdf. Accessed January 14, 2016.

61. American Geriatrics Society Panel on the Pharmacologic Management of Persistent Pain in Older Persons. Pharmacologic management of persistent pain in older persons. *J Am Geriatr Soc.* 2009;57:1331.

62. Budnitz DS, Lovegrove MC, Shehab N, et al. Emergency hospitalizations for adverse drug events in older Americans. *N Engl J Med.* 2011;365:2002.

63. Hadjistavropoulos T, Hadjistavropoulos HD. *Pain Management for Older Adults: A Self-Help Guide.* Washington, DC: American Psychological Association; 2015. Available at http://ebooks.iasp-pain.org/pain_management_for_older_adults/ See also International Association for the Study of Pain eBookstore. Available at http://ebooks.iasp-pain.org./ Accessed January 19, 2016.

64. Savage SR. Multidimensional care of chronic pain: reducing reliance on opioids for relief, June 2013. Webinar–American Medical Association. Available at http://eo2.commpartners.com/users/ama/session.php?id = 11044. Accessed January 19, 2016.

65. American Academy of Pain Medicine. Pain index. Pain intensity scales. Available at http://www.painmed.org/SOPResources/ClinicalTools/government-websites/. Accessed January 19, 2016.

66. Annon J. The PLISSIT model: A proposed conceptual scheme for the behavioral treatment of sexual problems. *J Sex Educ Ther.* 1996;2(2):1–15.

67. Wallace M. How to Try This; Sexuality Assessment. *Am J Nurs.* 2008;108(7):40–48.

68. Dowling-Castronovo A, Bradway C. Urinary incontinence. In: Boltz M, Capezuti E, Fulmer T, et al., (eds.), *Geriatric Nursing Protocols for Best Practice.* 4th ed., Chapter 18, pp. 393–387. New York, NY: Springer Publishing Company, LLC; 2012.

69. Dowling-Castronovo A, Specht JK. How to try this: Assessment of transient urinary incontinence in older adults. *AJN.* 2009;109(2):62–71.

70. Agency for Health Care Research and Quality: National Guideline Clearinghouse. Multiple guidelines related to urinary incontinence available. Available at http://www.guideline.gov/search/search.aspx?term=urinary+incontinence. Accessed January 20, 2016.

71. Centers for Disease Control and Prevention. Cigarette Smoking—United States, 2006–2008 and 2009–2010, Table 1. Prevalence of current smoking among persons aged 12–17 years, by selected characteristics—National Survey on Drug Use and Health, United States, 2006–2010, in CDC Health Disparities and Inequalities Report—United States, 2013. *MMWR.* 2016;Vol 62(3):82. Available at http://www.cdc.gov/mmwr/pdf/other/su6203.pdf. Accessed January 20, 2016.

72. National Institute on Aging. Age Page: Alcohol use in older people. Available at https://www.nia.nih.gov. Accessed January 20, 2016.

73. Centers for Disease Control and Prevention. Binge Drinking, United States, 2011- Table - Prevalence, frequency, and intensity of binge-drinking, by sex, age group, race/ethnicity, education, and disability—Behavioral Risk Factor Surveillance System, United States, 2011. in CDC Health Disparities and Inequalities Report—United States, 2013. *MMWR.* 2016;Vol 62(3):79. Available at http://www.cdc.gov/mmwr/pdf/other/su6203.pdf. Accessed January 20, 2016.

74. American Geriatrics Society. Alcohol use disorders in older adults. AGS clinical practice guidelines screening recommendation. *Ann Long Term Care.* 2006;14. Available at http://www.annalsoflongtermcare.com/article/5143. Accessed August 15, 2015.

75. Wilson SR, Knowles SB, Huang Q, et al. The prevalence of harmful and hazardous alcohol consumption in older U.S. adults: data from the 2005–2008 National Health and Nutrition Examination Survey (NHANES). *J Gen Intern Med.* 2014;29:312.

76. Bommersbach TJ, Lapid MI, Rummans TA, et al. Geriatric alcohol use disorder: a review for primary care physicians. *Mayo Clin Proc.* 2015;90:659.

77. Bradley KA, DeBenedetti AF, Volk RJ, et al. AUDIT-C as a brief screen for alcohol misuse in primary care. *Alcohol Clin Exp Res.* 2007;31(7):1208–1217.

78. Kaner E, Beyer F, Dickinson H, et al. Effectiveness of brief alcohol interventions in primary care populations. *Cochrane Database Syst Rev.* 2007;(2):CD004148.

79. Montreal Cognitive Assessment. 2015. Available at http://www.mocatest.org./ Accessed January 20, 2016.

80. Liew TM, Feng L, Gao Q, et al. Diagnostic utility of Montreal Cognitive Assessment in the Fifth Edition of Diagnostic and Statistical Manual of Mental Disorders: major and mild neurocognitive disorders. *J Am Med Dir Assoc.* 2015;16:144.

81. James PA, Oparil S, Carter BL, et al. 2014 Evidence-based guidelines for the management of high blood pressure in adults: report from the panel members appointed to the Eighth Joint National Committee (JNC8). *JAMA.* 2014; 311:507.

82. Kitzman DW, Taffet G. Chapter 74: Effects of aging on cardiovascular structure and function. In: Halter JB, Ouslander JG, Tinetti ME, et al., eds. *Hazzard's Geriatric Medicine and Gerontology,* 6th ed. New York, NY: McGraw-Hill; 2009.

83. Krakoff LR, Gillespie RL, Ferdinand KC, et al. 2014 hypertension recommendations from the Eighth Joint National Committee panel members raise concerns for elderly black and female populations. *J Am Coll Cardiol.* 2014;64:394.

84. Benetos A, Rossignol P, Cherubini A, et al. Polypharmacy in the aging patient: management of hypertension in octogenarians. *JAMA.* 2015;314:170.

85. Bangalore S, Gong Y, Cooper-DeHoff RM, et al. 2014 Eighth Joint National Committee panel recommendation for blood pressure targets revisited: results from the INVEST study. *J Am Coll Casrdiol.* 2014;64:784.

86. Weber MA, Bakris GL, Hester A, et al. Systolic blood pressure and cardiovascular outcomes during treatment of hypertension. *Am J Med.* 2013;126:501.

87. Freeman R, Wieling W, Axelrod FB, et al. Consensus statement on the definition of orthostatic hypotension, neutrally mediated syncope and the postural tachycardia syndrome. *Clin Auton Res.* 2011;21:69.

88. Vijayan J, Sharma VK. Neurogenic orthostatic hypotension—management update and role of droxidopa. *Ther Clin Risk Manag.* 2015;8:915.

89. Sathyapalan T, Aye MM, Atkin SL. Postural hypotension. *BMJ.* 2011:342:d3128.

90. Perlmuter LC, Sarda G, Casavant V, et al. A review of the etiology, associated comorbidities, and treatment of orthostatic hypotension. *Am J Ther.* 2013;20:279.

91. Lal H, Cunningham A, Olivier G, et al. Efficacy of an adjuvanted herpes zoster subunit vaccine in older adults. *N Engl J Med.* 2015; 372:2087.

92. Wilson JF. In the clinic. Herpes zoster. *Ann Intern Med.* 2011;154:ITC3.

93. Addis VM, DeVore HK, Summerfield ME. Acute visual changes in the elderly. *Clin Geriatr Med.* 2013;29:165.

94. Borooah S, Dhillon A, Dhillon B. Gradual loss of vision in adults. *BMJ.* 2015;350:h2093.

95. Liew G, Baker ML, Wong TY, et al. Differing associations of white matter lesions and lacunar infarction with retinal microvascular signs. *Int J Stroke.* 2014;9:921.

96. Wang JJ, Baker ML, Hand PJ, et al. Transient ischemic attack and acute ischemic stroke: associations with retinal microvascular signs. *Stroke.* 2011;42:404.

97. Vajaranant TS, Wu S, Torres M, et al. The changing face of primary open-angle glaucoma in the United States: demographic and geographic changes from 2011 to 2050. *Am J Ophthalmol.* 2012;154:303.

98. Weinreb RN, Aung T, Medeiros FA. The pathophysiology and treatment of glaucoma: a review. *JAMA.* 2014;311: 1901.

99. Ratnapriya R, Chew EY. Age-related macular degeneration-clinical review and genetics update. *Clin Genet.* 2013; 84:160.

100. Friedman PK, Kaufman LB, Karpas SL. Oral health disparity in older adults: dental decay and tooth loss. *Dent Clin North Am.* 2014;58:757.

101. Yellowitz JA, Schneiderman MT. Elder's oral health crisis. *J Evid Based Dent Pract.* 2014;14 Suppl:191.

102. Gibson PG, McDonald VM, Marks GB. Asthma in older adults. *Lancet.* 2010;376:803.

103. Goldberg LR. In the clinic. Heart failure. *Ann Intern Med.* 2010;152:ITC6–1.

104. Coffey S, Cox B, Williams MJ. The prevalence, incidence, progression, and risks of aortic valve sclerosis: a systematic review and meta-analysis. *J Am Coll Cardil.* 2014;63:2852.

105. Manning MJ. Asymptomatic aortic stenosis in the elderly: a clinical review. *JAMA.* 2013;310:1490.

106. Sandoval-Leon AC, Drews-Elger K, Gomez-Fernandez CR, et al. Paget's disease of the nipple. *Breast Cancer Res Treat.* 2013;141:1..

107. McDermott MM. Lower extremity manifestations of peripheral artery disease: the pathophysiologic and functional implications of leg ischemia. *Circ Res.* 2015;116:1540.

108. Miller KL, Baraldi CA. Geriatric gynecology: promoting health and avoiding harm. *Am J Obstet Bynecol.* 2012; 207:355.

109. Mathias S, Nayak US, Isaacs B. "Balance in elderly patient" The "Get Up and Go" Test. *Arch Phys Med Rehabil.* 1986;67:387.

110. Podsiadlo D, Richardson S. The Timed "Up and Go". *J Am Geriatr Soc.* 1991;39:142.

111. Borson S, Scanlan JM, Chen PJ, et al. The Mini-Cog as a screen for dementia: Validation in a population-based sample. *J Am Geriatr Soc.* 2003;51:1451–1454.

112. Borson S, Scanlan JM, Watanabe J, et al. Improving identification of cognitive impairment in primary care. *Int J Geriatr Psychiatry.* 2006;21:349–355.

113. Lessig M, Scanlan J, et al. Time that tells: Critical clock-drawing errors for dementia screening. *Int Psychogeriatr.* 2008 June;20(3):459–470.

114. Tsoi K, Chan J, et al. Cognitive tests to detect dementia: A systematic review and meta-analysis. *JAMA Intern Med.* 2015;E1–E9.

115. McCarten J, Anderson P, et al. Screening for cognitive impairment in an elderly veteran population: Acceptability and results using different versions of the Mini-Cog. *J Am Geriatr Soc.* 2011;59:309–213.

116. McCarten J, Anderson P, et al. Finding dementia in primary care: The results of a clinical demonstration project. *J Am Geriatr Soc.* 2012;60:210–217.

117. Scanlan J, Borson S. The Mini-Cog: Receiver operating characteristics with the expert and naive raters. *Int J Geriatr Psychiatry.* 2001;16:216–222.

118. Mahlknecht P, Kiechl S, Bloem BR, et al. Prevalence and burden of gait disorders in elderly men and women aged 60–97 years: a population-based study. *PLoS One.* 2013;8:e69627.

119. Lewis SJ. Neurological update: emerging issues in gait disorders. *J Neurol.* 2015;262:1590.

120. Stevens JA, Phelan EA. Development of STEADI: a fall prevention resource for health care providers. *Health Promot Pract.* 2013;14:706.

121. Tinetti ME, Kumar C. The patient who falls: "It's always a trade-off." *JAMA.* 2010;303:258.

122. Jankovic J. Gait disorders. *Neurol Clin.* 2015;33:249.

123. Lam R. Office management of gait disorders in the elderly. *Can Fam Physician.* 2011;57:765.

124. Odenheimer G, Funkenstein HH, Beckett L, et al. Comparison of neurologic changes in "successful aging" persons vs the total aging population. *Arch Neurol.* 1994;51:573.

125. Chahine LM, Stern MB. Diagnostic markers for Parkinson's disease. *Curr Opin Neurol.* 2011;24:309.

126. Parkinson's Disease Foundation. Statistics on Parkinson's. Available at http://www.pdf.org/en/parkinson_statistics. Accessed January 10, 2016.

127. Gestuvo MK. Health maintenance in older adults: combining evidence and individual preferences. *Mt Sinai J Med.* 2012;79:560.

128. Nicholas JA, Hall WJ. Screening and preventive services for older adults. *Mt Sinai J Med.* 2011;78:498.

129. Centers for Disease Control and Prevention, Administration on Aging, Agency for Healthcare Research and Quality, and Centers for Medicare and Medicaid Services. *Enhancing Use of Clinical Preventive Services Among Older Adults.* Washington, DC: AARP; 2011. Available at http://www.cdc.gov/aging/pdf/Clinical_Preventive_Services_Closing_the_Gap_Report.pdf. Accessed January 20, 2016.

130. Eckstrom K, Feeny DH, Walter LC, et al. Individualizing cancer screening in older adults: a narrative review and framework for future research. *J Gen Intern Med.* 2013;28:292.

131. Leipzig RM, Whitlock EP, Wolff TA, et al. Reconsidering the approach to prevention recommendations for older adults. *Ann Intern Med.* 2010;153:809.

132. American Geriatrics Society Expert Panel on the Care of Older Adults with Multimorbidity. Patient-centered care for older adults with multiple chronic conditions: a stepwise approach from the American Geriatrics Society: American Geriatrics Society Expert Panel on the Care of Older Adults with Multimorbidity. *J Am Geriatr Soc.* 2012;60:1957.

133. Hötting K, Röder B. Beneficial effects of physical exercise on neuroplasticity and cognition. *Neurosci Biobehav Rev.* 2013;37(9 Pt B):2243.

134. Buchman AS, Boyle PA, Yu L, et al. Total daily physical activity and the risk of AD and cognitive decline in older adults. *Neurology.* 2012;78:1323.

135. Lee L, Heckman G, Mohar FJ. Frailty: Identifying elderly patients at high risk of poor outcomes. *Can Fam Physician.* 2015;61:227.

136. Chou CH, Hwang CL, Wu YT. Effect of exercise on physical function, daily living activities, and quality of life in the frail older adults: a meta-analysis. *Arch Phys Med Rehabil.* 2012; 93:237.

137. American College of Sports Medicine. Exercise is Medicine–Summary Sheet for Healthcare Providers and Healthcare Providers Action Guide. Available at http://www.exerciseismedicine.org/support_page.php?p=8. Accessed January 20, 2016.

138. Crookham J. A guide to exercise prescription. *Prim Care.* 2013;40:801.

139. Centers for Disease Control and Prevention. Preventing falls in older adults. Updated September 23 2013. Available at http://www.cdc.gov/Features/OlderAmericans/ Accessed January 20, 2016.

140. Centers for Disease Control and Prevention. How much physical activity do older adults need?. Physical activity is essential to healthy aging. Updated June 4, 2015. Available at http://www.cdc.gov/physicalactivity/basics/older_adults/index.htm. Accessed January 17, 2016.

141. U.S. Preventive Services Task Force. Draft Recommendation Statement Impaired Visual Acuity in Older Adults: Screening, 2015. Available at http://www.uspreventiveservicestaskforce.org/Page/Document/draft-recommendation-statement161/impaired-visual-acuity-in-older-adults-screening. Accessed January 20, 2016.

142. Centers for Disease Control and Prevention. Vaccine information statements. Updated August 7, 2015. Available at http://www.cdc.gov/vaccines/hcp/vis./ Accessed January 17, 2016.

143. Kim DK, Bridges CB, Harriman KH. Advisory Committee on Immunization Practices recommended immunization schedule for adults aged 19 years or older: United States. *Ann Intern Med*. 2015;162:214.

144. Walter LC, Covinsky KE. Cancer screening in elderly patients—a framework for individualized decision making. *JAMA*. 2011;285:2750.

145. U.S. Preventive Services Task Force. Draft recommendation statement. Depression in adults: screening. 2015. Available at http://www.uspreventiveservicestaskforce.org/Page/Document/draft-recommendation-statement115/depression-in-adults-screening1. Accessed January 17, 2016.

146. Taylor WD. Depression in the elderly. *N Engl J Med*. 2014; 371:1228.

147. Maurer DM. Screening for depression. *Am Fam Physician*. 2012; 85:139.

148. Lin JS, O'Connor, E, Rossom RC, et al. Screening for cognitive impairment in older adults: an evidence update for the U.S. Preventive Services Task Force. 2013. Evidence Syntheses No. 107. Available at http://www.ncbi.nlm.nih.gov/books/NBK174643/. Accessed January 17, 2016.

149. Alzheimer's Association. 2015. Alzheimer's disease: facts and figures. Available at http://www.alz.org/facts/#prevalence. Accessed January 17, 2016.

150. Mayeux R. Early Alzheimer's disease. *N Engl J Med*. 2010; 362:2194.

151. Blass DM, Rabins PV. In the clinic. Dementia. *Ann Intern Med*. 2014;161:ITC-2.

152. Marcantonio ER. In the clinic. Delirium. *Ann Intern Med*. 2011;154:ITC6–1.

153. American Psychiatric Association. *Neurocognitive disorders, in Diagnostic and Statistical Manual of Mental Disorders*. 5th ed. Washington, DC: American Psychiatric Publishing; 2013:602.

154. Iverson DJ, Gronseth GS, Reger MA, et al. Practice Parameter update: evaluation and management of driving risk in dementia. Report of the Quality Standards Subcommittee of the American Academy of Neurology. *Neurology*. 2010;74:1316.

155. Martin AJ, Marottoli R, O'Neill D. Driving assessment for maintaining mobility and safety in drivers with dementia. *Cochrane Database Syst Rev*. 2013;8:CD006222.

156. Wang XM, Brisbin S, Loo T, et al. Elder abuse: an approach to identification, assessment and intervention. *CMAJ*. 2015; 187:575.

157. Acierno R, Hernandez MA, Amstadter AB, et al. Prevalence and correlates of emotional, physical, sexual, and financial abuse and potential neglect in the United States: the National Elder Mistreatment Study. *Am J Public Health*. 2010;100:292.

158. National Center of Elder Abuse, Administration on Aging. Elder abuse: the size of the problem. Available at http://www.ncea.aoa.gov/Library/Data/index.aspx. Accessed January 20, 2016.

159. U.S. Preventive Services Task Force. Final recommendation statement. Intimate partner violence and abuse of elderly and vulnerable Adults: screening, 2013. Available at http://www.uspreventiveservicestaskforce.org/Page/Document/UpdateSummaryFinal/intimate-partner-violence-and-abuse-of-elderly-and-vulnerable-adults-screening?ds = 1&s = elder abuse. Accessed January 20, 2016.

160. O'Sullivan R, Mailo K, Angeles R, et al. Advance directives: survey of primary care patients. *Can Fam Physician*. 2015;61:353.

161. Torke AM, Sachs GA, Helft PR, et al. Scope and outcomes of surrogate decision making among hospitalized older adults. *JAMA Intern Med*. 2014;174:370.

accommodation eye changes focus to see objects at various distances which occurs by changes in the shape of the lens.

achalasia failure to relax smooth muscles of the gastrointestinal tract.

acral pertaining to extremities.

actinic keratosis localized thickening of outer layers of the skin from prolonged sun exposure, precursor to skin cancer.

aerophagia swallowing of air.

afterload resistance to left ventricular ejection; the forces that impede the flow of blood out of the heart, that is, the compliance of the aorta and the volume of blood in the left ventricle.

akinesia loss or impairment of voluntary activity.

alae the cartilaginous flap on the outer side of each nostril.

alopecia hair loss.

anhedonia lack of pleasure in acts that are normally pleasurable.

anisocoria unequal pupil size.

aperture opening for the light.

arciform arcurate, bowed; shaped like an arc.

arcus lipoides a white ring around the limbus of the eye, due to lipid deposition in the peripheral cornea.

arthralgia pain in a joint.

articular pertaining to joints.

ataxia the loss of full control of bodily movements.

atelectasis a collapsed or airless condition of the lung.

aterixis a motor control disturbance with intermittent periods of involuntary movements.

atherosclerosis the formation of fibrofatty deposits in the intimal lining of large and medium arteries, which leads to hardening and narrowing of the arteries.

atraumatic without injury.

atrophy a wasting or decrease in size or physiologic activity of a part of the body.

bipolar disorder affective disorder in which the person has both manic and depressive episodes.

bradycardia slow heartbeat, usually less than 60 beats per minute.

bradykinesia extreme slowness of movement.

bronchitis inflammation of the mucous membrane of the bronchial airways, caused by irritation or infection.

bulbar conjunctiva thin and transparent covering of the sclera on the anterior of the eye.

canthi corners of the eyes; singular is canthus.

cephalagia pain in the head.

cerumen (earwax) a yellowish or brownish waxy substance secreted in the ear canal; helps to clean, lubricate, and protect from infections or insects.

cholestasis condition caused by a decrease in bile.

cibophobia fear of eating, or loathing for, food.

claudication pain with walking.

coitus sexual intercourse.

contractility the ability of the heart muscle fiber to stretch during ventricular filling; in the healthy heart the stretch is proportional to the force of the contraction; the intrinsic ability of cardiac muscle to develop force for a given muscle length.

convergence movement of two objects toward a common point.

coronal plane along the long axis of the body, dividing the body into anterior and posterior portions.

crepitus a crackling or rattling sound made by a part of the body, either spontaneously or during physical examination, for example, the grating of a joint in osteoarthritis.

crude touch sensation perceived as light touch but without accurate localization.

cryptorchidism undescended testicle.

cutdown a surgical procedure to insert a cannula into a vein or artery to administer fluids or drugs.

dermatome area of the body innervated by the sensory root of a single spinal nerve.

diaphoresis profuse sweating.

diopters measurement of the optical powers of a lens.

diplopia double vision.

disequilibrium loss or lack of equilibrium or stability.

dysarthria difficulty in articulating words.

dysdiadochokinesis impaired ability to perform rapid alternating movements.

dyslipidemia an abnormal concentration of lipids or lipoproteins in the blood.

dyspareunia abnormal pain during sexual intercourse.

dyspepsia chronic or recurrent discomfort or pain centered in the upper abdomen.

dysphagia difficulty swallowing.

dysplasia abnormal development of tissue.

dyspnea labored or difficult breathing, shortness of breath.

dysthymia loss of interest or pleasure in all usual activities or pastimes but not severe enough to meet major depressive episode criteria.

dysuria pain or difficulty voiding.

echoic imitation of a sound.

ectasia a dilated milk duct.

ectopy displacement.

ectropion eversion, usually of the eyelid.

edema abnormal accumulation of fluid in the intercellular spaces of the body.

edentulous without teeth.

embolus undissolved matter in the blood, such as a blood clot.

entropion turning inward, usually eyelid turns in toward the eye.

equilibrium state of balance.

erythema reddening of the skin; a nonspecific sign of skin inflammation, injury or irritation; caused by dilation of the skin capillaries.

euphoria a state of happiness.

evert turning outward of the foot.

facies the appearance of the face.

fascia fibrous connective tissue.

fasciculation involuntary contraction or twitching of muscle fibers, visible under the skin.

fever abnormal elevation in body temperature.

fibrillation uncoordinated electrical activity of the heart; quivering or spontaneous contraction of individual muscle fibers, which can be atrial or ventricular.

fibroadenoma small, solid, noncancerous lump composed of glandular and fibrous tissues.

flank pain pain in one side of the body between the upper abdomen and the back.

fossa a furrow or shallow depression.

frenulum a fold of mucous membrane extending from the floor of mouth to midline of the undersurface of the tongue or extending from the upper or lower lip to the gingiva.

fundus back portion of the interior of the eye, visible through the pupil using the ophthalmoscope.

gait the manner or style of walking.

glaucoma disease in which fluid builds up and causes damage to the optic nerve

granuloma small nodule, inflammation.

hematochezia bright red blood in feces.

hematuria blood in the urine.

hemianopsia inability to see half of the visual field, generally on one side.

hemolysis the destruction of red blood cells.

hemoptysis expectoration of blood that arises from the larynx, trachea, bronchi or lungs.

hertz a unit of frequency equal to one cycle per second.

hydrocele accumulation of serous fluid in a saclike cavity in the scrotum.

hyperacusis increased sensitivity to sounds.

hyperopia farsighted or inability of the eye to focus on objects close by.

hyperplasia abnormal proliferation of cells.

hyperreflexia overactive reflexes.

hyperresonance an increased resonance during percussion, caused by over inflation of the lungs as in emphysema or asthma.

hypertrophy increase in the size of an organ or body part, such as a muscle.

hypothermia decrease in temperature.

icterus jaundice, a generalized yellowing of the skin, often secondary to liver disease (Icteric is adjective).

insomnia inability to sleep or remain asleep.

inspissated thickened by dehydration, evaporation, or absorption.

intertriginous an area where two skin areas may touch or rub together.

kyphosis exaggerated outward or convex curvature of the thoracic spine.

lateral decubitus position side lying position.

leukoplakia precancerous change in mucous membrane (usually thick and white lesions).

lordosis exaggerated inward or concave curvature of the lumbar spine.

lymphedema swelling of a body part that is due to pooling of interstitial fluid caused by the blockage of a lymph node or vessel.

maceration the process of softening a solid by steeping in a fluid. Maceration of the skin occurs when it is consistently wet. The skin softens, turns white, and can easily get infected with bacteria or fungi.

malaise feeling of sickness or indisposition.

malignant progressive or deadly.

mania an emotional disorder characterized by euphoria or irritability, increased psychomotor activity, rapid speech, flight of ideas, decreased need for sleep, distractibility, grandiosity, and poor judgment; occurs in bipolar disorder.

mastitis infection of the breast resulting in pain, redness, swelling, and warmth.

mastoid hard, bony structure behind the ear.

melena black "tar" color and consistency to feces due to blood pigments.

microglossia abnormally small tongue.

micturition urination.

miosis excessive pupil constriction.

myalgia tenderness or pain in the muscles.

mydriasis prolonged pupil dilation.

myopia nearsighted or inability of the eye to focus on objects at a distance.

neoplasm a new and abnormal formation of tissue, as a tumor or growth, which serves no useful function. It may be benign or malignant.

nocturia urinary frequency at night.

normocephalic a person whose head and all major organs of the head are in a normal condition and without significant abnormalities.

nummular coin shaped.

obstipation intestinal obstruction; severe constipation.

obtunded reduced level of consciousness, responds slowly and somewhat confused.

odynophagia pain with swallowing.

ophthalmoplegia eyes not aligned.

orchitis inflammation of a testis.

orthopnea labored breathing that occurs when lying flat and is relieved by sitting up.

otitis externa inflammation of the skin of the ear canal.

otoscope a medical instrument consisting of a magnifying lens and light and used for examining the ear.

palpebral conjunctiva thick, opaque, vascular lining of the inner surface of the eyelids.

palpebral fissures opening between the upper and lower eyelids.

palpitations a sensation of rapid or irregular beating of the heart. The patient may describe the sensation as thudding, fluttering, or throbbing under the sternum.

palsy paralysis.

parenchyma the essential elements of an organ essential to its functioning, as distinct from the capsule that encompasses it and other supporting structures.

paresthesia sensation of numbness, prickling, or tingling.

paroxysmal nocturnal dyspnea (PND) sudden attacks of dyspnea that occur when patients are asleep in bed.

pedicle a small stalk or stalklike structure, supports or connects an organ or other body part.

pedunculated attached to a base by means of a *peduncle*, or slender stalk, for example, a skin tag or polyp.

percutaneous through the skin.

phobia irrational fear of an object, activity, or situation.

photophobia light sensitivity from excess light entering the eye, which may overstimulate the photoreceptors in the retina, which then stimulates the optic nerve.

pleximeter finger finger that receives the percussion strike from the opposite hand, usually the third finger of the nondominant hand.

plexor finger finger that strikes the finger pressing on the patient's body during percussion, usually the third finger of the dominant hand.

pneumothorax a collection of air in the pleural cavity, "collapsed lung."

polyuria significant increase in 24-hour urine.

postictal altered state of consciousness which occurs after a seizure and before return to baseline.

precordium the area on the anterior chest that overlies the heart and great vessels.

preload the end-diastolic stretch of a heart muscle fiber; end-diastolic volume.

presbyopia changes with age, farsightedness due to decreased elasticity in the lens.

presyncope experience of lightheadedness, muscular weakness, blurred vision, or feeling faint.

prodrome early symptom(s) before the onset of a disease.

proliferative growing or producing by multiplication of parts.

protuberant rounded.

ptosis drooping of the upper eyelid.

radicular pertaining to a spinal nerve root.

regurgitation a backward flowing, as in the return of solids or fluids to the mouth from the stomach or the back flow of blood through a defective heart valve.

resonance quality of the sound heard during percussion of the normal lung.

scaling removal of the surface.

scaphoid concave or hollowed.

scoliosis lateral curvature of the spine.

sebum a fatty secretion of the sebaceous glands of the skin.

serpiginous a term used to describe the shape or arrangement of lesions that have a wavy or serpent-like patter.

shotty small, hard, round, discrete nodules, resembling shotgun pellets.

somatoform has psychological symptoms that are similar to those of a physical disease.

speculum instrument for inserting into and holding open a cavity of the body, for example, the vagina.

stadiometer instrument to measure height, attach to the wall to insure accuracy.

stasis slowed or stopped flow, for example, blood flow in veins.

steatorrhea excess fat in the feces, oily or greasy appearance.

stenosis the constriction or narrowing of a passage or orifice, for example, a heart valve or blood vessel.

strabismus eyes are not directed at the same point; crossed eyes.

stroke volume the amount of blood ejected by the left ventricle with each contraction.

subluxation a partial dislocation of a joint.

symmetry opposite sides compared to assess equivalence in size, shape, and position.

syncope the transient and usually sudden loss of consciousness, accompanied by an inability to remain standing; fainting.

tachycardia an abnormally fast heartbeat, usually over 100 beats per minute.

tangential lighting lighting from the side to be able to better see small movements or pulsations of the body and decrease shadows.

tenesmus straining to defecate or urinate without results, often painful.

teres round and smooth; cylindrical; used to describe certain muscles and ligaments.

thelarche the beginning of breast development.

thrill a palpable vibration felt over the precordium or an artery due to blood turbulence, associated with grade 4 to 6 heart murmurs.

thrombophlebitis inflammation of a vein in conjunction with the formation of a thrombus.

thrombosis a blood clot that adheres to the wall of a blood vessel, usually a vein.

tinnitus a ringing or buzzing sound that is heard by the patient.

tophaceous pertaining to a tophus: a knobby swelling containing a deposit of sodium biurate seen in individuals with gout.

torticollis contraction of the muscles of the neck, which draw the head to one side.

transtentorial herniation uncal herniation, the inner part of the temporal lobe (uncus), is squeezed and pushes tentorium putting pressure on the brainstem.

traumatic brain injury (TBI) occurs when an outside force traumatically injures the brain.

tympany a clear hollow drum-like note heard during percussion over gas-filled organs, such as the stomach and bowels.

valgus bent; turned outward; the distal part of leg is deviated outward, that is, knock-kneed.

varus a term for the inward angulation of the distal segment of a bone or joint, that is, bowleg.

vertigo patients feel they or their surroundings are in a state of constant movement; usually due to a problem with the inner ear, but can also be caused by visual problems.

viscera internal organs enclosed within a cavity.

xanthelasma yellow, lipid-rich plaque present on the eyelids, associated with hyperlipidemia.

Note: Page numbers followed by b indicate in-chapter boxed material, those followed by t indicate end-of-chapter tables, and those followed by f indicate figures.

muscle groups, 616
physical examination, 617–620
inspection, 617
muscle strength test, 620
palpation, 617–619
range of motion, 619
Knock-knee pattern, children, 882
Knock-knees, 617
Koplik spots, 319t
Korotkoff sounds, weak/inaudible
arrhythmias, 133
hypertensive patient, 134
obese or very thin patient, 134
white coat hypertension, 134
Kussmaul breathing, 365t
Kyphosis, 602f, 933. *See also* Spine

L

Labial adhesions, in prepubertal children, 881
Labial frenulum, 290
Labia majora, 747, 747f
Labia minora, 747, 747f
Lacrimal apparatus, 251
Lacrimal gland, 237
Lacrimal puncta, 237
Lacrimal sac, 237
inflammation of (dacryocystitis), 267t
Landau reflex, 853b
Language barrier, interviewing patient with, 60–61
Language development
infants, 814
preschoolers, 854
school-aged children, 856
toddlers, 854
Large pupils, 738t
Laryngitis, cough in, 362t
Lateral collateral ligament (LCL), 617
Lateral condyle, of tibia, 615
Lateral epicondyle, of femur, 615
Lateral epicondylitis, 588
Lateral flexion
back, 606f, 606t
neck, 605t
Lateralization test, 299
Lateral lymph nodes, 540, 540f
Lateral malleolus, 621, 621f
Lateral nail folds, 176, 176f
Latissimus dorsi, 601, 601f
Lazy eye, 866
Leading questions, 49–50
Left atrial pressure, 378–379, 378f–379f
Left homonymous hemianopsia, 265t
Left lower quadrant, 474, 474f, 475–476, 475f
Left lower quadrant pain, 508
Left-sided heart failure
dyspnea in, 360t–361t
edema in, 390–391
physical findings in, 370t–371t
Left upper quadrant, 474, 474f, 475, 475f
Left ventricle, 375, 375f
Left ventricular failure
and cough, 362t
dyspnea in, 360t–361t
Left ventricular hypertrophy (LVH), 957
Left ventricular pressure, 377–379, 377f–379f
Leg-length discrepancy, 901
Legs, 451
arterial supply to, 460
deep veins of, 442

inspection of, 451–452
length measurement of, 626
palpation of, 452–457
dorsalis pedis pulse, 455
DVT, 454
edema, 452–453
femoral pulse, 454
popliteal pulse, 454–455
posterior tibial pulse, 456
swelling, 453–454
superficial veins of, 442, 442f
Length, infants, 822
Lens, 252
Lenses, effect of aging on, 932
Lesbian, gay, bisexual, and transgender (LGBT)
health care, 779
Leukoedema, 302
Leukokoria, 831
Leukoplakia, 319t, 323t
Leukorrhea, 749
Levator palpebrae, 237
Libido, 769
Lichenification, 199t
Lid lag, 255
Lid retraction, 266t
Lifestyle habits, 178, 245, 284, 289
Ligamentous laxity, 573
Ligaments, 568
Lighting and environment, 105–106
Light reaction, 240, 240f
Linear lesions, 195t
Lingual frenulum, 291
Lipomas, 528t
abdominal wall, 528t
Lips
abnormalities of, 315t–316t
physical examination of, 302
Listening
active, 49
in health assessment, 5
Literacy, low, interviewing patient with, 61
Liver
in children, 878b, 879
in infants, 843
Liver disease, 175, 205t
Liver enlargement, 531t
Lobar pneumonia, physical findings in, 370t–371t
Location, 13, 71
Lordosis, 602f. *See also* Spine
Loss of sensation, 682
Loss of smell, 687
Low back pain, 571–572, 636t
prevention of, 629–630
Low blood pressure, 133
Lower Extremity Amputation Prevention (LEAP)/
Semmes–Weinstein test, 718
Lower motor neurons, 673
Low literacy, interviewing patient with, 61
Lumbar concavity, 602f
Lumps
history of, 541, 563t–564t
palpation of, 550
Lumps and swellings, in eyes, 267t
Lung abscess
and cough, 362t
and hemoptysis, 362t
Lung cancer
cough in, 362t
hemoptysis in, 362t

Lungs. *See also* Thorax
aging on, effect of, 932
in children, 875
fissures and lobes, 329–330, 329f, 330f
Lung sounds. *See* Breath sounds
Lunula, 176
Lymphadenopathy, 456
in childhood, 873
in children, 916t
Lymphangitis, acute, 466t–467t
Lymphatic duct, right, 444
Lymphatic system and lymph nodes, 195–196, 195f
anatomy and physiology of, 443f, 444–445,
445f, 540–541, 540f
breast, 540, 540f
fluid exchange and capillary bed, 445–446
reproductive system
female, 749
male, 768
Lymphedema, 470t
Lymph nodes, 217–218, 443–445, 443f, 445f,
540, 540f
in children, 874
physical examination of, 220–222

M

Macrocephaly, 823, 829
Macroglossia, 833
Macula, 238
Macular degeneration, 259, 932, 956
Male breast, 539, 549
Male genitalia
in adolescents, 897–898
in children, 879–880, 880f
in infants, 843–844
Malocclusion of teeth, 303, 872
Malodor, 957
Mammary duct ectasia, 548
Mammography, 558, 559
Marginal gingivitis, 320t
Masseter, 577, 577f
Mastoiditis, acute, 869
Mastoid process, 278
Maxillary sinuses, 301
McBurney point, 507
Measles, 922t
Mechanical obstruction, 521t
Media
arteries, 439, 439f, 440
venous, 441–442
Medial collateral ligament (MCL), 616
Medial condyle, of tibia, 615
Medial epicondyle, of femur, 615
Medial epicondylitis, 588
Medial malleolus, 621, 621f
Median nerve, in carpal tunnel, 591, 591f
Mediastinal crunch, 369t
Medical records, review of, 40
Medications
older adults and, 946–947
in past history, 72
seeking care, 97
Medullated nerve fibers, 271t
Meibomian glands, 237
Melanin, 175
Melanoma, 955. *See also* Skin cancer
incidence of, 187–188
malignant, 204t
risk factors for, 188

Somatic nervous system, 670
Somatic pain, 141
Sore throat, 293
Spastic diplegias, 884
Spastic hemiparesis, 732t
Spasticity, 576, 742t
Specificity, of clinical findings, 34
Specula, 758
Speculum, 110
Speech, 123
  disorders of, 731t
Spermatic cord, 767
  abnormalities of, 782t
Spermatocele and cyst of epididymis, 782t
Spheroidal joints, 569, 570f, 570t
Sphygmomanometer, 111, 127
SPICES mnemonic (geriatric syndromes), 943
Spina bifida occulta, 845
Spinal cord, 669, 669f
  defect, 826
  lesions of, 727t
Spinal nerve, 671
Spinal nerve lesion, 728t
Spinal reflex
  deep tendon, 677–678, 678b
  muscle stretch reflex, 677–678, 678b
Spinal root lesion, 728t
Spine, 599–607
  bony structures, 599–600
  cervical and lumbar vertebrae, 599f
  joints, 600
  muscle groups, 601
  physical examination, 601–607
    inspection, 601–602
    palpation, 602–604
    range of motion and maneuvers, 604–607
Spinothalamic tract, 676
Spinous processes of vertebrae, 328, 328f
Spirituality
  assessment, 98–101
    Stoll's guidelines for, 100–101
  definitions of, 98
Spleen
  in children, 879
  in infants, 843
Splenic percussion sign, 501
Splenius capitis, 601, 601f
Splenius cervicis, 601, 601f
Splenomegaly, 501
  in children, 879
Spontaneous pneumothorax, dyspnea in, 360t–361t
Sports preparticipation screening evaluation, 902
SpPin, 34
Sputum
  mucoid, 335
  purulent, 335
Squamous cell carcinoma, 187, 203t, 955. See also
    Skin cancer
Stadiometer, 109
Staining of teeth, 872, 916t
Standard precautions, 113–114
Stasis ulcer, 200t
Stenotic valve, 381
Steppage gait, 732t
Stepping reflex, 853b
Stereognosis, 700
Stereotype, cultural, 90
Sternal angle, 326, 326f
Sternoclavicular joint, 579, 579f, 580, 582

Sternocleidomastoids, 332
Stethoscope, 111
  bell of, 404–405
  diaphragm of, 404
  heads for, 405, 405f
  "inching" of, 406, 406f
  use of, 405
Still murmur, in children, 876, 877b
Stoll's guidelines for spiritual assessment,
    100–101
Stone, renal, 489
Stool with red blood, 524t
Strabismus, 915t
  in children, 866
Stranger anxiety, in toddlers, 858
Streptococcal pharyngitis, 873, 916t
Streptococcal pneumonia, 358–359
Stress incontinence, 487, 489, 526t–527t
  nursing process for, 32
Stridor, 369t, 833
Stroke, 680, 720–725
  hemorrhagic, 720
  ischemic, 721
  prevention and patient education, 721b–722b
  primary prevention, 723–724b
  secondary prevention, 725
  transient ischemic attack and, 721
  types of, 729t–730t
  warning signs and symptoms, 722, 722b
Stroke volume, 380
Sty (Hordeolum), 267t
Subacromial bursa, 581, 581f. See also Shoulder
Subarachnoid hemorrhage, and headache, 79
Subcortical gray matter, lesions of, 727t
Subcutaneous tissues, 174, 175
Subjective data, 12
  obtaining, 13–14
  vs. objective data, 13t
Subjective information, 12
Submandibular gland, 221
Subscapular lymph nodes, 540, 540f
Subtalar joint, 621, 621f
Sudden arterial occlusion, 456
Sudden infant death syndrome (SIDS), 829
Summarization, in interviewing, 53
Sunscreen, regular use of, 189
Superficial phlebitis, 466t–467t
Superficial vein thrombosis, 466t–467t
Superior vena cava, 375, 375f, 442
Supernumerary nipples, 539, 539f
Supernumerary teeth, 832
Supination, elbow, 589t
Suprapatellar pouch, 619
Suprapubic pain, 488
Supraventricular premature contractions, 425t
Supraventricular tachycardia
  in children, 908t
Sustained hypertension
  in adolescents, 893
  in children, 864
S wave, 383, 383f
Sweat glands, anatomy and physiology, 176
Sympathetic nervous system, 670
Symphysis pubis, 607, 607f
Symptoms
  characteristic, 12
  as cone, 46
  in confusing patient, 55
  definition of, 12

identifying, 16–17
past occurrences of, 72
sequence and timing, 45
seven attributes of, 45, 71
vs. sign, 13t
Syncope, 682–683
  in elderly, 930
Synovial fluid, 568
Synovial joints, 568–569, 568t, 569f
  structure of, 569–570
Syphilis, congenital, 913t
Syphilitic chancre, 780t
Systemic lupus erythematosus, 205t
Systems review, 69t, 76–79
Systole
  extra heart sounds in, 409t, 429t
  jugular venous undulations in, 385, 385f
  pressures and heart sounds in, 376, 377–378,
    377f, 379f
Systolic aortic murmur, 934
Systolic blood pressure (SBP)
  in elderly, 930
  estimation, 129
  identification, 130
Systolic clicks, 429t
Systolic ejection sound, early, 378, 429t
Systolic heart sounds, 435t
Systolic murmurs, in adults, 409, 410
Systolic pressure, 129, 385, 385f

T

Tachypnea, 365t, 825
Tactile fremitus, 367t
  , assessment of, 350
Talkative patient, 57
Talus, 621, 621f
Tandem walking, 695
Tangential lighting, 106, 106f
Tanner sex maturity rating (SMR) stages
  in boys, 897b–898b
  in girls
    breasts, 895, 896b
    pubic hair, 899b–900b
Tanning beds and skin cancer, 188–189
Target lesions, 195t
Tarsal plates, 237
Teeth
  in children, 871–872, 872b
  in elderly, 932
  findings in, 320t–321t
    abrasion with notching, 321t
    attrition, 321t
    erosion, 321t
    Hutchinson teeth, 321t
  misalignment of, 872
  physical examination of, 302–303
  types and age of eruption, 872b
Telangiectatic nevus, 826
Temperature
  axillary, 137
  in elderly, 930
  in health promotion, 143
  in infants, 825
  oral, 136
  rectal, 136
  in school-aged children, 865
  temporal artery, 137
  tympanic membrane, 137
  vital signs and, 135–136